Second E

T0228143

ENDOCRINE DISRUPTORS

Effects on Male and Female Reproductive Systems

Second Edition

ENDOCRINE DISRUPTORS

Effects on Male and Female Reproductive Systems

EDITED BY

Rajesh K. Naz

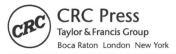

CRC Press
Taylor & Francis Group
Boca Raton London New York

CRC Press is an imprint of the
Taylor & Francis Group, an **informa** business

CRC Press
Taylor & Francis Group
6000 Broken Sound Parkway NW, Suite 300
Boca Raton, FL 33487-2742

©2005 by Taylor & Francis Group, LLC
CRC Press is an imprint of Taylor & Francis Group, an Informa business

First issued in paperback 2019

No claim to original U.S. Government works

ISBN-13: 978-0-367-45426-5 (pbk)
ISBN-13: 978-0-8493-2281-5 (hbk)

Visit the Taylor & Francis Web site at
http://www.taylorandfrancis.com

and the CRC Press Web site at
http://www.crcpress.com

Library of Congress Card Number 2004054449

Library of Congress Cataloging-in-Publication Data

Endocrine disruptors : effects on male and female reproductive systems / edited by Rajesh
K. Naz. -- 2nd ed.
    p. cm.
Includes bibliographical references and index.
ISBN 0-8493-2281-2 (alk. paper)
1. Reproductive toxicology. 2. Endocrine toxicology. I. Naz, Rajesh K.
[DNLM: 1. Endocrine Diseases--chemically induced. 2. Infertility--chemically induced.
3. Environmental Pollutants--adverse effects. 4. Estrogens--pharmacology. 5. Genital
Diseases, Female--chemically induced. 6. Genital Diseases, Male--chemically induced. WP
570 E556 2004]
RA1224.2.E63 2004
616.6'92—dc22   2004054449

Dedication

This book is dedicated to our pursuit of knowledge to make this planet free of environmental pollution.

Preface

The first edition of *Endocrine Disruptors: Effects on Male and Female Reproductive Systems* was published by CRC Press LLC in 1999. In the last five years, there has been tremendous progress in this field both from the academic perspective as well as the new emerging clinical manifestations of the endocrine disruptors, or "gender benders" as they are popularly called. Several previously unknown risks of the endocrine disruptors are being unfolded as research progresses. To name a few, recently estrogen replacement therapy has been shown to increase the incidence of endometrial cancer, novel androgens of anthropogenic origin in the environment were discovered in 2001, and the incidence of infertility, impotency, and neoplasms has shown to increase in men and women. The endocrine-disrupting environmental chemicals, both naturally occurring and man-made, have affected fish, wildlife, and humans, and have been implicated in causing feminization of male birds, alligators, and fish. The first edition was very well received and appreciated both by the scientific community as well as by the general public, and is on the best-selling list of CRC Press. Due to these pressing reasons, it became imperative to write the second edition of the book updating the knowledge and new insights gained during the last five years.

An alarming concern has been raised among the scientific community, policy makers, and the general public regarding the reproductive and health hazards of the endocrine-disrupting environmental chemicals. "Each man in this room is half the man his grandfather was." These were the words quoted during a Congressional hearing reporting the startling and controversial finding of a serious decline in the quality and quantity of human spermatozoa. Various reports have revealed a decline in sperm concentrations of healthy men from 113×10^6/ml in 1938 to 66×10^6/ml in 1990. Recently (2000), meta-analysis of 101 studies published during 1934–1996 indeed confirmed the declining trend in semen parameters in the United States and Europe, decreasing by 50% over the past 50 years. Although available data may be considered insufficient to deduce worldwide conclusions, the fact remains that infertility and erectile dysfunction (ED) are on the rise in the United States and other parts of the world. Similar concerns have been reported for women with an increased incidence of infertility, premature ovarian failure (POF), polycystic ovarian syndrome (PCOS), endometriosis, spontaneous abortions, early menopause, birth defects, and other postnatal structural and functional abnormalities. These findings have led scientists and environmentalists to believe that the human species is approaching a fertility crisis, while others think that the available data is insufficient to deduce worldwide conclusions. The topic of gonadotoxicity remains a real challenge and concern to almost everyone, both men and women. It has been the subject of a number of reviews, with a myriad of environmental agents now being classified

CRC Press
Taylor & Francis Group
6000 Broken Sound Parkway NW, Suite 300
Boca Raton, FL 33487-2742

©2005 by Taylor & Francis Group, LLC
CRC Press is an imprint of Taylor & Francis Group, an Informa business

First issued in paperback 2019

No claim to original U.S. Government works

ISBN-13: 978-0-367-45426-5 (pbk)
ISBN-13: 978-0-8493-2281-5 (hbk)

**Visit the Taylor & Francis Web site at
http://www.taylorandfrancis.com**

**and the CRC Press Web site at
http://www.crcpress.com**

Library of Congress Card Number 2004054449

Library of Congress Cataloging-in-Publication Data

Endocrine disruptors : effects on male and female reproductive systems / edited by Rajesh
    K. Naz. -- 2nd ed.
        p.   cm.
Includes bibliographical references and index.
ISBN 0-8493-2281-2 (alk. paper)
1. Reproductive toxicology. 2. Endocrine toxicology. I. Naz, Rajesh K.
[DNLM: 1. Endocrine Diseases--chemically induced. 2. Infertility--chemically induced.
3. Environmental Pollutants--adverse effects. 4. Estrogens--pharmacology. 5. Genital
Diseases, Female--chemically induced. 6. Genital Diseases, Male--chemically induced. WP
570 E556 2004]
RA1224.2.E63 2004
616.6′92—dc22   2004054449

resulting in POF, an early menopause. POF can cause an increased risk of osteoporosis, cardiovascular disease, and ovarian cancer (P. Devine and P.B. Hoyer). The fourth chapter describes how the environmental toxicants (*p,p'*-DDE and HCB) affect fetal and embryonic development (M. Edelbrock, M. Fernstrom, and K. Williams). The fifth chapter describes the estrogenic compounds called phytoestrogens that are present in plants, especially soy products, and thus can disrupt the endocrine milieu through dietary sources (H. Patisaul and P. Whitten). The sixth chapter discusses the effects and mechanisms of estrogens and xenoestrogens on the development of breast cancer (A. Soto and C. Sonnenschein). The seventh chapter reviews the genomic and nongenomic novel mechanisms of action of xenoestrogens through the estrogen receptor (ER)-dependent and ER-independent pathways (R. Bigsby, M. Mercado-Feliciano, and J. Mubiru). The last chapter in this section focuses on the effects and mechanisms of action of 2,3,7,8-tetrachlorodibenzo-*p*-dioxin (TCDD) and related environmental antiestrogens on tumorigenesis and breast cancer (S. Safe).

The second section of this book deals with the effects of endocrine disruption by various environmental toxicants on the male reproductive system, focusing on male fertility and development of benign prostate hyperplasia (BPH) and prostate cancer. This section includes five chapters. The first chapter describes the effects of endocrine disruptors on male fertility and discusses controversial issues regarding the global decline in fertility of men (S. Sikka, M. Kendirci, and R. Naz). The second chapter elegantly describes the effects and mechanism(s) of action of androgenic compounds and antiandrogens on sex differentiation and testicular function including androgen biosynthesis (E. Gray Jr., W. Kelce, and associates). This chapter describes how antiandrogens have the potential to alter male sexual differentiation and reproductive development, whereas the androgenic substances can masculinize and defeminize females. The third chapter in this section deals with the effects of endocrine disruptors (antiestrogens as well as antiandrogens) on ED in men (S. Sikka, M. Kendirci, and R. Naz). Fifty-two percent of men 40 to 70 years old experience some degree of ED, affecting 20 to 30 million men in the United States. The fourth chapter describes the role of natural and man-made estrogens in prostate development, discussing the opposite effects of low and high doses of estrogenic chemicals (C. Richter, B. Timms, and F. vom Saal). The last chapter in this section focuses on the effects of environmental metal ions on the development of BPH and prostate cancer (S.-M. Ho).

The second edition of the book is a unique and comprehensive treatise, offering up-to-date information on a topic that has become a major concern among the scientific community and general public. The authors of this book are expert investigators who are pioneers in their fields and have presented the data in a dynamic manner that undoubtedly establishes this edition as a model source of recent, updated, cutting-edge, authentic, vital, and viable scientific information. In conclusion, it is a must-have book. If you liked the first edition, you will love the second one.

Editor

Rajesh K. Naz, Ph.D., is Professor of Obstetrics and Gynecology, and Physiology, as well as Director of the Division of Research at the Medical College of Ohio in Toledo.

Dr. Naz received his B.S. and M.S. degrees in biochemistry in 1973 and 1975, respectively. He received his Ph.D. in immunology in 1980 from the prestigious All India Institute of Medical Sciences in New Delhi, under the guidance of the renowned reproductive endocrinologist G.P. Talwar. In 1984, following postdoctoral work in reproductive immunology at the University of Michigan Medical School in Ann Arbor and then at the Oregon Regional Primate Research Center at Beaverton, he was appointed Assistant Professor and Director of the *In Vitro* Fertilization and Andrology Laboratories at the George Washington University in Washington, D.C. He joined the Albert Einstein College of Medicine in 1987 and was promoted to Associate Professor and Director of Research in 1989. He moved to the Medical College of Ohio in 1996.

Dr. Naz is a member of the Society for Gynecologic Investigation, American Society of Biochemistry and Molecular Biology, American Society for the Immunology of Reproduction, International Society for the Immunology of Reproduction, American Society of Reproductive Medicine, American Society of Andrology, Society for the Study of Reproduction, Endocrine Society, American Association for the Advancement of Science, and the New York Academy of Sciences.

Dr. Naz has lectured on reproductive immunology at numerous national and international symposia and at various conferences. He has received many prestigious awards and honors, and is a scientific reviewer for various grant proposals and research manuscripts for journals. He also is the member of the editorial boards of seven journals including *Biology of Reproduction* and *Archives of Andrology*, and is the associate editor of *Frontiers in BioScience*, *Human Reproduction*, and *Molecular Reproduction and Development.*

He has served in several study sections of the National Institutes of Health, including chairman of the Special Emphasis Panel SBIR Study Section. He has also served as a regular member of NIH's Reproductive Endocrinology Study Section.

Dr. Naz has published over 160 articles in scientific journals, as well as authoring and editing four books: *Immunology of Reproduction, Male Reproductive Medicine: From Spermatogenesis to Sperm Function and Modulation of Fertility, Prostate: Basic and Clinical Aspects*, and *Endocrine Disruptors: Effects on Male and Female Reproductive Systems*. His current interests include the molecular mechanisms underlying endocrinologic and immunologic control of fertility and infertility, and benign prostate hyperplasia (BPH) and prostate cancer in humans. He is especially interested in how the endocrine disruptors and environmental toxins can modify the male and female reproductive systems.

Contributors

Peter Thomas and
Izhar A. Khan
The University of Texas at Austin
Marine Science Institute
Austin, TX

Retha R. Newbold and
Wendy Jefferson
Developmental Endocrinology
  Section
Laboratory of Molecular
  Toxicology
Division of Intramural Research
National Institute of
  Environmental Health Sciences,
  NIH, DHHS
Research Triangle Park, NC

Retha R. Newbold
National Institute of
  Environmental Health Sciences
Research Triangle Park, NC

Patrick J. Devine, Ph.D.
Institut Armand Frappier
Institut National de la Recherche
  Scientifique
Montreal, Quebec, Canada

Patricia B. Hoyer, Ph.D.
Department of Physiology
Arizona Health Sciences Center
University of Arizona
Tucson, AZ

Michael A. Edelbrock
Department of Biochemistry and
  Molecular Biology
Medical College of Ohio
Toledo, OH
Environmental, Safety, and Health
  Management
The University of Findlay
Findlay, OH

Martha J. Fernstrom
Department of Biochemistry and
  Molecular Biology
Medical College of Ohio
Toledo, OH

Kandace J. Williams
Department of Biochemistry and
  Molecular Biology
Medical College of Ohio
Toledo, OH

Heather B. Patisaul
Center for Behavioral Neuroscience
Emory University
Atlanta, Georgia

Patricia L. Whitten
Department of Anthropology
Emory University
Atlanta, GA

A.M. Soto and C. Sonnenschein
Tufts University School of Medicine
Department of Anatomy and
  Cellular Biology
Boston, MA

Robert M. Bigsby,
Minerva Mercado-Feliciano, and
Josephine Mubiru
Department of Obstetrics and
  Gynecology
Department of Pharmacology and
  Toxicology
Indiana University School of Medicine
Indianapolis, IN

Robert M. Bigsby, Ph.D.
Department of Obstetrics and
  Gynecology
Indiana University School of
  Medicine
Indianapolis, IN

Stephen H. Safe
Department of Veterinary Physiology
  and Pharmacology
Texas A&M University
College Station, TX

Suresh C. Sikka
Department of Urology
School of Medicine
Tulane University Health Sciences
  Center
New Orleans, LA

Muammer Kendirci
Department of Urology
School of Medicine
Tulane University Health Sciences
  Center
New Orleans, LA

Rajesh Naz
Division of Research
Department of OB/GYN and
  Physiology
Medical College of Ohio
Toledo, OH

L. Earl Gray Jr.
MD-72, Endocrinology Branch
Reproductive Toxicology Division
US Environmental Protection Agency
Research Triangle Park, NC

Vickie Wilson
MD-72, Endocrinology Branch
Reproductive Toxicology Division
US Environmental Protection Agency
Research Triangle Park, NC

Tammy Stoker
MD-72, Endocrinology Branch
Reproductive Toxicology Division
US Environmental Protection Agency
Research Triangle Park, NC

Christy Lambright
MD-72, Endocrinology Branch
Reproductive Toxicology Division
US Environmental Protection Agency
Research Triangle Park, NC

Johnathan Furr
MD-72, Endocrinology Branch
Reproductive Toxicology Division
US Environmental Protection Agency
Research Triangle Park, NC

Nigel Noriega
MD-72, Endocrinology Branch
Reproductive Toxicology Division
US Environmental Protection Agency
Research Triangle Park, NC

Phillip Hartig
MD-72, Endocrinology Branch
Reproductive Toxicology Division
US Environmental Protection Agency
Research Triangle Park, NC

Mary Cardon
MD-72, Endocrinology Branch
Reproductive Toxicology Division
US Environmental Protection Agency
Research Triangle Park, NC

Mitch Rosen
MD-72, Endocrinology Branch
Reproductive Toxicology Division
US Environmental Protection Agency
Research Triangle Park, NC

Gerald Ankley
Mid Continent Ecology Division
NHEERL
Duluth, MN

Andrew Hotchkiss
Department of Psychology
Ohio State University
Columbus, OH

Edward F. Orlando
St. Mary's College of Maryland
St. Mary's, MD

Louis J. Guillette
University of Florida
Zoology Dept.
Gainesville, FL

William R. Kelce
Safety Sciences-Kalamazoo
Pfizer Global Research and
  Development
Pfizer Corporation
Kalamazoo, MI

Suresh C. Sikka
Department of Urology
School of Medicine
Tulane University Health Sciences
  Center
New Orleans, LA

Muammer Kendirci
Department of Urology
School of Medicine
Tulane University Health Sciences
  Center
New Orleans, LA

Rajesh Naz
Division of Research
Department of OB/GYN and
  Physiology
Medical College of Ohio
Toledo, Ohio

Catherine A. Richter
Division of Biological Sciences
University of Missouri-Columbia
Columbia, MO

Barry G. Timms
Division of Basic Biomedical Sciences
University of South Dakota
School of Medicine
Vermillion, SD

Frederick S. vom Saal
Division of Biological Sciences
University of Missouri-Columbia
Columbia, MO

Shuk-Mei Ho
Department of Surgery
University of Massachusetts Medical
  School
Worcester, MA

Acknowledgments

I thank the reviewers for contributing to the second edition of this book in a timely manner. I am grateful to Dipa Valambhia for the kind consideration, happiness, and immense love that have helped to compile this book. Thanks to Abhi and Manu Naz for love and understanding.

I am indebted for the support from my department and medical school, and from the National Institutes of Health (HD24425) for making publication of this second edition possible.

Table of Contents

Section I

Effect on the Female Reproductive System

1 Disruption of Nongenomic Steroid Actions on Gametes and Serotonergic Pathways Controlling Reproductive Neuroendocrine Function by Environmental Chemicals

Peter Thomas and Izhar A. Khan

CONTENTS

0-8493-2281-2/05/$0.00+$1.50
© 2005 by CRC Press

3

1.1 INTRODUCTION

Over the last decade there has been a heightened awareness and concern among the scientific community, policy makers, and general public over the reproductive hazards of endocrine-disrupting environmental chemicals, particularly xenobiotic estrogens (xenoestrogens), to fish, wildlife, and humans [1, 2]. Feminization of male birds, alligators, and fish and the production of the estrogen-induced yolk precursor, vitellogenin, in male freshwater fish have been reported after environmental exposure to xenoestrogens such as o,p'-DDT and Kepone, and to kraftmill effluent and sewage containing nonylphenols [1, 3–5]. In humans, estrogenic effects of Kepone were detected in male workers at a pesticide manufacturing plant [1]. Xenoestrogens have also been implicated in the apparent increase in breast cancer, one of the leading causes of death in women [6], and in the purported decrease in average sperm counts in semen samples collected from men over the past 50 years [7]. However, to date clear evidence of direct effects of endocrine-disrupting chemicals on human health at levels measured in the general population is lacking [8].

Extensive research over the past decade has identified a rapidly growing list of environmental contaminants that disrupt reproductive processes in vertebrates, primarily by exerting estrogenic or antiestrogenic actions [1, 8–10]. Most of these estrogenic xenobiotics, such as DDT and its isomers, PCBs and their hydroxylated metabolites, Kepone, methoxychlor metabolites, and nonylphenol and bisphenyl A are considered to exert their estrogenic effects primarily by binding to nuclear estrogen receptors [8, 9, 11–15]. However, the genomic actions of estrogens can also be influenced by other signaling mechanisms (receptor cross-talk) such as growth factors [16, 17]. Dioxin (2,3,7,8-tetrachlorodibenzo-p-dioxin, TCDD) and related dibenzo-p-dioxins, dibenzo-furans, and PCBs are thought to induce antiestrogenic effects indirectly by binding to the arylhydrocarbon receptor (AhR) [18] and subsequent interference of estrogen receptor binding to DNA response elements [19].

However, there is recent evidence that AhR ligands can also exert estrogenic effects and that the agonist-activated AhR/Arnt heterodimer associates with estrogen receptors, resulting in recruitment of unliganded estrogen receptor and co-activator p300 to estrogen-responsive gene promoters and subsequent activation of transcription [20]. In addition, a variety of xenobiotic compounds are capable of binding to nuclear androgen and progesterone receptors [14, 21]. For example, vinclozolin metabolites and the DDT analog p,p'-DDE, are effective competitors of androgen binding to vertebrate androgen receptors and have antiandrogenic actions in mammals [14, 21–23].

Although interference with the genomic actions of steroid hormones is considered to be the principal mechanism of endocrine disruption by many xenobiotics, chemicals could potentially act via different mechanisms at other sites on the hypothalamus–pituitary–gonadal axis to disrupt reproductive function [24, 25]. Monoaminergic and amino acid neurotransmitter pathways in the hypothalamus modulate the synthesis and secretion of gonadotropin releasing hormone (GnRH), which in turn regulates the secretion of gonadotropins from the pituitary. Therefore, neuropharmacological and neurotoxic chemicals that alter hypothalamic neurotransmitter function [15, 26–28] could influence GnRH secretion [29] and secondarily alter gonadotropin secretion, resulting in disruption of the reproductive cycle. Alternatively, chemicals could exert direct effects on GnRH neuronal activity [30]. In addition, direct actions of heavy metals have been demonstrated at the pituitary to alter gonadotropin secretion [31, 32] and at the gonadal level to disrupt steroidogenesis [15, 33]. Xenobiotics could also potentially interfere with nongenomic actions of steroids mediated by binding to steroid membrane receptors on oocytes and sperm plasma membranes [34, 35] or interfere with binding of catecholestrogens to catecholamine receptors in the brain [36].

This chapter discusses some nontraditional sites and mechanisms of chemical interference with hypothalamus-pituitary-gonadal function, identified in a well-characterized vertebrate model of reproductive endocrine toxicology, the Atlantic croaker (*Micropogonias undulatus*). The characteristics of maturation-inducing steroid receptors on plasma membranes of oocytes and sperm and their physiological roles in the final maturation of gametes are described. New information on the cloning, sequencing, and characterization of these progestin membrane receptors, the first information on the identity of any steroid membrane receptor, is briefly summarized. Data indicating that they are unrelated to nuclear steroid receptors, but instead have features of G-protein coupled receptors, will be described. Evidence of binding of xenoestrogens to the membrane receptors and disruption of final gamete maturation is presented, and the potential susceptibility of steroid membrane receptors to interference by lipophilic xenobiotic estrogens is discussed.

In addition, some mechanisms of endocrine disruption by neurotoxic chemicals are described. Studies showing that a PCB mixture, Aroclor 1254, and lead, both of which are neurotoxic, can disrupt neuroendocrine function and gonadotropin secretion in croaker by inducing a decline in hypothalamic serotonin concentrations are reviewed. Evidence is presented that chronic Aroclor 1254 treatment causes a decrease in the activity of tryptophan hydroxylase (TPH), the rate limiting enzyme in serotonin synthesis that is associated with reduced hypothalamic levels of the enzyme. Preliminary studies suggest that the labile TPH protein undergoes peroxidative damage after exposure to the PCB mixture, resulting in the formation of malondialdehyde adducts and loss of enzymatic activity.

1.2 NONGENOMIC ACTIONS OF STEROIDS

The classic model of hormone action for all known classes of steroids and many xenoestrogens involves diffusion or transport of the steroid or xenoestrogen across the plasma membrane, its binding to intracellular receptors in target cells, activation of the receptor, and tight association of the hormone-receptor complex and associated proteins to specific nuclear binding sites, resulting in alteration of gene transcription [9, 37]. However, convincing evidence has recently been obtained by many different laboratories using a wide variety of animal and cell models that many steroid effects are too rapid to be explained by the classic genomic mechanism and that steroids can also act at the cell surface to induce rapid intracellular responses by binding to membrane-bound receptors [38–40]. Alterations in ion fluxes and intracellular concentrations of calcium and other ions have been observed within 1 min of steroid addition and activation of second messengers within a few minutes [41, 42].

Moreover, these rapid, cell-surface initiated steroid actions often do not involve alterations in gene transcription (nongenomic). The importance of nonclassical steroid actions has become more widely appreciated in the past few years as many additional rapid, nongenomic actions of steroids have been reported in a wide range of tissues and cell types. For example, estrogen causes rapid prolactin release from pituitary cell lines [43], rapid release of intracellular calcium in rat granulosa cells

[44], and short-term electrophysiological changes in various brain regions [45]. Progesterone also induces rapid effects such as calcium influx into human sperm [41, 46, 47] and dopamine release from the corpus striatum [48], whereas glucocorticoids have been shown to cause rapid electrophysiological effects on mammalian neurons [49], behavioral effects [50], and lysis of lymphoma cells [51]. Steroid membrane receptors have been positively identified in many tissues where rapid nongenomic steroid effects have been observed (38–40). Specific plasma membrane receptors for estrogens have been identified in rat pituitary, liver, and uterine tissues [52, 53] and in fish testes [54]; for glucocorticoids in liver, brain, and lymphoma cells [50, 55, 56]; for progesterone in rat brain and sperm membranes [57, 58] and in fish oocyte and sperm membranes [59, 60]; and for androgens in endothelial cells and in fish ovaries [61, 62].

1.2.2 ENDOCRINE DISRUPTION OF NONGENOMIC STEROID ACTIONS

Recent studies have shown that nongenomic steroid actions, such as genomic ones, are susceptible to interference by xenoestrogens at environmentally realistic concentrations [34, 54, 63–69]. Therefore, xenoestrogens and other environmental chemicals have the potential to influence a broad range of critical physiological and pathological processes in animals by this mechanism, including many processes that until now have been thought to be exclusively influenced by genomic steroid mechanisms. For example, hormone secretion appears to be susceptible to chemical disruption by this mechanism. Xenoestrogens have been shown to influence rapid estrogen-induced changes in the secretion of insulin [66], androgens [54], and prolactin [69], resulting in endocrine disturbances.

Evidence that nongenomic steroid actions, like genomic ones, are susceptible to interference by xenoestrogens was first obtained in a fish model [34, 70]. The observation that several xenoestrogens blocked the induction of oocyte maturation (OM) of Atlantic croaker oocytes *in vitro* by the maturation-inducing steroid (20β-S) provided initial evidence for this mechanism of endocrine disruption [34]. Oocytes that fail to mature are incapable of fertilization. Inhibition of OM was also observed *in vivo* after 2 weeks' exposure to low, realistic concentrations of water-soluble fractions of fuel oil and Aroclor 1254 and after injection of Kepone [71]. Similar antagonistic actions of xenoestrogens on progestogen induction of OM *in vitro* by a nongenomic mechanism were subsequently confirmed in an amphibian model, *Xenopus* [65]. Xenoestrogens, such as nonylphenol and *o,p'*-DDT, can mimic the nongenomic action of estrogens, causing calcium influx into rat smooth muscle cells [68].

Moreover, evidence has recently been obtained for interference of a nongenomic steroid action in humans. A xenoestrogen, genestein, disrupts the acrosome reaction in human sperm, a process induced by progesterone [72]. However, xenoestrogen interactions with the steroid membrane receptors thought to mediate these actions were not investigated or could not be demonstrated, so the mechanism of interference with these nongenomic steroid actions remained unclear.

Disruption of a nongenomic steroid action by a xenobiotic chemical binding to a steroid membrane receptor was first demonstrated for the maturation-inducing steroid (MIS) receptor mediating OM in a teleost model, the spotted seatrout [73]. Several xenoestrogens that antagonize MIS (17,20β-trihydroxy-4-pregnen-3-one, 20β-S) stimulation of sperm motility in Atlantic croaker are also effective competitors for 20-S binding to the sperm membrane receptor [35]. Xenoestrogens have also been shown to mimic the rapid, nongenomic actions of estrogens by binding to estrogen membrane receptors. Several xenoestrogens display relatively high binding affinities for the membrane estrogen receptor in Atlantic croaker testes, similar to their binding affinities for the nuclear estrogen receptor in this species [54, 74], and also mimic the inhibitory actions of estrogens on testicular androgen production [54]. In rats, the nongenomic action of a xenoestrogen, bisphenol A, on insulin secretion was associated with its binding to the membrane estrogen receptor [66].

It is concluded from these studies that rapid, nongenomic steroid actions are likely susceptible to disruption by xenobiotic chemicals via interference with receptor binding. Most of the evidence to date for this mechanism of endocrine disruption has been obtained for gamete maturation in fish models. Therefore, progestin induction of oocyte and sperm maturation, the membrane progestin receptors that mediate these nongenomic actions, and their interference by xenoestrogens are discussed in subsequent sections in greater detail.

1.2.3 OOCYTE MATURATION IN FISH AND AMPHIBIANS

1.2.3.1 Role of Oocyte Progestin Membrane Receptors

The nongenomic actions of progestin maturational steroids (MIS) on OM in amphibians and fishes and the roles of receptors on the oocyte plasma membrane as intermediaries in progestin action have been widely recognized for nearly two decades [75, 76] and currently are the most thoroughly characterized models of membrane receptor-mediated steroid action. The discovery that steroids could induce meiotic maturation of amphibian and teleostean oocytes in simple *in vitro* incubation systems stimulated intensive research on the natural MISs in these vertebrate groups and their mechanisms of action [75, 77]. It was shown that the amphibian MIS, progesterone, was ineffective in inducing OM when microinjected in *Xenopus laevis* and *Rana pipiens* oocytes [78, 79], but it was effective when applied externally bound to beads or in a polymer form [80, 81]. Identical results were obtained with the teleostean MIS, 17, 20-dihydroxy-4-pregnen-3-one (17, 20β-P) in goldfish oocytes [82].

Moreover, inhibitors of transcription did not prevent 17,20β-P-induced final OM in teleosts, which supports the concept that the action of the MIS is nongenomic [77]. The finding that increases in cyclic AMP levels by pharmacological agents block MIS stimulation of OM *in vitro* also suggests that the action of the MIS is nongenomic and instead involves a second messenger signal transduction pathway [77]. A decrease in cyclic AMP is required for MIS induction of final oocyte maturation in rainbow trout and spotted seatrout, which is mediated by activation of a pertussis toxin-sensitive inhibitory G-protein in the signal transduction pathway across the oocyte plasma membrane to the cytoplasm [77, 83]. A cytoplasmic factor, named maturation-promoting factor, composed of cdc 2 kinase and cyclin B, is formed and is the intracellular mediator of OM [77].

Direct evidence for the presence of a membrane receptor for the MIS and its involvement in final OM was first obtained in amphibians, *Xenopus* [76, 84, 85] and *Rana* [86], primarily using photoaffinity labeling with the synthetic progestin, R5020. The existence of a high-affinity ($K_d = 10^{-9}$M) progesterone receptor in the plasma membrane of *Xenopus* oocytes has since been confirmed using a membrane filtration technique [87], although it was found that the ligand used in earlier studies, R5020, recognizes a different binding site than the natural MIS.

1.2.3.2 Characteristics of Ovarian MIS Membrane Receptors in Fishes

The first convincing evidence for the existence of a high-affinity ($K_d = 10^{-9}$M), low-capacity ($10^{-3} - 10^{-12}$ mol/g ovary) membrane receptor for the teleost MIS was obtained in spotted seatrout (*Cynoscion nebulosus*) ovaries for 17, 20, 21-trihydroxy-4-pregnen-3-one (20β-S), the natural MIS in this species [59, 88]. Subsequently, specific binding of the salmonid MIS, 17,20β-P, and R5020 to ovarian and oocyte membrane preparations has been reported in brook trout and rainbow trout and in yellowtail [89, 90, 91] and for the perciform MIS, 20β-S, in striped bass [92]. The membrane receptor for the MIS in spotted seatrout ovaries shows the greatest steroid specificity, only structurally similar C21 steroids have similar binding affinities [59, 93], whereas most other MIS membrane receptors investigated to date also show significant binding to androgens and estrogens [87, 89, 90]. A close correlation has been demonstrated between the receptor binding affinities of steroids for the MIS membrane receptor in spotted seatrout ovaries and their agonist and antagonist activities in *in vitro* OM bioassays. The presence of hydroxyl groups at both the 17 and 20 positions on the progesterone nucleus appears to be essential for agonist activity in the seatrout OM bioassay, whereas hydroxyls at both the 20β and 21 positions are required for high-binding affinity for the receptor [93]. The presence of hydroxyls at all three positions (17α, 20, and 21 positions, i.e., 20-S) results in greatest affinity for the receptor and the most potent induction of oocyte maturation in the bioassay. The action of 20β-S is rapid: 1-min exposure to 20β-S is sufficient to induce OM, which is consistent with its rapid rate of association with the receptor.

Figure 1.1 shows the effects of incubating follicle-enclosed seatrout oocytes with the MIS (20β-S) in the presence of two steroids with high relative binding affinities (RBAs) for the receptor, but lacking maturation-inducing activity, 20β, 21-dihydroxy-4-pregnen-3-one (20β,21-P) and pregnenolone. Germinal vesicle breakdown (GVBD, i.e., disappearance of the nucleus) was used as the end point in the OM bioassay [94]. Induction of GVBD by 1-min exposure to 5 nM and 50 nM 20β-S was inhibited by coincubation with 300 nM 20, 21-P, which has hydroxyls on the 20 and 21 positions of the progesterone nucleus (RBA 50%) and 300 nM pregnenolone, which has a hydroxyl on the 3β position (RBA 96%). Other steroids that displaced 50% or more of the bound, tritiated 20β-S from its receptor at a concentration of 300 nM also

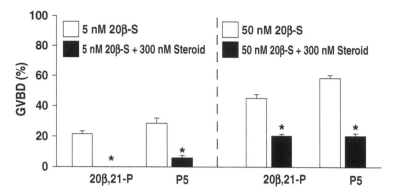

FIGURE 1.1   Effects of coincubating 20β,21-dihydroxy-4-pregnen-3-one (20β,21-P) and pregnenolone (P5) with 20β-S for 1 min. on subsequent final maturation of spotted seatrout oocytes *in vitro*. % GVBD: percentage of oocytes that completed germinal vesicle breakdown. Asterisks denote treatments significantly different from corresponding 20β-S treatment alone (N = 6).

significantly inhibited 20β-S-induced GVBD [93]. Only one other steroid, 17, 20β-P, caused significant induction of OM after 1-min exposure; but its potency was much lower than that of 20β-S, which is consistent with its low RBA (< 1.0%). These studies demonstrate that the 1-min GVBD *in vitro* bioassay with seatrout oocytes is highly specific for the natural MIS, 20β-S. No other steroids are capable of inducing GVBD at physiological concentrations. The ability of the bioassay to detect antagonism of MIS action by other steroids also indicates its potential for examining the consequences of interference of 20β-S action on the oocyte membrane receptor by xenobiotic chemicals.

1.2.3.3 Xenoestrogen Binding to the Ovarian MIS Membrane Receptor in Fish

Although a broad range of xenobiotic organic compounds have been shown to disrupt early development as well as endocrine and reproductive functions in vertebrates by binding to nuclear steroid receptors, little information is currently available on whether these organic compounds can also bind to steroid membrane receptors and disrupt steroid action at the level of the plasma membrane. Xenobiotic interactions with steroid membrane receptors cannot be predicted from their affinities for nuclear receptors because their steroid ligand specificities differ, especially for synthetic antihormones [95]. For example, the steroid specificity of the nuclear progestogen receptor in seatrout ovarian tissue, which mediates 20β-S induction of ovulation, differs considerably from that of the seatrout ovarian 20β-S membrane receptor [59, 93–96, 97].

The development of a reliable filter assay for the 20β-S membrane receptor and the availability of large amounts of starting material (seatrout ovaries weigh up to 1 kg) has permitted detailed investigations of the interactions of xenobiotics with steroid membrane receptors to be conducted. The displacement of 5 nM ^{3}H-20β-S

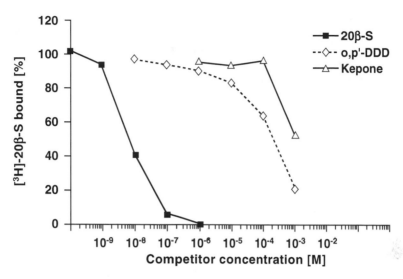

FIGURE 1.2   Competition by the xenoestrogens o,p'-DDD and Kepone for ^{3}H-20β-S binding to the spotted seatrout ovarian MIS membrane receptor. Binding is expressed as a percentage of total binding (binding suppressed by 300 nM 20β-S).

by the organochlorines Kepone, methoxychlor, o,p'-DDD, and o,p'-DDE over a broad range of concentrations (1 nM – 1 mM) was investigated in competition assays. The organochlorines were added to the assay buffer dissolved in ethanol (final concentration 1%), which did not affect receptor binding. The ovarian membrane preparations were incubated with the organochlorines and ^{3}H-20β-S for 30 min at 4°C before separation of bound from free by filtration through glass microfiber filters. All the organochlorines displaced the ^{3}H-20β-S in a concentration-dependent manner [73]. Displacement curves for o,p'-DDD and Kepone are shown in Figure 1.2. Significant displacement of 20β-S was observed with o,p'-DDD at a concentration of 100:M. Kepone had a lower binding affinity in this assay, although in several other receptor assays binding affinity was tenfold higher [73]. To determine if this decrease in ^{3}H-20β-S binding is due to disruption of the plasma membrane and loss of binding sites, membrane preparations were incubated with o,p'-DDD, Kepone, or buffer alone for 30 min and subsequently washed thoroughly four times to remove any of the compounds prior to conducting the 20β-S receptor assay. It was found that prior exposure to these compounds did not alter the [^{3}H]-20β-S binding capacity of the membrane receptor preparation, thereby indicating that they did not destroy binding sites and that the inhibition of receptor binding is reversible.

To determine whether inhibition of binding by Kepone was competitive, Scatchard plot analyses of ^{3}H 20β-S binding were performed in the presence of Kepone [73, 98]. Different concentrations of Kepone (0.2, 1, and 10:M) altered the K_D value of ^{3}H-20β-S binding to the receptor without changing the B_{max}, which suggests that the binding is competitive. However, Scatchard analysis with other organochlorines suggests that xenobiotic binding to the receptor is often noncompetitive. Recent studies indicate that a broad range of xenobiotic organic compounds, including many that are estrogenic, are capable of displacing ^{3}H-20β-S from the membrane receptor. Estrogenic hydroxylated PCB congeners such as 2',5'-PCB-3-OH cause 50% displacement of 20β-S from the receptor at a concentration of 10:M, similar to their affinities for the seatrout hepatic nuclear estrogen receptor (unpubl. obs.). Nonylphenol and the mycotoxin estrogen, zearalenone, diethylstilbestrol, and several other synthetic estrogens and antiestrogens have tenfold higher relative binding affinities for the receptor, causing significant displacement in the high nanomolar concentration range. Estradiol has a similar binding affinity, displacing 13% of ^{3}H-20β-S at a concentration of 300 nM [93]. We conclude therefore that the seatrout progestin membrane receptor is susceptible to interference by a variety of xenoestrogens.

1.2.3.4   Xenoestrogen Interference with MIS Induction of Oocyte Maturation

Bioassays of OM were conducted with xenoestrogens that bound to the seatrout receptor to determine whether they displayed agonist activities or antagonized the actions of 20β-S. Ovarian tissue from Atlantic croaker, a closely related species belonging to the same family as seatrout, was used for the *in vitro* bioassays. Approximately 50 follicle-enclosed oocytes were preincubated for 9 hours in culture medium in the presence of gonadotropin to induce maturational competence, that is, the ability of oocytes to undergo final maturation in response to the MIS [94, 99]. One critical component of this process induced by the periovulatory surge in gonadotropin secretion is upregulation of the oocyte membrane MIS receptor [99–102]. The culture medium was removed at the end of the preincubation period and replaced with fresh medium containing either 20β-S alone or 20β-S in combination with various concentrations of Kepone or *o,p'*-DDD (dissolved in ethanol, final concentration 0.1%), and the "primed" oocytes were incubated for an additional 12 hours to allow them to complete final maturation. Dissolution of the nucleus or germinal vesicle (germinal vesicle breakdown) was scored by visual examination under low-power magnification at the end of the incubation.

Nearly all of the oocytes had completed GVBD after incubation in 29 or 290 nM 20β-S alone (Figure 1.3), the lipid globules in the ooplasm had fused, and the oocytes were fully hydrated. Maturation of the majority of the oocytes in response to 290 nM 20β-S was inhibited by exposure to 100:M Kepone or *o,p'*-DDD for 12 hours [34]. Maturation was abnormal and arrested at early stages in most of the oocytes. The oocytes in the xenoestrogen-exposed groups that completed GVBD had an abnormal appearance; incomplete clearing of the ooplasm, hydration, and oil droplet formation were often observed [34]. The inhibition of GVBD by Kepone and *o,p'*-DDD in response to 290 nM 20β-S was concentration dependent, significant inhibition occurring at concentrations of 1 and 10 nM (Figure 1.3). Almost identical concentration-response relationships were observed when seatrout oocytes were incubated with these xenoestrogens (results not shown). The two xenoestrogens did not act as agonists on GVBD at any of the concentrations tested. A variety of other organochlorine xenoestrogens including methoxychlor, DDT derivatives, and hydroxylated PCBs also inhibited GVBD of croaker and seatrout oocytes in a concentration-dependent manner (unpublished observation).

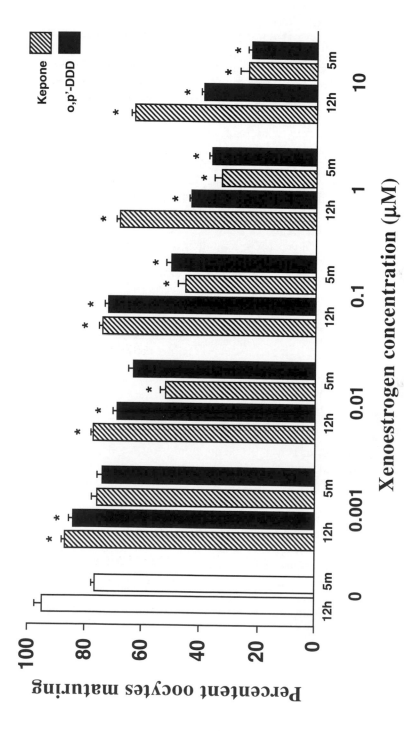

FIGURE 1.3 Concentration-dependent effects of Kepone and *o,p′*-DDD on 20β-S-induced GVBD of primed Atlantic croaker oocytes *in vitro*. Oocytes were exposed for 12 h to both xenobiotics in the presence of 290 nM 20β-S or for 5 min in the presence of 29 nM 20β-S, or 20β-S alone (clear bars). Bars represent means ± S.E.M. of six observations. Asterisks denote means significantly different from controls (p < 0.05, Tukey's HSD test). (From Ghosh, S. and Thomas, P., *Mar. Environ. Res.* 39, 159, 1995. With permission.)

The finding that some of the oocytes underwent GVBD even at the highest Kepone and o,p'-DDD concentrations tested (100:M) suggests that the xenobiotics are not merely toxic to the oocytes but instead may antagonize the actions of 20β-S. Association of 20β-S with the membrane receptor is rapid with a t_j of less than 2 min [59]. Consequently, incubation of maturationally competent croaker oocytes with 20β-S for 1 to 5 min is sufficient to induce GVBD [93]. Short-term incubations were therefore conducted with the xenobiotics to limit the possible contribution of nonspecific toxic actions to the effects observed. Co-incubation of the oocytes with 29 nM 20β-S and o,p'-DDD or Kepone for 5 min followed by 5 min of repeated washing and an additional 12-hour incubation in media alone resulted in a concentration-dependent inhibition of GVBD (Figure 1.3). The functional integrity of the oocytes was not impaired after exposure to the xenobiotics, because subsequent exposure to 20β-S completely restored the ability of the oocytes to undergo GVBD. Pronounced inhibitory effects of Kepone and o,p'-DDD on GVBD induced by 29 nM 20β-S were observed after only 5 min exposure (Figure 1.3).

Although the concentration-dependent inhibition of GVBD by the xenobiotics in these bioassays is consistent with an antagonistic action mediated by the membrane receptor, additional experiments will be required to confirm this mechanism of endocrine disruption. Recent refinements have increased the sensitivity of the bioassay, with significant induction of GVBD occurring after 1 min exposure to 5 nM 20β-S, close to its K_d [59]. Thus, it is now possible to investigate xenobiotic antagonism with steroid action at the membrane receptor over a broader range of 20β-S concentrations.

1.2.3.5 Significance of Receptor Location in Plasma Membrane

The finding that the majority of xenoestrogens that bind to the membrane progestin receptor in seatrout ovaries display little or no affinity for the nuclear progestin receptor in this species [97] suggests that localization of the receptor in the plasma membrane may be important for xenobiotic binding activity. Many of the xenoestrogens tested are highly lipophilic and readily interact with biological membranes, which are rich in lipids [103, 104]. Techniques to solubilize the membrane receptor and measure competition with 20β-S binding to the solubilized protein were developed to investigate this possibility. Removal of the receptor from the plasma membrane by solubilization did not alter the binding affinities of natural and synthetic steroids, whereas it resulted in a complete loss of binding to a variety of xenoestrogens such as DDT analogs and hydroxylated PCBs. In a separate study, the binding of organic compounds lacking estrogenic activity with different degrees of lipophilicity (octanol/water coefficients) to the membrane receptor was investigated in competition assays. The two most lipophilic compounds, dibenzofuran and biphenyl, caused significant displacement of ^{3}H-20β-S at a concentration of 100 nM, whereas none of the other organic compounds were effective competitors at this concentration (unpublished observation).

In conclusion, these studies demonstrate that the MIS membrane receptor is susceptible to interference by xenoestrogens and also by highly lipophilic nonestrogenic organic compounds. These xenobiotics act as antagonists, blocking the induction of OM in response to 20β-S. The finding that localization of the receptor in the plasma membrane is a requirement for binding to xenobiotic antagonists, but not for binding to steroids, suggests that the binding sites for these two classes of ligands differ. However, information on the primary structure of steroid membrane receptors will be required to model likely binding sites for natural and xenobiotic ligands. Finally, these results suggest that steroid membrane receptors are potentially susceptible to interference by lipophilic organic compounds, particularly xenoestrogens, and may be additional targets for these compounds.

1.2.4 SPERM ACTIVATION IN MAMMALS AND FISH

1.2.4.1 Rapid Actions of Progesterone on Sperm Membranes in Mammals

Studies over the past decade have demonstrated that progesterone exerts direct and rapid nongenomic actions on human sperm, resulting in hyperactive motility and induction of the acrosome reaction, increased binding to the zona pellucida, and fusion with the oocyte [47, 58, 105, 106]. This activation of sperm by progesterone has been shown by several laboratories to be mediated by an influx of calcium [47, 107–109]. Moreover, the increase in intracellular calcium concentrations is rapid, occurring within seconds, and is concentration dependent [46, 110, 111], which suggests that progesterone exerts a nongenomic action by binding to a specific cell-surface receptor on sperm [58, 107, 109]. The increase in calcium in sperm after exposure to progesterone activates phospholipase C [46], resulting in rapid changes in swimming direction (hyperactivation) and the acrosome reaction. One of the possible functions of hyperactive motility in mammalian sperm is to provide increased thrust necessary for the penetration of the oocyte zona [112].

Although this receptor has not yet been fully characterized, several other lines of evidence also suggest the existence of a specific progesterone membrane receptor on mammalian sperm. Progesterone is still able to increase sperm calcium concentrations and calcium influx when it is bound to bovine serum albumin (BSA) and unable to traverse the plasma membrane, suggesting a cell-surface site of action [113, 47]. Histological studies using fluorescein-isothiocyanate labelling of the progesterone–BSA complex have confirmed that the binding sites are on the plasma membrane of the sperm head [114, 115]. Studies on the structure-activity relationships for calcium influx and the acrosome reaction have suggested that the steroid specificity of the putative progesterone membrane receptor differs considerably from that of the classical nuclear progesterone receptor [107, 116, 117, 118]. However, the steroid binding of this putative receptor has not been fully characterized.

1.2.4.2 Characteristics of Sperm MIS Membrane Receptor in Fishes

Recently, MIS receptors were identified and fully characterized on plasma membranes of spotted seatrout and Atlantic croaker sperm [60, 119], using a modification

TABLE 1.1

Characteristics of Atlantic Croaker 20-S Sperm Membrane Receptor

Receptor Criteria	Binding Characteristics
1. High affinity, single receptor site	K_d = 25.5nM, single class binding sites (by Scatchard analysis)
2. Low capacity, saturable binding	B_{max} = 0.085 nM ml^{-1} milt; saturated with 20nM [^{3}H]-20β-S
3. Displaceable binding	Association T1/2 = 2 min., dissociation T1/2 = 2.5 min.
4. High steroid specificity	RBA[1]: 17,20β-P, Prog., S-<0.11; T-<0.11;T-<0.01; E$_2$, F no binding
5. Tissue specificity[2]	Sperm, testis, ovary, liver, not in gill
6. Biological validation	1.5–2.5 x increase receptor conc. after incubation with GtH

[1] Relative binding affinity, calculated from concentration of 20β-S causing 50% displacement.

[2] Data also from Patiño and Thomas (1990) in spotted seatrout tissue.

of the protocol developed for assaying the ovarian membrane MIS receptor in these species [59, 93]. Saturation analysis showed the presence of saturable 20β-S binding in the membrane fractions of seatrout and croaker sperm and testes; complete saturation was achieved with approximately 20 nM 20β-S [60, 119] (Table 1.1). Scatchard analyses indicated the presence of a single class of high-affinity (K_d = 18–22 nM), low-capacity (B_{max} = 0.09–0.003 nM ml^{-1}milt), binding sites, in the membrane preparations (Figure 1.4). The ^{3}H-20β-S binding was readily displaced with excess cold 20β-S. The rates of association and dissociation were extremely rapid; each had a t$_{\int}$ of less than 2.5 min. These rapid rates of association and dissociation are characteristic of plasma membrane receptors. The binding was highly specific for 20β-S (Figure 1.5); all the other C21 steroids tested had relative binding affinities of less than 15% for the seatrout receptor (Figure 1.5). The binding affinity of testosterone was two orders of magnitude lower, whereas estradiol and cortisol were ineffective at displacing 20β-S from the binding sites on croaker sperm [119].

Estradiol had a slightly higher affinity for the seatrout sperm and testes receptor (RBA 0.4%, Figure 1.5), but the specificities of the receptors for the other steroids were practically identical [60]. This pattern of steroid-binding affinity is similar to that of the ovarian MIS membrane receptor [59, 93] but differs remarkably from that of the nuclear progestin receptor in seatrout testes in which several C21 steroids display higher affinities [96, 97]. Specific 20β-S binding was limited primarily to reproductive tissues with small amounts also present in the liver (Table 1.1).

The final criterion that needs to be satisfied for a binding moiety to be designated as a receptor is that changes in receptor abundance are consistent with its proposed physiological functions. In male fish the prespawning surge in plasma gonadotropin levels causes increases in MIS production and milt volume. It was found that hormonal stimulation of gonadotropin secretion by GnRH injection caused a two- to threefold increase in sperm 20β-S concentrations 2 days later, which was accompanied by an increase in milt volume. Similarly, incubation of minced croaker and

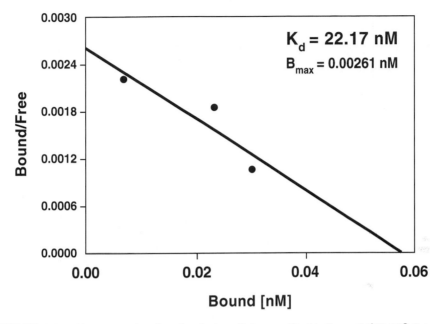

FIGURE 1.4 Representative Scatchard plot of the specific binding of [³H]-20β-S to a spotted seatrout spermatozoa plasma membrane extract, K_d = 22.17 nM, B_{max} = 0.00261 nmol mL⁻¹ milt. (From Thomas, P., Breckenridge-Miller, D., and Detweiler, C., *Fish Physiol. Biochem.* 17, 109, 1997. With permission.)

seatrout testicular tissues with gonadotropin for 18 hours increased sperm receptor levels severalfold compared to controls [60, 119]. Therefore, sperm membrane 20β-S binding in both species fulfills all the criteria for their designation as hormone receptors.

1.2.4.3 Role of Sperm MIS Membrane Receptor in Sperm Motility

The majority of teleosts are egg laying (oviparous) and have external fertilization. Unlike mammalian sperm, the sperm of oviparous teleost species are immotile in the seminal fluid and are activated by changes in osmotic pressure when they are released into the external medium [120]. However, many basic features of the acquisition of sperm motility in teleosts are similar to those of mammals. For example, calcium influx via calcium channels and elevated cyclic AMP levels also appear to be involved in the final activation of sperm in teleost species [121–123]. Calcium is a potent stimulator of sperm motility in teleosts [123, 124] and increases the velocity and turning rate of sperm, similar to hyperactivation of mammalian sperm. However, calcium does not induce the acrosome reaction in fish sperm, since fish sperm lack this structure and instead enter the oocyte via a specialized channel, the micropyle. These calcium-induced changes in sperm motility are considered to be necessary for optimum fertilization capacity.

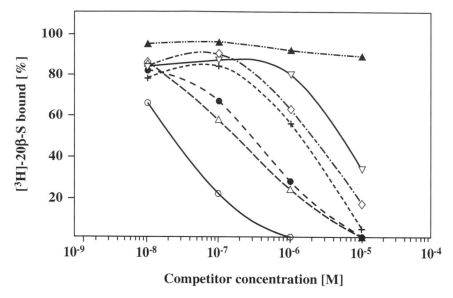

FIGURE 1.5   Steroid binding specificity of spotted seatrout testicular plasma membrane preparations. Membranes were incubated for 30 min with 20 nM]³H]-20β-S and 10 nM-10 :M competitor: o – o 20β-S, △ – △ 17,20β-P, • – • progesterone, + – + 11-deoxycortisol, ▲ – ▲ cortisol, ∇ – ∇ estradiol, ◊ – ◊ testosterone. (From Thomas, P., Breckenridge-Miller, D. and Detweiler, C., *Fish Physiol. Biochem.* 17, 109, 1997. With permission.)

Several lines of evidence suggest the MIS receptor on croaker sperm is an important intermediary on sperm activation. Incubation of sperm with 20β-S, but not with other steroids, increases the percentage that are motile as well as sperm velocity and their turning rate. This stimulatory effect of 20β-S is concentration dependent and is enhanced if 20β-S receptor concentrations on croaker sperm are upregulated by prior *in vivo* treatment with LHRH [125]. Incubation with 20β-S also causes rapid increases in intrasperm free calcium concentrations [125]. These studies suggest, therefore, that 20β-S activates croaker sperm by elevating intracellular free calcium levels and that the process is dependent upon sufficient numbers of MIS sperm membrane receptors and functional calcium channels. Thus, it is proposed that the basic mechanism of sperm activation by progestins in the male reproductive tract of a teleost species with external fertilization is similar to that induced by progesterone in the female tract of a vertebrate group with internal fertilization, the mammals.

1.2.4.4   Xenoestrogen Binding to Sperm MIS Membrane Receptor

The ability of the xenoestrogens, Kepone, *o,p′*-DDE and 2′4′6′-PCB-4-OH, and a mycotoxin estrogen, zearalenone, to displace ³H-20β-S from the croaker sperm membrane MIS receptor was examined in competitive binding assays [35, 60]. Sperm membrane preparations were incubated in the presence of ³H-20β-S with or without

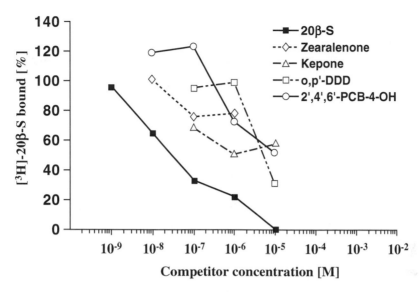

FIGURE 1.6 Competition by xenoestrogens, Kepone, *o,p'*-DDE and 2',4',6'-PCB-4-OH, and a mycotoxin estrogen, zearalenone for ^{3}H-20β-S binding to the Atlantic croaker sperm MIS membrane receptor. Binding is expressed as a percentage of total binding (binding suppressed by 300 nM 20β-S). (From Thomas, P., Breckenridge-Miller, D., and Detweiler, C., *Mar. Environ. Res.* 46, 163, 1998. With permission.)

various amounts of unlabelled 20β-S or the estrogenic compounds (concentration range: 10 nM–1 mM) for 30 to 60 min. at 4°C. Maximum specific binding was expressed as the binding suppressed by 100-fold excess unlabeled 20β-S.

All four estrogenic compounds were effective competitors for ^{3}H-20β-S binding to the sperm membrane MIS receptor (Figure 1.6). Zearalenone and Kepone caused significant displacement at a concentration of 100 nM. None of the estrogenic compounds were capable of completely displacing 20β-S from the receptor and only one, *o,p'*-DDE, caused more than 50% displacement under these assay conditions. In addition, the slopes of their competition curves were not parallel to that of 20β-S, which suggests that the xenobiotic binding is of the noncompetitive type.

1.2.4.5 Effects of Xenobiotics on Sperm Motility

In a preliminary study, Kepone caused a concentration-dependent decrease in the motility of croaker sperm after incubation with sperm *in vitro* for 1 to 2 minutes, with significant impairment of motility at a concentration of 200 μM [35]. Recently, a variety of xenoestrogens (e.g., *o,p'*-DDT and *o,p'*-DDE) and other xenobiotic compounds (e.g., atrazine) at low, environmentally realistic concentrations (0.1–0.01 μM), after 5 minutes' treatment *in vitro*, were shown to block the increase in the motility of croaker sperm in response to 20β-S treatment [125]. Interestingly, the xenobiotic compounds at these concentrations did not alter basal, unstimulated sperm motility, which suggests that their inhibitory actions are solely on hormone stimulation of sperm motility, presumably by binding to the sperm 20β-S membrane receptor. Increasing the hormone concentrations should overcome the inhibitory actions of receptor antagonists, because binding of agonists and antagonists to steroid receptors is readily displaceable and competitive. Therefore, the finding that a tenfold increase in 20β-S concentrations completely reverses the inhibitory action of the xenobiotic compounds on sperm motility is further evidence that they act via binding to the 20β-S membrane receptor [125].

Decreases in sperm motility have been observed in fish exposed to a variety of xenobiotic compounds, and inhibition of the acrosome reaction in human sperm exposed to genestein [72] is associated with declines in fertilization capacity. Interestingly, decreases in sperm motility and abnormal sperm have previously been reported in factory workers exposed to Kepone, which was thought to be a primary cause of their decreased fertility [12]. Taken together, these studies on fish and humans suggest that sperm function may be particularly sensitive to disruption by xenoestrogens. The experiments with croaker sperm provide the first evidence, to our knowledge, of binding of xenoestrogens to a steroid membrane receptor on vertebrate sperm. Clearly, the progestin membrane receptor on vertebrate sperm is a potential site of interference by estrogenic xenobiotics and other endocrine-disrupting chemicals.

1.2.4.6   Current Issues in Endocrine Disruption of Nongenomic Steroid Actions

Evidence has been obtained in a vertebrate model that a variety of xenoestrogens are effective competitors of progestins for binding to plasma membrane receptors on both oocytes and sperm. Several of these xenobiotics can antagonize the actions of the progestin, 20β-S, thereby disrupting the processes of final gamete maturation. Localization of the receptor in the plasma membrane appears to be necessary for receptor binding to these lipophilic xenobiotic chemicals. However, further investigations on endocrine disruption of nongenomic steroid actions will be required to determine their broad toxicological significance. Currently, the extent of nongenomic steroid endocrine disruption is unknown. To date, the effects of a limited number of xenobiotic chemicals on only a few nongenomic steroid actions have been investigated. Information on which nongenomic steroid actions are particularly sensitive to chemical interference by this mechanism is required, as well as the effective chemical concentrations. The development of bioassays that measure earlier responses in the steroid-signaling pathway, such as activation of intracellular second messengers, are likely to be more specific and sensitive than the gamete maturation assays.

Additional research is also needed on the nature of endocrine disruption and the role of membrane localization of the receptor on its disruption by lipophilic xenobiotic compounds. Knowledge of the molecular mechanisms involved in xenobiotic chemical/steroid membrane receptor interactions will be required to model the binding sites and develop QSARs. However, the current complete lack of information on the structures of steroid membrane receptors and their steroid binding sites have prevented the development of experimental and theoretical approaches to determine their interactions with xenobiotic chemicals at the molecular level.

Recently, a novel gene, unrelated to any previously characterized in vertebrates, with the major characteristics of a membrane progestin receptor, was discovered in our laboratory in a well-characterized reproductive endocrine model, spotted seatrout [42]. Subsequently, 13 closely related genes were identified and completely sequenced in other vertebrates, and could be separated into three clades on the basis of sequence identity and phylogenetic analysis, called α, β, and γ subtypes (126). These studies providing the first information on the structures of any steroid receptors unrelated to nuclear steroid receptors are briefly summarized below.

1.2.5 CLONING, IDENTIFICATION, AND CHARACTERIZATION OF PROGESTIN MEMBRANE RECEPTORS IN FISH AND OTHER VERTEBRATES

A combination of protein purification, antibody screening, and molecular approaches was used to clone the 20β-S from a seatrout ovarian library [83]. DEAE chromatography of a solubilized seatrout ovarian membrane extract produced a partially purified membrane progestin receptor fraction with significant 20β-S binding activity containing a single, major protein band of 40 kDa. This fraction was used to immunize mice. Hybridomas were established, and positive monoclonal antibodies that recognized seatrout ovarian membrane proteins in the 20 to 100 kDa range and bound the solubilized receptor in a double-antibody receptor-capture assay developed in our laboratory were identified [83]. The positive antibodies were considered to recognize portions of the membrane progestin receptor and, therefore, suitable for screening a seatrout ovarian cDNA expression library. A positive clone, a 1.4-Kb fragment, was completely sequenced and appeared to be a novel gene, unrelated to any previously characterized vertebrate gene. The following eight criteria were satisfied for designation of the novel seatrout gene as a membrane steroid receptor.

Plausible structure: Structural analysis of the deduced amino acid sequence of the gene using a variety of computer programs that predict the subcellular localization, hydrophilicity profile, and structure indicates the protein is localized in the plasma membrane and has seven transmembrane domains, characteristic of a major class of membrane receptors, GPCRs [42]. A proposed model for the insertion of the seatrout protein in the plasma membrane is shown in Figure 1.7. Thus, the structure of the novel seatrout protein is plausible for a membrane receptor. Other studies described below with the seatrout receptor are consistent with the hypothesis that it is coupled to an inhibitory G-protein ($G_{i/o}$).

Tissue specificity: Northern blot analyses show the seatrout mRNA (4.0 kb) is only present in reproductive tissues, the ovary and testis, with lesser amounts in the brain and pituitary, and is not detected in other tissues including heart, gill, liver, kidney, muscle, spleen, and intestine.

Subcellular localization: Western blot analysis of tissues and immunocytochemical labeling of seatrout ovarian sections using a polyclonal antibody to a synthetic peptide derived from the first extracellular domain demonstrates exclusive localization of the protein (40 kDa) in the plasma membrane of oocytes. No immunoreactivity was detected in the oocyte cytosolic fraction or in the follicle cells. A slightly larger molecular weight band was also detected on Western blots of sperm membrane

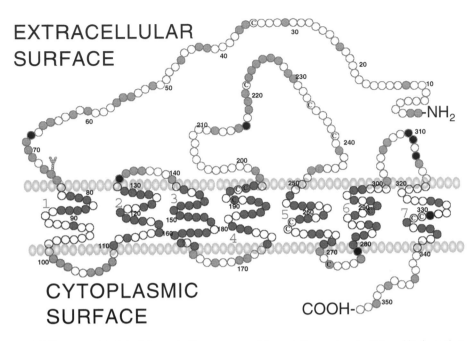

FIGURE 1.7   Model of the probable structure of the putative seatrout mPR and its insertion in the plasma membrane based on hydrophilicity and amino acid residue charge analyses. Amino acid residues that are identical in the six mPRαs identified in vertebrates are shaded and those diagnostic of the α clade in black. Cysteine residues (c) and a possible glycosylation site (Y) are shown. (From Zhu, Y., Rice,C.D., Pang, Y., Pace, M., and Thomas, P. *Proc. Natl. Acad. Sci. USA* 100, 2231, 2003. Copyright Proceedings of the National Academy of Sciences USA, 2003.)

fractions. The localization of the putative receptor protein on the plasma membranes of oocytes and sperm is consistent with our earlier biochemical receptor studies that demonstrated the presence of membrane progestin receptors on these germ cells.

Steroid binding: One of the most critical criterion to meet is that the recombinant protein produced in an expression system demonstrates steroid binding characteristics typical of steroid receptors. The cell membranes of human breast cancer cells (MDA-MB-231 cells) stably transfected with the putative progestin membrane receptor have high-affinity (Kd: 7.5 nM), saturable, low-capacity (Bmax: 0.026 nM) specific, single 20β-S binding site by saturation and Scatchard analyses. No specific 20β-S binding was observed to plasma membranes of untransfected breast cancer cells or cells transfected with an empty vector or reversed mSR insert (specific binding < 1% that of the transfected cells). The kinetics of association/dissociation of [^{3}H] progesterone binding to the recombinant protein are rapid with t$_{1/2}$ s of 2 to 8 minutes, which is typical of steroid membrane receptors. The steroid binding was specific for progestins; estradiol, cortisol, and testosterone had very low or no affinity for the receptor. To our knowledge this is the first report of a protein structurally unrelated to nuclear steroid receptors that has the binding characteristics of a steroid receptor.

Signal transduction: Progesterone and 20β-S altered two signal transduction pathways in human breast cancer (MDA-MB-231) cells stably transfected with the seatrout cDNA and expressing the recombinant protein on the plasma membrane, but were ineffective in cells transfected with the empty carrier vector or a reversed cDNA insert [42]. Adenylate cyclase activity was reduced within 5 minutes of progestin addition and recovered within 30 minutes. The progestin-induced decrease in intracellular cAMP levels was blocked by pretreatment with pertussis toxin, an inhibitor of $G_{i/o}$-mediated signaling pathways.

In contrast, the progestins activated MAP kinase; Erk1 and Erk2 were activated within 5 minutes of stimulation by progesterone and 20β-S, and their activities subsequently declined by 15 minutes. Alteration of intracellular signal transduction pathways upon addition of progestin hormones to a cell line transfected with the seatrout gene indicates it is coupled to these pathways, a requirement for steroid membrane receptors whose signal is initiated at the cell surface. Recently, direct evidence has been obtained that the receptor activates an inhibitory G-protein and therefore may be a GPCR.

Hormonal regulation: In vitro treatment of ovarian tissues with 20β-S caused an disregulation of both the seatrout receptor mRNA and its protein in seatrout oocytes [42]. Receptor protein levels were also increased after gonadotropin treatment coincident with the onset of oocyte maturational competence.

Biological relevance: Receptor protein levels were higher in oocytes undergoing meiotic maturation than in oocytes at earlier stages of maturation in seatrout captured on their spawning grounds and were lowest in ovulated oocytes [42]. These patterns of receptor protein changes during OM, both during natural spawning and hormonal induction in the laboratory studies, are very similar to those observed previously in the biochemical binding studies with the seatrout 20β-S receptor [101] and provide further evidence of an involvement of the seatrout receptor protein in meiotic maturation of oocytes in this species. The coupling of the receptor to a pertussis toxin-sensitive inhibitory G-protein is also consistent with its identity as the membrane receptor regulating oocyte maturation.

Finally, the demonstration that microinjection of zebrafish oocytes with two types of antisense oligonucleotides to the homologous gene in zebrafish blocked MIS induction of oocyte maturation, whereas control injections with mis-antisense or sense oligos were ineffective [42], provides direct evidence of the physiological importance of this novel gene and its homologue in zebrafish in the progestin induction of meiotic maturation of fish oocytes.

Multiplicity: Thirteen closely related cDNAs have been identified in other fish, amphibian, and mammalian species, including humans [126]. The cDNAs have been classified into three subtypes that have distinct tissue distributions in the gonads, brain, and kidney in humans. It is noteworthy that the recombinant proteins of the three mammalian genes that have been produced in *E.coli* also bind progestins and have characteristics of membrane progesterone receptors.

1.3 REPRODUCTIVE NEUROENDOCRINE TOXICITY

The regulation of GnRH neuronal activity and gonadotropin secretion is under complex control by monoaminergic and amino acid neurotransmitter systems and has been extensively characterized both in mammals and fish [127–133]. Although both stimulatory and inhibitory influences of one of these neurotransmitters, serotonin (5-hydroxytryptamine; 5-HT), on GnRH and LH secretion have been reported in mammals, depending on their developmental stage, most studies have shown that 5-HT exerts a stimulatory action on GnRH neurons to increase LH secretion [127, 134–138]. Similarly, 5-HT stimulates LH secretion in Atlantic croaker and goldfish, the two teleosts in which effects of 5-HT have been investigated in detail, by acting on the GnRH system in the preoptic-anterior hypothalamic area (POAH) and at the pituitary gland [130, 139–142]. The selective degeneration of serotonergic nerve terminals in the ventromedial region of the hypothalamus with the administration of 5,7-dihydroxytryptamine, a 5-HT neurotoxin, causes a reduction in LH levels in rats [143]. Therefore, one potential mechanism of impairment of the stimulatory 5-HT-GnRH neuroendocrine pathway controlling LH secretion in vertebrates by environmental chemicals could be by inducing lesions in the hypothalamic 5-HT system.

1.3.1 STIMULATORY 5-HT-GnRH NEUROENDOCRINE PATHWAY CONTROLLING LH SECRETION IN FISH

The schematic diagram in Figure 1.8 shows possible sites of 5-HT action on the GnRH-LH system in fish. 5-HT neurons arising mainly from the hypothalamus regulate GnRH function and LH secretion. The 5-HT nerve terminals impinging on a GnRH cell body in the POAH and on GnRH terminals in the POAH and pituitary, as well as directly on a gonadotrope, are indicated. In addition, steps in 5-HT synthesis and catabolism are shown in a magnified 5-HT nerve terminal.

One specialized feature of the 5-HT system in croaker and other fish species is the presence of 5-HT neurons in the hypothalamic area (reproductive part) of the brain in addition to those in the posterior brain Raphe region [129, 141, 144]. In higher vertebrates, including mammals, the 5-HT neuronal cell bodies are present in the Raphe region and send their projections to all parts of the brain to regulate a variety of other 5-HT-dependent functions, in addition to influencing the reproductive neuroendocrine system [145]. On the other hand, in fish neuroendocrine function is regulated by 5-HT neurons present in the hypothalamic region that stimulate the GnRH-LH system in the POAH and pituitary. This unique feature of the serotonergic system controlling reproductive neuroendocrine function in fishes greatly facilitates investigations on the sites and mechanisms of PCB neuroendocrine toxicity.

For example, the neuroendocrine influence of the serotonergic system can be assessed independently from other serotonergic functions by investigating it in the fish hypothalamus and directly relating it to neuroendocrine function after PCB exposure. The GnRH released from its nerve terminals in the pituitary in response to a highly coordinated neurotransmitter input, including the stimulatory action of 5-HT, binds to GnRH receptors present on the membranes of gonadotropes. This leads to activation of a cascade of intracellular events leading to the regulation of

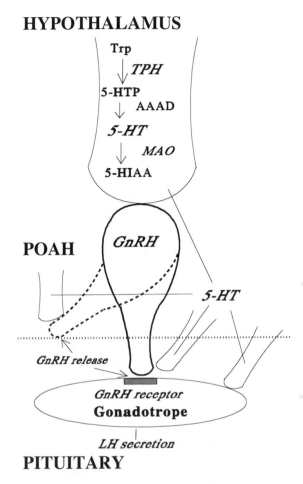

FIGURE 1.8 Schematic diagram showing multiple 5-HT nerve terminals impinging on a GnRH cell body in the preoptic area and GnRH nerve terminals in the anterior hypothalamus and pituitary to indicate possible sites of 5-HT action on the GnRH system in fish. 5-HT could also act directly at the level of pituitary gonadotropes to stimulate LH secretion. AAAD: aromatic amino acid decarboxylase; 5-HIAA: 5-hydroxyindolacetic acid; 5-HT: 5-hydroxytryptamine; 5-HTP: 5-hydroxytryptophan; MAO: monoamine oxidase; POAH: preoptic-anterior hypothalamus; Trp: tryptophan; TPH: tryptophan hydroxylase. Abbreviations in *italics* indicate biochemical measures included in the present study.

the synthesis and secretion of the two gonadotropins, FSH and LH. In addition, GnRH up-regulates GnRH receptors in the pituitary to further increase the gonadotropic response to GnRH stimulation.

Therefore, disruption of even one of the components of this stimulatory neuroendocrine (5-HT-GnRH) system controlling LH secretion is likely to result in adverse reproductive consequences. The series of experiments described below examine alterations in different components of the 5-HT-GnRH-LH pathway after treatments with PCB and neuropharmacological agents in order to establish linkages between PCB-induced disruption of the 5-HT system and LH secretion observed previously in croaker [28, 146].

1.3.2 NEUROENDOCRINE TOXICITY OF AROCLOR 1254

Evidence has accumulated that one major class of contaminants, PCBs, impairs the function of serotonergic and other monoaminergic neurotransmitter systems in vertebrate brains. Several laboratory studies have shown that PCBs at sub-lethal concentrations influence dopamine (DA), norepinephrine (NE), 5-HT, and their metabolite concentrations in discrete brain areas of rats and primates [27, 28, 147–151]. The decrease in DA concentrations by PCBs in rats appears to be due to inhibition of tyrosine hydroxylase, although the mechanism of this inhibition in unknown [152]. PCBs have been shown to reduce 5-HT concentrations and increase the metabolite (5-hydroxyindolacetic acid, 5-HIAA) to 5-HT ratio both in rats [151, 153] and croaker [28]. In a recent study in rats, we have demonstrated that the Aroclor 1254-induced decrease in 5-HT concentrations is associated with a decrease in its synthetic enzyme, tryptophan hydroxylase [154].

In addition to their effects on neurotransmitter metabolism, PCBs impair LH secretion in rats [155, 156] and Atlantic croaker, which is accompanied by inhibition of gonadal growth in croaker [146]. Furthermore, PCB exposure inhibits LH secretion in croaker in response to stimulation by a GnRH analog (GnRHa) both *in vivo* and *in vitro* [28, 142, 157]. These results suggest that PCB-induced disruption of the hypothalamic 5-HT system is associated with the impairment of LH secretion in croaker because 5-HT exerts stimulatory influences on LH secretion in this species [130, 131, 142).

1.3.2.1 Effects of Aroclor 1254 on Hypothalamic Tryptophan Hydroxylase and Monoamine Oxidase Activities

The neurotransmitter 5-HT is synthesized from the amino acid tryptophan in the presence of the rate-limiting enzyme, tryptophan hydroxylase, and catabolized by monoamine oxidase (MAO) to its inactive metabolite, 5-hydroxyindolacetic acid (Figure 1.8). To determine whether the decrease in 5-HT levels is caused by changes in TPH or MAO activity, we measured both enzymes after exposure of croaker to the PCB mixture during the recrudescence phase of the gonadal cycle. PCB exposure resulted in a significant reduction (38%) in hypothalamic TPH activity, whereas MAO activity was not significantly altered [142].

The results demonstrate for the first time in any vertebrate species that impairment of the hypothalamic 5-HT system by PCB involves a decrease in TPH activity. The decline in hypothalamic TPH activity was accompanied by a significant decrease in the *in vivo* gonadotropin (LH) response to stimulation by a GnRH analog [142, 157]. These *in vivo* results are consistent with our previous *in vitro* findings, in which LH release from pituitary fragments was assessed after fish were exposed to PCB in the diet [28, 146]. The lower hypothalamic 5-HT levels resulting from reduced 5-HT synthesis could be responsible for the decrease in the LH response to GnRHa, because 5-HT exerts a stimulatory control on LH secretion in croaker [130, 131].

Similarly, 5-HT and its precursor, 5-hydroxytryptophan (5-HTP), stimulate GnRH and LH release in mammals, including humans [127, 136, 137], and the degeneration of serotonergic nerve terminals by the 5-HT neurotoxin, 5,7-dihydroxytryptamine, results in reduced LH levels in rats [143]. Therefore, lesions in the 5-HT system induced by PCB or other agents can impair the stimulatory 5-HT–GnRH-LH pathway in vertebrates. It is concluded from these studies that the decrease in hypothalamic 5-HT concentrations after PCB exposure involves impairment of TPH activity and is associated with the disruption of GnRHa-induced LH secretion.

1.3.2.2 Effects of PCB, PCPA, and PCB+5-HTP on Hypothalamic TPH Activity and 5-HT Concentrations

The possible association between impaired TPH activity and serotonergic function after PCB exposure was explored using serotonergic drugs. Para-chlorophenylalanine (PCPA), an irreversible TPH inhibitor [158], was used to mimic the effect of PCB on TPH activity and 5-HT concentrations. In addition, 5-hydroxytryptophan (5-HTP), the intermediate in 5-HT synthesis, was used to bypass the TPH-dependent hydroxylation step in 5-HT synthesis and restore neuronal 5-HT levels, because 5-HTP is readily converted into 5-HT by endogenous aromatic amino acid decarboxylase [159]. PCPA administration significantly reduced hypothalamic TPH activity and 5-HT concentrations to levels similar to those induced by PCB exposure (Figure 1.9). Moreover, 5-HTP treatments in combination with PCB restored hypothalamic 5-HT concentrations, while TPH activity remained low compared to the controls [142]. In conclusion, PCPA treatment can mimic the effects of PCB on TPH activity and 5-HT concentrations, and 5-HTP co-treatment can prevent the PCB-induced decline in 5-HT concentrations, thereby providing further evidence that PCB impairs the TPH-dependent hydroxylation step in 5-HT biosynthesis.

1.3.2.3 Effects of PCB, PCPA, and PCB+5-HTP on GnRH Content in the POAH and Pituitary

To determine whether a decrease in hypothalamic TPH activity results in impairment of the gonadotropin response to GnRHa by interfering with the GnRH system, we measured GnRH content in the POAH and pituitary gland after treatment with PCB and PCPA. Both PCB and PCPA treatments elicited a significant decrease in GnRH content in the POAH (PCB: 86.5%; PCPA 72.6%; Figure 1.10A). Moreover, 5-HTP treatment prevented the PCB-induced decline in GnRH content in the POAH (Figure 1.10A). Changes in pituitary GnRH were not statistically significant. One interpretation of these results is that disruption of the stimulatory 5-HT input leads to impairment of GnRH synthesis. These results clearly demonstrate that the disruption of hypothalamic TPH activity by both PCB and PCPA results in impairment of GnRH function, and bypassing the TPH-dependent hydroxylation with 5-HTP prevents the PCB-induced decline in GnRH content in the POAH.

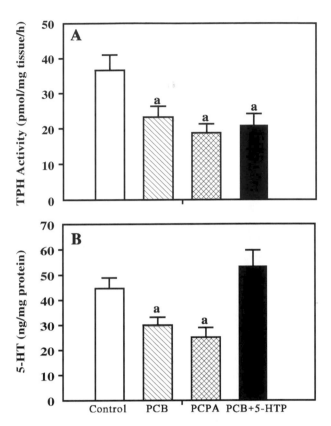

FIGURE 1.9　Effects of PCB, PCPA, and PCB+5-HTP on the hypothalamic TPH activity (A) and 5-HT concentrations (B). Each bar represents mean ± SEM of eight observations. [a]Significantly different from the respective control. (From Khan, I.A. and Thomas, P., *Biol. Reprod.* 64, 955, 2001. With permission.)

1.3.2.4　Effects of PCB, PCPA, and PCB+5-HTP on Basal and 5-HT-Induced GnRH Release from the POAH and Pituitary Slices Incubated *In Vitro*

To test the functional integrity of the neurons to release GnRH in response to 5-HT stimulation, the POAH and pituitary slices were challenged *in vitro* with 5-HT (20 μg/ml). 5-HT significantly (two- to threefold) stimulated GnRH release from both POAH and pituitary slices [142] in all the treatment groups, which shows that the GnRH neurons are still responsive to the high 5-HT concentrations *in vitro* after *in vivo* PCB treatment. However, the PCB and PCPA treatments caused significant attenuation of both spontaneous (unstimulated) and 5-HT-induced GnRH release from POAH slices [142]. In contrast, spontaneous and 5-HT-induced GnRH release from POAH slices in the PCB+5-HTP group was comparable to that in the control group. The ability of PCPA to mimic the effects of PCB on the GnRH system, and that of 5-HTP treatments to reverse these effects, indicates that the decrease in

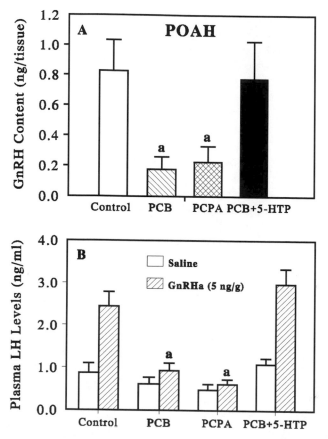

FIGURE 1.10   Effects of PCB, PCPA, and PCB+5-HTP on the GnRH content in the POAH (A), and the basal (saline) and GnRHa-induced LH secretion (B). Each bar represents mean ± SEM of eight to ten observations. [a]Significantly different from the respective control group. (Adapted from Khan, I.A. and Thomas, P., *Biol. Reprod.* 64, 955, 2001. With permission.)

hypothalamic TPH activity is at least partially responsible for the PCB-induced impairment of the GnRH system.

1.3.2.5   Effects of PCB, PCPA, and PCB+5-HTP on Basal and GnRHa-Induced LH Secretion

In order to determine whether alterations in the 5-HT and GnRH components are accompanied by changes in LH secretion, we examined both basal and GnRHa-induced LH secretion after treatments with PCB and the serotonergic pharmacological agents. PCPA mimicked the inhibitory effect of PCB on GnRHa-induced LH secretion, whereas 5-HTP treatments in combination with PCB exposure prevented the disruption of LH secretion (Figure 1.10B). Interestingly, the LH response to GnRHa in the three treatment groups followed exactly the patterns of the hypothalamic 5-HT concentrations (Figure 1.9). The excellent correlation observed between the decreases in hypothalamic TPH activity and 5-HT concentrations and impairment of LH secretion is likely due to the presence of 5-HT neurons in this neuroendocrine center of the brain that controls LH secretion (129, 141, 142).

These findings provide strong evidence that the PCB-induced disruption of LH secretion involves impairment of 5-HT synthesis via inhibition of the rate-limiting enzyme, TPH. Similar to our results in croaker, PCPA abolishes the daily LH surge in estrogen-treated ovariectomized rats, and 5-HTP treatment restores the surge [160]. These findings demonstrate a parallelism in PCPA and 5-HTP effects on LH secretion between a fish and mammalian species. In addition, 5-HTP enhances LH secretion during the follicular phase in women, possibly via stimulation of GnRH neurons [137]. Further, there is epidemiological evidence for neuroendocrine and reproductive dysfunction, including reduced LH secretion, in women exposed to PCBs occupationally or in the diet [161, 162]. Therefore, PCBs may disrupt LH secretion in rats [155, 156] and humans [162] via similar mechanisms of neuroendocrine toxicity as those identified in croaker.

1.3.2.6　Effects of PCB and GnRH Replacement Therapy on GnRH Receptors and LH Secretion

Finally, we examined whether PCB-induced impairment of the LH response to GnRHa was due to a decrease in the number of pituitary GnRH receptors (GnRH-R). In addition, slow-release GnRHa implants were used in combination with PCB in an attempt to prevent the possible decrease in the GnRH-R concentrations. PCB exposure of croaker during the gonadal recrudescence phase resulted in a decrease in pituitary GnRH-R concentration (Figure 1.11A), which was accompanied by a reduced LH response to GnRHa *in vivo* (Figure 1.11B). The lower dose implants of GnRHa (5 ng/g) in combination with the PCB exposure restored GnRH-R concentrations to control values (Figure 1.11A).

In contrast, the higher dose (50 ng/g) failed to restore GnRH-R concentrations and instead slightly reduced (40% decrease) them compared to those in the PCB treatment group alone. In a second similar experiment, low-dose GnRHa implants increased circulating LH levels in PCB-treated fish as well as restored the LH response to GnRHa injections (10 ng/g BW, 1 h before termination of the experiment) to that observed in the control group (Figure 1.11B). However, the high-dose GnRHa implants resulted in a complete loss of the LH response to GnRHa stimulation. Pituitary GnRH-R concentrations vary during the reproductive cycle in both mammals and fish [163, 164], and gradually increase during gonadal recrudescence in goldfish [164] and croaker [165]. Moreover, there is evidence that GnRH regulates GnRH-R concentrations in these two fish species [142, 164].

Therefore, one of the reasons for the lower pituitary GnRH-R concentrations observed in PCB-exposed croaker [142] might be insufficient GnRH release from the pituitary nerve terminals, resulting in reduced up-regulation of the GnRH-R. The finding that the low-dose GnRHa implants up-regulated GnRH-R, increased basal LH secretion, and fully restored the LH response to GnRHa in PCB-exposed croaker is consistent with a mechanism of PCB toxicity involving decreased GnRH secretion. On the other hand, the complete loss of the LH response to further stimulation by

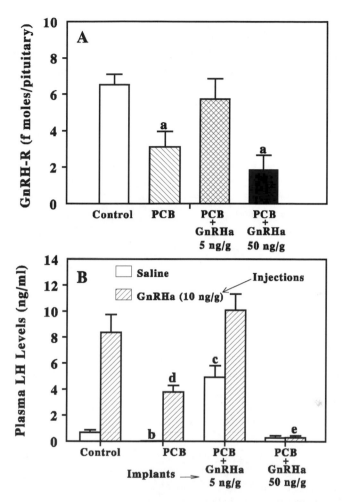

FIGURE 1.11 Effects of PCB alone and in combination with the GnRHa implants on the GnRH receptor (GnRH-R) content (A), and on the basal (saline) and GnRHa-induced LH secretion (B). The number of GnRH-R was determined by single point assays (N = 5; 20 pituitaries/group) using membrane fractions of one pituitary equivalent and 7.5×10^{-10} M [^{125}I]mGnRH/tube in duplicate in the presence or absence of 10^{-6} M-mGnRH. The bars for plasma LH levels represent mean ± SEM of 10 observations. [a]Significantly lower than the control group in panel A. [b]Significantly lower than the saline-injected control. [c]Significantly higher than the saline-injected control. [d]Significantly lower than the GnRHa-injected control. [e]Significantly lower than the other GnRHa-injected groups. (From Khan, I.A. and Thomas, P., *Biol. Reprod.* 64, 955, 2001. With permission.)

GnRHa in fish with high-dose GnRHa implants was likely due to down-regulation of GnRH-R or depletion of pituitary LH stores. The efficacy of low-dose GnRHa implants in restoring the LH response to GnRHa clearly indicates disruption of GnRH machinery by PCB, and demonstrates that the GnRH therapy can ameliorate PCB-induced disruption of LH secretion.

In conclusion, the results of our investigations on the effects of Aroclor 1254 on the stimulatory 5-HT-GnRH neuroendocrine pathway controlling LH secretion are summarized in Figure 1.12 and clearly identify TPH as one of the targets of neuroendocrine disruption by the PCB mixture. In addition, the finding that GnRH content was drastically reduced in the POAH of fish exposed to PCB suggests possible inhibition of GnRH synthesis. Moreover, the decreases in GnRH release from the POAH and the number of GnRH receptors in the pituitary, together with the lack of a reduction in pituitary GnRH content (GnRH stored in nerve terminals), point to the impairment of GnRH release as an additional site of neuroendocrine disruption by PCB. Thus, PCB at environmentally realistic concentrations [28] can impair neuroendocrine function in croaker. Although the exact mechanisms by which Aroclor 1254 reduces hypothalamic TPH activity are not fully understood, recent evidence suggests it may involve a decrease in TPH protein content, which appears to be associated with oxidative damage [166]. More detailed studies are in progress to determine the type and extent of damage to TPH protein and whether antioxidants can prevent PCB-induced destruction/inactivation of the enzyme and resultant neuroendocrine disruption.

1.3.3 EFFECT OF LEAD ON HYPOTHALAMIC MONOAMINERGIC SYSTEMS AND NEUROENDOCRINE FUNCTION

There is extensive literature on the reproductive toxicity and neurotoxicity of lead in vertebrates [167, 168]. The effects of chronic lead exposure on reproductive endocrine function were investigated in Atlantic croaker. Administration of lead (0.5 and 1.5 mg/100 g body wt./day) in the diet for 30 days caused a marked suppression of ovarian steroidogenesis and ovarian growth [169]. The preliminary results suggested that the suppressive effects of lead were mediated in part by an impairment of gonadotropin secretion. Previous studies had shown that lead influences monoamine metabolism in both mammals and fish [170, 171], and the neuroendocrine axis is a major target of the metal in mammals [24, 25]. Therefore, in a subsequent experiment hypothalamic monoamine concentrations and gonadotropin secretion were measured in male croaker receiving the same lead treatment regime. Lead caused only minor changes in the hypothalamic concentrations of the biogenic amines epinephrine, norepinephrine, dopamine, and serotonin and their metabolites 3,4 dihydroxyphenylacetic acid, 3-methoxytyramine, homovanillic acid, and 5-hydroxyindol acetic acid (5-HIAA) [15]. The effects of the lead treatments on the concentrations of 5-HT and its metabolite 5-HIAA in the hypothalamus are shown in Figure 1.13A.

There was a trend of a decrease in 5-HT concentrations and an increase in the content of its metabolite in both hypothalamic areas after lead exposure, but these changes were not significant. However, the hypothalamic 5-HIAA to 5-HT ratio, a measure of serotonin metabolism or turnover, was significantly elevated in the lead-treated fish (Figure 1.13A). Chronic exposure to the higher dose of lead also significantly inhibited both basal and GnRHa-induced LH secretion from pituitary fragments *in vitro* (Figure 1.13B). The attenuation of the LH response to GnRHa was similar to

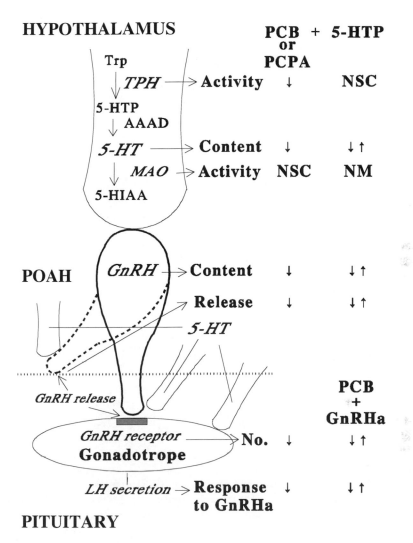

FIGURE 1.12 Summary of the results incorporated into the schematic diagram in Figure 1.1 showing all the biochemical indices measured in this study after the pharmacological manipulations indicated. GnRHa: GnRH analog; NM: not measured; No.: number of GnRH receptors in pituitary membrane preparations; NSC: no significant change; PCB: Aroclor 1254; PCPA: para-chlorophenylalanine; see Figure 1.1 legend for other abbreviations.

that observed after treatment with the 5-HT$_2$ receptor antagonist, ketanserin [130]. Thus, these results provide preliminary evidence that the effects of lead on gonadotropin secretion may be partially mediated by decreases in hypothalamic serotonergic activity. The decrease in gonadotropin secretion after exposure to lead was accompanied by a dose-related inhibition of gonadal growth and decreased circulating levels of androgens [15]. Recent evidence in croaker suggests disruption of GnRH function

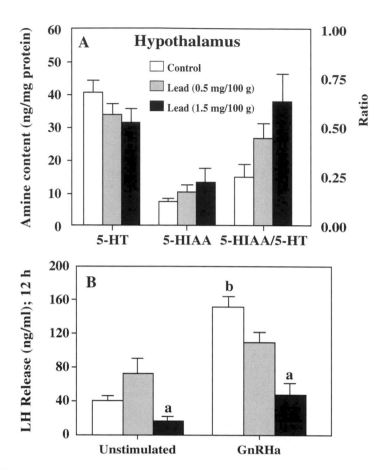

FIGURE 1.13 Lead-induced alterations in serotonin metabolism in the hypothalamus (A), and *in vitro* LH release in response to a GnRH analog (GnRHa) from the pituitaries of control and lead-exposed fish. Bars represent means ± standard error of mean of 10 to 12 observations. [a]Significantly different from the respective control group. [b]Significantly different from the unstimulated control group. 5-HIAA: 5-hydroxy indolacetic acid. (Adapted from Thomas, P. and Khan, I.A., in *Chemically Induced Alterations in Functional Development and Reproduction of Fishes*, 1997, 29. With permission from SETAC.)

by a similar lead exposure (unpublished observations), which may at least partially account for the lead-induced impairment of LH secretion described above.

The studies with croaker suggest that the serotonergic system in hypothalamic areas of the brain controlling gonadotropin secretion is sensitive to interference by Aroclor 1254 and lead, representatives of two different classes of neurotoxic and reproductive toxic chemicals. The toxic mechanisms of these two chemicals on the hypothalamic serotonergic system are thought to differ and are currently being investigated. Possible estrogenic actions of Aroclor 1254 metabolites mediated by nuclear estrogen receptors in the hypothalamus shall also be considered. A large body of evidence, mostly circumstantial, suggests that many other chemicals, including mercury, organochlorine, and organophosphorous pesticides, xenobiotic estrogens, and central nervous system drugs impair reproductive endocrine function at the hypothalamic level in vertebrates [12, 24, 146, 171–173]. More comprehensive studies will be required, however, to determine whether alteration of neurotransmitter function is a widespread mechanism of neuroendocrine disruption by environmental chemicals.

1.4 SUMMARY

Vertebrate reproduction is an intricate process involving extensive physiological coordination, which is primarily controlled by the hormones secreted by the hypothalamus–pituitary–gonadal axis. The overall complexity of the reproductive endocrine system, and the integrated nature of its response to environmental stimuli, have complicated investigations of its disruption by xenobiotic chemicals. Chemicals can potentially exert their effects at multiple sites on the hypothalamus–pituitary–gonadal axis and by a variety of mechanisms to interfere with reproductive endocrine function [21, 22]. This chapter describes toxic actions of xenobiotics in the hypophysiotropic region of the hypothalamus, at the pituitary, ovary, oocytes, and sperm, resulting in disruption of endocrine function. Evidence for chemical interference with the nongenomic actions of steroids via binding to steroid membrane receptors is reviewed. In addition, studies showing that representative neurotoxic chemicals can impair neuroendocrine reproductive function by disrupting hypothalamic serotonergic systems are summarized. These novel mechanisms of endocrine disruption warrant further investigation in different vertebrate models and target tissues.

ACKNOWLEDGMENTS

This research was supported by Public Health Service grants ESO4214 and ESO7672, and EPA STAR grant R-82902401.

REFERENCES

1. Colborn, T., Vom Saal, F. S., and Soto, A. M., Developmental effects of endocrine-disrupting chemicals in wildlife and humans, *Environ. Health. Perspect.,* 101, 378, 1993.
2. Twonbly, R., Assault on the male, *Environ. Health Perspect.,* 103, 802, 1995.
3. Davis, W. P. and Bartone, S. A., Effects of kraft mill effluent on the sexuality of fishes: an environmental early warning, in *Chemically Induced Alterations in Sexual and Functional Development: The Wildlife/Human Connection,* Colborn, T. and Clement, C., Eds., Princeton Scientific Publ., Princeton, NJ, 1992, 113.
4. Jobling, S., Sumpter, J. P., Detergent components in sewage effluent are weakly oestrogenic to fish: an *in vitro* study using rainbow trout (*Oncorhynchus mykiss*) hepatocytes, *Aquat. Toxicol.,* 27, 361, 1993.
5. Raloff, J., The gender binders: are environmental hormones emasculating wildlife, *Science News,* 145, 24, 1994.

6. Davis, D. L., Bradlow, H. L., Wolff, M., W., Woodruff, T., Hoel, D. G., and Anton-Culver, H., Medical hypothesis: xenoestrogens as preventable causes of breast cancer, *Environ. Health Perspec.,* 101, 372, 1993.

7. Sharpe, R. and Skakkebaek, N. E., Are oestrogens involved in falling sperm counts and disorders of the male reproductive tract, *Lancet,* 341, 1392, 1993.

8. International Programme on Chemical Safety, *Global Assessment of the State of the Science of Endocrine Disruptors.* Damstra, T., Barlow, S., Bergman, A., Kavlock, R., and Van Der Kraak, G., Eds. International Programme For The Sound Management Of Chemicals, World Health Organization, 179pp, 2002.

9. McLachlan, J. A., Functional toxicology: a new approach to detect biologically active xenobiotics, *Environ. Health Perspect.,* 101, 386, 1993.

10. Jobling, S., Reynolds, T., White, R., Porter, M. G., and Sumpter, J. P., A variety of environmentally persistent chemicals, including some phthalate plasticizers are weakly estrogenic, *Environ. Health Perspect.,* 103, 582, 1995.

11. Nelson, J. A., Effects of dichlorodiphenyltrichlorethane (DDT) analogs and polychlorinated biphenyl mixtures on 17b[^{3}h] estradiol binding to rat uterine receptor, *Biochem. Pharmacol.,* 23, 447, 1973.

12. Bulger, W. H. and Kupfer, D., Estrogenic activity of pesticides and other xenobiotics on the uterus and male reproductive tract, in *Endocrine Toxicity,* Thomas, J. A., Korach, K. S., and McLachlan, J. A., Eds., Raven Press, New York, 1985, 1.

13. Korach, K. S., Sarver, P., Chae, K., McLachlan, J.A., and McKinney, J. D., Estrogen receptor-binding activity of polychlorinated hydroxybiphenyls conformationally restricted structural probes, *Mol. Pharmacol.,* 37, 120, 1987.

14. Gray, E. L., Jr., Monosson, E., and Kelce, W. R., Emerging issues: the effects of endocrine disruptors on reproductive development, in *Interconnections Between Human and Ecosystem,* Guilio, R. T. and Monosson, E., Eds., Chapman and Hall, 1996, 46.

15. Thomas, P. and Khan, I. A., Mechanisms of chemical interference with reproductive endocrine function in sciaenid fishes, in *Chemically Induced Alterations in Functional Development and Reproduction of Fishes,* Rolland, R. M., Gilbertson, M., and Peterson, R. E., Eds., SETAC Technical Publications Series, 1997, 29.

16. Lee, A. V., Weng, C.-N., Jackson, J. G., and Yee, D., Activation of estrogen receptor-mediated gene transcription by IGF-1 in human breast cancer cells, *J. Endocrinol.,* 152, 39, 1997.

17. Ignar-Trowbridge, D. M., Pimentel, M., Parker, M. G., McLachlan, J. A., and Korach, K. S., Peptide growth factor cross-talk with the estrogen receptor requires the A/B domain and occurs independently of protein kinase C or estradiol, *Endocrinology,* 137, 1735, 1996.

18. Safe, S., Astroff, B., Harris, M., Zacharaewski, T., Dickerson, R., Romkes, M., and Biegel, L., 2,3,7,8-tetrachlorodibenzo-*p*-dioxin (TCDD) and related compounds as antiestrogens: characterization and mechanism of action, *Pharmacol. Toxicol.,* 64, 400, 1991.

19. Khara, I., Saatcioglu, F., Antiestrogenic effects of 2,3,7,8-tetracholorodibenzo-*p*-dioxin are mediated by direct transcriptional interference with the liganded estrogen receptor, *J. Biol. Chem.,* 271, 10533, 1996.

20. Ohtake, F., Takeyama, K., Matsumoto, T., Kitagawa, H., Yamamoto, Y., Nohara, K., Tohyama, C., Krust, A., Mimura, J., Chambon, P., Yanagisawa, J., Fuji-Kuriyama, Y., and Kato, S., Modulation of oestrogen receptor signaling by association with the activated dioxin receptor, *Nature,* 423, 545, 2003.

21. Lundholm, C. E., The effects of DDE, PCB and chlordane on the binding of progesterone to its cytoplasmic receptor in eggshell gland mucosa of birds and the endometrium of mammalian uterus, *Comp. Biochem. Physiol.*, 89C, 361, 1988.

22. Kelce, W. R., Stone, C. R., Laws, S. C., Gray, L. E., Kemppainen, J. A., and Wilson, E. M., Persistent DDT metabolite *p,p'*-DDE is a potent androgen receptor antagonist, *Nature*, 375, 581, 1995.

23. Sperry, T. and P. Thomas, Identification of two nuclear androgen receptors in kelp bass (*Paralabrax clathratus*) and their binding affinities for xenobiotics: comparison with Atlantic croaker (*Micropogonias undulatus*) androgen receptors, *Biol. Reprod.*, 61, 1152, 1999.

24. Mattison, D. R., Gates, A. H., Leonards, A., Wide, M., Hemminki, K., and Copius Peereboom-Stegeman, J. H. J., Reproductive and developmental toxicity of metals: female reproductive system, in *Reproductive and Developmental Toxicity of Metals,* Clarkon, T. W., Norberg, G. N., Sager, P. R., Eds., Plenum Press, New York, 1983, 41.

25. Thomas, P., Teleost model for studying the effects of chemicals on female reproductive endocrine function, *J. Exp. Zool.*, 4, 126, 1990.

26. Uphouse, L., Effects of chlordecone on neuroendocrine function of female rats, *Neurotoxicology*, 6, 191, 1985.

27. Seegal, R. F., Brosch, C. O., and Bush, B., Regional alterations in serotonin metabolism induced by oral exposure of rats to polychlorinated biphenyls, *Neurotoxicology*, 7, 155, 1986.

28. Khan, I. A. and Thomas, P., Aroclor 1254-induced alterations in hypothalamic monoamine metabolism in the Atlantic croaker (*Micropogonias undulatus*): correlation with pituitary gonadotropin release, *Neurotoxicology*, 18, 553, 1997.

29. Cicero, T. J., Badger, T. M., Wilcox, C. E., Bell, R. D., and Meyer, E. R., Morphine decreases luteinizing hormone by an action on the hypothalamic-pituitary axis, *J. Pharmacol. Exp. Ther.*, 203, 548, 1977.

30. Klein, D., Wan, Y. Y., Kamyab, S., Okuda, H., and Sokol, R. Z., Effects of toxic levels of lead on gene regulation in the male axis: increase in messenger ribonucleic acids and intracellular stores of gonadotrops within the central nervous system, *Biol. Reprod.*, 50, 802, 1994.

31. Thomas, P., Effects of cadmium on gonadotropin secretion from Atlantic croaker pituitaries incubated *in vitro, Mar. Environ. Res.*, 35, 141, 1993.

32. Cooper, R. A., Goldman, J. M., Rehnberg, G. L., McElroy, W. K., and Hein, J. F., Effects of metal cations on pituitary hormone secretion *in vitro, J. Biochem. Toxicol.*, 2, 241, 1987.

33. Singhal, R. L., Vijayvargia, R., and Shukla, G. S., Toxic effects of cadmium and lead on reproductive functions, in *Endocrine Toxicology*, Thomas, J. A., Korach, K. S., MaLachlan, J. A., Eds., Raven Press, New York, 1985, 149.

34. Ghosh, S. and Thomas, P., Antagonistic effects of xenobiotics on steroid-induced final maturation of Atlantic croaker oocytes *in vitro, Mar. Environ. Res.*, 39, 159, 1995.

35. Thomas, P., Breckenridge-Miller, D., and Detweiler, C., The teleost sperm membrane progestogen receptor: interactions with xenoestrogens, *Mar. Environ. Res.*, 46, 163, 1998.

36. Metzgan, D. A., Nontraditional sites of estrogen action, *Environ. Health Persp.*, 5, 39, 1995.

37. Tsai, M. J. and O'Malley, B. W., Molecular mechanisms of action of steroid/thyroid receptor superfamily members, *Annu. Rev. Biochem.*, 63, 451, 1994.

38. Watson, C.S. and Gametchu, B., Membrane-initiated steroid actions and the proteins that mediate them, *Proc. Soc. Exp. Biol. Med.*, 220, 9, 1999.

39. Falkenstein, E., Tillman H.-S., Christ, M., Feuring, M. and Wehling, M., Multiple actions of steroid hormones — a focus on rapid, nongenomic effects, *Pharmacol. Rev.,* 52, 513, 2000.

40. Revelli, A., Massobrio, M., and Tesarik, J., Nongenomic actions of steroid hormones in reproductive tissues, *Endocr. Rev.,* 19, 3, 1998.

41. Blackmore, P.F., Rapid non-genomic actions of progesterone stimulate Ca^{2+} influx and the acrosome reaction in human sperm, *Cell. Signal.,* 5(5), 531, 1993.

42. Zhu, Y., Rice, C.D., Pang, Y., Pace, M., and Thomas, P., Cloning, expression, and characterization of a membrane progestin receptor and evidence it is an intermediary in meiotic maturation of fish oocytes, *Proc. Natl. Acad. Sci. USA, 100*, 2231, 2003a.

43. Pappas, T. C., Gametchu, B., Yannariello-Brown, J., Collins, T. J., and Watson, C. S., Membrane estrogen receptors in GH3/B6 cells are associated with rapid estrogen-induced release of prolactin, *Endocrine, 2,* 813, 1994.

44. Morley, P., Whitfield, J. F., Vanderhyden, B. C., Tsang, B. K., and Schwartz, J., A new, nongenomic estrogen action: the rapid release of intracellular calcium, *Endocrinology,* 131, 1305, 1992.

45. Nabekura, J., Oomura, Y., Minami, T., Mizuno, Y., and Fukudo, A., Mechanism of the rapid effect of 17-estradiol on medial amygdala neurons, *Science,* 233, 226, 1986.

46. Thomas, P. and Meizel, S., Phosphatidylinositol 4,5-biphosphate hydrolysis in human sperm stimulated with follicular fluid or progesterone is dependent upon Ca^{++} influx, *Biochem. J.,* 264, 539, 1989.

47. Blackmore, P. F., Neulen, J., Lattanzio, F., and Beebe, S. J., Cell surface-binding sites for progesterone mediate calcium uptake in human sperm, *J. Biol. Chem.,* 266, 18655, 1991.

48. Dluzen, D. E. and Ramirez, V. D., Progesterone effects upon dopamine release from the corpus striatum of female rats, II. Evidence for a membrane site of action and the role of albumin, *Brain Res.,* 476, 338, 1989.

49. Hua, S. Y. and Chen, Y. Z., Membrane receptor-mediated electrophysiological effects of glucocorticoid on mammalian neurons, *Endocrinology,* 124, 687, 1989.

50. Orchinik, M., Murray, T. F., and Moore, F. L., A corticosteroid receptor in neuronal membranes, *Science,* 252, 1848, 1991.

51. Gametchu, B., Glucocorticoid receptor-like antigen in lymphoma cell membranes: correlation to cell lysis, *Science,* 236, 456, 1987.

52. Pappas, T.C., Gametchu, B., and Watson, C. S., Membrane estrogen receptors identified by multiple antibody and impeded ligand labeling, *FASEB J.,* 9, 404, 1995.

53. Pietras, R. and Szego, C. M., Estrogen receptors in uterine plasma membrane, *J. Steroid Biochem.,* 2, 1471, 1979.

54. Loomis, A.K. and Thomas, P. Effects of estrogens and xenoestrogens on androgen production by Atlantic croaker testes *in vitro*: evidence for a nongenomic action mediated by an estrogen membrane receptor, *Biol. Reprod.,* 62, 995, 2000.

55. Suyemitsu, T. and Terayama, H., Specific binding sites for natural glucocorticoids in plasma membranes of rat liver, *Endocrinology,* 96, 1499, 1975.

56. Ke, F.-C. and Ramirez, V. D., Binding of progesterone to nerve cell membranes of rat brain using progesterone conjugated to ^{125}I bovine serum albumin as a ligand, *J. Neurochem.,* 54, 467, 1990.

57. Lan, N. C., Chen, J.S., Belelli, D., Pritchett, D. B., Seeburg, P. H., and Gee, K. W., A steroid recognition site is functionally coupled to an expressed $GABA_A$-benzodiazepene receptor, *Europ. J. Pharmacol.,* 188, 403, 1994.

58. Baldi, F., Luconi, M., Bonaccorsi, L., Maggi, M., Francavilla, S., Gabriela, A., Properzi, G., and Forti, G., Nongenomic progesterone receptor on human spermatozoa; biochemical aspects and clinical implications, *Steroids,* 64, 143, 1999.

59. Patiño, R. and Thomas, P., Characterization of membrane receptor activity for 17α,20β,21-trihydroxy-4-pregnen-3-one in ovaries of spotted seatrout (*Cynoscion nebulosus*), *Gen. Comp. Endocrinol.,* 78, 204,1990.

60. Thomas, P., Breckenridge-Miller, D. and Detweiler, C., Binding characteristics and regulation of the 17α, 20β,21-trihydroxy-4-pregen-3-one (20β-S) receptor on testicular and sperm membranes of spotted seatrout (*Cynocscion nebulosus), Fish Physiol. Biochem.,* 17,109, 1997.

61. Liu, D. and Dillon, J. S., Dehydroepandrosterone activates endothelial cell nitric oxide synthetase by a specific plasma membrane receptor coupled to $G\alpha_{12,3}$, *J. Biol. Chem.,* 277, 21379, 2002.

62. Braun A. and Thomas, P., Androgens inhibit estradiol-17β synthesis in Atlantic croaker (*Micropogonias undulatus*) ovaries by a nongenomic mechanism initiated at the cell surface, *Biol. Reprod.,* 69, 1642, 2003.

63. Thomas, P. Chemical interference with genomic and nongenomic actions of steroids in fishes: role of receptor binding, *Mar. Environ. Res.,* 50, 127, 2000.

64. Watson, C. S., Pappas, T. C. and Gametchu, B. The other estrogen receptor in the plasma membrane—implications for the actions of environmental estrogens. *Environ. Health Perspect.,* 103, Suppl. 7, 41, 1995.

65. Pickford, D. B. and Morris, I. D., Effects of endocrine-disrupting contaminants on amphibian oogenesis: methoxychlor inhibits progesterone-induced maturation of *Xenopus laevis* oocytes *in vitro, Environ. Health Perspect.,* 107(4):285, 1999.

66. Nadal, A., Ropero, A. B., Laribi, O., Maillet, M., Fuentes, E., and Soria, B., Nongenomic actions of estrogens and xenoestrogens by binding at a plasma membrane receptor unrelated to estrogen receptor alpha and estrogen receptor beta, *Proc. Natl. Acad. Sci. USA,* 97, 11603, 2000.

67. Thomas, P., Chemical interference with the genomic and nongenomic actions of steroids in fishes: role of receptor binding, *Mar. Environ. Res.,* 50:127, 2000.

68. Ruehlmann, D. O., Steinert, J. R., Valverde, M. A., Jacob, R., and Mann, G. E., Environmental estrogenic pollutants induce acute vascular relaxation by inhibiting L-Type Ca2 channels in smooth muscle cells, *FASEB J.,* 12, 613, 1998.

69. Watson, C. S., C. H. Campbell, and B. Gametchu. Membrane estrogen receptors on rat pituitary tumor cells: immuno-identification and responses to oestradiol and xenoestrogens, *Exp. Physiol.,* 84, 1013, 1999.

70. Thomas, P., Nontraditional sites of endocrine disruption by chemicals on the hypothalamus-pituitary-gonadal axis: interactions with steroid membrane receptors, monoaminergic pathways and signal transduction systems, in *Endocrine Disruptors: Effects on Male and Female Reproductive Systems,* R. K. Naz, Ed., CRC Press, Boca Raton, FL, 1999, 3.

71. Thomas, P. and Budiantara, L., Reproductive life history stages sensitive to oil and naphthalene in Atlantic croaker, *Mar. Environ. Res.,* 39, 147, 1995.

72. Kumi-Diaka J. and Townsend, J., Toxic potential of dietary Genistein isoflavone and beta-Lapachone on capacitation and acrosome reaction of epididymal spermatozoa, *J. Med. Food,* 6, 201, 2003.

73. Das, S. and Thomas, P., Pesticides interfere with the nongenomic action of a progestogen on meiotic maturation by binding to its plasma membrane receptor on fish oocytes, *Endocrinology,* 140(4), 1953, 1999.

74. Loomis, K. and Thomas, P., Binding characteristics of estrogen receptor (ER) in Atlantic croaker (*Micropogonias undulatus*) testis: different affinity for estrogens and xenobiotics from that of hepatic ER, *Biol. Reprod.*, 61:51, 1999.

75. Masui, Y. and Clarke, H. J., Oocyte maturation, *Int. Rev. Cytol.*, 57, 185, 1979.

76. Sadler, S. E. and Maller, J. L., Identification of a steroid receptor on the surface of *Xenopus* oocytes by photoaffinity labeling, *J. Biol. Chem.*, 257, 355, 1982.

77. Nagahama, Y., Yoshikuni, M., Yamashita, M., and Tanaka, M., Regulation of oocyte maturation in fish, in *Fish Physiology, Vol. XIII, Molecular Endocrinology of Fish*, Sherwood, N. M. and Hew, C. L., Eds., Academic Press, San Diego, 1994, 393.

78. Masui, Y. and Markert, C. L., Cytoplasmic control of nuclear behavior during meiotic maturation of frog oocytes, *J. Exp. Zool.*, 177, 129, 1971.

79. Smith, L. D. and Ecker, R. E., The interaction of the steroids with *Rana pipens* oocytes in the induction of maturation, *Develop. Biol.*, 25, 232, 1971.

80. Ishikawa, K., Hanaoka, Y., Kondo, Y., and Imai, K., Primary action of steroid hormone at the surface of amphibian oocyte in the induction of germinal vesicle breakdown, *Mol. Cell. Endocrinol.*, 9, 91, 1977.

81. Godeau, J. F., Scharder-Slatkine, S., Hubert, P., and Baulieu, F. F., Induction of maturation in *Xenopus laevis* oocytes by a steroid linked to a polymer, in *Proc. Natl. Acad. Sci. USA*, 75, 2353, 1978.

82. Nagahama, Y., 17α,20β-dihydroxy-4-pregnen-3-one: a teleost maturation-inducing hormone, *Develop. Growth Diff.*, 29, 1, 1987.

83. Thomas, P., Zhu, Y., and Pace, M., Progestin membrane receptors involved in the meiotic maturation of teleost oocytes: a review with some new findings, *Steroids,* 67, 511–517, 2002.

84. Sadler, S. E., Bower, M. A., and Maller, J. L., Studies of a plasma membrane steroid receptor in *Xenopus* oocytes using the synthetic progestin RU486, *J. Steroid Biochem.*, 22, 419, 1985.

85. Blondeau, J. P. and Baulieu, E. E., Progesterone receptor characterized by photoaffinity labelling in the plasma membrane of *Xenopus laevis* oocytes, *Biochem. J.*, 219, 785, 1984.

86. Kostellow, A. B., Weinstein, S. P., and Morill, G. A., Specific binding of progesterone to the cell surface and its role in the meiotic divisions in *Rana* oocytes, *Biochim. Biophys. Acta,* 720, 356, 1982.

87. Liu, Z. and Patiño, R., High-affinity binding of progesterone to the plasma membrane of *Xenopus* oocytes: characteristics of binding and hormonal and developmental control, *Biol. Reprod.*, 78, 980, 1993.

88. Thomas, P. and Trant, J. M., Evidence that 17α,20β,21-trihydroxy-4-pregnen-3-one is a maturation-inducing steroid in spotted seatrout, *Fish Physiol. Biochem.*, 7, 185, 1989.

89. Maneckjee, A., Idler, D. R., and Weisbart, M., Demonstration of putative membrane and cytosol steroid receptors for 17α,20β-dihydroxy-4-pregnen-3-one in brook trout, *Salvelinus fontinalis*, during terminal stages of oocyte maturation, *Fish. Physiol. Biochem.*, 6, 19, 1991.

90. Yoshikuni, M., Shibata, N., and Nagahama, S., Specific binding of [³H]17α,20β-dihydroxy-4-pregnen-3-one to oocyte cortices of rainbow trout (*Oncorhynchus kisutch*), *Fish Physiol. Biochem.*, 1, 15, 1993.

91. Rahman, M., Ohta, K., Yoshikuni, M., Nagahama, Y., Chuda, H., and Matsuyama, M., Characterization of ovarian membrane receptor for 17, 20β-dihydroxy-4-pregnen-3-one, a maturation inducing hormone in yellowtail, *Seriola quinqueradiata*. *Gen.Comp. Endocrinol.* 127, 71, 2002.

92. W. V., Ghosh, S., Thomas, P., and Sullivan, C. V., A receptor for the oocyte maturation-inducing hormone, 17α,20β,21-trihydroxy-4-pregnen-3-one, on ovarian membranes of striped bass, *Biol. Reprod.*, 56, 266, 1997.

93. Thomas, P. and Das, S., Correlation between binding affinities of C21 steroids for the maturation-inducing steroid membrane receptor in spotted seatrout ovaries and their agonist and antagonist activities in an oocyte maturation bioassay, *Biol. Reprod.*, 57, 999, 1997.

94. Trant, J. M. and Thomas, P., Structure-activity relationships of steroids in inducing germinal vesicle breakdown of Atlantic croaker oocytes *in vitro*, *Gen. Comp. Endocrinol.*, 71, 307, 1988.

95. Towle, A. C. and Sze, P. Y., Steroid binding to synaptic plasma membrane: differential binding of glucocorticoids and gonadal steroids, *J. Steroid Biochem.*, 18, 135, 1983.

96. Pinter, J., and Thomas, P., Characterization of a progestogen receptor in the ovary of the spotted seatrout *Cynoscion nebulosus*, *Biol. Reprod.*, 52, 667, 1995a.

97. Pinter, J. and Thomas, P., The ovarian progestogen receptor in the spotted seatrout, *Cynoscion nebulosus*, demonstrates steroid specificity intermediate between progesterone and glucocorticoid receptors in other vertebrates, *J. Steroid Biochem. Molec. Biol.*, 60, 113, 1997.

98. Scatchard, G., The attractions of proteins for small molecules and ions, *Ann. N. Y. Acad. Sci.*, 51, 660, 1949.

99. Thomas, P. and Patiño, R., Changes in 17α,20β,21-trihydroxy-4-pregnen-3-one membrane receptor concentrations in ovaries of spotted seatrout during final oocyte maturation, in *Proc. 4th Int. Symp. Reproductive Physiology of Fish,* Scott, A.P., Sumpter, J., Kime, D., and Rolfe, M.S., Eds., University of East Anglia Press, 1991, 122.

100. Patiño, R. and Thomas, P., Effects of gonadotropin on ovarian intrafollicular processes during the development of oocyte maturational competence in a teleost, the Atlantic croaker: Evidence for two distinct stages of gonadotropic control of final oocyte maturation, *Biol. Reprod.*, 43, 818, 1990b.

101. Thomas, P., Pinter, J., and Das, S., Upregulation of the maturation-inducing steroid membrane receptor in spotted seatrout ovaries by gonadotropin during oocyte maturation and its physiological significance, *Biol. Reprod.*, 64, 21, 2001.

102. Thomas, P., Hormonal control of final oocyte maturation in sciaenid fishes, in *Perspectives in Comparative Endocrinology*, Davey, K. G., Peter, R. E., and Tobe, S. S., Eds., *Nat. Res. Council Can.*, 1994, 619.

103. Birnbaum, C. S. The role of structure in the disposition of halogenated aromatic xenobiotics, *Environ. Health. Persp.*, G1, 11, 1985.

104. Antunes-Madeira, M. C., Almeida, L. M., and Madeira, V. M. C., Depth-dependent effects of DDT and lindane on the fluidity of native membranes and extracted lipids: implications for mechanisms of toxicity, *Bull. Environ. Contam. Toxicol.*, 51, 787, 1993.

105. Osman, R. A., Andria, M. L., Jones, A. D., and Meizel, S., Steroid induced exocytosis: the human sperm acrosome reaction, *Biochem. Biophys. Res. Commun.*, 168, 828, 1989.

106. Sueldo, C. E., Oehinger, S., Subias, E., Mahony, M., Alexander, N. J., Burkman, L. J., and Acosta, A. A., Effect of progesterone on human zona pellucida sperm binding and oocyte penetrating capacity, *Fertil. Steril.*, 60, 137, 1993.

107. Blackmore, P. F., Fisher, J. F., Spilman, C. H., and Bleasdale, J. E., Unusual steroid specificity of the cell surface progesterone receptor on human sperm, *Mol. Pharmacol.*, 49, 727, 1996.

108. Baldi, E., Casano, R., Falseti, C., Krausz, C., Maggi, M., and Forti, G., Intracellular calcium accumulation and responsiveness to progesterone in capacitating human spermatozoa, *J. Andrology*, 12, 323, 1991.

109. Sabeur, K., Edwards, D. P., and Meizel, S., Human sperm plasma membrane progesterone receptor(s) and the acrosome reaction, *Biol. Reprod.*, 54, 993, 1996.

110. Baldi, E., Falsetti, C., Krausz, C., Gervasi, G., Carloni, V., Casano, R., and Forti, G., Stimulation of platelet-activating factor synthesis by progesterone and A23187 in human spermatozoa, *Biochem. J.*, 292, 209, 1993.

111. Blackmore, P. F., Rapid non-genomic actions of progesterone stimulate Ca^{2+} influx and the acrosome reaction in human sperm, *Cell. Signal.*, 5, 531, 1993.

112. Suarez, S. S. and Pollard, J. W., Capacitation, the acrosome reaction, and motility in mammalian sperm, in *Controls of Sperm Motility: Biological and Clinical Aspects*, Gagnon, C., Ed., CRC Press, Boca Raton, FL, 1990, 77.

113. Aitken, R. J., Buckingham, D. W., and Irvine, D. S., The extragenomic action of progesterone on human spermatozoa: evidence for a ubiquitous response that is down-regulated, *Endocrinology*, 137, 3999, 1996.

114. Meizel, S. and Turner, K. O., Progesterone acts at the plasma membrane of human sperm. *Mol. Cell. Endocrinol.*, 11, R1, 1991.

115. Blackmore, P. F. and Lattanzio, F. A., Cell surface localization of a novel non-genomic progesterone receptor on the head of human sperm, *Biochem. Biophys. Res. Commun.*, 181, 331, 1991.

116. Tesarik, J., Mendoza, C., Moos, J., and Carreras, A., Selective expression of a progesterone receptor on the human sperm surface, *Fertil. Steril.*, 58, 784, 1992.

117. Uhler, M. L., Leung, A., Chan, S. Y. W., and Wang, C., Direct effects of progesterone and antiprogesterone on human sperm hyperactivated motility and acrosome reaction, *Fert. Steril.*, 58, 1191, 1992.

118. Yang, J., Serres, C., Philibert, D., Robel, P., Baulieu, E. E., and Jouannet, P., Progesterone and RU486: opposing effects on human sperm, *Proc. Nat. Acad. Sci. USA*, 1994, 529.

119. Thomas, P., Das, S., Breckenridge-Miller, D., and Detweiler, C., Characterization and regulation of a progestin receptor on Atlantic croaker sperm membranes, in *Advances in Comparative Endocrinology, Volume II*, Kawashima, S. and Kikuyama, S., Eds., Monduzzi Editore S.p.A., 1997, 1381

120. Billard, R. and Cosson, M. P., The energetics of fish sperm motility, in *Controls of Sperm Motility: Biological and Clinical Aspects*, Gagnon, C., Ed., CRC Press, Boca Raton, FL, 1990, 153.

121. Miura, T., Yamauchi, K., Takahashi, H., and Nagahama, Y., The role of hormones in the acquisition of sperm motility in salmonid fish, *J. Exp. Zool.*, 261, 359, 1992.

122. Billard, R. and Cosson, M. P., Some problems related to the assessment of sperm motility in freshwater fish, *J. Exp. Zool.*, 261, 122, 1992.

123. Cosson, M. P., Billard, R., and Letellier, L., Rise of internal Ca^{2+} accompanies the initiation of trout sperm motility, *Cell. Motil. Cytoskel.*, 14, 424, 1989.

124. Detweiler, C. and Thomas, P., The role of ions and ion channels in the regulation of Atlantic croaker sperm motility, *J. Exp. Zool.*, 281, 139, 1998.

125. Thomas, P., Rapid, nongenomic steroid actions initiated at the cell surface: lessons from studies with fish, *Fish Physiol. Biochem.*, in press.

126. Zhu, Y., Bond, J. and Thomas, P., Identification, classification, and partial characterization of genes in humans and other vertebrates homologous to a fish membrane progestin receptor. *Proc. Natl. Acad. Sci. USA*, 100, 2237, 2003.

127. Vitale, M. L., Parisi, M. N., Chiocchio, S. R., and Tramezzani, J. H., Serotonin induces gonadotropin release through stimulation of LH-releasing hormone release from the median eminence, *J. Endocrinol.*, 111, 309, 1986.

128. Malven, P.V., Gonadotropins in the female, Chapter 11, in *Mammalian Neuroendocrinology*, CRC Press, Boca Raton, FL, 1993, 181.

129. Kah, O., Anglade, I., Lepretre, E., Dubourg, P., and de Monbrison, D., The reproductive brain in fish, *Fish Physiol. Biochem.*, 11, 85, 1993.

130. Khan, I. A. and Thomas, P., Stimulatory effects of serotonin on maturational gonadotropin release in the Atlantic croaker, *Micropogonias undulatus*, *Gen. Comp. Endocrinol.*, 88, 388, 1992.

131. Khan, I. A. and Thomas, P., Seasonal and daily variations of plasma gonadotropin II response to a LHRH analog and serotonin in the Atlantic croaker (*Micropogonias undulatus*): Evidence for mediation by 5-HT$_2$ receptors, *J. Exp. Zool.*, 269, 531, 1994.

132. Khan, I. A. and Thomas, P., GABA exerts stimulatory and inhibitory influences on gonadotropin II secretion in the Atlantic croaker (*Micropogonias undulatus*), *Neuroendocrinology*, 69, 261, 1999.

133. Blázquez, M., Bosma, P. T., Fraser, E. J., Van Look, K. J. W., and Trudeau, V. L., Fish as models for the neuroendocrine regulation of reproduction and growth, *Comp. Biochem. Physiol.*, C119, 345, 1998.

134. Arias, P., Szwaecfarb, B., de Rondina, D. C., Carbone, S., Sverdlik, R., and Moguilevsky, J. A., *In vivo* and *in vitro* studies on the effect of serotonergic system on luteinizing hormone and luteinizing hormone-releasing hormone secretion in prepubertal and peripubertal female rats, *Brain Res.*, 523, 57, 1990.

135. Li, S. and Pelletier, G., Involvement of serotonin in the regulation of GnRH gene expression in the male rat brain, *Neuropeptides*, 29, 21, 1995.

136. Fink, G., Dow, R. C., McQueen, J. K., Bennie, J. G. and Carroll, S. M., Serotonergic 5-HT$_{2A}$ receptors are important for the oestradiol-induced surge of luteinizing hormone-releasing hormone in the rat, *J. Neuroendocrinol.*, 11, 63, 1999.

137. Lado-Abeal, J., Rey, C., Cabezas-Agricola, J. M., Rodriguez, A., Camarero, E., and Cabezas-Serrato, J., L-5-hydroxytryptophan amplifies pulsatile secretion of LH in the follicular-phase of normal women, *Clin. Endocrinol.*, 47, 555, 1997.

138. Hery, M., Francois-Bellan, A. M., Hery, F., Deprez, P., and Becquet, D., Serotonin directly stimulates luteinizing hormone-releasing hormone release from GT1 cells via 5-HT$_7$ receptors, *Endocrine*, 7, 261, 1997.

139. Somoza, G. M. and Peter, R. E., Effects of serotonin on gonadotropin and growth hormone release from *in vitro* perifused goldfish pituitary fragments, *Gen. Comp. Endocrinol.*, 82, 103, 1991.

140. Yu, K. L., Rosenblum, P. M. and Peter, R. E., *In vitro* release of gonadotropin-releasing hormone from the brain preoptic-anterior hypothalamic region and pituitary of female goldfish, *Gen. Comp. Endocrinol.*, 81, 256, 1991.

141. Khan, I. A. and Thomas, P., Immunocytochemical localization of serotonin and gonadotropin-releasing hormone in the brain and pituitary gland of the Atlantic croaker, *Micropogonias undulates*, *Gen. Comp. Endocrinol.*, 88, 388, 1993.

142. Khan, I. A. and Thomas, P., Disruption of neuroendocrine control of luteinizing hormone secretion in Atlantic croaker by Aroclor 1254 involves inhibition of hypothalamic tryptophan hydroxylase activity, *Biol. Reprod.*, 64, 955, 2001.

143. Van de Kaar, L. D., Lorens, S. A., Vodraska, A., Allers, G., Green, M., Van Orden, D. E., and Van Orden, L. S. 3rd, Effects of selective midbrain and diencepahlic 5,7-dihydroxytryptamine lesions on serotonin content in individual preoptico-hypothalamic nuclei and on serum luteinizing hormone levels, *Neuroendocrinology*, 31, 309, 1980.

144. Kah, O. and Chambolle, P., Serotonin in the brain of the goldfish, *Carassius auratus*: An immunocytochemical study, *Cell Tissue Res.*, 234, 319, 1983.

145. Jacobs, B. L. and Azmitia, E. C., Structure and function of the brain serotonin system, *Physiol. Rev.*, 72, 165, 1992.

146. Thomas, P., Effects of Aroclor 1254 and cadmium on reproductive endocrine function and ovarian growth in Atlantic croaker, *Mar. Environ. Res.*, 28, 499, 1989.

147. Seegal, R. F., Bush, B., and Brosch, K. O., Polychlorinated biphenyls induce regional changes in brain norepinephrine concentrations in adult rats, *Neurotoxicology*, 6, 13, 1985.

148. Seegal, R. F., Bush, B., and Shain, W., Lightly chlorinated *ortho*-substituted PCB congeners decrease dopamine in non-human primate brain and in tissue culture, *Toxicol. Appl. Pharmacol.*, 106, 136, 1990.

149. Seegal, R. F., Bush, B., and Brosch, K. O., Sub-chronic exposure of the adult rat to Aroclor 1254 yields regionally-specific changes in dopaminergic function, *Neurotoxicology*, 12, 55, 1991.

150. Seegal, R. F., Bush, B., and Shain, W., Neurotoxicology of *ortho*-substituted polychlorinated biphenyls, *Chemosphere*, 23, 1941, 1991.

151. Chu, I., Villeneuve, D. C., Yagminas, A., Lacavalier, P., Poon, R., Feeley, M., Kennedy, F. W., Seegal, R. F., Hakånsson, H., Ahlborg, U. G., Valli, V. E., and Bergman, Å., Toxicity of 2,2',4,4',5,5'-hexachlorobiphenyl in rats: Effects following 90-day oral exposure, *J. Appl. Toxicol.*, 16, 121, 1996.

152. Choski, N. Y., Kodavanti, P. R. S., Tilson, H. A., and Booth, R. G., Effects of polychlorinated biphenyls (PCBs) on brain tyrosine hydroxylase activity and dopamine synthesis in rats, *Fund. Appl. Toxicol.*, 39, 76, 1997.

153. Seegal, R. F., Epidemiological and laboratory evidence of PCB-induced neurotoxicity, *Crit. Rev. Toxicol.*, 26, 709, 1996.

154. Khan, I. A. and Thomas, P., Aroclor 1254 inhibits tryptophan hydroxylase activity in rat brain, *Arch. Toxicol.*, in press.

155. Desaulniers, D., Leingartner, K., Wade, M., Fintelman, E., Yagminas, A., and Foster, W. G., Effects of acute exposure to PCBs 126 and 153 on anterior pituitary and thyroid hormones and FSH isoforms in adult Sprague Dawley male rats, *Toxcol. Sci.*, 47, 158, 1999.

156. Jansen, H. T., Cooke, P. S., Porcelli, J., Liu, T. C., and Hansen, L. G., Estrogenic and antiestogenic actions of PCBs in the female rat: *In vitro* and *in vivo* studies, *Reprod. Toxicol.*, 7, 237, 1993.

157. Khan, I. A. and Thomas, P., Lead and Aroclor 1254 disrupt reproductive neuroendocrine function in Atlantic croaker, *Marine Environ. Res.*, 50, 119, 2000.

158. Jequier, E., Lovenberg, W., and Sjoerdsma, A., Tryptophan hydroxylase inhibition: the mechanism by which *p*-chlorophenylalanine depletes rat brain serotonin, *Mol. Pharmacol.*, 3, 274, 1967.

159. Fuller, R. W., Drugs altering serotonin synthesis and metabolism, in *Neuropharmacology of Serotonin*, Green, A. R., Ed., Oxford University Press, New York, 1985, 1.

160. Coen, C. W. and MacKinnon, P. C. B., Serotonin involvement in the control of phasic luteinizing hormone release in the rat: Evidence for a critical period, *J. Endocrinol.*, 82, 105, 1979.

161. Medola, P., Buck, G. M., Server, L. E., Zieiezny, M., and Vena, J. E., Consumption of PCB-contaminated freshwater fish and shortened menstrual cycle length, *Am. J. Epidemiol.,* 146, 955, 1997.

162. Gerhard, I., Daniel, V., Link, S., Monga, B., and Runnebaum, B., Chlorinated hydrocarbons in women with repeated miscarriages, *Environ. Health Persp.,* 106, 675, 1998.

163. Clayton, R. N., Solano, A. R., Garcia-Vela, A., Dufau, M., and Catt, K. J., Regulation of pituitary receptors for gonadotropin-releasing hormone during the rat estrous cycle, *Endocrinology,* 107, 699, 1980.

164. Habibi, H. R., De Leeuw, R., Nahorniak, C. S., Goss, H. J. Th., and Peter, R. E., Pituitary gonadotropin-releasing hormone (GnRH) receptor activity in goldfish and catfish: Seasonal and gonadal effects, *Fish. Physiol. Biochem.,* 7, 109, 1989.

165. Khan, I. A., Mathews, S., Okuzawa, K., Kagawa, H., and Thomas, P., Alterations in the GnRH-LH system in relation to gonadal stage and Aroclor 1254 exposure in Atlantic croaker, *Comp. Biochem. Physiol.,* 129B: 251, 2001.

166. Khan, I. A. and Thomas, P., Vitamin E co-treatment reduces Aroclor 1254-induced impairment of reproductive neuroendocrine function in Atlantic croaker. *Marine Environ. Res.,* in press.

167. Abel, E. L., *Lead and Reproduction, a Comprehensive Bibliography,* Greenwood Press, London, Conn., 1984, 117.

168. Pounds, J. G., Cory-Slechta, D. A., and Cranmer, J. M., Eds., *New Dimensions of Lead Neurotoxicity: Redefining Mechanisms and Effects,* Intox Press, Little Rock, 1993.

169. Thomas, P., Reproductive endocrine function in female Atlantic croaker exposed to xenobiotics, *Mar. Environ. Res.,* 24, 179, 1988.

170. Singh, A. and Ashraf, M., Neurotoxicity in rats sub-chronically exposed to low levels of lead, *Vet. Hum. Toxicol.,* 31, 21, 1989.

171. Katti, S. R. and Sathyanesan, A. G., Lead nitrate induces changes in brain constituents of the freshwater fish *Clarias batrachus* (L), *Neurotoxicology,* 7, 45, 1986.

172. Müller, W. F., Hobson, W., Fuller, G. B., Knauf, W., Coulston, F., and Konte, F., Endocrine effects of chlorinated hydrocarbons in rhesus monkeys, *Ecotox. Environ. Saf.,* 2, 161, 1978.

173. Wilson, C. A. and Leigh, A. J., Endocrine toxicology of the female reproductive system, in *Endocrine Toxicology,* Atterwill, C. K. and Flack, J. D., Eds., Cambridge University Press, 1992, 313.

2 Developmental and Reproductive Abnormalities Associated with Environmental Estrogens: Diethylstilbestrol (DES) as an Example

Retha R. Newbold and Wendy Jefferson

CONTENTS

0-8493-2281-2/05/$0.00+$1.50
© 2005 by CRC Press

2.1 INTRODUCTION

Over the last decade, concern has increased that widespread adverse effects are occurring in humans, domestic animals, and wildlife populations as a result of exposure to environmental chemicals that possess endocrine-disrupting activity (1–3). A number of pesticides, industrial byproducts, manufactured products, such as plastics, pharmaceuticals, and natural chemicals have been implicated in disrupting the mammalian endocrine system. These chemicals are collectively referred to as endocrine-disrupting chemicals (EDCs). Initial concern focused only on chemicals with estrogenic activity but now chemicals with any hormone-like activity are included. Some of these chemicals do not easily break down and are known to persist and bio-accumulate in the environment, hence the reason for concern.

Adverse long-term health consequences have been proposed to be linked to exposure to these endocrine-modulating chemicals; in women, increased cancer rates in the breast, ovary, and uterus, as well as other reproductive tract abnormalities (endometriosis, fibroids, and subfertility/infertility) have been reported; in men, increased prostatic and testicular cancer, and poor semen quality associated with subfertility or infertility have been suggested. Similar concerns of adverse effects in domestic animals and wildlife have focused on observations regarding reproductive disorders involving endpoints such as: reduced fertility, reduced egg hatchability, reduced viability of offspring, slow growth rates, wasting and lower rates of activity in neonates, impaired hormone activity, and modified adult sexual behavior observed in various species including birds, fish, alligators, panthers, and mink; immune dysfunction has also been reported in dolphins, whales, and turtles (3). These abnormalities may have a common etiology and be caused by disruption of normal endocrine function as a result of exposure to environmental chemicals that mimic the actions of naturally occurring hormones (4, 5).

In mammals and other vertebrates, hormones provide an important role in regulating normal reproductive tract development and function (6). During differentiation and periods of high mitotic activity, such as during the proliferative phase of the estrous cycle or in preparation for pregnancy, hormones aid cell-to-cell communications; in addition, specific and coordinated cellular responses are directed by hormones in their target tissues. It is well established that hormones produced by one group of cells have the ability to direct and signal the course of development and response of another group of cells. Thus, steriod hormones have been identified as major players in regulating developmental processes in target tissues such as the reproductive tract. Hormones accomplish their function of stimulating or inhibiting various cellular pathways by binding with receptor molecules. The hormone/receptor complex then interacts with DNA and with second-messenger systems to produce specific actions such as protein synthesis and cAMP turnover. Environmental chemicals that mimic hormones can (a) duplicate the normal hormone process, or (b) interact with the receptor causing an aberrant function, (c) interact additively or synergistically with natural hormones, causing an exaggerated response, or (d) interact with the receptor and block hormone/receptor interactions, resulting in decreased or blocked function.

Disruption of normal endocrine function has moved to the center of many toxicological studies focusing on reproductive toxicants. A key issue involved with the recent concern of adverse effects of environmental endocrine-disrupting chemicals is that such affects may be caused by exposure to relatively small doses during a "unique window of vulnerability" for the fetus or neonate during development, and that the effects may not show up until much later in life (7). These low-dose exposures will be discussed in further detail. Developmental exposures, in particular, are very difficult to monitor since chemicals may exert their effects only at a specific time in differentiation and then disappear. Therefore, using even the most sophisticated analytical procedures to detect minute amounts of chemicals may not associate a particular chemical exposure with an adverse outcome.

Further difficulty in identifying suspect chemicals is complicated by the vast number of compounds that have been reported to have endocrine-disrupting effects (4). For example, many man-made or generated chemicals used in industrial and household products including pesticides and plasticizers, pharmaceuticals, and dietary supplements, as well as some naturally occurring substances such as phytoestrogens found in plants have endocrine modulating activity.

Although difficulties exist in identifying chemicals and in showing an association with specific long-term effects, ample concern remains that chemicals with endocrine modulating activity are adversely affecting reproductive tract development and function. Some investigators have assumed that after sexual maturity, exposure to endocrine disrupters does not permanently alter the function of hormone-responsive tissues and are therefore not important; however, permanent changes in brain (8) and vaginal tissues (9) have been shown in mature experimental animals following administration of estrogenic chemicals. Thus, chronic, low-level exposure to estrogenic chemicals in the environment, even after maturity, can possibly have adverse effects in humans similar to those observed in estrogen-treated laboratory animals. These chemicals may, therefore, pose a health risk even at low levels of adult exposure. Although adult exposure is indeed important, the focus of our chapter is on exposure of the fetus or neonate because of the increased susceptibility of this stage of development to environmental insults.

2.2 DEVELOPMENTAL BASIS OF ADULT DISEASE

In the late 1980s, reports surfaced that suggested the fetal environment, as reflected by low birth size and poor nutrition, were related to increased risk of non-communicable diseases later in adult life. This association was first described for coronary heart disease, but it quickly extended to include type 2 diabetes, osteoporosis, and metabolic and endocrine dysfunction. These findings led to the development of the "fetal origins of adult disease" paradigm in which a substantial research effort now focuses on life-long consequences of perinatal influences on chronic disease (10, 11). Perinatal effects are no longer viewed in terms of just teratogenic changes or acute birth injury such as the thalidomide-induced limb malformations, but whether changes induced in early development (preimplantation through early childhood stages) may lead to life-long consequences. Many of these changes are not obvious and cannot be detected until much later in life. Although it is generally recognized that adaptive plastic responses during early development often have consequences for function in adult life, it is still controversial whether developmental consequences actively contribute to the burden of human adult disorders.

Difficulties exist in looking at the role of chemical exposures during development and their relationship to adult disease. Considering what is currently known about chemicals that can disrupt the endocrine system, their effects (1) may be manifested differently, and with permanent consequences, in the embryo, fetus, and neonate as compared to effects resulting from exposure to adults; (2) can alter the course of development for the exposed organism, with the outcome dependent on the specific developmental exposure periods; and (3) are often delayed and not recognized until the organism reaches maturity or perhaps even later in life, even though the critical period of exposure occurred during embryonic, fetal, or neonatal life. In spite of these difficulties, research findings continue to add support to the idea that environmental chemicals, in particular those with estrogenic activity, can have endocrine-disrupting effects that result in long-term health consequences.

As an example, the profound effects of estrogens on the developing reproductive tract have been demonstrated by prenatal exposure to the synthetic estrogen, diethylstilbestrol (DES) (12). These DES effects were well recognized and firmly documented long before the proposed "developmental basis of adult disease" paradigm; however, DES clearly points out that chemical exposure, in addition to nutrition and other perinatal factors, can significantly alter the developing organism and cause long-term effects.

2.3   DES AS A PROTOTYPE ENVIRONMENTAL ESTROGEN

DES, a non-steroidal compound with properties similar to the natural female sex hormone estradiol, was synthesized in 1938; it was specifically designed for its potent estrogenic activity and its easy solubility. Like many of today's environmental estrogens, DES was not structurally similar to natural estrogens (4). In fact, early research with DES showed that compounds with diverse structures could exhibit similar biological functions associated with estrogens. A historical account of the development and use of DES and the early search for compounds with estrogenic activity has been summarized (13). DES also demonstrated another significant point, the potential toxic effects of estrogens. The well-documented adverse effects in DES-exposed humans justify the concern of developmental exposure to other environmental estrogens and endocrine disruptors. Of particular significance are the reports that prenatal DES exposure may result in health consequences for multiple generations (14–17).

For almost 30 years, physicians prescribed DES to women with high-risk pregnancies to prevent miscarriages and other complications of pregnancy. Unfortunately, in 1971, a report associated DES with a rare form of reproductive tract cancer termed "vaginal adenocarcinoma," which was detected in a small number (< 0.1%) of adolescent daughters of women who had taken the drug while pregnant. Later, DES was also linked to more frequent benign reproductive tract problems in an estimated 95% of the DES-exposed daughters; reproductive organ dysfunction, abnormal pregnancies, reduction in fertility, immune system disorders, and periods of depression have been subsequently reported.

Similarly, DES-exposed male offspring demonstrated structural, functional, and cellular abnormalities following prenatal exposure; hypospadias, microphallus, retained testes, inflammation, and decreased fertility have all been reported (12). DES became the first example of an *in utero* estrogenic toxicant in humans; it was shown to cross the placenta and induce a direct effect on the developing fetus. DES is no longer used clinically to prevent miscarriage, but a major concern remains that when DES-exposed women age, and reach the time at which the incidence of reproductive organ cancers normally increase, they will show a much higher incidence of cancer than unexposed individuals.

Further, the possibility of second-generation effects has been reported (14–17), which puts still another generation at risk for developing problems associated with DES treatment of their grandmothers. Thus, the DES episode continues to have serious health consequences and serves as an unfortunate reminder of the toxicities that can be caused by hormonally active chemicals.

Questions of the mechanisms involved in DES-induced teratogenic and carcinogenic effects prompted us to develop an experimental animal model to study the adverse effects of estrogens and other endocrine-disrupting chemicals on reproductive tract development and differentiation. The murine animal model has successfully duplicated and predicted many adverse effects observed in humans with similar DES-exposure (Table 2.1). These findings provide useful endpoints pertinent to the evaluation of the possible adverse effects of other environmental estrogenic compounds.

TABLE 2.1
Similar Developmental Effects of Prenatal Exposure to DES in Mice and Humans

	Male Offspring	Female Offspring
Reproductive Tract Dysfunction	Subfertility/Infertility Decreased Sperm Counts	Subfertility/Infertility Poor Reproductive Outcome
Structural Malformations	Microphallus and Hypospadias Retained Hypoplastic Testes Retained Mullerian Remnants (anatomical feminization)	Oviduct, Uterus, Cx, Vagina Paraovarian Cysts of Mesonephric Origin Retained Mesonephric Remnants

Cellular Abnormalities	Testicular Tumors
	Tumors in Retained Mullerian
	  Remnants
	Epididymal Cysts
	Prostatic Lesions and Inflammation
		Proliferative Epithelial Lesions of
		  the Oviduct
		Vaginal Adenomyosis and
		  Adenocarcinoma

2.4   DES ANIMAL MODELS TO STUDY HUMAN DISEASE

For the prenatal DES exposure model, pregnant outbred CD-1 mice were treated by subcutaneous injections of DES dissolved in corn oil on days 9 to 16 of gestation. The doses of DES ranged from 0.01 to 100 µg/kg maternal body weight; the highest dose of DES is equal to or less than that given therapeutically to pregnant women, and the lower doses are comparable to exposure to weak environmental estrogens. Pregnant mice delivered their young on day 19 of gestation, and their offspring were followed for up to 24 months of age. The time of *in utero* DES-exposure for the offspring encompassed the major period of organogenesis of the genital tract in the mouse.

While many developmental events in the genital tract continue into neonatal life for the mouse, similar differentiation events occur entirely *in utero* in humans (18). In both species, however, early in the normal development of the reproductive tract of an embryo, there is an undifferentiated stage in which the sex of the embryo cannot be determined. At this stage, the gonads have not developed into either testis or ovary, and all embryos have a double set of genital ducts, Müllerian (paramesonephric) and Wolffian (mesonephric) ducts. In the female, as sex differentiation occurs, the Müllerian ducts differentiate into the oviduct, uterus, cervix, and upper vagina, while the mesonephric duct regresses.

In the male, under the influence of testicular secretions, the mesonephric ducts form the epididymis, vas deferens, and other tissues such as the seminal vesicles, while the Müllerian duct regresses. Exposure to DES during this critical period of sex differentiation resulted in alterations in both the female and male reproductive tract, including the partial or complete retention of the opposite duct system in both sexes. Although adverse effects are demonstrated in both sexes, only changes in developmentally DES-exposed females will be further discussed because of space constraint. Resulting abnormalities in the females include structural, functional, and long-term changes throughout all regions of the reproductive tract (19, 20).

2.4.1   EARLY REPRODUCTIVE SENESCENCE AND DYSFUNCTION

Poor reproductive outcome has been reported in prenatal DES exposed women (12); in addition, subfertility and infertility have also been reported in animals (21) following developmental exposure to DES. For mice, reproductive tract dysfunction was assessed in the DES-exposed animal model by breeding prenatal DES-exposed female mice to control untreated male mice using a continuous breeding protocol (21). The breeding study showed that prenatal exposure to varying doses of DES (0.01 to 100 µg/kg maternal body weight) resulted in a striking dose-related decrease in the fertility of the offspring (21). Over the 32-week breeding period, the effects ranged from minimal subfertility (90% of controls at the lowest DES dose) to essential sterility at the two highest DES doses (10 and 100 µg/kg). It was interesting to note that exposure to DES at the lowest dose (0.01 µg/kg maternal body weight) which was chosen as an environmentally relative dose, showed a decrease in fertility approximately midway through the study (21). This early reproductive senescence at low dose exposure is currently being investigated. At the higher DES doses, the mechanisms responsible for the subfertility were the result of multiple factors: oviductal malformation; ovarian dysfunction; altered uterine environment and reproductive tract secretions; uterine, cervical, and vaginal structural alterations. Taken together, these alterations establish the fact that exposure to DES, even at relatively low levels, impairs reproductive capacity throughout the animal's lifetime. Numerous reports of altered pregnancy outcomes in young women exposed *in utero* to DES, as well as accidental DES exposure to wildlife resulting in infertility, demonstrate the importance of similar findings in the DES-exposed mouse model, and suggest that other environmental estrogens may also play a role in decreased female fertility. Specific effects in reproductive tract tissues are discussed in more detail.

2.4.2 OVARIAN TOXICITY

Unquestionably, the ovary is a target for perturbation by DES and other environmental estrogenic compounds. Increased inflammation, early depletion of follicles, multi-ovular follicles, decreased number of corpora lutea, altered gonadotropin levels, increased number of ovarian cysts, increased interstitial compartment and ovarian tumors were observed in the developmentally exposed DES mice and were likely contributors to reproductive dysfunction in this animal model. These data of ovarian toxicity in the prenatal DES experimental animal model support the contention that chemical endocrine disrupters may indeed be related to decreases in fertility later in life. It also raises the possibility that there is an association with developmental exposure to endocrine disrupting chemicals and ovarian tumors reported to be on the rise in the general population. While the ovary is itself a direct target for these toxicants (22–24), the hypothalamic/pituitary axis may also be disturbed by exposure to DES and manifest as ovarian/reproductive tract dysfunction.

2.4.3 OVIDUCTAL TOXICITY

Differentiation of the oviduct was altered following prenatal DES exposure (25). Malformations of the oviduct were observed in 100% of the females treated *in utero* with 100 μg/kg of DES but not in any control mice. Animals exposed to doses < 100 μg/kg showed less extensive malformation with fewer oviductal "coils" being the most prominent feature; the lowest DES dose did not result in any apparent structural changes in the oviduct although this dose was associated with early reproductive senescence as previously discussed. Oviductal malformations observed in the high DES-dosed mice persisted throughout life and permanently distorted the anatomical relationship of the uterus, oviduct, and ovary. Retention of this fetal oviductal phenotype into adulthood was termed "developmentally arrested oviduct" (25).

The experimental DES-exposed animal model clearly established the oviduct as a target for the teratogenic effects of DES. Moreover, the arrest in development resulting from prenatal exposure to DES suggests a role for estrogens in the normal morphogenesis of the oviduct. It is possible that an increase in estrogen levels during oviductal development may play a role in the ultimate structural or functional integrity of this tissue in humans, as well as, mice. In fact, some of the more important features of the "developmentally arrested oviduct" in mice exposed prenatally to DES, such as decreased oviductal length, relative lack of fimbriae, and abnormal anatomical location have been described in women exposed to DES during gestation (26). Thus, altered or arrested development of the mammalian oviduct appears to be a general biological consequence of prenatal exposure to DES. A recent report has described molecular mechanisms associated with this developmental arrest (27, 28). Estrogens were shown to regulate the expression of important homeobox genes during development; expression of the homeobox gene Hoxa-9 corresponds to oviductal, Hoxa-10 corresponds to cervical, and Hoxa-11 corresponds to uterine differentiation events. DES was demonstrated to down-regulate the expression of these homeobox genes during Mullerian duct differentiation resulting in malformed reproductive structures (27, 28). Other environmental estrogens may similarly down-regulate these specific genes if exposure occurs during critical stages of differentiation leading to malformations of the reproductive tract.

Functional alterations were also characteristic of the malformed oviducts (25). Prenatal DES exposure resulted in lack of development of an uterotubal value at the junction of the oviduct and uterus so that fluids could readily pass from the uterus into the oviduct and ovarian bursa. This valve is a missing barrier in the mouse that is certainly a factor in the increased inflammation observed in the ovary and oviduct of aged mice (22).

Cellular defects in the oviduct of DES-exposed mice likely contributed to functional abnormalities. In DES-treated mice, the columnar cells lining the oviductal lumen and the mucosal folds were irregularly arranged as compared to controls. Further, "gland formation" was observed in the oviduct of DES-exposed animals that extended through the muscularis, a histological feature never observed in control mice (29). Hyperplasia of the epithelial compartment was often noted, and inflammatory changes were more prevalent in all segments of the DES oviduct compared to controls.

Histologic changes in DES-exposed mice, that is, epithelial hyperplasia and gland formation (diverticuli) of the oviductal mucosa that extend into the muscle wall, resemble the clinically described lesion, salpingitis isthmica nodosa (SIN). Since its description in the late 1800s, the etiology and pathogenesis of SIN had been the subject of much debate. Clinically, this lesion had been related to ectopic tubal pregnancy and infertility. The data obtained from our experimental DES-exposed animal models raise the possibility that clinically noted cases of SIN can result from an altered hormonal environment during early development. This is supported by the finding of SIN in the oviduct of young women prenatally exposed to DES (30).

Although the observed cellular changes appear to reside in the epithelium, it is not clear whether the epithelium is responding independently or in combination with factors from the underlying stroma. Since the connective tissue in these DES-treated mice is relatively thin and hypoplastic, there may be a defect in the stromal compartment that modifies the epithelial response.

Considering these observations in the DES oviduct, the proliferative capacity of Müllerian duct derived tissues (oviduct, uterus, cervix, and upper vagina) may be determined by hormonal exposure during development. If estrogen levels are significantly elevated, as with prenatal DES treatment of animals and humans, the proliferative capacity of the reproductive tract epithelium may be permanently altered.

2.4.4 UTERINE (FIBROIDS AND ADENOCARCINOMA) AND VAGINAL TOXICITY

In addition to the oviduct, structural changes were observed in other regions of the reproductive tract. The uterus was a frequent target of DES-induced structural changes. Following prenatal exposure to the high DES dose (100 μg/kg), the uterus of prepubescent animals was smaller in diameter and length with compared with control females of the same age. Histological changes in the prepubescent DES-exposed uterus included a poorly organized muscle compartment and decreased gland formation. In response to estrogen stimulation, prepubescent mice exposed to high doses of DES during prenatal development displayed decreased uterine growth response, decreased uterine luminal fluid quantity and protein concentration, alterations in specific uterine luminal proteins, and altered cellular differentiation (squamous metaplasia). (Altered cellular responses were also observed in lower DES dose groups, but the responses were different than in high dose groups; this is discussed in more detail in Section V of this chapter.) Structural hypoplasia of the uterus and decreased responsiveness of the uterus to an estrogen challenge remained common features throughout life of the high dose prenatally DES-exposed animals. In aged prenatal DES-exposed females, cystic endometrial hyperplasia and squamous metaplasia in hypoplastic uterine structures were frequently found. Also, a low incidence of benign (leiomyomas) and malignant (adenocarcinoma, stromal cell sarcoma) tumors was observed in prenatally DES-exposed mice (31).

The low incidence of malignant uterine tumors following prenatal DES exposure was in sharp contrast to the high prevalence of adenocarcinoma seen after exposure to DES on neonatal days 1 to 5. Modifying the murine animal model to test for sensitivity in the neonatal period, a time which corresponds to developmental events that are still occurring prenatally in humans, resulted in ~95% of the mice ($\geq$ 18 months of age) developing uterine neoplasia. The incidence of leiomyomas was also higher in neonatally treated mice as compared to prenatal treatment but the number was low compared to adenocarcinoma. Lesions of the epithelium have traditionally received the most attention for DES-induced toxic effects, however, the findings of increased incidence of leiomyomas in the experimental mouse model (32), combined with similar findings in DES exposed women (33), suggest that other tissue compartments are adversely affected resulting in tumors. Since the etiology of uterine fibroids (leiomyomas) is unknown, it is possible that exposure to environmental estrogenic compounds or increased levels of circulating estrogens during development may indeed contribute to the development of fibroids.

In the cervico-vaginal region of prenatally DES-exposed mice, striking structural abnormalities were also observed as seen in the uterus. The vaginal fornix was shallower and, in some cases, completely absent, as compared to controls (34). Urethral openings were often observed to be abnormally located anterior to the vulva (persistent urogenital sinus) in some of the animals exposed prenatally to 100 μg/kg of DES (female hypospadias). "Gland-like structures" associated with this abnormality were assumed to be of urothelial origin.

In addition to structural malformations, prenatal DES-treated animals (100 μg/kg) had excessive vaginal keratinization. In some animals, increased keratinization combined with basal cell hyperplasia resulted in irregular pegs of epithelium that extended into the subadjacent stroma. In 25% of the 12- to 18-month-old prenatal DES mice, epidermoid tumors of the vagina were observed. Excessive keratinization, epithelial pegs, and epidermoid tumors were not usually observed in the vagina of animals exposed to doses of DES lower than 100 μg/kg and were never observed in control untreated animals.

The benign lesion, vaginal adenosis, was seen in 75% of the mice exposed to DES on days 1 to 5 of neonatal life, but it was not a common finding in mice treated prenatally with DES (34). The often-cited DES-associated neoplastic lesion, vaginal adenocarcinoma, was observed after prenatal DES exposure but not after neonatal exposure. Although vaginal adenocarcinoma is an extremely rare tumor in both animals and humans, it is considered a hallmark lesion of DES exposure (12). The development of vaginal adenocarcinoma has been thought to originate from an alteration in the cellular differentiation of the Müllerian duct epithelium. However, the relationship of vaginal adenosis and adenocarcinoma remains unclear. Since neonatal mouse studies show a high incidence of vaginal adenosis but no cases of vaginal adenocarcinoma, the demonstration of vaginal adenocarcinoma in the prenatal DES-exposed animal model which shows a low incidence of adenosis suggests that the stage of cellular differentiation at the time of DES exposure may be the most critical event in the final expression of these abnormalities. By necessity, experimental animal models that are developed to study toxicity of various chemicals should encompass both prenatal and neonatal reproductive tract differentiation especially since the corresponding developmental events occur entirely prenatally in humans.

Taken together, the alterations observed throughout all regions of the murine reproductive tract demonstrate that exposure to estrogenic compounds during critical stages of sex differentiation results in adverse structural, functional, and long-term consequences. The long-term changes in these tissues include various lesions, some of which are neoplastic. The natural history and the mechanisms involved in the induction and progression of the lesions are critical issues for continued study.

In summary, developmentally DES-exposed mouse models, both prenatal and neonatal exposure, have provided some useful comparisons to similarly DES-exposed women (20). The finding of the extremely rare lesion, vaginal adenocarcinoma, in prenatally DES-exposed mice, in particular recommends the mouse model for the study of human disease. Continued investigation into the range of DES-induced abnormalities observed in the mouse model using prenatal and/or neonatal exposures will offer a better understanding of the developmental events and the mechanisms involved in the chemical disruption of reproductive tract differentiation and resulting toxicities.

2.5 LOW-DOSE EFFECTS

The concern of low-dose effects rises from the number of chemicals that potentially have endocrine-disrupting activity. Over 80,000 chemicals are currently registered for commercial use in the United States and an estimated 2000 new ones are introduced annually, so the potential for this number of substances to have an environmental impact is great. It is generally assumed that little risks exist because exposures are normally low and hormonal activity is weak, but the full extent of the effects of most of these chemicals is unknown and untested. Further, exposure occurs to multiple chemicals that may act additively or synergistically. Recognizing that the developing organism is uniquely sensitive to perturbation by chemicals with estrogenic and/or endocrine disrupting activity (7), we sought to determine if exposure to very low doses of these chemicals during critical stages of genital tract differentiation would permanently alter the developmental program of target tissues, so that they respond atypically to further stimuli at puberty. Although DES is a potent estrogenic compound, effects observed at very low doses can be used to predict potential adverse effects of weaker environmental estrogens (35–38).

Using the neonatal exposure model, pups were treated by subcutaneous injections of DES (0.0001 to 1,000 µg/kg, Sigma Chemical Co., St. Louis, Mo.) in corn oil or corn oil alone (Control) once per day on neonatal days 1–5. Mice were weaned at 17 days of age, housed 4/cage, and challenged with 3 daily subcutaneous doses of 17β-estradiol (Sigma, 500 µg/kg) or DES (Sigma, 10 µg/kg) on days 17 to 19. (These doses were previously determined to cause maximum uterine wet weight response in prepubescent mice (39)). On the fourth day, mice were sacrificed, and body and uterine weights were determined. Care was taken not to loose uterine luminal fluid.

Neonatal DES treatment resulted in altered uterine response to estrogen challenge in prepubescent mice (Table 2.2). Mice treated with low neonatal doses of .001 and .01 µg/kg and challenged with estrogen at puberty had increased body weights and elevated uterine wet weights relative to controls challenged with estrogen. In contrast, mice treated with (10 to 1000 µg/kg) neonatal doses had reduced uterine weights (Table 2.2) as we previously described following prenatal DES exposure (40). After adjusting for body weight differences by analysis of covariance (ANCOVA), uterine weight changes remained statistically significant ($p < 0.05$ by Dunnett's test) in the .01, 10, and 100 µg/kg groups. Challenge with DES or estradiol at equal estrogenic doses caused similar dose-response patterns.

In unchallenged mice, no significant effect of neonatal DES on uterine weight in any dose group was seen except for the high dose (1000 µg/kg) group, which was less than controls (.0045 ± .0003 g versus .0128 ± .0015 g, respectively).

To determine if fluid retention was solely responsible for altered uterine wet weight responses and to investigate potential mechanisms involved in the observed altered responses, uterine tissues were examined for morphological alterations and immunohistochemical localization of estrogen receptor (ER) α. (ER was evaluated but protein levels were extremely low in the uterus and difficult to detect any change with estrogen treatment). Tissue from unchallenged low dose (neonatal DES.01

TABLE 2.2
Summary of Uterine Wet Weight Responses in Prepubescent Mice Treated with DES During Neonatal Life

Neonatal DES Dose (μg/kg)	Challenge[a]	N	Body Weight (g)	Uterine Weight (g)	Adjusted Ut. Weight[b]
0	+	11	9.42 ± 0.53	0.077 ± 0.009	0.084 ± 0.009
0.0001	+	12	9.01 ± 0.40	0.064 ± 0.007	0.078 ± 0.006
0.001	+	12	11.25 ± 0.29*	0.103 ± 0.007*	0.083 ± 0.005
0.01	+	12	10.79 ± 0.38*	0.123 ± 0.008*	0.111 ± 0.005*
0.1	+	8	9.71 ± 0.21	0.084 ± 0.008	0.079 ± 0.004
1	+	8	9.96 ± 0.43	0.074 ± 0.005	0.066 ± 0.008
10	+	3	9.00 ± 0.46	0.030 ± 0.004*	0.030 ± 0.009*
100	+	4	9.02 ± 0.15	0.033 ± 0.005*	0.033 ± 0.003*
1,000	+	4	5.17 ± 0.21*	0.009 ± 0.001*	c
0	–	8	9.87 ± 0.35	0.0128 ± 0.0015	0.0120 ± 0.0014
0.0001	–	12	9.17 ± 0.50	0.0114 ± 0.0001	0.0123 ± 0.0014
0.001	–	12	9.98 ± 0.35	0.0128 ± 0.0014	0.0121 ± 0.0011
0.01	–	12	9.96 ± 0.23	0.0125 ± 0.0010	0.0119 ± 0.0009
0.1	–	8	9.25 ± 0.15	0.0092 ± 0.0003	0.0109 ± 0.0004
1	–	8	9.53 ± 0.20	0.0108 ± 0.0010	0.0120 ± 0.0005
10	–	4	9.60 ± 0.16	0.0082 ± 0.0003	0.0096 ± 0.0003
100	–	4	9.19 ± 0.21	0.0075 ± 0.0005	0.0096 ± 0.0004
1,000	–	4	6.64 ± 0.72	0.0045 ± 0.0003*	c

[a] Challenged at 17 days of age with 3 daily subcutaneous injections of DES (10 μg/kg); challenge with 17β-estradiol (500 μg/kg) gave similar results.
[b] Adjusted for body weight.
[c] Because of the marked reduction in body weight, this group was excluded from the ANCOVA.
* $p < 0.05$ vs. controls (Dunnett's test). Data are presented as mean ± S.E.

Data summarized from Newbold, et al. 2004.

μg/kg) group showed enhanced ERα immunoreactivity in all tissue compartments (luminal and glandular epithelium, and stroma, Table 2.3), whereas ERα immunoreactivity was similar or lower in the neonatal high dose (1000 μg/kg) group when compared the unchallenged controls (38). Pathological changes in the uterus of the high dose group showed pseudostratified luminal epithelium and disorganized epithelial, stromal, and smooth muscle compartments as reported following prenatal treatment with DES (31). These data showed that, not only was uterine wet weight altered, but both ERα levels and cellular localization within uterine tissue were also changed following developmental exposure to DES.

Another group of mice were treated neonatally with DES (.01 or 1000 μg/kg) or corn oil as controls and challenged just prior to puberty with a single dose of estrogen to provide additional support that levels of ERα were altered. Western blots verified that ERα was significantly higher (p <0.05) in the low-dose neonatal DES

TABLE 2.3
ERα, Lactoferrin, and c-fos Expression *in Uteri* from Prepubescent Mice Neonatally Exposed to DES

Treatment[a]	ERα Intensity[b]	LF Intensity[c]	c-fos Intensity[d]
Control	134.2 ± 16.7	119.27 ± 15.15	11.77 ± 4.33
DES 0.01	202.1 ± 4.1*	227.70 ± 3.95*	80.93 ± 5.85*
DES 1,000	164.3 ± 12.5	209.07 ± 4.99	38.03 ± 6.10

[a] Mice (4 per group) were exposed to DES at 0.01 and 1,000 μg/kg dissolved in corn oil or corn oil alone (Control) on days 1–5 of neonatal life.

[b] At 17 days of age, ERα levels were determined in the uteri of unchallenged mice (n = 4).

[c] At 17 days of age, LF levels were determined in the uteri of mice (n = 4) that were challenged with a single injection of estrogen and collected 18 hrs. later.

[d] At 17 days of age, c-fos levels were determined in the uteri of mice (n = 4) that were challenged with a single injection of estrogen and collected 18 hrs. later.

Intensity of each endpoint was quantitated by image analysis software (Image Pro). The intensity scale is from 0 (not detectable) to 250 (most intense).

* $p < 0.05$ vs. controls (Dunnett's test). Data are presented as mean ± S.E.

Data summarized from Newbold, et al. 2004.

group as compared to controls; the slight increase in ERα intensity in the high-dose group was not significant (Table 2.3), but histological examination of the high dose group showed altered cellular phenotypes in uterine tissues. Since ER levels in estrogen target tissues are set during differentiation and development, change in these levels caused by xenoestrogen exposure could be expected to alter subsequent ER-associated response pathways. Therefore, we evaluated several ER-mediated responses.

Using proliferating nuclear antigen (PCNA) labeling of the tissue sections as a marker of cell proliferation, the low dose DES (.01μg/kg) had a higher uterine epithelial labeling index as compared to controls (49.6 ± 2.3 versus 21.2 ± 1.1). Further, RPA of uterine tissues (10 μg total RNA per sample) from mice treated neonatally with DES showed an increase in ER- mediated responses such as lactoferrin (LF), an estrogen-inducible mRNA in the uterus (41), compared to controls; c-fos was also increased in the low dose DES group but not in control and high DES groups. Quantitation of LF and c-fos intensity by image analysis is shown in Table 2.3. These ER-associated responses are consistent with high levels of ER in the low-dose group and lower levels in the high-dose groups.

To determine if these effects were permanent, an additional group of mice were treated with neonatal DES (0.001 to 10 μg/kg) and housed until 4 to 5 months of age. These adult mice were ovariectomized and challenged 7 days later as described for the prepubescent mice. A similar pattern of response (enhanced uterine wet weight response at the low dose of .01 μg/kg and dampened response at the high dose of 10 μg/kg) was seen. The similarities of response between prepubertal and adult animals show that uterine responses are permanently altered by developmental exposure to estrogens.

These data show that exposure to DES during critical stages of development can permanently imprint the uterus to respond abnormally to estrogen at puberty and later in life. One mechanism responsible for the abnormal uterine response involves increased levels of ERα prior to challenge after low dose exposure to neonatal DES (.01 μg/kg), and ER-mediated morphological and biochemical responses including induction of c-fos, PCNA, and LF after challenge; at high doses, the altered response involved pathological changes in the uterine tissue as evidenced by the data showing reduced uterine weight with the neonatal 1000 μg/kg dose, but little difference in ERα, LF, and c-fos in this group when compared with controls. It is quite possible other endocrine-disrupting chemicals may have similar effects and that other differentiating tissues can be similarly imprinted. Further, this alteration may occur at very low levels of exposure, doses to which people are typically exposed. We are in the process of testing other environmental estrogens for altered uterine responses at puberty.

The evidence of biological effects at low doses was confirmed by this study and supports the conclusions summarized in the NTP Report of the Low Dose Review (42, 43) that low dose effects are indeed possible. The significance of this data to human health is uncertain and requires more study. However, toxicological studies using experimental animal models have established an increased prevalence of reproductive tract neoplasia with developmental exposure to low doses of environmental estrogens (31), and an association of elevated ER levels with the development of uterine neoplasia later in life (44).

2.6 MECHANISMS OF REPRODUCTIVE TOXICITY

Numerous studies have demonstrated that developmental exposure to DES interferes with the normal differentiation of the Müllerian duct and the regression of the Wolffian duct. Although the mechanisms are not completely understood, a molecular component in the malformation of the tissues and perhaps in the cellular changes may be responsible. Studies discussed earlier suggest a molecular mechanism responsible for the structural alterations observed in oviduct, uterus, cervix, and vagina (27, 28). Cellular changes may also be closely linked to these structural alterations. Furthermore, permanent abnormal gene imprinting has been described (28) in which neonatal exposure to DES causes demethylation of an estrogen-responsive gene in the mouse uterus. The relationship of this finding to tumor induction is continuing to be investigated.

The role of the estrogen receptor in the induction of abnormalities and tumors following developmental exposure to DES, has also been studied by using transgenic mice which overexpress ER (MT-mER). Transgenic ER mice were treated with DES during neonatal life and followed as they aged. It was hypothesized that because of the abnormal expression of the ER, the reproductive tract tissues of the MT-mER mice may be more susceptible to tumors after neonatal exposure to DES. In fact, it is interesting to note that mice overexpressing the ER were at a higher risk of developing abnormalities, including uterine adenocarcinoma in response to neonatal DES when compared with DES-treated wild type mice; at 8 months, 73% of the DES-treated MT-mER mice compared to 46% of the DES-treated wild type mice had uterine adenocarcinoma. Further, these abnormalities occurred at an earlier age as compared to wild type DES mice (44). The transgenic mouse studies suggest that the level of ER present in a tissue may be a determining factor in the development of estrogen-related tumors. The specific role in the induction and progression of the lesions requires additional study. Additional transgenic mouse models that express variant forms of the ER or the ER knockout, as well as experimental models constructed with the new ERβ, will also aide in determining the role of the ER in the development of these reproductive lesions. Since various estrogenic compounds have been reported to bind preferentially to either ERα or ERβ, these models will be essential in extrapolating human health risks to environmental estrogen exposures.

2.7 SUMMARY AND CONCLUSION

Sufficient evidence has been accumulated through the years by many laboratories to show that exposure of the developing fetus to exogenous estrogens adversely affects the differentiation of the genital tract. Data demonstrate that reproductive tract structure and function are altered, and long-term changes occur including both benign and malignant cellular abnormalities. Cellular changes were seen in aged DES-exposed females at all doses examined; the degree of severity of specific lesions was dose related. Although fertility was decreased in mice in a dose-dependent manner after developmental estrogen exposure at all doses tested, a decrease in fertility was observed in low dose estrogen-exposed animals only later in life. These data suggest that fertility may not be a sensitive marker of reproductive toxicants in mice exposed to low levels of endocrine disrupters until they age. Similarly, male offspring exposed developmentally to low doses of DES did not show altered fertility early in life but were still susceptible to increased reproductive tract tumors later in life (16). In combination, these data suggest that estrogenic substances occurring in the environment at low levels may adversely effect fertility later in life, but of further concern, they may have additional long-term consequences, including increases in benign and malignant lesions that warrant attention. The DES animal model provides the opportunity to further study this possibility.

While animal studies must be considered carefully if extrapolation to humans is to follow, the DES-exposed mouse model has provided some interesting comparisons to similarly exposed humans. The model has duplicated and predicted many of the lesions observed in DES-exposed women. Although DES is a potent estrogen, it continues to provide markers of the adverse effects of exposure to estrogenic and other endocrine-disrupting substances during development, whether these exposures come from naturally occurring chemicals, synthetic, or environmental contaminants, or from pharmaceutical agents. Although chemicals not associated with hormone-mimicking activity may be involved indirectly or directly in reproductive tract toxicities, by far, the most common culprits are those substances demonstrating endocrine-modulating effects. Furthermore, mature animals may experience adverse effects to these chemicals, but the developing organism is particularly sensitive to perturbation by these compounds and often experience permanent long-lasting consequences. Ongoing mechanistic studies will help identify potential female reproductive toxicants and will help better access the risks of exposure to endocrine-disrupting chemicals in the environment if chemical exposures occur during critical stages of development.

ACKNOWLEDGMENTS

The authors are greatly indebted to Elizabeth Padilla-Burgos for skillful technical expertise in the conduct of the DES experiments in the preparation of this paper. Also, the authors wish to thank Dr. Bill Bullock, Wake Forest University School of Medicine, for his diagnosis in pathology over the years.

REFERENCES

1. Colborn, T. and Clement, C. Chemically-Induced Alterations in Sexual and Functional Development: The Wildlife/Human Connection. Princeton, NJ: Princeton Scientific, 1992.
2. Colborn, T., vom Saal, F. S., and Soto, A. M. Developmental effects of endocrine-disrupting chemicals in wildlife and humans. *Environ. Health Perspect.*, 101: 378–384, 1993.
3. Colborn, T., Dumanski, D., and Myers, J. P. Our Stolen Future. New York: Penguin Books, Inc., 1996.
4. McLachlan, J. A. Estrogens in the Environment. New York: Elsevier Science Publishing Co., 1985.
5. McLachlan, J. A. Functional toxicology: a new approach to detect biologically active xenobiotics. *Environ. Health Perspect.*, 101: 386–387, 1993.
6. George, F. W. and Wilson, J. D. Sex determination and differentiation. In: E. Knobil, J. D. Neil, L. L. Ewing, G. S. Greenwald, C. L. Markert, and D. W. Pfaff (eds.), The Physiology of Reproduction, pp. 3–26. New York Raven Press, 1988.
7. Bern, H. The Fragile Fetus. In: T. Colborn and C. Clement (eds.), Chemically-Induced Alterations in Sexual and Functioal Development: The Wildlife/Human Connection. Princeton, NJ: Princeton Scientific Publishing Co., 1992.
8. Brawer, J. R., Naftolin, F., Martin, J., and Sonnenschein, C. Effects of a single injection of estradiol valerate on the hypothalamic arcuate nucleus and on reproductive function in the female rat. *Endocrinology*, 103: 501–512, 1978.
9. Adler, A. J. and Nelson, J. F. Aging and chronic estradiol exposure impair estradiol-induced cornification but not proliferation of vaginal epithelium in C57BL/6J mice. *Biol. Reprod.*, 38: 175–182, 1988.
10. Gluckman, P. D. Intrauterine growth retardation: future research directions. *Acta Paediatr. Suppl.*, 388: 96–99, 1993.
11. Barker, D. J., Eriksson, J. G., Forsen, T., and Osmond, C. Fetal origins of adult disease: strength of effects and biological basis. *Int. J. Epidemiol.*, 31: 1235–1239, 2002.

12. Herbst, A. L. and Bern, H. A. Developmental Effects of Diethylstilbestrol (DES) in Pregnancy. New York: Thieme-Stratton, 1981.

13. Newbold, R. R. and McLachlan, J. A. Transplacental hormonal carcinogenesis: diethylstilbestrol as an example. In: J. Huff, J. Boyd, and J. C. Barrett (eds.), Cellular and Molecular Mechanisms of Hormonal Carcinogenesis: Environmental Influences, pp. 131–147. New York: Wiley-Liss, 1996.

14. Turusov, V. S., Trukhanova, L. S., Parfenov Yu, D., and Tomatis, L. Occurrence of tumours in the descendants of CBA male mice prenatally treated with diethylstilbestrol. *Int. J. Cancer*, 50: 131–135, 1992.

15. Walker, B. E. and Haven, M. I. Intensity of multigenerational carcinogenesis from diethylstilbestrol in mice. *Carcinogenesis*, 18: 791–793, 1997.

16. Newbold, R. R., Hanson, R. B., Jefferson, W. N., Bullock, B. C., Haseman, J., and McLachlan, J. A. Proliferative lesions and reproductive tract tumors in male descendants of mice exposed developmentally to diethylstilbestrol. *Carcinogenesis*, 21: 1355–1363, 2000.

17. Newbold, R. R., Hanson, R. B., Jefferson, W. N., Bullock, B. C., Haseman, J., and McLachlan, J. A. Increased tumors but uncompromised fertility in the female descendants of mice exposed developmentally to diethylstilbestrol. *Carcinogenesis*, 19: 1655–1663, 1998.

18. Tuchmann-Duplessis, H. and Haegel, P. Illustrated Human Embryology. New York: Springer Verlag, 1982.

19. Newbold, R. R. and McLachlan, J. A. Diethylstilbestrol associated defects in murine genital tract development. In: J. A. McLachlan (ed.), Estrogens in the Environment II: Influences in Development, pp. 288–318. New York: Elsevier, 1985.

20. Newbold, R. Cellular and molecular effects of developmental exposure to diethylstilbestrol: implications for other environmental estrogens. *Environ. Health Perspect.*, 103 Suppl 7: 83–87, 1995.

21. McLachlan, J. A., Newbold, R. R., Shah, H. C., Hogan, M. D., and Dixon, R. L. Reduced fertility in female mice exposed transplacentally to diethylstilbestrol (DES). *Fertil. Steril.*, 38: 364–371, 1982.

22. Newbold, R. R., Bullock, B. C., and Mc Lachlan, J. A. Exposure to diethylstilbestrol during pregnancy permanently alters the ovary and oviduct. *Biol. Reprod.*, 28: 735–744, 1983.

23. Haney, A. F., Newbold, R. R., and McLachlan, J. A. Prenatal diethylstilbestrol exposure in the mouse: effects on ovarian histology and steroidogenesis *in vitro*. *Biol Reprod.*, 30: 471–478, 1984.

24. Davis, B. and Newbold, R. R. Ovarian toxicology. In: P. W. Harvey, K. Rush, and A. Cockburn (eds.), Endocrine and Hormonal Toxicology, pp. 111–124. New York: John Wiley and Sons, 1999.

25. Newbold, R. R., Tyrey, S., Haney, A. F., and McLachlan, J. A. Developmentally arrested oviduct: a structural and functional defect in mice following prenatal exposure to diethylstilbestrol. *Teratology*, 27: 417–426, 1983.

26. DeCherney, A. H., Cholst, I., and Naftolin, F. Structure and function of the fallopian tubes following exposure to diethylstilbestrol (DES) during gestation. *Fertil. Steril.*, 36: 741–745, 1981.

27. Ma, L., Benson, G. V., Lim, H., Dey, S. K., and Maas, R. L. Abdominal B (AbdB) Hoxa genes: regulation in adult uterus by estrogen and progesterone and repression in mullerian duct by the synthetic estrogen diethylstilbestrol (DES). *Dev. Biol.*, 197: 141–154, 1998.

28. Li, S., Ma, L., Chiang, T., Burow, M., Newbold, R. R., Negishi, M., Barrett, J. C., and McLachlan, J. A. Promoter CpG methylation of Hox-a10 and Hox-a11 in mouse uterus not altered upon neonatal diethylstilbestrol exposure. *Mol. Carcinog.*, 32: 213–219, 2001.

29. Newbold, R. R., Bullock, B. C., and McLachlan, J. A. Diverticulosis and salpingitis isthmica nodosa (SIN) of the fallopian tube. Estrogen-induced diverticulosis and SIN of the mouse oviduct. *Am. J. Pathol.*, 117: 333–335, 1984.

30. Shen, S. C., Bansal, M., Purrazzella, R., Malviya, V., and Strauss, L. Benign glandular inclusions in lymph nodes, endosalpingiosis, and salpingitis isthmica nodosa in a young girl with clear cell adenocarcinoma of the cervix. *Am. J. Surg. Pathol.*, 7: 293–300, 1983.

31. McLachlan, J. A., Newbold, R. R., and Bullock, B. C. Long-term effects on the female mouse genital tract associated with prenatal exposure to diethylstilbestrol. Cancer Research, 40: 3988–3999, 1980.

32. Newbold, R. R., Moore, A. B., and Dixon, D. Characterization of uterine leiomyomas in CD-1 mice following developmental exposure to diethylstilbestrol (DES). *Toxicol. Pathol.*, 30: 611–616, 2002.

33. Baird, D. and Newbold, R. Increased incidence of leiomyomas in DES exposed women. Environ. Health Perspect., submitted.

34. Newbold, R. R. and McLachlan, J. A. Vaginal adenosis and adenocarcinoma in mice exposed prenatally or neonatally to diethylstilbestrol. *Cancer Res.*, 42: 2003–2011, 1982.

35. Sheehan, D. M. and vom Saal, F. S. Low dose effects of endocrine disruptors — a challenge for risk assessment. Risk Policy Report, September 19, 1997.

36. vom Saal, F. S., Timms, B. G., Montano, M. M., Palanza, P., Thayer, K. A., Nagel, S. C., Dhar, M. D., Ganjam, V. K., Parmigiani, S., and Welshons, W. V. Prostate enlargement in mice due to fetal exposure to low doses of estradiol or diethylstilbestrol and opposite effects at high doses. *Proc. Natl. Acad. Sci. USA*, 94: 2056–2061, 1997.

37. Welshons, W. V., Nagel, S. C., Thayer, K. A., Judy, B. M., and vom Saal, F. S. Low-dose bioactivity of xenoestrogens in animals: fetal exposure to low doses of methoxychlor and other xenoestrogens increases adult prostate size in mice. *Toxicol. Ind. Health*, 15: 12–25, 1999.

38. Newbold, R., Jefferson, W. N., Padilla-Banks, E., and Haseman, J. Developmental exposure to diethylstilbestrol (DES) alters uterine response to estrogens in prepubescent mice: low verses high dose effects. Reproductive Toxicology, 2004.

39. Padilla-Banks, E., Jefferson, W. N., and Newbold, R. R. The immature mouse is a suitable model for detection of estrogenicity in the uterotropic bioassay. *Environ. Health Perspect.*, 109: 821–826, 2001.

40. Maier, D. B., Newbold, R. R., and McLachlan, J. A. Prenatal diethystilbestrol exposure alters murine uterine responses to prepubertal estrogen stimulation. *Endocrinology*, 116: 1878–1886, 1985.

41. Jefferson, W. N., Padilla-Banks, E., and Newbold, R. R. Lactoferrin is an estrogen responsive protein in the uterus of mice and rats. *Reprod. Toxicol.*, 14: 103–110, 2000.

42. National Toxicology Program's Report of the Endocrine Disruptors Low-Dose Peer Review. Research Triangle Park: National Toxicology Program, Department of Health and Human Services, 2001.

43. Melnick, R., Lucier, G., Wolfe, M., Hall, R., Stancel, G., Prins, G., Gallo, M., Reuhl, K., Ho, S., Brown, T., Moore, J., Leaky, J., Haseman, J., and Kohn, M. Summary of the National Toxicology Program's Report of the Endocrine Disruptors Low Dose Peer Review. *Environ. Health Perspect.*, 110: 427–431, 2002.

44. Couse, J. F., Davis, V. L., Hanson, R. B., Jefferson, W. N., McLachlan, J. A., Bullock, B. C., Newbold, R. R., and Korach, K. S. Accelerated onset of uterine tumors in transgenic mice with aberrant expression of the estrogen receptor after neonatal exposure to diethylstilbestrol. *Mol. Carcinog.*, 19: 236–242, 1997.

3 Ovotoxic Environmental Chemicals: Indirect Endocrine Disruptors

Patrick J. Devine, Ph.D. and
Patricia B. Hoyer, Ph.D.

CONTENTS

3.1 INTRODUCTION

Reproductive function in women can be compromised by exposure to toxic chemicals.[1] Couples are postponing the start of a family because of the increasing number of women pursuing a career. These recent trends have enhanced an awareness of chemicals in the workplace and the environment, and their impact on the life span of reproductive function. A variety of considerations can affect fertility in women who are older when beginning a family, and women with fertility problems may not discover them until their reproductive life span is waning. In addition to a generally reduced quality of oocytes with age,[2] more years of exposure to environmental influences can also have a potential effect. In considering the risk of environmental exposures on reproductive function and women's health, special attention should be paid to those chemicals with the potential to impair ovarian function, because the ovary is critical to normal reproduction.

The ovary performs two important roles, development and delivery of the female gamete (oocyte), and production of ovarian hormones such as inhibin and the female sex steroids, estrogen and progesterone.[3,4] Whereas the oocyte is required for fertilization, ovarian hormone output is required for oocyte development, feedback signaling to the hypothalamus and pituitary, and establishment and early maintenance of pregnancy.

Reproductive toxicants can affect ovarian function in a variety of ways. Indirect effects on ovarian function might result from altered pituitary output of gonadotropins (follicle-stimulating hormone, FSH, and luteinizing hormone, LH). Such alterations could be caused by chemicals that disrupt neuroendocrine feedback by estrogen and progesterone. Alternatively, reproductive toxicants can have direct ovarian effects on steroid hormone production. The estrogens are responsible for oocyte development, whereas progesterone is required for implantation and early maintenance of pregnancy. Therefore, xenobiotic exposure that alters ovarian steroid hormone production or metabolism could affect oocyte development and ovulation, as well as neuroendocrine feedback, reproductive tract function, and pregnancy. By a different route, reproductive toxicants can disrupt ovarian function through destruction of oocytes. Extensive destruction of oocytes depletes the ovary of follicles, which also eliminates steroid hormone production. The ultimate result of complete follicular destruction in a woman is ovarian failure (menopause). Following ovarian failure, steroid hormone production (especially estradiol) becomes greatly reduced, neuroendocrine feedback is disrupted, and circulating levels of gonadotropins rise. Therefore, oocyte destruction ultimately disrupts endocrine balance by causing a reduction in estrogen and progesterone, and an elevation in FSH and LH.

In summary, endocrine disruption can be caused by reproductive toxicants via direct alterations in steroid hormone production (ovary) or by interference with steroid hormone action (hypothalamus, pituitary, reproductive tract). Alternatively, endocrine disruption can be indirect, resulting from ovarian failure caused by extensive oocyte destruction. Early reproductive failure in women has been linked to increased risks of arthritis, urinary tract infections, osteoporosis, [5,6] cardiovascular disease,[7] depression,[8] and Alzheimer's disease.[9,10] There is also a known increase in the incidence of ovarian cancer.[11] This observation has been well supported in animal studies.[12] Therefore, loss of reproductive potential can have a severe health impact. Thus, in addition to reduced fertility resulting from ovotoxicity in females, there are long-term health risks associated with premature ovarian failure (early menopause). Because of these health risks, the subject of this chapter is chemicals that destroy ovarian follicles.

3.2 OVARIAN FUNCTION

3.2.1 FOLLICULAR DEVELOPMENT

One of the primary functions of the ovary is to provide mature oocytes for successful reproduction. Development and maturation of oocytes occurs within ovarian follicles. Immediately following formation during fetal development, follicles enter the most immature stage of development, termed primordial. Successful ovulation requires appropriate follicular development, during which the follicle has passed through a number of distinct developmental stages.[4] Primordial follicles provide the pool for recruitment of developing follicles; therefore, they are the fundamental reproductive unit within the ovary.

3.2.1.1 Prenatal Development

During fetal development, primordial germ cells (oogonia) that are formed invade the indifferent gonad and undergo rapid hyperplasia. Oogonia become oocytes, once they stop dividing and become arrested at the diplotene stage (prophase) of the first meiotic division. The oocyte does not commence meiosis again unless triggered to ovulate, should that occur. As a result, the lifetime supply of oocytes is set at the time of birth. Around the time of birth, individual oocytes within the ovary become surrounded by a single layer of flattened somatic cells (pre-granulosa cells) and a basement membrane to form primordial follicles.[4] Association of the granulosa cells with the oocyte is critical at all subsequent times for maintenance of viability, and follicle growth and development.[13]

3.2.1.2 Follicular Development in Adults

3.2.1.2.1 Primordial Follicles

In humans, 1 to 2 pre-ovulatory follicles develop approximately every 28 days, whereas in rats 6 to 12 follicles develop every 4 to 5 days.[3] Primordial follicles form the pool from which these follicles develop. Throughout the reproductive life span, the total number of primordial follicles that become ovulated is small compared to the total population. Instead, the vast majority of follicles are lost to attrition in various early stages of development by a process called atresia. The exact determinant for selection of a follicle for ovulation is not understood, but is believed to be under intra-ovarian control.[3]

3.2.1.2.2 Primary Follicles

The first sign of oocyte growth in primordial follicles is alteration of surrounding squamous (flattened) granulosa cells into cuboidal shaped cells, followed by initiation of proliferation of these cells.[4] Once a follicle makes the transition from primordial to primary, other structural changes occur such as development of the zona pellucida, a protective glycoprotein matrix.[3,4] At this stage, another layer of specialized somatic cells begin to proliferate outside the basement membrane enclosing the oocyte and granulosa cell layer, designated theca interna cells. Theca cells provide two important functions: (1) attachment of arterioles for the development of an independent blood supply, and (2) secretion of the steroid progestin and androgen hormones to regulate follicle development.[4]

3.2.1.2.3 Large Pre-antral Follicles

As follicles continue to develop, the layers of granulosa cells surrounding the oocyte increase rapidly to become large pre-antral, growing follicles, with diameters 250 µm. The somatic cells acquire receptors for follicle-stimulating hormone to enhance follicle growth, and develop steroidogenic capacity for synthesis of androgens, estrogens, and progesterone.

3.2.1.2.4 Antral Follicles

The number of follicles that reach the final stage of development is quite small compared to those that began development from the primordial pool. In women, only one follicle per menstrual cycle is usually chosen as the dominant follicle destined for ovulation. As the follicle develops beyond the pre-antral stage, it acquires a fluid-filled cavity, antrum, formed by separations within the granulosa cell layers. During the final period of development, a pre-ovulatory follicle becomes more sensitive to the gonadotropins FSH and LH than were smaller antral and preantral follicles.[3] Theca cells within the follicle contain receptors for LH, and respond to hormonal input with synthesis and secretion of androgens. Conversely, granulosa cells contain receptors for FSH and respond to hormonal input with expression of the enzyme aromatase. In this capacity, granulosa cells can directly convert the androgens secreted by theca cells to estrogens. Prior to ovulation, granulosa cells also begin to express receptors for LH in readiness for receiving a signal from the LH surge as a trigger for ovulation and luteinization.[4] Prior to ovulation and after the LH surge, the oocyte will be signaled to continue meiotic progression through to the second meiotic division. The second meiotic division is only completed if fertilization of the oocyte occurs.

3.2.2 FOLLICULAR ATRESIA

The number of oocytes present in ovaries is dynamic and varies with age. The total number of oocytes peaks during embryonic development. In humans, that number, about 7 million, occurs at five months gestation; at birth the number has dropped to 2 million, 250,000 to 400,000 at puberty, and none remain at menopause.[4,14] During the lifetime of a woman, ovulation only accounts for 400 to 600 oocytes. Therefore, the others have been lost at various stages of development by the process of atresia. Thus, atresia is the natural fate of the vast majority of ovarian follicles (> 99%), since only a select few follicles that develop will ever be ovulated.[4]

3.2.2.1 Apoptosis as Atresia

The ultimate event associated with follicular atresia is the mechanism of physiological cell death, apoptosis.[15] Apoptosis is used by many tissues to delete unwanted cells.[16,17] In distinct contrast to apoptosis, cell death by necrosis is a passive form of cell death that usually occurs in response to injury and elicits an inflammatory response in the surrounding tissue. The ultimate decisive features used to distinguish between apoptosis and necrosis are based upon morphological characteristics.[16] The earliest definitive changes of a cell undergoing apoptosis is compaction of chromatin into dense masses (margination) along the nuclear membrane, condensation of the cytoplasm, and reduction in nuclear size, retained membrane integrity of cytoplasmic organelles. As the process continues, multiple apoptotic bodies (membrane-enclosed structures containing both nuclear and cytoplasmic components) separate from the dying cell, which are quickly phagocytosed by healthy neighboring cells. Contrary to this, necrosis involves organelle and cytoplasmic swelling caused by a destruction of plasma membrane integrity, followed by release of lysosomal enzymes that accelerate membrane disintegration and damage to surrounding cells.

Apoptosis and necrosis can also be distinguished by certain biochemical features. Apoptosis often depends on ligand-receptor interactions (e.g., Fas/Fas ligand) and is an active, energy-requiring process. Triggering of apoptosis leads to altered localization of bcl-2 family members or activation of certain Caspases (Caspase 2, 3, 8, and 9), which in turn activate proteolytic and DNA-degrading enzymes.[18] Through studies involving gene-deficient mice, some genes such as Bax and Bcl-2 have been shown to influence follicle numbers by altering apoptosis.[19] In most cell types, genomic DNA is degraded in a specific internucleosomal pattern to produce low molecular weight fragments (180 base pairs) that appear as a characteristic "ladder" formation on agarose gels.[17] However, this pattern of DNA fragmentation is not observed in all cells undergoing apoptosis, including granulosa cells from immature (small pre-antral) ovarian follicles, in which DNA is degraded in a non-specific, random pattern.[20] This is because these cells do not express the specific endonuclease necessary to produce the normal pattern of DNA laddering in rats.[21] Thus, morphological evaluation remains the most reliable distinction between apoptotic and necrotic mechanisms of cell death.[22]

3.2.3 MENOPAUSE

Depletion of functional primordial follicles from the ovary is the underlying cause of ovarian failure (menopause), because this dormant follicle pool represents the cohort for recruitment of all developing follicles. Absence of primordial follicles ultimately leads to the complete loss of follicles of all sizes. As a result, estrogen-producing (granulosa) cells in pre-ovulatory follicles also become depleted. Besides the loss of fertility, menopause has been associated with a variety of health problems in women, as previously mentioned. It is felt that these adverse health risks are the result of loss of estrogen. Thus, identifying and protecting against environmental or occupational exposures that may induce menopause earlier in women becomes even more critical.

3.3 IMPACT OF XENOBIOTIC-INDUCED DAMAGE ON OVARIAN FUNCTION

Multiple aspects of specific chemical exposures determine overall effects on female reproduction. These include the level and duration of exposure, the metabolic capacity of the ovary and other tissues to activate or detoxify the chemical, and the age or reproductive status of the individual exposed. Together, these variables greatly influence whether or not a chemical has detrimental effects on ovarian function.

The level of exposure to an environmental chemical required to produce ovarian damage is of particular importance. It is under rare, accidental circumstances that individuals are acutely exposed to toxic levels of reproductive toxicants, and the effects of these exposures can usually be detected and evaluated. However, the possible effects of chronic exposure to low levels of reproductive toxicants are more difficult to determine. Biochemical markers for detecting ovarian damage are lacking. Therefore, fertility problems caused by low levels of ongoing environmental exposures may go unrecognized for years. Extensive loss of primordial follicles has the potential for causing early menopause or, still later, development of ovarian cancer. Because of the insidious nature of primordial follicle loss, low-level exposures can cause 'silent' damage and are of the most concern. As an example of this, mice treated with a single dose of cyclophosphamide (CPA) that causes depletion of approximately 50% of primordial follicles remain reproductively fertile.[23] Thus, extensive damage of this follicle population has not yet caused physiological signaling of the onset of premature ovarian failure that will likely ensue.

Another factor related to the effect of exposure of a woman to a reproductive toxicant is the developmental stage in her reproductive life span at the time of exposure (Figure 3.1). Chemical-induced destruction of some or all germ cells during fetal development, childhood, or adult years can lead to sterility or reduced reproductive years. Temporary infertility may be manifest in the adult cyclic woman, whereas exposure during childhood can delay or accelerate puberty. During

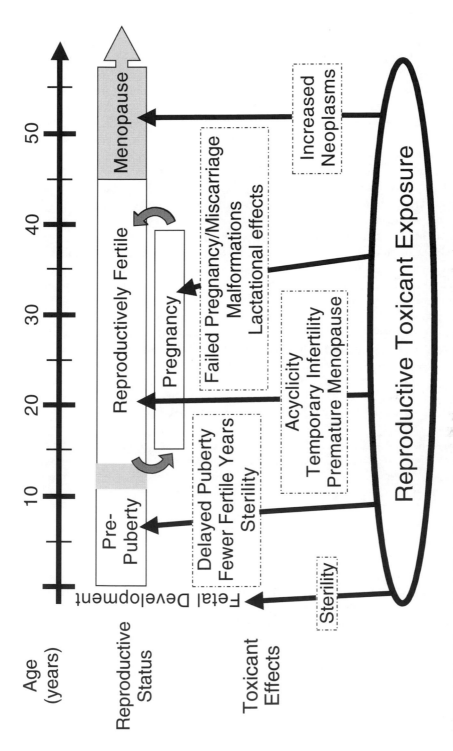

FIGURE 3.1 Potential age-related effects of reproductive toxicants in females. The impact(s) of reproductive toxicants are partially dependent upon the age or reproductive status of the exposed individual. In most cases, direct ovarian toxicity can lead to premature ovarian failure and infertility (menopause).

pregnancy, xenobiotic exposures can cause detrimental effects, such as miscarriages or failed pregnancies, resulting from ovarian effects.

For chemicals that destroy oocytes, the stage of development at which the follicle is destroyed determines the impact that exposure to the chemical will have on reproduction. Chemicals which selectively damage large growing or antral follicles only temporarily interrupt reproductive function because these follicles can be replaced by recruitment from the greater pool of primordial follicles if exposure ceases. Thus, these chemicals produce acyclicity (amenorrhea in women), a readily reversible form of infertility that is manifest relatively soon after exposure.[24–26] Conversely, chemicals that extensively destroy oocytes contained in primordial and primary follicles can cause permanent infertility and premature ovarian failure (early menopause in women) since once a primordial follicle is destroyed, it cannot be replaced. Destruction of oocytes contained in primordial follicles may have a delayed effect on reproduction until such a time that recruitment for the number of growing and antral follicles can no longer be supported.[24, 27]

Although direct destruction of ovarian follicles may not immediately alter circulating hormone levels, the loss of ovarian hormone regulation results in eventual disruption of negative feedback at the level of the hypothalamus and pituitary. Follicle-stimulating hormone, produced in the anterior pituitary, regulates follicular development and is under a negative feedback regulation of release by ovarian hormones, such as estrogen, progesterone, and inhibin.[28] The mechanism by which chemicals are ovotoxic could be to disrupt this feedback loop of endocrine regulation, directly altering the system at the level of the hypothalamus or pituitary. Conversely, a primary effect at the ovarian level might cause a later disruption of this regulatory axis. In the latter case, ovarian failure would produce rather than result from changes in circulating FSH levels, and FSH levels would increase due to loss of negative feedback from ovarian hormones.

Such increases in circulating FSH levels have been observed in long-term studies in both female mice and rats treated with the occupational chemicals, 4-vinylcyclo-hexene (VCH) and its ovotoxic metabolite, 4-vinylcyclohexene diepoxide, respectively, for 30 days (age 28 to 58 days) and then observed for up to 1 year.[27,29] In spite of a selective loss of the majority of primordial and primary follicles measured by 30 days, FSH levels were only increased above control animals at 240 days in mice and 120 days in rats. This corresponded with a time point at which numbers of antral follicles were significantly decreased in the rat.[29] Therefore, ovarian changes preceded the rise in circulating FSH levels. In spite of such ovarian damage, vaginal cytology still displayed evidence of ovarian cyclicity in VCH-treated mice at 240 days. By 360 days (from the onset of 30 days of dosing), unlike control animals, treated animals of both species displayed complete ovarian failure, as determined by increased circulating levels of FSH, loss of estrous cyclicity, the complete absence of ovarian follicular or luteal structures, and marked ovarian atrophy. Furthermore, at 360 days there was histological evidence of pre-neoplastic changes in ovaries of treated mice. From these studies, it was concluded that the ovarian failure and pre-neoplastic changes that occur long after cessation of chemical exposure are indirect consequences resulting from the depletion of small, pre-antral follicles.

3.4 EFFECTS OF SPECIFIC OVOTOXIC CHEMICALS

3.4.1 PRE-ANTRAL FOLLICLE DAMAGE

Destruction of oocytes contained in ovarian primordial follicles can be caused by a variety of environmental chemicals.[12] Exposures that extensively destroy primordial and primary follicles can cause irreversible infertility (premature menopause in women), since once destroyed, they cannot be replaced. Furthermore, destruction of primordial follicles will have a delayed effect on cyclicity that is undetected until there are no follicles left to be recruited for development.[24,27]

3.4.1.1 Ionizing Radiation

Radiation therapy is one of the most common human exposures with a high potential to destroy germ cells. This type of therapy is designed to be toxic to rapidly dividing cells, specifically cancerous cells, but target specificity remains relatively poor. Thus, permanent infertility has become a common side-effect of these treatments in patients.[30] Exposure to irradiation is known to produce rapid destruction of oocytes contained in primordial follicles, followed by increased follicular atresia, stromal hypertrophy, and loss of ovarian weight.[31] These effects are suspected in humans because of reports of amenorrhea and sterility in women undergoing therapeutic irradiation.[32,33] The age of patients greatly influences their sensitivity to radiation, with younger women appearing more resistant to ovarian toxicity. In animal studies, Mattison and Schulman[14] noted that prenatal exposure to ionizing radiation also affects the number of oocytes and reproductive capacity of female offspring. Unlike oocytes in young women, rapidly dividing primordial germ cells and oogonia present during fetal development in all species are highly sensitive to destruction by ionizing radiation.[31]

3.4.1.2 Chemotherapeutic Agents

Roughly 25 females per 1000 will develop some type of cancer before the age of 35 (Statistics Canada), and approximately 1 in 1000 adults are survivors of childhood cancers.[34] Concerns over side-effects of chemotherapy have increased as survival rates of cancer patients improve (currently ~56% overall survival rate[30]). Since antineoplastic therapy was first used to treat various malignancies, the ability of these agents to produce ovarian failure has been documented. Effects of chemotherapeutic exposures on reproductive function in patients are primarily a concern for those under the age of 40 who may wish to have children; however, undergoing early reproductive failure also increases the risks for developing other diseases. In addition to chemotherapy for cancer, alkylating agents such as cyclophosphamide are also used in treatments of autoimmune disorders. Thus, significant numbers of people are exposed to these agents. Nitrogen mustard, chlorambucil, and vinblastine have all been reported to cause sterility in women.[32,33,35] CPA has also been shown to cause premature ovarian failure and secondary tumors in women.[36,37] The induction of permanent infertility following chemotherapy is thought to depend predominantly on the type of treatment and on the age of the patient,[38] with estimated frequencies of reproductive failure varying widely (20 to 60%). Children exposed to chemotherapy prior to puberty are less likely to become permanently infertile than adults.[39] Yet, retention of ovarian function does not mean ovarian damage did not occur, and premature menopause is still a possibility.

These observed effects in humans have motivated a variety of studies in rodents to better elucidate chemotherapeutic-induced ovotoxicity, predominantly using CPA. Mice treated with low levels of CPA for 1 year demonstrated specific ovarian toxicity, including acyclicity, reduced numbers of oocytes (especially primordial), and corpora lutea, and developed cysts/tumors in the ovarian germinal epithelium.[40] In multiple short-term studies involving rats and mice, susceptibility to CPA was greatest in primordial follicles in exposed animals.[41,42] These results were in contrast to reports in which loss of larger growing[43] or antral ovarian follicles[44] was not associated with a loss of primordial follicles in SD rats injected with CPA. Plowchalk and Mattison[45] observed a time- and dose-dependent relationship between CPA and ovarian toxicity by looking at changes in ovarian structure and function. In C57BL/6N mice given a single injection (i.p.) of CPA (75, 200, or 500 mg/kg), primordial follicle numbers were significantly reduced to 73%, 42%, and 38% of controls, respectively. The loss of primordial follicles was essentially complete at 3 days and the estimated ED50 (concentration that produced 50% follicle loss) was 122 mg/kg body weight. From these results it appears that premature ovarian failure in women treated with CPA is likely to be, via destruction of primordial follicles.

3.4.1.3   Cigarette Smoking

Many epidemiological studies performed over the last 5 decades have shown that cigarette smoke is a reproductive toxicant, demonstrating a strong relationship between smoking and impaired fertility. One study reported that rates of pregnancy were reduced to 57% in heavy smokers and 75% in light smokers when compared with non-smokers; furthermore, the time to conception for smokers was 1 year longer than for non-smokers.[46] Women smokers have also been reported to experience a 1- to 4-year earlier age at the onset of menopause.[47,48] Thus, a significant amount of data exists to demonstrate a relationship between smoking and reduced fertility, but the mechanism is not well understood.[49] Along with the impact on fertility, there are also effects of cigarette smoke on pregnancy and the fetus. Prenatal exposure to cigarette smoke has been associated with retarded intra-uterine growth and premature deliveries.[50] Additionally, conception in women whose mothers smoked while pregnant was significantly reduced when compared with women whose mothers did not smoke.[51] In animal studies, exposure of mice *in utero* to cigarette smoke resulted in a reduced number of ovarian primordial follicles in female offspring.[52]

There are several possible mechanisms by which cigarette smoke might be involved in the earlier onset of menopause among smokers. Cigarette smoke is a complex mixture of alkaloids (nicotine), polycyclic aromatic hydrocarbons (PAHs), nitroso compounds, aromatic amines, and protein pyrolysates, many of which are carcinogenic.[53] Nicotine acting on the central nervous system might affect secretion of hormones involved in regulation of ovarian function.[48] Smoking women have been shown to have significantly decreased follicular levels of estradiol, compared with non-smokers.[54] Furthermore, extracts of cigarette smoke significantly decreased estradiol secretion by human granulosa cells in culture.[55] Alternatively, cigarette smoke can induce certain liver-metabolizing enzymes, which may also accelerate metabolism of steroid hormones.[48,56] However, because of the logical association between early menopause and oocyte destruction, some of the effects of cigarette smoke on fertility are likely to be due to damage to small pre-antral follicles.

3.4.1.4 Polycyclic Aromatic Hydrocarbons

Due to the prevalence of polycyclic aromatic hydrocarbons in cigarette smoke and in the environment from various combustion processes (including automobile exhaust), many animal studies have examined the potential of PAHs to cause ovarian damage or inhibit fertility.[47] Three PAHs, benzo[a]pyrene (BaP), 3-methylcholanthrene (3-MC), and 9:10-dimethyl-1:2-benzanthracene (DMBA), have all been demonstrated to cause ovarian damage. In one set of studies, Krarup reported that DMBA depletes oocytes and produces ovarian tumors in mice.[57,58] The three PAHs, BaP, 3-MC, and DMBA, destroyed oocytes in small follicles of Sprague-Dawley rats and in D2 and B6 mice, within 14 days following a single i.p. injection,[59] with mice being more susceptible to ovotoxicity than rats.

Related to the mechanisms of these effects, BaP produced chromosomal aberrations in CHO cells and mouse oocytes,[60] and 3-MC produced a destruction of oocytes that ultrastructurally resemble the physiological process of atresia.[61] Following single high-level i.p. injections of PAHs in mice, the relative toxicities causing oocyte destruction in primordial follicles was observed to be DMBA > 3MC > BaP.[62] This was similar to the relative toxicities determined for these compounds in experiments exposing mice and rats to multiple doses at lower levels of these compounds.[63] In this study, it was determined that mice were more sensitive than rats to these compounds and that ovarian damage from repeated exposures occurred at much lower doses than occurred following single doses. Furthermore, results suggested that there is variable sensitivity and target follicle specificity between species among the chemicals tested.

Exposure to these chemicals during pregnancy can also affect reproductive potential of offspring. Daily oral exposure in mice *in utero* between 7 and 16 days of gestation with BaP caused severely compromised fertility of female offspring (10 mg/kg).[64] A direct relationship between the dose of PAHs and destruction of primordial follicles has been shown in the mouse ovary.[62] In a subsequent study, mice given single intraperitoneal (i.p.) doses ranging from 1 to 100 mg/kg of BaP demonstrated an ED50 of 15 mg/kg for oocyte destruction in B6 mice.[65] Interestingly, significant oocyte destruction was demonstrated following a single high dose of BaP (100 mg/kg), whereas the same level of oocyte loss was observed with a low dose (10 mg/kg) given daily for 10 days.[66] This observation provides support for a cumulative ovotoxic effect of chronic exposures to low doses.

3.4.1.5   Occupational Chemicals

Due to the detrimental effects on the ozone layer caused by chlorofluorocarbons and the ban on their use, 1- and 2-bromopropane (BP) had been proposed as substitute propellants and cleaning solvents. These chemicals were found to have detrimental effects on both male and female workers in a Korean factory.[67,67] Sixteen of twenty-five exposed women were found to have amenorrhea, high levels of FSH and LH, and ten women complained of hot flashes. Ovaries in six of these women were found to range from atrophic to almost normal upon follow-up laparoscopic examination.[68] Later studies in rats demonstrated both neurological and reproductive effects.[69–71] Several recent studies have focused on the reproductive effects of 1- and 2-bromopropane. There were decreased ovarian follicles in multiple stages of development,[72,73] but time course and morphological studies performed in rats have suggested that 2-BP initially targets primordial follicles.[74] In contrast, 1-BP was reported to have no effect on primordial follicle numbers following prolonged inhalation exposures.[75] There is also evidence for antral follicle damage in women and rodents caused by these industrial chemicals.[72,75]

1,3-butadiene (BD) and the related olefins, isoprene and styrene, are released during the manufacture of synthetic rubber and thermoplastic resins, and the estimated annual occupational exposure of U.S. employees is 3,700 to 1,000,000 people.[76] These chemicals have also been reported in cigarette smoke and automobile exhaust.[76,77] Chronic inhalation studies have shown that carcinogenesis for BD is higher in mice than rats.[78] Animals exposed to BD and its metabolites by inhalation at concentrations of 62.5 ppm demonstrated that target tissues in mice (heart, lung, fat, spleen, and thymus) contained significantly greater amounts of BD epoxides than those same tissues in rats.[78] At lower doses, female mice exposed daily by inhalation for up to 2 years exhibited ovarian atrophy, granulosa cell hyperplasia, and benign and malignant granulosa cell tumors.[77] Therefore, reproductive effects were observed following chronic exposure to low doses.

Because of the ability of these compounds to become epoxidated, they have the potential to be ovotoxic and carcinogenic. In one study, the metabolite of BD, 1,3-butadiene monoepoxide (1.43 mmole/kg), depleted small follicles by 98% and growing follicles by 87% in female B6C3F1 mice dosed daily for 30 days compared with control animals.[79] At a much lower dose, 0.14 mmole/kg, the diepoxide of 1,3-butadiene depleted small follicles by 85% and growing follicles by 63%. The results of this study support that a diepoxide formed in the metabolism of BD is more potent than the monoepoxide at inducing follicle loss. Additionally, isoprene was reported to be ovotoxic, whereas styrene and its monoepoxide did not reduce mouse ovarian follicle numbers.[79]

There are mixed opinions as to the risk of human exposure to BD-induced toxicity. According to Bond et al.,[80] there is not enough evidence for an association between occupational exposure and human lymphatic and hematopoietic cancers. They have shown that the metabolic activation of the carcinogenic form occurs to a greater extent in mice than in rats and humans. Furthermore, they concluded that because concentrations likely to be encountered in the environment or workplace are usually below 2 ppm, there is not likely a carcinogenic risk to humans. However, the potential cumulative effect of long-term exposure to low concentrations over the course of years was not discussed. This is particularly important when the target cells are of a non-renewing type (for instance, ovarian follicles).

The dimerization of 1,3-butadiene forms 4-vinylcyclohexene, VCH. The VCH family of compounds are occupational chemicals released at low concentrations during the manufacture of rubber tires, plasticizers, and pesticides.[76,81] VCH has been shown in mice to 1) produce selective destruction of primordial and primary follicles,[82] 2) cause premature ovarian failure,[27,29] 3) increase the risk for development of ovarian tumors,[83] and 4) affect normal ovarian development of female offspring exposed *in utero*.[84] The metabolite, 4-vinylcyclohexene diepoxide (VCD), was shown to cause selective destruction of primordial and primary follicles in both mice and rats,[82,85] and premature ovarian failure in rats.[29] Because no significant effects on other tissues have been reported in studies with this class of compounds, the damage they produce appears to be highly specific and does not involve widespread toxicity. Ovarian damage caused by VCH and its related epoxide metabolites has been demonstrated by a variety of exposure routes, including dermal,[86] oral,[84] inhalation,[87] and i.p. injection.[82] It is, therefore, important to understand the mechanism(s) by which this damage, shown to have such selective yet far-reaching effects, is initiated. The overall sequence of events associated with VCH- and VCD-induced ovarian toxicity is shown in Figure 3.2. Logically, gaining a detailed understanding of the mechanisms of ovotoxicity of these chemicals requires focusing on the primary events associated with the destruction of primordial and primary follicles. Dosing of mice with VCH (800 mg/kg) for 30 days destroyed about 90% of ovarian small pre-antral (primordial and primary) follicles.[27,82] Follicle loss was not seen at 10 days, but was significant following 15 days of daily dosing.[82] The loss of follicles within 30 days of daily dosing was sufficient to cause premature ovarian failure within 1 year, as evidenced by loss of cyclicity, ovarian atrophy, and pre-neoplastic changes in ovarian cells.[27] In the longer term, two years of dosing with VCH resulted in development of rare ovarian neoplasms in female mice.[83] Another study evaluated the effects of a 2-year dermal application of VCD.[86] These results showed an increase in neoplasms of the skin in male and female mice at the site of application and an additional increase in the development of ovarian follicular atrophy and tubular hyperplasia in female mice.

3.4.1.6 Other Ovotoxic Agents

The alkylating agents 1,4-di(methanesulfonoxy)-butane (Myleran), trimethylene-melamin (TEM), and isopropyl methanesulfonate (IMS) have been shown to destroy oocytes in small follicles in SECXC57BL/F1 mice following a single i.p. injection.[24] This destruction was observed within 3 days of dosing with TEM and IMS, and within 14 days with Myleran. Daily oral administration of nitrofurazone over 2 years caused ovarian lesions, including development of benign mixed tumors and granulosa cell tumors in mice.[88] The results of an *in vitro* mutagenicity study in E. coli using a number of industrial and laboratory chemicals demonstrated a high correlation between alkylating activity and increased mutagenicity.[89] In addition

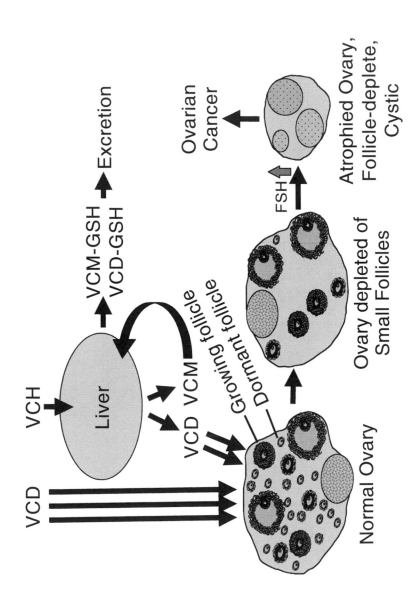

FIGURE 3.2 Effects associated with repeated *in vivo* exposures to VCH or VCD. VCH is metabolized to VCM and VCD in the liver, which is transported in the blood to the target site, the ovary. The active metabolite, VCD, induces depletion of the smallest ovarian follicles, causing eventual loss of all follicle types and leading to ovarian failure. These alterations subsequently cause ovarian atrophy and increased circulating FSH levels, followed by possible formation of cysts or neoplasms.

to the chemicals discussed so far, Dobson and Felton [31] reported a variety of other compounds that were capable of producing significant primordial follicle loss in mice. These chemicals included methyl and ethyl methanesulfonate, busulfan, and urethane. Additionally, of a number of fungal toxins and antibiotics tested, procarbazine HCl, and 4-nitroquinoline-1-oxide were ovotoxic. Finally, dibromochloropropane, urethane, N-ethyl-N-nitrosourea, and bleomycin demonstrated primordial follicle killing, with bleomycin being the most potent. In general, all of these ovotoxic chemicals are also known to possess mutagenic-carcinogenic effects. Thus, these studies have further provided a correlation between ovotoxicity and subsequent development of tumorigenesis. How these two events are linked is not clearly understood at this time. Hexachlorobenzene (HCB), a persistent halogenated hydrocarbon in the environment, has been identified as a contaminant in human follicular fluid.[90] This is of particular concern in view of the ability of HCB to destroy primordial follicles in Rhesus and cynomolgus monkeys.

3.4.2 ANTRAL FOLLICLE DAMAGE

Selective damage by toxicants to large growing or antral follicles may cause interruption of cyclicity by impacting on ovarian steroid production and ovulation. This effect is generally reversible because if exposure to the toxicant ceases, more follicles can ultimately be recruited for development from the pool of primordial follicles that remains.

3.4.2.1 Chemotherapeutic Agents

In addition to widespread destruction of primordial follicles by cyclophosphamide in ovaries of rats and mice, growing follicles have also been reported to be affected. Ataya et al. described specific losses of follicles > 30 μm in rhesus monkeys given multiple doses of cyclophosphamide.[91] The immediate precursors of phosphoramide mustard (the bioactive form of CPA) given to mice were observed to reduce antral follicle numbers, and cause loss of ovarian volume and uterine weight.[42] Also, in rats, dosing with CPA caused destruction of antral follicles at doses that did not affect primordial follicles.[44] In contrast, under conditions that completely destroyed primordial follicles in mice, only partial destruction of antral follicles was observed.[45] This demonstrated the greater sensitivity of primordial germ cells to this compound in mice. However, in both studies in rats and mice, lower ovarian weight, reduced follicular and luteal volume, and lower circulating 17-β estradiol levels were most highly associated with the loss of antral follicles.[44,45] The effect on antral follicle numbers in both studies was reversible. Thus, whereas ovotoxicity that impacts the primordial follicle pool causes irreversible effects, damage to larger follicles can have a temporary impact on cyclicity.

3.4.2.2 Polycyclic Aromatic Hydrocarbons

An effect of DMBA and BaP on antral follicles has been observed in mice.[92] DMBA decrease numbers of small follicles initially, with a secondary effect on large follicles. In a morphological assessment of ovaries collected from mice that were dosed with PAHs, Mattison [93] reported that BaP, 3-MC, and DMBA all destroyed primordial follicles; however, only DMBA impacted antral follicles. Yet, in a subsequent study in mice, BaP decreased numbers of corpora lutea, and this effect was reversible.[94] These observations are consistent with targeting of BaP to antral follicles and subsequent disruption of ovulation. Although there are discrepancies in findings between the two studies, it is apparent that under certain conditions, PAH damage to antral follicles can occur.

3.4.2.3 Phthalates

One class of chemicals that has received recent attention in reproductive toxicology is the phthalates. Detrimental reproductive effects have been reported in both human epidemiological studies and rodent studies.[95] These chemicals, which are diesters of o-phthalic acid, are utilized in the plastics industry to enhance the flexibility of polyvinyl chloride products. They are included in such products as cosmetics, lubricants, plastic tubing, medical devices, vinyl upholstery, surgical gloves, toys, solvents, and pesticides. Phthalates can leach out of plastics into air, water, or food.[96]

Di-(2-ethylhexyl)phthalate (DEHP) and other diester phthalates are widely used in the production of many polyvinyl chloride-based plastics, including medical and food packages. Because they are not covalently linked to the plastic resin, phthalates can contaminate the surrounding environment.[26] In a reference human population, multiple phthalate metabolites were detected in urine of approximately 75% of those tested,[97] demonstrating that humans are exposed to significant levels. Daily exposures may vary greatly among individuals, but are estimated to be 2 mg/day for DEPH alone.[98] Correlations were identified between urinary phthalate levels in humans and pregnancy complications[99] or rates of successful pregnancies.[100] Di-(2-ethylhexyl)phthalate and its monoester metabolite (MEHP) are likely the most widely studied of the phthalate esters. A recent study in female SD rats reported that repeated oral exposure to DEHP caused disruptions of reproductive function.[26] These disruptions included delayed ovulations; reduced granulosa cell size in antral follicles; decreased circulating estradiol, progesterone, and LH levels; and increased FSH. Mechanistic analyses have linked effects of phthalates to peroxisome proliferator-activated receptors (PPARs) (reviewed in [101]). It is known that multiple phthalates can induce hepatic 17β-hydroxysteroid dehydrogenase (17β–HSD IV), which metabolizes estradiol to estrone.[102] Further evidence suggests that this upregulation of 17β-HSD occurs through the PPAR-α receptor. In addition to activating PPAR-α, MEHP can also activate PPAR-γ, which suppresses expression of aromatase in granulosa cells of antral follicles.[103,104] Overall, these observations demonstrate that the direct effect of this class of chemicals on the ovary is specific for antral follicle stages.

3.4.2.4 Halogenated Aryl Hydrocarbons

Endocrine disrupters that display estrogenic/anti-estrogenic effects have been actively studied for their ability to induce *in utero* developmental alterations. The intracellular mechanisms of these disruptions are only beginning to be understood. The pesticide, 2,3,7,8-tetrachlorodibenzo-*p*-dioxin (TCDD) has been the subject of many studies related to sexual development and fertility.[105] However, a few recent studies have reported that TCDD can also cause direct ovarian effects. The effect of a single oral dose of TCDD on numbers of oocytes ovulated and estrous cyclicity was observed in female rats.[106] Exposure to TCDD prolonged the diestrous stage, and reduced the time in proestrus and estrus. Additionally, there was a reduction in the number of oocytes ovulated in treated rats. These findings provide strong evidence that TCDD impairs ovulation. TCDD was further studied for its effect on hormone-induced follicular development and ovulation.[107] The data from this study were consistent with reduced ovulation via a hypothalamic-pituitary effect. However, ovulation was also reduced in hypophysectomized animals, suggesting a direct ovarian effect as well. As regards the mechanisms involved, an *in vitro* study observed that TCDD significantly reduced 17-β-estradiol production in human luteinized granulosa cells in culture.[108] Further investigation demonstrated that TCDD produced these effects via interactions with the EGF linked-mitotic signaling pathway involving mitogen-activated protein kinases and protein kinase A.

The polychlorinated biphenyl, 3,3′,4,4′-tetrachlorobiphenyl (TCB), has been shown to have teratogenic effects in mice[109] and to be embryolethal in rats.[110] A transplacental effect of TCB on ovarian development in fetal mice has also been reported.[111] By 28 days of age in female mice exposed to TCB *in utero* on day 13 of gestation, there was a 40 –to 50% loss of follicles in all stages of development. However, this reduction did not adversely affect reproductive capacity during a 5-month period of testing.

Thus, it appears that direct endocrine disrupters may exert their reproductive and developmental effects at a variety of different sites. Even though an initial impact on endocrine balance may cause some of the observed effects, there is growing evidence to suggest that direct ovarian effects are produced, as well.

3.4.1.5 Occupational Chemicals

The effects of 1- and 2-BP were also observed on antral follicle development in rats. For 1-BP, reproductive studies of long-term inhalation exposures (400 to 800 ppm) suggest that growing and antral follicles, and not primordial follicles, are the target of this chemical.[75] 2-BP (500, 1000 mg/kg, i.p., once every 2 to 3 days, for 15 to 17 days) was found to prolong estrous cycles, decrease ovulations, and alter pre-ovulatory follicle morphology.[72] Rats exposed to 1- or 2-BP (up to 1000 ppm by inhalation, 8 hours/day, 21 days) had no significant changes in the number of abnormally long estrous cycles, ovarian or uterine weights, or numbers of ovulated oocytes, but significant changes were observed in these endpoints following 1,2-dibromopropane exposures (100 to 200 ppm).[73] Direct effects of 2-BP on the oocyte might also occur, as suggested by increased micronuclei and decreased cell numbers observed in preimplantation mouse embryos following exposures to 2-BP.[112]

3.5   OVARIAN METABOLISM

The ovary contains enzymes responsible for biotransformation and detoxification of many xenobiotics. Both the rat and mouse ovary contain epoxide hydrolase, glutathione-S-transferases, and cytochromes P-450 that metabolize known ovarian toxicants.[113-115] Therefore, biotransformation of chemicals may occur within the ovary. Immunohistochemical localization of enzymes suggests differential expression among the various ovarian structures, thereby providing significantly different exposures through region-specific bioactivation or detoxification of ovotoxicants near certain classes of oocytes.

3.5.1   BIOACTIVATION

Reproductive toxicants can compromise ovarian function via destruction of oocyte-containing follicles.[1,12] Many xenobiotic chemicals are metabolized once they have been taken into the body. In some cases, the chemical form that is introduced must be metabolized to a more reactive intermediate to produce toxic effects. This conversion often represents metabolism of the parent compound, by Phase I classes of enzymes, such as the family of cytochrome P450-associated enzymes. Expression of these enzymes may be under hormonal control, as demonstrated by increased content of microsomal cytochrome P-450 in rat ovaries as the animals developed toward puberty, with even greater increases in pregnant rats.[114] These results are complicated, however, by the fact that some cytochrome P-450 enzymes (aromatase or CYP19, P450 side chain cleavage or P450scc/CYP11a1, 17-hydroxylase 17,20-lyase or P450c17) are involved in steroidogenesis and may not be important for metabolism of xenobiotics. In the ovary, expression of cytochrome P-450s 2A, 2B, and 2E1 was significantly increased in target follicles in response to exposures to VCH or VCD (i.p.), and activity of 2E1 was increased by VCH in total ovarian tissue.[116] Whereas bioactivation of various parent compounds can occur directly in the ovary or in metabolically active tissues such as liver, ovarian expression of various cytochrome P-450 enzymes suggests that the ovary is capable of xenobiotic metabolism.

3.5.2   DETOXIFICATION

Phase I enzymes, including the cytochrome P450 enzymes, often generate activated metabolites of xenobiotics, and Phase II classes of enzymes generally cause detoxification during xenobiotic metabolism. This formation of non-toxic metabolites usually also enhances their solubility for excretion. Major enzymatic pathways for detoxification of xenobiotic epoxides are hydration to corresponding diols (catalyzed by microsomal epoxide hydrolase, EH), and conjugation with glutathione (catalyzed by glutathione-S-transferase, GST). Detoxification reactions catalyzed by EH and GST occur in many tissues including the ovary.[114,117] Expression of the specific isoforms of GSTs in rat ovaries was found to be age-dependent and hormonally regulated.[118] In human ovaries, specific isoenzymes were regionally compartmentalized.[119] Activities of EH, GST, and P450s in rats were high in the neonate, decreased by 2 weeks of age, reached a maximum near the onset of puberty, and were even further elevated in pregnant rats.[114] These data are suggestive of hormonal induction of ovarian detoxification enzymes.

3.5.3 METABOLISM OF SPECIFIC CHEMICALS

3.5.3.1 Chemotherapeutic Agents

Chemotherapy is one of the most toxic exposures to humans as regards germ cell destruction.[120] Cyclophosphamide has been studied more thoroughly than most due to its widespread use as a chemotherapeutic agent. CPA induces loss of primordial follicles and can cause sterility. Phosphoramide mustard has been determined to be the antineoplastic and ovotoxic form of this chemical.[42,121] Mice were dosed with chemicals capable of forming specific metabolites of cyclophosphamide (phosphoramide mustard, phosphoramide mustard cyclohexylamine salt or trans-4-phenylcyclophosphamide; or acrolein, didechlorocyclophosphamide and allyl alcohol). Only those chemicals that released phosphoramide mustard induced ovarian toxicity. The greater potency of phosphoramide mustard-producing chemicals compared to CPA in mice was attributed to a bypassing of detoxification steps, allowing more toxic metabolite to reach the ovary.[42] Metabolism of cyclophosphamide is thought to occur in the liver with uptake of the reactive metabolites from the blood to the ovary.[121] However, the possibility exists for detoxification of toxic metabolites in specific regions of the ovary, which might explain the follicle-stage-specific toxicity.

3.5.3.2 Polycyclic Aromatic Hydrocarbons

Polycyclic aromatic hydrocarbons are persistent organic chemicals generated as products of combustion. Many animal studies have demonstrated ovotoxic effects of these compounds. Polycyclic aromatic hydrocarbons are not directly ovotoxic, but require metabolic activation to reactive metabolites.[122] Oocyte destruction by PAHs may involve distribution of the parent compound to the ovary, where ovarian enzymes involved in PAH biotransformation metabolize the compound to reactive intermediates (e.g., through aryl hydrocarbon hydroxylase or epoxide hydrolase).[65,123] However, enzymes capable of activating PAHs have been identified in ovarian tissue in mice and rats,[65] monkeys,[124] and humans.[125]

As regards bioactivation, BaP is metabolized initially by microsomal cytochrome P450 enzymes to arene oxides,[126] which may then spontaneously form phenols and subsequently be converted to the trans-dihydrodiol by epoxide hydrolase. The diol epoxide, 7,8-dihydrodiol-9,10-epoxide, displays the greatest degree of mutagenicity, carcinogenicity, and ovotoxicity.[65] Mattison and Nightingale[66] showed that B6 mice were more susceptible to BaP than D2 mice, whereas both strains were equally susceptible to the arene oxide metabolite.[127] Furthermore, inhibition of PAH metabolism with α–naphthoflavone prevented PAH-induced oocyte destruction observed in mice.[62,65] Detoxification of the diol epoxide involves further hydrolysis to the tetrol or conjugation to glucuronides, sulfate, or glutathione. Other PAHs, DMBA and 3-MC, follow similar metabolic pathways.[126] Sub-chronic low-dose exposures of mice and rats to BAP, DMBA, and 3-MC, however, caused reductions in different follicle populations for each of these chemicals,[63] suggesting that differences in metabolism or follicle susceptibility may exist.

The involvement of ovarian enzymes in bioactivation was demonstrated in studies that employed direct intra-ovarian injections of BaP.[128] The enzyme responsible for the initiation of PAH metabolism is a cytochrome P450-dependent microsomal mono-oxygenase, aryl hydrocarbon hydroxylase (AHH).[127] AHH has been studied in detail to determine the relationship between metabolism of PAHs and ovotoxicity.[65] The inducibility of AHH varied between different mouse strains, and the ovotoxicity of 3-MC was related to AHH inducibility, whereas ovotoxicity of DMBA or BAP was not.[129] DMBA metabolism by cytochrome P450-dependent DMBA mono-oxygenase activity has been measured in enriched granulosa/theca cell fractions isolated from ovaries collected from rats,[116] monkeys,[124] and humans.[125] Increased ovarian DMBA hydroxylase activity was measured during proestrus and estrus in rats, suggesting induction of enzyme expression by estradiol or gonadotropins. Taken together, these data provide evidence that bioactivation of PAHs can be directly performed within the ovary. Overall, it is the combined processes of bioactivation, distribution, and detoxification both throughout the body and locally in the ovary that determine ovarian susceptibility to these compounds.

3.5.3.3   4-Vinylcyclohexene

Multiple chemicals have been demonstrated to be bioactivated to the diepoxide form, including the occupational chemicals 2-bromopropane, 1,3-butadiene, and 4-vinylcyclohexene. The role of biotransformation in VCH-induced ovarian toxicity has been well established. Following 30 days of daily dosing of female B6C3F1 mice and Fischer 344 rats with VCH, primordial and primary follicles were reduced in ovaries of mice, but not rats.[82] Cytochrome P450 enzymes convert VCH to two possible monoepoxides (4-vinylcyclohexene monoepoxide, VCME), the 1,2-VCME, and 7,8-VCME forms, then further metabolize them to the diepoxide, VCD. Structure-activity studies determined that the ultimate ovotoxic form, with the lowest ED_{50}, is VCD.[79] Similar studies have provided evidence that the diepoxide of butadiene is also the ultimate ovarian toxicant.[79] The greater sensitivity of mice compared to rats was partly due to different capabilities for bioactivation of VCH. This was demonstrated by measurable blood levels of 1,2-VCME in VCH-exposed mice but not rats,[130] a 4 to 6x greater metabolism of VCH to 1,2-VCME by hepatic microsomes from mice versus from rats,[131] and a 56-fold higher V_{max} for conversion of VCH to 1,2-VCME in mouse liver as opposed to rat liver.[132] Specific induction of CYP2A and CYP2B was seen in response to VCH or 1,2-VCME exposures in mice but not rats.[133] In purified human microsomes, only CYP2E1 and CYP2B6 were capable of bioactivation of VCH to epoxides. Thus, these results demonstrate that epoxidation of VCH represents bioactivation, and it was concluded that the species variation in susceptibility to VCH was, in part, due to differences in the capacity of mice and rats to form VCD.

3.5.3.4 Vinylcyclohexene Diepoxide

The greater sensitivity of rats versus mice to the ovotoxicity of VCD suggested that detoxification of VCD may also play a role in species-specific sensitivity to VCH-induced ovotoxicity. It was shown that the rat had greater capacity for conversion of VCD to its inactive tetrol, as compared with the mouse, and that only rats possessed detectable ovarian VCD-hydrolytic enzymatic activity.[132] Similar results have been reported for epoxides of butadiene.[134] Therefore, the greater susceptibility of mice over rats relates to both enhanced bioactivation and reduced detoxification of the ovotoxic epoxides. Both microsomal epoxide hydrolase (mEH) and cytosolic GST, which are likely to be involved in metabolism of VCD, are expressed in the ovary.[114] Evidence that VCD is metabolized by EH has been provided in studies with rabbit liver microsomes.[135] Exposure of mice or rats to VCD caused significant depletion of hepatic glutathione levels,[136] whereas ovarian levels in rat were unaffected.[137] This may reflect glutathione conjugation to VCD through glutathione transferase activity.

Pre-antral follicles isolated from rat ovaries were capable of converting VCD to the inactive tetrol metabolite.[138] Following *in vitro* incubation, the smallest follicles displayed a lower capacity to convert VCD to the tetrol than did larger pre-antral follicles. These results provide evidence that the rat ovary can directly detoxify VCD, but that the smallest follicles targeted for ovotoxicity have a reduced capacity for this conversion.

3.6 MECHANISMS OF OVOTOXICITY

The mechanism(s) by which ovotoxic chemicals act directly on the ovary are generally not well understood but might be due to one of several possible mechanisms. In each case, ovarian follicles and oocytes are the underlying targets. Oocyte destruction can result from a toxic chemical causing direct damage to the oocyte. Alternatively, chemicals may interfere with the critical inter-cellular interactions between oocytes and granulosa cells necessary at all stages of follicular development either through direct toxicity to granulosa cells[13] or through disruption of cell-cell communication. Lastly, environmental chemicals might cause follicle loss by accelerating the overall rate of atresia, the normal and poorly understood mechanism by which the majority of follicles degenerate during development.

3.6.1 Cell Death

Only a select few follicles in the ovary will ever develop fully and be ovulated.[4] Instead, the vast majority begin development but are lost by a process of cell death, called atresia. Atretic follicles at all stages of development can be morphologically distinguished from healthy ones. Follicular atresia in mammals has been shown to occur via a mechanism of physiological cell death, apoptosis.[15,139]

It has been proposed that most forms of xenobiotic-induced premature ovarian failure are due to increased rates of atresia.[1] However, there appears to be a relationship between the dose given of a chemical, the duration of treatment, and the type of cell death that follows. In general, it has been found that low doses of toxic chemicals typically induce apoptosis, whereas higher doses often cause necrosis.[140,141] Furthermore, a temporal relationship between apoptosis and necrosis has also been reported, with apoptosis being induced rapidly (1 to 7 hours) following a single dose of the hepatotoxicant dimethylnitrosamine, and necrosis occurring at a later time (12 to 24 hours).[142,143] Taken together, these results suggest that mild cellular damage can induce a program for death, apoptosis; whereas more severe damage results in uncontrolled cell death through necrosis.[144] These trends were also observed in studies investigating ovotoxicity in rats and mice, with morphological evidence consistent for both types of cell death reported. Ovaries collected from mice given a relatively high dose of cyclophosphamide (500 mg/kg) demonstrated necrotic damage, specifically in oocytes of primordial follicles containing granulosa cells.[45,94] Conversely, atretic changes in primordial follicles were reported at lower doses (100 mg/kg). Antral follicles demonstrated evidence of atresia at the higher dose in mice (500 mg/kg),[45] as well as in rats dosed with 150 mg/kg CPA.[44]

In mice treated with PAHs (80 mg/kg BaP, 3-MC, or DMBA), oocyte morphology consistent with necrosis was observed in primordial follicles.[93] These changes caused by 3-MC and BaP were seen in the absence of visible effects in the associated granulosa cells. However, DMBA produced more visible toxicity by destroying oocytes and follicles more extensively and disrupting ovarian architecture. Morphological evidence consistent with increased atresia in small pre-antral follicles was also reported in ovaries collected from rats dosed daily for 10 days with the occupational chemical, 4-vinylcyclohexene diepoxide (VCD, 80 mg/kg; [145]). In rats treated with the phthalate, DEHP, antral follicle damage was observed in association with retarded ovulation.[26] The morphological changes in these follicles were also consistent with atresia.

Many reports have provided examples of xenobiotic-induced apoptosis. In recent years there has been an increase in the investigation of apoptotic cell death following treatment with toxic chemicals.[144] Hepatotoxicants such as thioacetamide, acetaminophen, and dimethylnitrosamine induce apoptosis *in vivo* and *in vitro*.[146,147] The halogenated aromatic hydrocarbon, tetrachlorodibenzo-*p*-dioxin (TCCD), can induce apoptosis in immature thymocytes.[148] The PAH, DMBA, induced internucleosomal cleavage (apoptosis) in mouse thymocytes and spleen cells.[149] Although there are examples of morphological evidence of ovotoxicity consistent with atresia, few reports have classified the specific type of cell death induced by reproductive toxicants in the ovary as apoptosis. Distinguishing characteristics associated with apoptosis were observed in primordial and primary follicles in ovaries from rats dosed with the occupational chemical, VCD.[20] Furthermore, there was no evidence of necrosis, such as cellular or organelle swelling or infiltration of macrophages, in ovaries from treated rats. Even at the ultrastructural level, no signs of necrosis or alterations in the atretic process were observed at any follicle stage.[29]

Multiple internal or external signals can trigger apoptosis, using multiple possible pathways.[139] Molecular markers of apoptosis examined following VCD exposures have supported that VCD-induced ovotoxicity is via apoptosis. The Bcl-2 family of proteins, which have members that are both pro- and anti-apoptotic, and apoptosis-related signaling pathways were found to be altered in isolated follicles from enzyme-dissociated ovaries of control and VCD-treated rats (summarized in Figure 3.3). Elevated levels of mRNA encoding the pro-apoptotic gene, *bax*, were measured in isolated fractions of small pre-antral follicles collected from rats following repeated exposures to VCD (80mg/kg/d, 15 d).[150] The pro-apoptotic protein, Bad, was increased specifically in those follicles.[151] Furthermore, Bcl-x$_{long}$ was translocated from the mitochondria (its site of anti-apoptotic action) to the cytoplasm, and the mitochondrial ratio of this protein to the pro-apoptotic Bax was significantly reduced to favor apoptosis. VCD also induced another pro-apoptotic event, mitochondrial cytochrome C diffusion into the cytoplasm. Activity and protein levels of Caspases 8, 9, and 3, enzymes involved in apoptotic signaling pathways, were also elevated following VCD dosing.[152] All of these effects were specific for the small follicles targeted by VCD, and were not seen in large pre-antral follicles or hepatocytes (non-target tissues). The importance of Bax in VCD-induced follicle loss was confirmed by determination that Bax-deficient mice were resistant to follicle depletion by VCD. In contrast, primordial follicles in mice lacking acid sphingomyelinase (enzyme that produces pro-apoptotic ceramide), the aryl hydrocarbon receptor, or Caspases 2 or 3 were just as sensitive to VCD exposures as wild-type animals,[153] although primary follicles were partially protected against VCD-induced follicle loss in Caspase 2- or 3-deficient mice. Taken together, these results support the idea that VCD-induced follicular atresia involves increased activation of the Bcl-2 pro-apoptotic signaling pathways.

3.6.2 Sites of Cellular Damage

Intracellular sites that are targeted by ovotoxic chemicals are still unknown for most chemicals. Many epoxide-containing compounds have been associated with increased mutagenicity (in *in vitro* bacterial assays),[154] DNA adducts, and sister chromatin exchanges.[155,156] Also, many ovotoxic compounds also cause an increased incidence of ovarian tumors.[12] However, whether DNA damage is the event that initiates ovotoxicity has not been determined for these chemicals. Nor is it understood why oocytes would be especially sensitive to DNA damage in such a cell-selective manner. To examine the follicle-stage-dependent chromosomal sensitivity of oocytes, several studies have determined the timing of oocyte damage following chemical exposures. By examining chromosomal anomalies in eggs or embryos and success of mating at different times after exposures, results correspond to effects at different stages of oocyte development.[157,158] Chromosomal damage was only detected in ovulated oocytes shortly after butadiene diepoxide exposures in superovulated mice.[159] Meirow et al. (2001) identified differences in follicle stage-dependent effects on reproductive success in mice following single exposures to cyclophosphamide (75 mg/kg),[158] which is thought to act through covalent DNA conjugation and cross-linking.

In contrast to DNA damage, it has been proposed that plasma membrane damage is more highly correlated with ovotoxicity that DNA damage.[31] This observation was supported by comparing alkylating properties with genetic activity in a variety

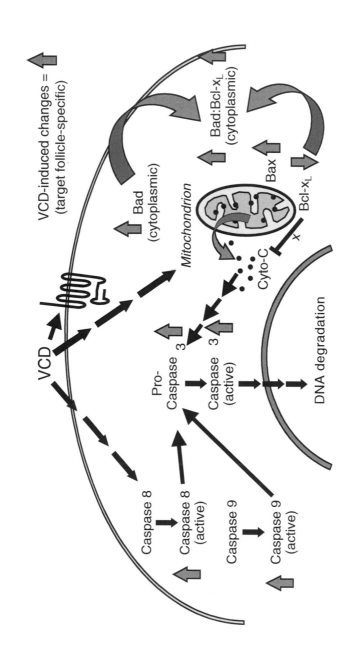

FIGURE 3.3 Mechanistic alterations caused by repeated VCD exposures induced specifically in target (primordial and primary) ovarian follicles leading to follicular atresia (apoptosis). One or more Caspase-dependent signal transduction pathways are activated, mitochondrial changes in localization of Bcl-2-related proteins induce release of cytochrome C from mitochondria, further promoting cells to undergo apoptosis. Gray arrows represent quantitative alterations in expression or localization.

of epoxide-containing chemicals.[160] Thus, the cellular event(s) initiated directly by ovotoxic chemicals may be at the level of proteins involved in signaling pathways or regulatory mechanisms associated with cell death/viability determination, rather than as a direct result of DNA damage.

3.7 SUMMARY

In summary, environmental chemicals that impact ovarian function can directly disrupt endocrine balance by decreasing production of ovarian hormones and interfering with ovulation. These effects are rather immediate, target large antral follicles, and can be reversed once there is no longer exposure to the chemical. On the other hand, ovarian function can be impaired by exposure to chemicals that destroy small pre-antral follicles. This produces an indirect disruption of endocrine balance, once hormonal feedback mechanisms have been affected. The manifestation of this type of ovarian toxicity is delayed until irreversible ovarian failure has occurred. This type of damage is of particular concern in women because of the health risks known to be associated with menopause. Future research should be aimed at understanding specific mechanisms of ovotoxicity and improving our ability to predict human risk from the wide variety of exposures to these chemicals in the environment.

REFERENCES

1. Mattison, D.R., *Reproductive Toxicology*, Raven Press, New York, 1985, 109.
2. Hollier, L.M., Leveno, K.J., Kelly, M.A., McIntire, D.D., and Cunningham, F.G., Maternal age and malformations in singleton births., *Obstet. Gynecol.*, 96, 701, 2000.
3. Richards, J.S., Maturation of ovarian follicles: actions and interactions of pituitary and ovarian hormones on follicular cell differentiation, *Physiol. Rev.*, 60, 51, 1980.
4. Hirshfield, A.N., Development of follicles in the mammalian ovary, *Int. Rev. Cytol.*, 124, 43, 1991.
5. Christiansen, C., Christensen, M.S., McNair, P., Hagen, C., Stocklund, K.E., and Transbol, I., Prevention of early postmenopausal bone loss: controlled 2-year study in 315 normal females, *Eur. J. Clin. Invest.*, 10, 273, 1980.
6. Bruning, P.F., Pit, M.J., de Jong-Bakker, M., van den Ende, A., Hart, A., and van Enk, A., Bone mineral density after adjuvant chemotherapy for premenopausal breast cancer, *Br. J. Cancer*, 61, 308, 1990.
7. Oparil, S., Arthur C. Corcoran Memorial Lecture. Hormones and vasoprotection, *Hypertension*, 33, 170, 1999.
8. Dhar, H.L., Gender, aging, health and society, *J. Assoc. Physicians India*, 49, 1012, 2001.
9. Paganini-Hill, A. and Henderson, V.W., Estrogen deficiency and risk of Alzheimer's disease in women, *Am. J. Epidemiol.*, 140, 256, 1994.
10. Sowers, M.R. and La Pietra, M.T., Menopause: its epidemiology and potential association with chronic diseases, *Epidemiol. Rev.*, 17, 287, 1995.
11. Mant, J.W.F. and Vessey, M.P., *Trends in cancer incidence and mortality*, Cold Spring Harbor Laboratory Press, Plainview, NY, 1994, 19, 287.
12. Hoyer, P.B. and Sipes, I.G., Assessment of follicle destruction in chemical-induced ovarian toxicity, *Annu. Rev. Pharmacol. Toxicol.*, 36, 307, 1996.

13. Buccione, R., Schroeder, A.C., and Eppig, J.J., Interactions between somatic cells and germ cells throughout mammalian oogenesis, *Biol. Reprod.*, 43, 543, 1990.

14. Mattison, D.R. and Schulman, J.D., How xenobiotic compounds can destroy oocytes, *Contemporary OB/GYN*, 15, 157, 1980.

15. Tilly, J.L., Kowalski, K.I., Johnson, A.L., and Hsueh, A.J., Involvement of apoptosis in ovarian follicular atresia and postovulatory regression, *Endocrinology*, 129, 2799, 1991.

16. Wyllie, A.H., Kerr, J.F., and Currie, A.R., Cell death: the significance of apoptosis, *Int. Rev. Cytol.*, 68, 251, 1980.

17. Compton, M.M., A biochemical hallmark of apoptosis: internucleosomal degradation of the genome, *Cancer Metastasis Rev.*, 11, 105, 1992.

18. Morita, Y. and Tilly, J.L., Oocyte apoptosis: like sand through an hourglass, *Dev. Biol.*, 213, 1, 1999.

19. McNatty, K.P., Fidler, A.E., Juengel, J.L., Quirke, L.D., Smith, P.R., Heath, D.A., Lundy, T., O'Connell, A., and Tisdall, D.J., Growth and paracrine factors regulating follicular formation and cellular function, *Mol. Cell. Endocrinol.*, 163, 11, 2000.

20. Springer, L.N., McAsey, M.E., Flaws, J.A., Tilly, J.L., Sipes, I.G., and Hoyer, P.B., Involvement of apoptosis in 4-vinylcyclohexene diepoxide-induced ovotoxicity in rats, *Toxicol. Appl. Pharmacol.*, 139, 394, 1996.

21. Boone, D.L., Yan, W., and Tsang, B.K., Identification of a deoxyribonuclease I-like endonuclease in rat granulosa and luteal cell nuclei, *Biol. Reprod.*, 53, 1057, 1995.

22. Payne, C.M., Bernstein C., and Bernstein H., Apoptosis overview emphasizing the role of oxidative stress, DNA damage and signal-transduction pathways, *Leuk. Lymphoma*, 19, 43, 1995.

23. Meirow, D., Lewis, H., Nugent, D., and Epstein, M., Subclinical depletion of primordial follicular reserve in mice treated with cyclophosphamide: clinical importance and proposed accurate investigative tool, *Hum. Reprod.*, 14, 1903, 1999.

24. Generoso, W., Stout, S.K., and Huff, S.W., Effects of alkylating chemicals on reproductive capacity of adult female mice, *Mutat. Res.*, 13, 171, 1971.

25. Jarrell, J.F., Bodo, L., Younglai, E.V., Barr, R.D., and O'Connell, G.J., The short-term reproductive toxicity of cyclophosphamide in the female rat, *Reprod. Toxicol.*, 5, 481, 1991.

26. Davis, B.J., Maronpot, R.R., and Heindel, J.J., Di-(2-ethylhexyl) phthalate suppresses estradiol and ovulation in cycling rats, *Toxicol. Appl. Pharmacol.*, 128, 216, 1994.

27. Hooser, S.B., Douds, D.P., DeMerell, D.G., Hoyer, P.B., and Sipes, I.G., Long-term ovarian and gonadotropin changes in mice exposed to 4-vinylcyclohexene., *Reprod. Toxicol.*, 8, 315, 1994.

28. Hedge, G.A., Colby, H.D., and Goodman, R.L., *Clinical Endocrine Physiology*, Saunders, Philadelphia, 1987, 189.

29. Mayer, L.P., Pearsall, N.A., Christian, P.J., Devine, P.J., Payne, C.M., McCuskey, M.K., Marion, S.L., Sipes, I.G., and Hoyer, P.B., Long-term effects of ovarian follicular depletion in rats by 4- vinylcyclohexene diepoxide, *Reprod. Toxicol.*, 16, 775, 2002.

30. Byrne, J., Long-term genetic and reproductive effects of ionizing radiation and chemotherapeutic agents on cancer patients and their offspring, *Teratology*, 59, 210, 1999.

31. Dobson, R.L. and Felton, J.S., Female germ cell loss from radiation and chemical exposures, *Am. J. Ind. Med.*, 4, 175, 1983.

32. Chapman, R.M., Gonadal injury resulting from chemotherapy, *Am. J. Ind. Med.*, 4, 149, 1983.

33. Damewood, M.D. and Grochow, L.B., Prospects for fertility after chemotherapy or radiation for neoplastic disease, *Fertil. Steril.*, 45, 443, 1986.

34. Revel, A. and Laufer, N., Protecting female fertility from cancer therapy, *Mol. Cell. Endocrinol.*, 187, 83, 2002.

35. Sobrinho, L.G., Levine, R.A., and DeConti, R.C., Amenorrhea in patients with Hodgkin's disease treated with antineoplastic agents, *Am. J. Obstet. Gynecol.*, 109, 135, 1971.

36. Warne, G.L., Fairley, K.F., Hobbs, J.B., and Martin, F.I., Cyclophosphamide-induced ovarian failure, *N. Engl. J. Med.*, 289, 1159, 1973.

37. Koyama, H., Wada, T., Nishizawa, Y., Iwanaga, T., and Aoki, Y., Cyclophosphamide-induced ovarian failure and its therapeutic significance in patients with breast cancer, *Cancer*, 39, 1403, 1977.

38. Thomson, A.B., Critchley, H.O., Kelnar, C.J., and Wallace, W.H., Late reproductive sequelae following treatment of childhood cancer and options for fertility preservation., *Best Pract. Res. Clin. Endocrinol. Metab.*, 16, 311, 2002.

39. Blumenfeld, Z., Dann, E., Avivi, I., Epelbaum, R., and Rowe, J.M., Fertility after treatment for Hodgkin's disease, *Ann. Oncol.*, 13, 138, 2002.

40. Miller, J.J. 3rd and Cole, L.J., Changes in mouse ovaries after prolonged treatment with cyclophosphamide, *Proc. Soc. Exp. Biol. Med.*, 133, 190, 1970.

41. Shiromizu, K., Thorgeirsson, S.S., and Mattison, D.R., Effect of cyclophosphamide on oocyte and follicle number in Sprague-Dawley rats, C57BL/6N and DBA/2N mice, *Pediatr. Pharmacol. (New York)*, 4, 213, 1984.

42. Plowchalk, D.R. and Mattison, D.R., Phosphoramide mustard is responsible for the ovarian toxicity of cyclophosphamide, *Toxicol. Appl. Pharmacol.*, 107, 472, 1991.

43. Ataya, K.M., McKanna, J.A., Weintraub, A.M., Clark, M.R., and LeMaire, W.J., A luteinizing hormone-releasing hormone agonist for the prevention of chemotherapy-induced ovarian follicular loss in rats, *Cancer Res.*, 45, 3651, 1985.

44. Jarrell, J., Lai, E.V., Barr, R., McMahon, A., Belbeck, L., and O'Connell, G., Ovarian toxicity of cyclophosphamide alone and in combination with ovarian irradiation in the rat, *Cancer Res.*, 47, 2340, 1987.

45. Plowchalk, D.R. and Mattison, D.R., Reproductive toxicity of cyclophosphamide in the C57BL/6N mouse: 1. Effects on ovarian structure and function, *Reprod. Toxicol.*, 6, 411, 1992.

46. Baird, D.D. and Wilcox, A.J., Cigarette smoking associated with delayed conception, *JAMA*, 253, 2979, 1985.

47. Everson, R.B., Sandler, D.P., Wilcox, A.J., Schreinemachers, D., Shore, D.L., and Weinberg, C., Effect of passive exposure to smoking on age at natural menopause, *Br. Med. J. (Clin. Res. Ed.)*, 293, 792, 1986.

48. Jick, H., Porter, J., and Morrison, A.S., Relation between smoking and age of natural menopause, *Lancet*, 1, 1354, 1977.

49. Shiverick, K.T. and Salafia, C., Cigarette smoking and pregnancy I: ovarian, uterine and placental effects, *Placenta*, 20, 265, 1999.

50. Mattison, D.R., Plowchalk, B.S., Meadows, M.J., Miller, M.M., Malek, A., and London, S., The effect of smoking on oogenesis, fertilization, and implantation, *Semin. Reprod. Endocrinol.*, 7, 291, 1989.

51. Weinberg, C.R., Wilcox, A.J., and Baird, D.D., Reduced fecundability in women with prenatal exposure to cigarette smoking, *Am. J. Epidemiol,*, 129, 1072, 1989.

52. Vahakangas, K., Rajaniemi, H., and Pelkonen, O., Ovarian toxicity of cigarette smoke exposure during pregnancy in mice, *Toxicol. Lett.*, 25, 75, 1985.

53. Stedman, R.L., The chemical composition of tobacco and tobacco smoke, *Chem. Rev.*, 68, 153, 1968.
54. Van Voorhis, B.J., Syrop, C.H., Hammitt, D.G., Dunn, M.S., and Snyder, G.D., Effects of smoking on ovulation induction for assisted reproductive techniques, *Fertil. Steril.*, 58, 981, 1992.
55. Barbieri, R.L., McShane, P.M., and Ryan, K.J., Constituents of cigarette smoke inhibit human granulosa cell aromatase, *Fertil. Steril.*, 46, 232, 1986.
56. Yeh, J. and Barbieri, R.L., Effects of smoking on steroid production, metabolism, and estrogen related diseases, *Semin. Reprod. Endocrinol.*, 7, 326, 1989.
57. Krarup, T., 9:10-dimethyl-1:2-benzantracene induced ovarian tumours in mice, *Acta Pathol. Microbiol. Scand.*, 70, 241, 1967.
58. Krarup, T., Oocyte destruction and ovarian tumorigenesis after direct application of a chemical carcinogen (9:0-dimethyl-1:2-benzanthrene) to the mouse ovary, *Int. J. Cancer*, 4, 61, 1969.
59. Mattison, D.R., Difference in sensitivity of rat and mouse primordial oocytes to destruction by polycyclic aromatic hydrocarbons, *Chem. Biol. Interact.*, 28, 133, 1979.
60. Basler, A. and Rohrborn, G., Chromosome aberrations in oocytes of NMRI mice and bone marrow cells of Chinese hamsters induced with 3,4-benzpyrene, *Mutat. Res.*, 38, 327, 1976.
61. Gulyas, B.J. and Mattison, D.R., Degeneration of mouse oocytes in response to polycyclic aromatic hydrocarbons, *Anat. Rec.*, 193, 863, 1979.
62. Mattison, D.R. and Thorgeirsson, S.S., Ovarian aryl hydrocarbon hydroxylase activity and primordial oocyte toxicity of polycyclic aromatic hydrocarbons in mice, *Cancer Res.*, 39, 3471, 1979.
63. Borman, S.M., Christian, P.J., Sipes, I.G., and Hoyer, P.B., Ovotoxicity in female Fischer rats and B6 mice induced by low-dose exposure to three polycyclic aromatic hydrocarbons: comparison through calculation of an ovotoxic index, *Toxicol. Appl. Pharmacol.*, 167, 191, 2000.
64. MacKenzie, K.M. and Angevine, D.M., Infertility in mice exposed *in utero* to benzo(a)pyrene, *Biol. Reprod.*, 24, 183, 1981.
65. Mattison, D.R., Shiromizu, K., and Nightingale, M.S., Oocyte destruction by polycyclic aromatic hydrocarbons, *Am. J. Ind. Med.*, 4, 191, 1983.
66. Mattison, D.R. and Nightingale, M.R., The biochemical and genetic characteristics of murine ovarian aryl hydrocarbon (benzo[a]pyrene) hydroxylase activity and its relationship to primordial oocyte destruction by polycyclic aromatic hydrocarbons, *Toxicol. Appl. Pharmacol.*, 56, 399, 1980.
67. Park, J., Kim, Y., Park, D., Choi, K., Park, S., and Moon, Y., An outbreak of hematopoietic and reproductive disorders due to solvents containing 2-bromopropane in an electronic factory, South Korea: Epidemiological survey, *J. Occup. Health*, 39, 138, 1997.
68. Koh, J.M., Kim, C.H., Hong, S.K., Lee, K.U., Kim, Y.T., Kim, O.J., and Kim, G.S., Primary ovarian failure caused by a solvent containing 2-bromopropane, *Eur. J. Endocrinol.*, 138, 554, 1998.
69. Takeuchi, Y., Ichihara, G., and Kamijima, M., A review of toxicity of 2-bromopropane: mainly on its reproductive toxicity, *J. Occup. Health*, 39, 191, 1997.
70. National Toxicology Program (NTP), NTP-CERHR Expert Panel Report 2-BP-02, U.S. Department of Health and Human Services, Public Health Service National Institutes of Health Public Information, Research Triangle Park, NC, 2002.

71. National Toxicology Program (NTP), NTP-CERHR Expert Panel Report 1-BP-02, U.S. Department of Health and Human Services, Public Health Service National Institutes of Health Public Information, Research Triangle Park, NC, 2002.
72. Sekiguchi, S., Asano, G., Suda, M., and Honma, T., Influence of 2-bromopropane on reproductive system—short-term administration of 2-bromopropane inhibits ovulation in F344 rats, *Toxicol. Ind. Health*, 16, 277, 2001.
73. Sekiguchi, S., Suda, M., Zhai, Y.L., and Honma, T., Effects of 1-bromopropane, 2-bromopropane, and 1,2-dichloropropane on the estrous cycle and ovulation in F344 rats, *Toxicol. Lett.*, 126, 41, 2002.
74. Yu, X.Z., Kamijima, M., Ichihara, G., Li, W., Kitoh, J., Xie, Z., Shibata, E., Hisanaga, N., and Takeuchi, Y., 2-Bromopropane causes ovarian dysfunction by damaging primordial follicles and their oocytes in female rats, *Toxicol. Appl. Pharmacol.*, 159, 185, 1999.
75. Yamada, T., Ichihara, G., Wang, H., Yu, X., Maeda, K., Tsukamura, H., Kamijima, M., Nakajima, T., and Takeuchi, Y., Exposure to 1-bromopropane causes ovarian dysfunction in rats, *Toxicol. Sci.*, 71, 96, 2003.
76. IARC (International Agency for Research on Cancer), Report No. 60, IARC monographs on the evaluation of carcinogenic risks to humans: some industrial chemicals, Lyon, France, 1994.
77. Melnick, R.L. and Huff, J., 1,3-Butadiene: toxicity and carcinogenicity in laboratory animals and humans, *Rev. Environ. Contam. and Tox.*, 124, 111, 1992.
78. Thornton-Manning, J.R., Dahl, A.R., Bechtold, W.E., Griffith, W.C. Jr., and Henderson, R.F., Disposition of butadiene monoepoxide and butadiene diepoxide in various tissues of rats and mice following a low-level inhalation exposure to 1,3-butadiene, *Carcinogenesis*, 16, 1723, 1995.
79. Doerr, J.K., Hooser, S.B., Smith, B.J., and Sipes, I.G., Ovarian toxicity of 4-vinylcyclohexene and related olefins in B6C3F1 mice: role of diepoxides, *Chem. Res. Toxicol.*, 8, 963, 1995.
80. Bond, J.A., Recio, L., and Andjelkovich, D., Epidemiological and mechanistic data suggest that 1,3-butadiene will not be carcinogenic to humans at exposures likely to be encountered in the environment or workplace, *Carcinogenesis*, 16, 165, 1995.
81. Rappaport, S.M. and Fraser, D.A., Air sampling and analysis in a rubber vulcanization area, *Am. Ind. Hyg. Assoc. J.*, 38, 205, 1977.
82. Smith, B.J., Mattison, D.R., and Sipes, I.G., The role of epoxidation in 4-vinylcyclohexene-induced ovarian toxicity, *Toxicol. Appl. Pharmacol.*, 105, 372, 1990.
83. National Toxicology Program (NTP), NTP Technical Report No. 303, U.S. Department of Health and Human Services, Public Health Service National Institutes of Health Public Information, Research Triangle Park, NC, 1986.
84. Grizzle, T.B., George, J.D., Fail, P.A., Seely, J.C., and Heindel, J.J., Reproductive effects of 4-vinylcyclohexene in Swiss mice assessed by a continuous breeding protocol, *Fundam. Appl. Toxicol.*, 22, 122, 1994.
85. Kao, S.-W., Sipes, I.G., and Hoyer, P.B., Early effects of ovotoxicity induced by 4-vinylcyclohexene diepoxide in rats and mice, *Reprod. Toxicol.*, 13, 67, 1999.
86. National Toxicology Program (NTP), NTP Technical Report No. 362, U.S. Department of Health and Human Services, Public Health Service National Institutes of Health Public Information, Research Triangle Park, NC, 1989.
87. Bevan C., Keller, D.A., Panepinto, A.S., and Bently, K.S., Effect of 4-vinylcyclohexene on micronucleus formation in the bone marrow of rats and mice, *Drug Chem. Toxicol.*, 24, 273, 2001.

88. Kari, F.W., Huff, J.E., Leininger, J., Haseman, J.K., and Eustis, S.L., Toxicity and carcinogenicity of nitrofurazone in F344/N rats and B6C3F1 mice, *Food Chem. Toxicol.*, 27, 129, 1989.

89. Hemminki, K., Falck, K., and Vainio, H., Comparison of alkylation rates and mutagenicity of directly acting industrial and laboratory chemicals: epoxides, glycidyl ethers, methylating and ethylating agents, halogenated hydrocarbons, hydrazine derivatives, aldehydes, thiuram and dithiocarbamate derivatives, *Arch. Toxicol.*, 46, 277, 1980.

90. Sevcik, M.L. and Jarrell, J.F., *Comprehensive Toxicology*, 10, Elsevier Press, Oxford, 1997, 369.

91. Ataya, K., Rao, L.V., Lawrence, E., and Kimmel, R., Luteinizing hormone-releasing hormone agonist inhibits cyclophosphamide-induced ovarian follicular depletion in rhesus monkeys., *Biol. Reprod.*, 52, 365, 1995.

92. Krarup, T., Oocyte survival in the mouse ovary after treatment with 9,10-dimethyl-1,2-benzanthracene, *J. Endocrinol.*, 46, 483, 1970.

93. Mattison, D.R., Morphology of oocyte and follicle destruction by polycyclic aromatic hydrocarbons in mice, *Toxicol. Appl. Pharmacol.*, 53, 249, 1980.

94. Swartz, W.J. and Mattison, D.R., Benzo(a)pyrene inhibits ovulation in C57BL/6N mice, *Anat. Rec.*, 212, 268, 1985.

95. Kavlock, R., Boekelheide, K., Chapin, R., Cunningham, M., Faustman, E., Foster, P., Golub, M., Henderson, R., Hinberg, I., Little, R., Seed, J., Shea, K., Tabacova, S., Tyl, R., Williams, P., and Zacharewski, T., NTP Center for the Evaluation of Risks to Human Reproduction: phthalates expert panel report on the reproductive and developmental toxicity of di(2-ethylhexyl) phthalate, *Reprod. Toxicol.*, 16, 529, 2002.

96. Lan, Z.J., Gu, P., Xu, X., Jackson, K.J., DeMayo, F.J., O'Malley, B.W., and Cooney, A.J., GCNF-dependent repression of BMP-15 and GDF-9 mediates gamete regulation of female fertility, *EMBO J.*, 22, 4070, 2003.

97. Blount, B.C., Silva, M.J., Caudill, S.P., Needham, L.L., Pirkle, J.L., Sampson, E.J., Lucier, G.W., Jackson, R.J., and Brock, J.W., Levels of seven urinary phthalate metabolites in a human reference population, *Environ. Health Perspect.*, 108, 979, 2000.

98. Fay, M., Donohue, J.M., and De Rosa, C., ATSDR evaluation of health effects of chemicals. VI. Di(2-ethylhexyl)phthalate. Agency for Toxic Substances and Disease Registry, *Toxicol. Ind. Health*, 15, 651, 1999.

99. Tabacova, S., Little, R., and Balabaeva, L., Maternal exposure to phthalates and complications of pregnancy, *Epidemiology*, 10, S127, 1999.

100. Aldyreva, M.V., Klimova, T.S., Iziumova, A.S., and Timofeevskaia, L.A., [The effect of phthalate plasticizers on the generative function], *Gig. Tr. Prof. Zabol.*, 25, 1975.

101. Lovekamp-Swan, T. and Davis, B.J., Mechanisms of phthalate ester toxicity in the female reproductive system, *Environ. Health Perspect.*, 111, 139, 2003.

102. Fan, L.Q., Cattley, R.C., and Corton, J.C., Tissue-specific induction of 17 beta-hydroxysteroid dehydrogenase type IV by peroxisome proliferator chemicals is dependent on the peroxisome proliferator-activated receptor alpha, *J. Endocrinol.*, 158, 237, 1998.

103. Lovekamp, T.N. and Davis, B.J., Mono-(2-ethylhexyl) phthalate suppresses aromatase transcript levels and estradiol production in cultured rat granulosa cells, *Toxicol. Appl. Pharmacol.*, 172, 217, 2001.

104. Lovekamp-Swan, T., Jetten, A.M., and Davis, B.J., Dual activation of PPARalpha and PPARgamma by mono-(2-ethylhexyl) phthalate in rat ovarian granulosa cells, *Mol. Cell. Endocrinol.*, 201, 133, 2003.

105. Safe, S. and Krishnan, V., Chlorinated hydrocarbons: estrogens and antiestrogens, *Toxicol. Lett.*, 82-83, 731, 1995.
106. Li, X., Johnson, D.C., and Rozman, K.K., Effects of 2,3,7,8-tetrachlorodibenzo-*p*-dioxin (TCDD) on estrous cyclicity and ovulation in female Sprague-Dawley rats, *Toxicol. Lett.*, 78, 219, 1995.
107. Li, X., Johnson, D.C., and Rozman, K.K., Reproductive effects of 2,3,7,8-tetrachlorodibenzo-*p*-dioxin (TCDD) in female rats: ovulation, hormonal regulation, and possible mechanism(s), *Toxicol. Appl. Pharmacol.*, 133, 321, 1995.
108. Moran, F.M., Conley, A.J., Corbin, C.J., Enan, E., VandeVoort, C., Overstreet, J.W., and Lasley, B.L., 2,3,7,8-tetrachlorodibenzo-*p*-dioxin decreases estradiol production without altering the enzyme activity of cytochrome P450 aromatase of human luteinized granulosa cells *in vitro*, *Biol. Reprod.*, 62, 1102, 2000.
109. Lucier, G.W., Davis, G.J., and McLachlan, J.A., *Hanford Biology Symposium Monograph*, Oak Ridge Technical Information Centre, 1977, 188.
110. Wardell, R.E., Seegmiller, R.E., and Bradshaw, W.S., Induction of prenatal toxicity in the rat by diethylstilbestrol, zeranol, 3,4,3′,4′,-tetrachlorobiphenyl, cadmium, and lead, *Teratology*, 26, 229, 1982.
111. Ronnback, C. and de Rooij, D.G., Effects of 3,3′,4,4′-tetrachlorobiphenyl on foetal germ cells in two mouse strains after repeated treatment of the dams during and after pregnancy, *Pharmacol. Toxicol.*, 74, 287, 1994.
112. Ishikawa, H., Tian, Y., and Yamauchi, T., Induction of micronuclei formation in preimplantation mouse embryos after maternal treatment with 2-bromopropane, *Reprod. Toxicol.*, 15, 81, 2001.
113. Bengtsson, M. and Rydstrom, J., Regulation of carcinogen metabolism in the rat ovary by the estrous cycle and gonadotropin, *Science*, 219, 1437, 1983.
114. Mukhtar, H., Philpot, R.M., and Bend, J.R., The postnatal development of microsomal expoxide hydrase, cytosolic glutathione S-transferase, and mitochondrial and microsomal cytochrome P-450 in adrenals and ovaries of female rats, *Drug Metab. Dispos.*, 6, 577, 1978.
115. Mukhtar, H., Philpot, R.M., and Bend, J.R., Epoxide-metabolizing enzyme activities and cytochrome P-450 content of rat ovaries during pregnancy, *Biochem. Biophys. Res. Commun.*, 81, 89, 1978.
116. Bengtsson, M., Reinholt, F.P., and Rydstrom, J., Cellular localization and hormonal regulation of 7,12-dimethylbenz[a]anthracene mono-oxygenase activity in the rat ovary, *Toxicology*, 71, 203, 1992.
117. Heinrichs, W.L. and Juchau, M.R., *Extrahepatic metabolism of drugs and other foreign compounds*, SP Medical and Scientific Books, New York, 1980, 1, 319.
118. Toft, E., Becedas, L., Soderstrom, M., Lundqvist, A., and Depierre, J.W., Glutathione transferase isoenzyme patterns in the rat ovary, *Chem. Biol. Interact.*, 108, 79, 1997.
119. Tiltman, A.J. and Haffajee, Z., Distribution of glutathione S-transferases in the human ovary: an immunohistochemical study, *Gynecol. Obstet. Invest.*, 47, 247, 1999.
120. Meirow, D. and Nugent, D., The effects of radiotherapy and chemotherapy on female reproduction, *Hum. Reprod. Update*, 7, 535, 2001.
121. Anderson, D., Bishop, J.B., Garner, R.C., Ostrosky-Wegman, P., and Selby, P.B., Cyclophosphamide: review of its mutagenicity for an assessment of potential germ cell risks, *Mutat. Res.*, 330, 115, 1995.
122. Sims, P., The metabolic activation of chemical carcinogens, *Br. Med. Bull.*, 36, 11, 1980.
123. Mattison, D.R., Singh, H., Takizawa, K., and Thomford, P.J., Ovarian toxicity of benzo(a)pyrene and metabolites in mice, *Reprod. Toxicol.*, 3, 115, 1989.

124. Bengtsson, M. and Mattison, D.R., Gonadotropin-dependent metabolism of 7,12-dimethylbenz(a)anthracene in the ovary of rhesus monkey, *Biochem. Pharmacol.*, 38, 1869, 1989.

125. Bengtsson, M., Hamberger, L., and Rydstrom, J., Metabolism of 7,12-dimethyl-benz(a)anthracene by different types of cells in the human ovary, *Xenobiotica*, 18, 1255, 1988.

126. Mumtaz, M.M., George, J.D., Gold, K.W., Cibulas, W., and DeRosa, C.T., ATSDR evaluation of health effects of chemicals. IV. Polycyclic aromatic hydrocarbons (PAHs): understanding a complex problem, *Toxicol. Ind. Health*, 12, 742, 1996.

127. Sims, P., Epoxides as reactive intermediates in aromatic hydrocarbon metabolism, *Biochem. Soc. Trans.*, 3, 59, 1975.

128. Shiromizu, K. and Mattison, D.R., The effect of intraovarian injection of benzo(a)pyrene on primordial oocyte number and ovarian aryl hydrocarbon, *Toxicol. Appl. Pharmacol.*, 76, 18, 1984.

129. Mattison, D.R. and Nightingale, M.S., Oocyte destruction by polycyclic aromatic hydrocarbons is not linked to the inducibility of ovarian aryl hydrocarbon (benzo(a)pyrene) hydroxylase activity in (DBA/2N X C57BL/6N) F1 X DBA/2N backcross mice, *Pediatr. Pharmacol. (New York)*, 2, 11, 1982.

130. Smith, B.J., Carter, D.E., and Sipes, I.G., Comparison of the disposition and *in vitro* metabolism of 4-vinylcyclohexene in the female mouse and rat, *Toxicol. Appl. Pharmacol.*, 105, 364, 1990.

131. Smith, B.J., Mattison, D.R., and Sipes, I.G., *Biological Reactive Intermediates IV*, Plenum Press, New York, 1990, 465.

132. Keller, D.A., Carpenter, S.C., Cagen, S.Z., and Reitman, F.A., *In vitro* metabolism of 4-vinylcyclohexene in rat and mouse liver, lung, and ovary, *Toxicol. Appl. Pharmacol.*, 144, 36, 1997.

133. Fontaine, S.M., Hoyer, P.B., Halpert, J.R., and Sipes, I.G., Role of induction of specific hepatic cytochrome P450 isoforms in epoxidation of 4-vinylcyclohexene, *Drug Metab. Dispos.*, 29, 1236, 2001.

134. Csanady, G.A., Guengerich, F.P., and Bond, J.A., Comparison of the biotransformation of 1,3-butadiene and its metabolite, butadiene monoepoxide, by hepatic and pulmonary tissues from humans, rats and mice, *Carcinogenesis*, 13, 1143, 1992.

135. Watabe, T., Hiratsuka, A., Isobe, M., and Ozawa, N., Metabolism of d-limonene by hepatic microsomes to non-mutagenic epoxides toward Salmonella typhimurium, *Biochem. Pharmacol.*, 29, 1068, 1980.

136. Giannarini, C., Citti, L., Gervasi, P.G., and Turchi, G., Effects of 4-vinylcyclohexene and its main oxirane metabolite on mouse hepatic microsomal enzymes and glutathione levels, *Toxicol. Lett.*, 8, 115, 1981.

137. Devine, P.J., Sipes, I.G., and Hoyer, P.B., Effect of 4-vinylcyclohexene diepoxide dosing in rats on GSH levels in liver and ovaries, *Toxicol. Sci.*, 62, 315, 2001.

138. Flaws, J.A., Salyers, K.L., Sipes, I.G., and Hoyer, P.B., Reduced ability of rat preantral ovarian follicles to metabolize 4-vinyl-1-cyclohexene diepoxide *in vitro*, *Toxicol. Appl. Pharmacol.*, 126, 286, 1994.

139. Johnson, A.L., Intracellular mechanisms regulating cell survival in ovarian follicles, *Anim. Reprod. Sci.*, 78, 185, 2003.

140. Ray, S.D., Sorge, C.L., Raucy, J.L., and Corcoran, G.B., Early loss of large genomic DNA *in vivo* with accumulation of Ca2+ in the nucleus during acetaminophen-induced liver injury, *Toxicol. Appl. Pharmacol.*, 106, 346, 1990.

141. Collins, R.J., Harmon, B.V., Gobe, G.C., and Kerr, J.F., Internucleosomal DNA cleavage should not be the sole criterion for identifying apoptosis, *Int. J. Radiat. Biol.*, 61, 451, 1992.

142. Pritchard, D.J. and Butler, W.H., Apoptosis—the mechanism of cell death in dimethylnitrosamine-induced hepatotoxicity, *J. Pathol.*, 158, 253, 1989.

143. Hirata, K., Ogata, I., Ohta, Y., and Fujiwara, K., Hepatic sinusoidal cell destruction in the development of intravascular coagulation in acute liver failure of rats, *J. Pathol.*, 158, 157, 1989.

144. Corcoran, G.B., Fix, L., Jones, D.P., Moslen, M.T., Nicotera, P., Oberhammer, F.A., and Buttyan, R., Apoptosis: molecular control point in toxicity, *Toxicol. Appl. Pharmacol.*, 128, 169, 1994.

145. Springer, L.N., Flaws, J.A., Sipes, I.G., and Hoyer, P.B., Follicular mechanisms associated with 4-vinylcyclohexene diepoxide-induced ovotoxicity in rats, *Reprod. Toxicol.*, 10, 137, 1996.

146. Shen, W., Kamendulis, L.M., Ray, S.D., and Corcoran, G.B., Acetaminophen-induced cytotoxicity in cultured mouse hepatocytes: correlation of nuclear Ca2+ accumulation and early DNA fragmentation with cell death, *Toxicol. Appl. Pharmacol.*, 111, 242, 1991.

147. Faa, G., Ambu, R., Congiu, T., Costa, V., Ledda-Columbano, G.M., Coni, P., Curto, M., Giacomini, L., and Columbano, A., Early ultrastructural changes during thioacetamide-induced apoptosis in rat liver, *J. Submicrosc. Cytol. Pathol.*, 24, 417, 1992.

148. McConkey, D.J., Hartzell, P., Nicotera, P., Wyllie, A.H., and Orrenius, S., Stimulation of endogenous endonuclease activity in hepatocytes exposed to oxidative stress, *Toxicol. Lett.*, 42, 123, 1988.

149. Burchiel, S.W., Davis, D.A., Ray, S.D., Archuleta, M.M., Thilsted, J.P., and Corcoran, G.B., DMBA-induced cytotoxicity in lymphoid and nonlymphoid organs of B6C3F1 mice: relation of cell death to target cell intracellular calcium and DNA damage, *Toxicol. Appl. Pharmacol.*, 113, 126, 1992.

150. Springer, L.N., Tilly, J.L., Sipes, I.G., and Hoyer, P.B., Enhanced expression of *bax* in small preantral follicles during 4-vinylcyclohexene diepoxide-induced ovotoxicity in the rat, *Toxicol. Appl. Pharmacol.*, 139, 402, 1996.

151. Hu, X., Christian, P.J., Sipes, I.G., and Hoyer, P.B., Expression and redistribution of cellular Bad, Bax, and Bcl-X(L) protein is associated with VCD-induced ovotoxicity in rats, *Biol. Reprod.*, 65, 1489, 2001.

152. Hu, X.M., Christian, P.J., Thompson, K.E., Sipes, I.G., and Hoyer, P.B., Apoptosis induced in rats by 4-vinylcyclohexene diepoxide is associated with activation of the caspase cascades, *Biol. Reprod.*, 65, 87, 2001.

153. Takai, Y., Canning, J., Perez, G.I., Pru, J.K., Schlezinger, J.J., Sherr, D.H., Kolesnick, R.N., Yuan, J., Flavell, R.A., Korsmeyer, S.J., and Tilly, J.L., Bax, caspase-2, and caspase-3 are required for ovarian follicle loss caused by 4-vinylcyclohexene diepoxide exposure of female mice *in vivo*, *Endocrinology*, 144, 69, 2003.

154. Wade, M.J., Moyer, J.W., and Hine, C.H., Mutagenic action of a series of epoxides, *Mutat. Res.*, 66, 367, 1979.

155. Citti, L., Gervasi, P.G., Turchi, G., Bellucci, G., and Bianchini, R., The reaction of 3,4-epoxy-1-butene with deoxyguanosine and DNA *in vitro*: synthesis and characterization of the main adducts, *Carcinogenesis*, 5, 47, 1984.

156. de Raat, W.K., Induction of sister chromatid exchanges by styrene and its presumed metabolite styrene oxide in the presence of rat liver homogenate, *Chem. Biol. Interact.*, 20, 163, 1978.

157. Albanese, R., Induction and transmission of chemically induced chromosome aberrations in female germ cells, *Environ. Mol. Mutagen.*, 10, 231, 1987.

158. Meirow, D., Epstein, M., Lewis, H., Nugent, D., and Gosden, R.G., Administration of cyclophosphamide at different stages of follicular maturation in mice: effects on reproductive performance and fetal malformations, *Hum. Reprod.*, 16, 632, 2001.

159. Tiveron, C., Ranaldi, R., Bassani, B., and Pacchierotti, F., Induction and transmission of chromosome aberrations in mouse oocytes after treatment with butadiene diepoxide, *Environ. Mol. Mutagen.*, 30, 403, 1997.

160. Turchi, G., Bonatti, S., Citti, L., Gervasi, P.G., and Abbondandolo, A., Alkylating properties and genetic activity of 4-vinylcyclohexene metabolites and structurally related epoxides, *Mutat. Res.*, 83, 419, 1981.

4 p, p'-DDE and HCB: Mechanisms of Toxicity to Fetal and Embryonic Mammalian Cells

Michael A. Edelbrock, Martha J. Fernstrom, and Kandace J. Williams

CONTENTS

0-8493-2281-2/05/$0.00+$1.50
© 2005 by CRC Press

4.1 INTRODUCTION: *P, P'* – DDE (1,1-DICHLORO-2,2-BIS(*P*-CHLOROPHENYL)ETHYLENE) AND HCB(HEXACHLOROBENZENE)

Persistent organic pollutants, as classified by the Environmental Protection Agency (EPA), have now been detected in virtually all ecosystems throughout the world, including the few remote environments that do not have any history of direct exposure. Because of the stability and persistence of these man-made chemicals within the environment, long-distance transport can include atmospheric, terrestrial/freshwater, and marine pathways. Additionally, long-term lipid storage of these hydrophobic chemicals has resulted in bioaccumulation and biomagnification within the worldwide food chain.[1]

In this chapter, we focus primarily on two persistent organochlorine pollutants; *p, p'*–DDE (1,1-dichloro-2,2-*bis*(*p*-chlorophenyl)ethylene) and HCB (hexachlorobenzene) and their effects on mammalian systems, with specific emphasis on embryonic and fetal cells. There is significant evidence for endocrine disruption activities by each of these chemicals or specific metabolites. However, the wide range of physiological dysfunction that has been attributed to these persistent organochlorines indicate additional mechanisms of toxicity within the cell. The most sensitive target tissue is the growing embryo or fetus that has not yet developed mature defense mechanisms against these xenobiotics. Moreover, the process of rapid growth and development of sensitive organs and tissues, if perturbed, can have life-long consequences. Immature organ systems that are believed to be most sensitive to chronic exposure to these chemicals, evidenced by epidemiological and basic research, include the nervous system, immune response, reproductive tissue, liver enzymes, kidney function, and adrenal and thyroid glands.[1,2]

This chapter contains a summary of both known and hypothetical mechanisms of toxicity of these two persistent organic pollutants, some of which is still in debate. Further, we describe specific genotoxic and cytotoxic effects of these chemicals on immature cells at low environmental concentrations, both separately and as a mixture. Despite what is currently known, there is much yet to understand in regard to toxic effects of environmental doses of individual chemicals and of mixtures at the molecular, cellular, and whole organism level. Accurate predictions of risk cannot be established for individuals and populations as a whole until much more is understood in regard to all of the mechanisms of action of these persistent organic pollutants.

4.1.1 Description of DDT and DDE

DDT (1,1,1-trichloro-2,2-*bis*-(*p*-chlorophenyl)ethane) is a chlorinated organic pesticide that has been used extensively to control mosquitoes and other insects from the early 1940s throughout the 1960s. The use of DDT was banned in the United States in 1972 by the EPA because of mounting concerns over long-term effects of animal and human exposure. However, the use of DDT to combat malaria and other insect vector-borne diseases still continues in third-world countries. The most active isomer, *p, p′*-DDT, is classified as a persistent organic pollutant by the EPA. The International Agency for Research on Cancer (IARC) has also classified this isomer of DDT into Group 2B: possibly carcinogenic to humans.

The molecular structure of DDE (1,1-dichloro-2,2-*bis*(*p*-chlorophenyl)ethylene) is of an aromatic organochloride consisting of two benzene rings joined to an ethene moiety located between the rings. Each of the two phenyl groups contains one substituted chlorine, and the ethene moiety contains two chlorines. DDE exists primarily as different isomeric metabolites of DDT. These different isomeric forms of DDE exist based upon the position of the chloro-substituted benzenes. Similar to other aromatic organochlorides, DDE is soluble in organic solvents and lipids, but not in water. This review primarily focus on the *p, p′*-DDE isomer (hereafter DDE) derived from *p, p′*-DDT.

The phenyl groups of both the parent molecule, DDT, and metabolite, DDE, confer high stability to these compounds. The lipophilic nature and low volatility of these persistent organochlorines allow for long-term soil adherence. Within soil, DDT and DDE are exceedingly resistant to microbial degradation, with an estimated half-life of DDT of 2 to 15 years or longer, based upon soil matrix conditions and microbial content.[3] In contrast, within the air, both DDT and DDE are degraded rapidly by sunlight (UV radiation).

4.1.2 Description of HCB

HCB is an aromatic organochloride, consisting of a benzene ring substituted with chlorine in each of the six ring carbons. This configuration gives HCB a very stable chemical structure, low water solubility, and a highly lipophilic nature. These properties contribute to long-term stability of HCB in soil, air, water, and lipophilic environments. The estimated half-life of HCB in air and water is 2.6 to 6 years and in soil can be 6 years or longer.[4] The physical and chemical properties of HCB are well suited to its former uses, primarily as a wood preservative and fungicide from the 1940s through the 1980s. The lipophilic nature combined with low volatility allow for adherence and prolonged contact when applied to grain during fumigation operations. Unfortunately, these same properties confer onto HCB the ability to disperse throughout the environment and bioaccumulate through the worldwide food chain. For these reasons, HCB is classified as a persistent organic pollutant by the EPA. In addition, IARC has classified HCB into Group 2B: possibly carcinogenic to humans.

4.2   DDE: OVERVIEW OF TOXIC MECHANISMS AND EFFECTS

Over the past 60 years, DDT, and especially DDE, have been bioaccumulating throughout the worldwide food chain. Concentrations within human and animal tissue have been measured since the late 1960s by the National Human Monitoring Program and in the early 1970s by the National Human Adipose Tissue Survey. These programs have documented steadily declining, but still detectable, concentrations in all tissues examined. Liver, kidney, nervous system, and adipose tissue are the main storage sites for DDT and its metabolites.[2] Moreover, preferential accumulation in adipose tissue, breast milk, and serum have been correlated to virtually all geographic areas, but are generally higher in Africa, Asia, and Latin America as compared to Europe or the USA.[5] This comes as no surprise given the current widespread use of DDT in areas of the former group of countries.

Human exposure to acute doses of DDT targets the central and peripheral nervous system, manifesting as tremors, excitability, dizziness, malaise, convulsions, and nausea.[2] These effects have been documented for known human exposure occurring primarily in the pesticide application and chemical manufacturing environments. However, there has been one remarkable study, conducted in the 1940s, in which oral doses were given to human volunteers with similar results.[6] Studies using animal models have demonstrated similar effects to the nervous system, with high doses of DDT resulting in convulsions and death from respiratory distress. It is not known what role the metabolite, DDE, may play in acute toxicity from exposure to DDT.[3]

Chronic exposure to DDT and its metabolite, DDE, have been associated with liver and kidney toxicity, carcinogenesis, immune response disruption, reproductive effects, and endocrine disruption.[3] Environmental concentrations of DDE within prenatal and postnatal populations throughout the world have been repeatedly established by measurements of DDE in cord blood, as well as maternal serum, lipids, and breast milk.[5,7-9] Animal models have demonstrated the transfer of DDE from mother to infant during prenatal development.[10] The preferential accumulation of DDE in lipid-rich areas of the body, combined with mobilization of lipids during lactation, support the hypothesis of increased postnatal exposure associated with breastfeeding. Postpartum exposure to DDE through lactation is likely the cause of high infant body burdens, and this is supported by both rodent and human studies. In one rat model, the transplacental transfer of DDE has been compared to lactational transfer.[10] These experiments have demonstrated an estimated 50 times higher concentration of DDE in the livers of pups exposed through lactation when compared with DDE concentrations during *in utero* exposure. Likewise, in humans, DDE concentrations are estimated to progressively increase in lactating infants, peaking at 6 months postpartum. The average 6-month North American postpartum DDE concentration range is estimated to be from 14.5 µg/kg to 187.4 µg/kg.[11] These reports clearly indicate that DDE is readily obtained from the environment, accumulated, and then transferred from mother to infant through lipid components of the milk.

Nevertheless, the effects of chronic environmental DDE exposure to the human fetus are not well characterized. Several researchers have demonstrated, however, that prenatal exposure to DDE in mammalian models can result in developmental defects. In particular, feminization of male rats exposed to DDE has been measured by a reduction in the anogenital distance and increased retention of thoracic nipples.[12,13] Other developmental effects of DDE exposure to prenatal rats include reduced sperm production, delayed onset of puberty, and reduced seminal vesicle, prostate, and testicular weight.[12,14] The ability of DDE to act as an antiandrogen has been experimentally demonstrated by both *in vitro* and *in vivo* studies.[12,15] In these experiments, DDE was demonstrated to bind to the androgen receptor (AR) with high affinity and competitively inhibit the expression of androgen-regulated genes. Other experiments have shown that DDE is antiandrogenic by its ability to attenuate the effects of testosterone propionate.[16]

The metabolism of DDT is carried out through dechlorination and dehydrocholorination, while DDE metabolism is by methylsulfonation events. A multi-step mechanism has been described based upon rodent studies using radioisotope labels.[17,18] It has been proposed that DDD is first formed by dechlorination of DDT, followed by oxygenation and eventual formation of 2,2 *bis*(*p*-chlorophenyl)acetic acid (DDA). *In vitro* studies using rat liver microsomes have demonstrated a predominance of the metabolite DDD over DDE during DDT metabolism.[19] While not all of the intermediate metabolites in these studies have been measured in humans, it has been presumed that the metabolic breakdown of DDT is similar to that found in rodents, with DDA the presumed endpoint for urinary elimination.[3] These studies, and others, have raised several questions regarding the role of DDE during the metabolism of DDT. Although clearly associated with the metabolism of DDT, it appears that DDE does not play an essential role within the elimination pathway of DDT by the body. Further, formation of DDE from DDT may actually prolong xenobiotic removal, as further metabolism of DDE to an excretable alcohol or acetic acid derivative is not readily accomplished. Indeed, administration of DDT or DDD has been demonstrated to result in excretable DDA formation, whereas administration of DDE did not appreciably metabolize to DDA.[3] This may indicate that DDE is not a predominant pathway of DDT metabolism, and therefore the deposition and presence of DDE in human tissues is evidence of an alternative and less-efficient metabolic pathway.

One likely pathway for the further metabolism of DDE involves the formation and bioactivation of methylsulfonyl-DDE (MeSO$_2$-DDE). Methylsulfonyl conjugates are present in the metabolism of several different organochlorines, and MeSO$_2$-DDE has been isolated in humans and several animals species.[20-22] Interestingly, this metabolite was first isolated from seal blubber in the Baltic region.[6] As well, there have been measurable levels of MeSO$_2$-DDE in human milk samples collected in Stockholm.[20] It is thought that MeSO$_2$-DDE can induce damage through conjugation reactions with cellular proteins and may specifically target adrenal tissue. Studies with mice have demonstrated a p450-induced mitochondrial degeneration and subsequent cellular necrosis of adrenal tissue by MeSO$_2$-DDE.[23] This has also been demonstrated to occur during fetal development.[24,25] Similarly, p450-catalyzed binding of MeSO$_2$-DDE within human adrenal tissue has been reported.[26] Similar binding effects of methylsulfonyl metabolites of other organochloride pollutants (notably polychlorinated biphenyls [PCBs]) are also subject to increasing investigation.[27]

These studies raise concerns for developmental damage due to deregulation of adrenal hormones and cytotoxic damage.

Many pesticides, including DDT, specifically target the liver and induce hepatotoxic effects. Human data are still limited as to the exact contribution of low environmental body burdens of DDT and DDE in regard to hepatotoxicity. Epidemiological evidence that organochlorines, including DDT, can increase human liver enzyme function has been suggested by several investigators.[3] Similar to other xenobiotic hydrocarbon derivatives, metabolism of both DDT and DDE appears to take place primarily in the hepatic cytochrome p450 (CYP) pathway. DDT administered to rodents has resulted in dose-dependent effects such as altered liver enzyme function and increased liver weights. Specifically, DDT, DDE, and DDD have been shown to induce rat hepatic cytochrome p450 content.[28,29] Interestingly, investigators have measured a sex-dependent induction of specific cytochrome p450 proteins (CYPs 2B and 3A) by DDT.[30] This raises the possibility that endocrine disruption by DDT may be, in part, mediated through induction of CYP isoenzyme expression.

Neither carcinogenic potential nor mechanisms of action of DDE in humans have been resolved at this time, even though IARC has categorized DDT as possibly carcinogenic to humans. This designation is based primarily on animal (rodent) studies. Evidence for the carcinogenic potential of DDT and DDE in rodents surfaced in the late 1970s in studies using mouse and hamster models. In one study, DDE has been shown to induce liver tumors in mice.[31] In addition, both male and female mice administered DDE developed a significant increase in hepatocellular carcinomas during studies conducted through the National Toxicology Program.[32] Further evidence of the carcinogenicity of DDE and DDT has been determined in hamsters administered either DDE or DDT; however, only DDE caused a significantly higher incidence of hepatocellular tumors within these studies. However, hyperplastic foci in liver tissue, as well as adrenocortical adenomas, were more frequent in hamsters given either DDE or DDT, as compared to controls.[33] In yet another study, the exposure of neonatal rats to high doses of DDE, and other organochlorines, resulted in a significant increase in methylnitrosourea (MNU)-induced mammary tumors.[34] Unfortunately, the investigators used a combination of DDE, DDT, and PCBs as the putative promoters; therefore, the individual tumor-promoting effects of DDE and DDT were not determined. However, DDT and its metabolites may play a specific role in cellular gap junctional mechanisms of communication during tumor promotion. Gap junctional communication is believed to signal cell homeostasis and therefore may act as a tumor-suppressing mechanism. Researchers have shown that DDT can interfere with the expression (and possibly phosphorylation) of connexin43 in rat epithelial cells and that this is concentration dependent.[35] Thus, DDT and its metabolite, DDE, may act as both an initiator and a promoter in rodents, depending on the dose and duration of exposure.

The genotoxic effects of DDT and DDE have been examined by both *in vivo* and *in vitro* studies since the early 1970s. Chromosomal aberrations have been demonstrated to occur within human lymphocytes, as well as in rat liver cells after exposure to these chemicals. Similarly, *in vitro* mammalian cell systems have demonstrated chromosomal aberrations after exposure to either DDE or DDT.[3] Moreover, DDE has been demonstrated to initiate double-strand DNA breaks in Chinese hamster cells.[36]

To date, there has not been a direct link between DDT or DDE body burden from chronic environmental exposure and human carcinogenesis. Several epidemiological studies have attempted to correlate DDE exposure and body burden to an increased risk of breast cancer. Many of these studies did not find correlation between DDE or DDT levels and tumorigenesis.[37-39] Other studies, however, have found an association of DDE or other organochlorine levels with breast cancer risk or metastasis to lymph nodes.[40-42] Additionally, researchers have implicated DDT in the promotion of estrogen-responsive tumors.[43,44] Many of these studies are difficult to evaluate as there is limited knowledge in regard to magnitude, route, or duration of exposure for the women surveyed.

Collectively, these and other studies have demonstrated a potential association of DDT, DDE, or other metabolites with the cancer process. Genotoxic effects of this persistent organic pollutant may lead to damage or alterations in gene expression and initiate cell transformation. As well, epigenetic effects such as interference with gap junctional communication, disruption of estrogen signaling, or other mechanisms may serve to prevent apoptosis, promote clonal expansion, and therefore contribute to the carcinogenic process. Further investigation is clearly needed to elucidate the mechanistic involvement of DDT and DDE and other metabolites in the cancer process.

4.2.1 EFFECTS OF DDE ON FETAL AND EMBRYONIC MAMMALIAN CELLS AT LOW ENVIRONMENTAL CONCENTRATIONS

Concentrations of DDE (specifically p, p -DDE) used in the research described below were determined by the mean concentration measured in human newborn cord blood samples. These blood samples were obtained from an ethnic group living an indigenous life-style in a geographic area within the Arctic. This population has, therefore, not been directly exposed to DDT.[45] Thus, the relatively low, but nonetheless consistently detectable, concentrations of DDE (but not DDT) measured in this human population most likely derive from a combination of biotransformation and bioaccumulation through the worldwide food chain. Each table or figure within this section containing the term "1X DDE" is the arithmetic mean of measured cord blood concentrations and is equal to 0.35 μg DDE per liter of media, "10X DDE" is equal to 3.5 μg DDE per liter of media, etc.[45]

DDE exposure to immature mammalian cells was investigated to determine whether relevant environmental concentrations of this persistent organic pollutant had any measurable short- or long-term toxic effects. Fibroblasts were chosen for this study as they are relatively unspecialized and represent the majority of cells within an embryo or fetus that do not have any significant capacity to further metabolize DDE. These immature cells are also unlikely to contribute significantly to potential endocrine-mediated effects of this metabolite of DDT. Thus, by decreasing the effects of cellular metabolic or endocrine activity to the smallest amount possible, we have been able to study mechanisms of direct toxicity of this persistent organic pollutant within mammalian cells. Potential toxic effects other than endocrine disruption resulting from the ongoing global accumulation of these organic pollutants are especially important to understand with regard to embryonic and fetal cells still in the process of undergoing programmed development, as these are the most vulnerable cells that are directly exposed to these ubiquitous chemicals.

Two cell types were chosen for these studies. NIH 3T3 cells are an immortal aneuploid murine embryonic fibroblast cell line. WS1 cells are primary human fetal fibroblasts with a normal chromosome number. Inclusion of these two distinct immature cell types in this study gave us the ability to identify the common effects of DDE on different immature mammalian cells as well as those effects unique to either cell type.

4.2.2 SHORT-TERM EFFECTS OF DDE TOXICITY ON IMMATURE MAMMALIAN CELLS

We initially observed that NIH 3T3 cells exhibited a decrease in total number of cells per plate in both 1X and 10X DDE treated samples by 2 to 4 hours exposure, as compared to control plates exposed to the acetone vehicle alone (results not shown).[45] By 24 hours, however, all plates were confluent, indicating the number of NIH 3T3 cells on all plates were similar. We similarly observed that WS1 cells exposed to 1X or 10X DDE for 2 to 4 hours exhibited a decrease in cell number in comparison to controls. In contrast to the NIH 3T3 cells, we did not find a recovery in the number of DDE-treated WS1 cells equal to control plates by the 24-hour time point.[45] Therefore, we measured cell viability by trypan blue assay to determine if observed decreases in cell number were the result of cell death.

The percentages of viable NIH 3T3 and WS1 cells that result from exposure to 1X or 10X DDE for 2 or 4 hours are depicted in Table 4.1. As compared to controls, there was a significant decrease in the percent of viable NIH 3T3 cells after 2 and 4 hours exposure to both 1X and 10X DDE ($p < 0.05$). However, at 6 to 12 hours (data not shown) there were no significant differences between the amount of cell death found on control NIH 3T3 plates or those plates treated with 1X or 10X DDE. Interestingly, WS1 cells treated with 1X or 10X DDE for 2, 4 (Table 4.1), or 6 hours (results not shown) exhibited no increase in cell death as compared to controls.[45] This indicates that the decrease in cell number after DDE exposure to WS1 cells are not due to cell death, unlike NIH 3T3 cells.

The "comet assay"[46] was then performed to determine if exposure to 1X or 10X DDE resulted in chromosomal damage. When assayed by alkaline electrophoresis, DNA damage, specifically single-strand breaks, result in an increased displacement between the leading edge of chromosomal DNA and the end of the tail (comet) and is apparent by an increase in total length of chromosomal DNA as measured within individual cells. Table 4.2 contains the average measurements from comet assays of NIH 3T3 and WS1 cells exposed to acetone alone (control), 1X or 10X DDE for 4 hours. When compared to controls, there was a significant increase in NIH 3T3 chromosomal DNA length after 4 hours exposure to both 1X and 10X DDE ($p < 0.05$), although the increased length within each treatment group was not significantly different from each other. In contrast, the chromosomal DNA lengths of WS1 cells treated with acetone alone (control), 1X, or 10X DDE for 4 hours were not significantly different from each other. Thus for NIH 3T3 cells, the decreased

TABLE 4.1
DDE: SHORT-TERM CELL VIABILITY[a]

Cell Type	Treatment	Percent (%) of Viable Cells	
		2h	4h
NIH 3T3	Control	97.6%	90.7%
	1X DDE	93.6%[b]	86.1%[b]
	10X DDE	91.1%[b]	82.6%[b]
WS1	Control	94.4%	93.3%
	1X DDE	96.1%	93.7%
	10X DDE	96.5%	93.3%

[a] Non-viable cells were identified by permeability to 0.4% trypan blue, as compared to impermeable viable cells. The number of non-viable cells was determined as a percentage (%) of the total number of cells counted and then subtracted from 100 to express the % of viable cells. Total number of cells counted was ≥ 1000 for all time points and treatments.

[b] Significant increase ($p < 0.05$) in cell death, by 2 or 4 hours of 1X or 10X DDE treatment, as compared to NIH 3T3 control cells exposed to the acetone vehicle alone, as determined by one-way ANOVA and Schiffe's comparisons. (Modified from Simonetti, J., Berner, J. and Williams, K., *Toxicology in Vitro*, 15, 169, 2001. With permission.)

percentage of viable cells might be the result of increased cytotoxicity due to DNA damage after DDE exposure.

The effects of 1X and 10X DDE on the progression of NIH 3T3 and WS1 cells through the cell cycle are shown in Figure 4.1. Flow cytometric results reveal no significant differences between the percentage of dividing cells (S phase) in the control, 1X, or 10X DDE-treated NIH 3T3 cells at the time points tested between 0 hour and 30 hours (Figure 4.1A).

WS1 control cells have a similar cell cycle profile as NIH 3T3 cells, in that cells begin to divide by 4 hours after exposure to acetone vehicle alone (Figure 4.1B). In contrast, 1X DDE-treated WS1 cells did not begin to divide until 6 hours after the initiation of DDE exposure. Furthermore, the 1X DDE-treated cells maintain the 2-hour lag in the number of cells entering S phase for at least 30 hours after the chemical has been added. WS1 cells treated with 10X DDE could not be measured by this flow cytometric technique, as this treatment group of cells could not survive the combined flow cytometric protocol plus exposure to 10X DDE. Clearly, the WS1 cells' ability to slow or arrest their cell cycle after exposure to DDE contributes toward the decreased cell number we initially observed. This ability to alter cell

TABLE 4.2
DDE: CHROMOSOMAL DAMAGE[a]

Cell Type	Treatment 4h	Total DNA Length
NIH 3T3	Control	15.9 ± 1.4 mm
	1X DDE	18.7 ± 1.8 mm[b]
	10X DDE	19.7 ± 2.7 mm[b]
WS 1	Control	14.7 ± 3.5 mm
	1X DDE	14.6 ± 4.2 mm
	10X DDE	14.2 ± 3.3 mm

[a] The comet assay was performed to determine if a 4-hour exposure to 1X or 10X DDE resulted in DNA damage. Single- and double-strand breaks within chromosomal DNA of individual cells results in an increased ability of the DNA to migrate through agarose during electophoresis and is observed as an increase in total DNA length. The total DNA length (the displacement between the leading edge of the chromosomal DNA and the end of the tail) of a minimum of 50 cells per treatment was measured and the average length calculated.

[b] Significant increase ($p < 0.05$) in DNA migration, indicating increased strand breakage, as compared to NIH 3T3 control cells, as determined by one-way ANOVA and Schiffe's comparisons. (From Simonetti, J., Berner, J. and Williams, K., *Toxicology in Vitro*, 15, 169, 2001. With permission.)

cycle kinetics may also contribute toward the increased percent of viable cells, due to increased time for DNA repair, when compared with NIH 3T3 cells.

We performed one additional short-term assay to investigate the effects of DDE on the intracellular redox state, by measuring alterations in cellular glutathione concentrations. Overall, cellular glutathione concentrations were altered more significantly in WS1 cells than in NIH 3T3 cells.[45] Others have noted, however, that alteration in glutathione concentrations within NIH 3T3 cells is not measurable under a variety of different circumstances (Clontech personal communication). Overall, reduced glutathione concentrations (GSH) in WS1 cells exposed to 1X or 10X DDE were significantly increased by 2 hours, followed by a significant decrease by 4 hours, with a return to normal levels by 6 hours after DDE exposure (results not shown).[45] Either increased oxidation of cellular substances requiring reduction by the GSH pathway is occurring to a larger extent in WS1 cells, or NIH 3T3 cells do not have effective use of their GSH reduction pathway (a possible metabolic defect leading to increased cell death within NIH 3T3 cells as compared to WS1 cells).

DDE: CELL CYCLE KINETICS

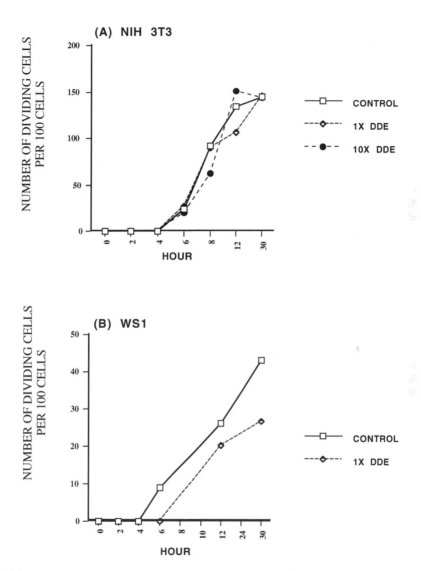

FIGURE 4.1 NIH 3T3 (A) and WS1 (B) cells were exposed to media containing BrdU, deoxycytidine, and either acetone alone (control), 1X, or 10X DDE. Samples (in duplicate) were harvested by trypsinization at the indicated time points and underwent BrdU–Hoescht flow cytometric analysis for number of dividing cells per 100 living cells. Data points representing WS1 cells exposed to 10X DDE are absent, as despite repeated trials, these cells could not survive both the cytometric protocol and DDE exposure. (From Simonetti, J., Berner, J., and Williams, K., *Toxicology in Vitro*, 15, 169, 2001. With permission.)

4.2.3 Long-Term Effects of DDE Toxicity on Immature Mammalian Cells

As indicated by Table 4.3, both 1X and 10X DDE had significant effects on the number of individual NIH 3T3 cells surviving to form colonies ($p < 0.05$). Exposure to DDE at both 1X and 10X concentrations resulted in a similarly significant decrease in the number of colonies formed per plate as compared to NIH 3T3 control cells. In contrast, neither 1X nor 10X DDE had an effect on the number of WS1 cells surviving to form colonies when compared with control cells. Therefore, the significant alteration of cell cycle kinetics of WS1 cells by DDE, as well as protective effects of the GSH/GSSG redox pathway, are likely protective effects for these immature human cells at these low environmental concentrations of DDE.[45]

A neoplastic transformation assay was also performed to determine if exposure to DDE affected the number of transformed foci arising within a population of NIH 3T3 cells. No significant difference was found between the number of NIH 3T3 foci formed within control plates or DDE exposed NIH 3T3 cells treated with up to 100X DDE, indicating that direct DDE exposure to these embryonic cells is not in and of itself carcinogenic (results not shown).[45] These results agree well with the literature, as discussed above, in that DDE does not appear to be a complete carcinogen in and of itself at low environmental concentrations. Therefore, it appears that the increased genotoxicity within NIH 3T3 cells observed by the comet assay (Table 4.2) contributes more significantly to cytotoxicity, resulting in cell death, than genotoxicity resulting in neoplastic transformation.

TABLE 4.3
DDE: COLONY FORMING ABILITY

Cell Type	Treatment	Percent (%) of Controls
NIH 3T3	1X DDE	57%*
	10X DDE	53%*
WS1	1X DDE	101%
	10X DDE	98%

Long-term survival of NIH 3T3 and WS1 cells chronically exposed to DDE was determined by the total number of subsequent colonies successfully formed after 10 days. Cell survival per treatment is expressed as a percentage (%) of the number of surviving colonies on the control plates. Percentages represent the average percentage survival from three independent experiments. Asterisk (*) indicates a significant difference from acetone alone (control) cells by one-way ANOVA ($p < 0.05$). (From Simonetti, J., Berner, J. and Williams, K., *Toxicology in Vitro*, 15, 169, 2001. With permission.)

4.3 HCB: OVERVIEW OF TOXIC MECHANISMS AND EFFECTS

Because of the long history of HCB manufacture and use, both acute and chronic health effects of this chemical in humans have been documented. During the late 1950s thousands of people in Turkey were acutely exposed to large quantities of HCB by the ingestion of bread produced from grain treated with HCB. This incident has provided the most solid evidence of acute effects of HCB exposure to humans. Primary acute health effects noted were porphryia cutanea tarda (PCT), which manifested as dermal lesions, areas of hyperpigmentation, and enlargement of the liver, thyroid, and lymph nodes.[47] The potential for human exposure has been greatly reduced during the past 20 years largely because of a reduction in the manufacture and use of HCB in the 1970s. Due to its environmental persistence, however, entry of HCB into the global environment still occurs from past polluted sites[48] and also as a chemical intermediate during the manufacture of other petroleum derivatives such as plastics and solvents. The primary exposure route in humans is through ingestion of contaminated foods and secondarily by inhalation of airborne HCB. Even subpopulations in Arctic regions have consistently measurable concentrations of HCB, thought to be derived mostly from biomagnification through the worldwide food chain.[49] As to be expected, even higher body burdens have been detected in regional areas near chemical manufacturing and in waste areas.[50-52] Although a general decline in human exposure and pollution levels has been evident in recent years, the EPA has drafted a national plan for reduction of the persistent bioaccumulative toxic pollutants (PBTs) to further assess and reduce exposure pathways to HCB and other PBT chemicals.

The danger of exposure to infants and neonatal populations has been established through measurements of HCB in newborn cord blood, maternal serum, breast milk, and lipids. The mobilization of lipids during lactation, combined with the propensity of HCB to accumulate in lipid-rich areas of the body, lend strong support to the hypothesis of exposure through these routes. In agreement with these recent studies, a significant number of breast-fed infants whose mothers ate the HCB-contaminated bread in Turkey subsequently died, presumably of complications from secondary exposure to HCB. More recent evidence of the transplacental uptake of HCB by the fetus[7,53] and subsequent uptake through breast feeding [54] has been characterized through cord blood analyses, and serum levels of the infant and mother. Advances in analytical methods have led to increased ability to accurately detect very low levels of HCB within these studies. For example, HCB cord blood concentrations in one study were reported in the range of 0.13 to 5.77 ng/ml, while maternal blood was 0.36 to 20.78 ng/ml.[53] The wide range of concentrations in this study resulted from a subset of mothers and newborns in the Spanish village of Flix where unusually high exposure to HCB contamination from organochloride production within close proximity to the village has been documented. Studies using rodent models provide additional evidence that HCB is capable of crossing the placenta during fetal development.[55] In these studies, dosing of hamsters and guinea pigs with HCB resulted in subsequent detection in all maternal and fetal tissues analyzed.

Although studies of neonates and mothers exposed to HCB have supported the transfer of HCB from mother to fetus, little information is available regarding the effect of chronic low-level exposure to the newborn. Neonatal developmental measurements collected at birth have demonstrated potential correlation to HCB cord blood concentrations. In one study, crown to heel measurements were negatively associated with HCB cord blood concentrations, although there was no association of body weight or head circumference to HCB levels.[56] Although physiological effects of prenatal exposure to low environmental concentrations of HCB have shown small differences in human and animal studies as compared to controls, behavioral effects are harder to quantify. The ability of lipophilic chemicals to cross the blood-brain barrier may increase the likelihood of HCB to affect behavior and sensorimotor skills. Evidence of hyperactivity, as measured by negative geotaxic reflex, olfactory discrimination, and exploratory behavior, has been evident in Sprague-Dawley pups exposed to HCB by maternal transfer *in utero*. However, there appeared to be no significant differences in learning and motor activity with regard to HCB exposure.[57] Similarly, no significant differences were reported in locomotor activity and active avoidance learning in WistarWU rats subjected to controlled behavior testing.[58]

Although the toxic effects of HCB (and other dioxin-like chemicals) have been mainly ascribed to direct interaction with the aryl hydrocarbon receptor (AhR),[50,59] mechanisms of action and subsequent effects of HCB or individual metabolites within the cell are areas of intense investigation. The cytochrome p450 pathway is the primary pathway by which most organic pollutants are targeted for elimination. Indeed, HCB appears to be targeted to cytochrome p450 pathways for xenobiotic transformation within several different tissues. Generally, persistent organic pollutants such as HCB are transformed to polar derivatives to allow for better urinary elimination. Polar derivatives have increased solubility in the aqueous cellular environment and removal through the urinary tract can be accomplished more readily. However, reactive oxygen species during metabolism is responsible for increased cellular oxidative stress and is a mechanism of toxicity for many chemicals that become bioactivated by this route.

HCB appears to undergo oxidative transformation to a pentachloro-epoxide intermediate, which subsequently becomes hydroxylated to form pentachlorophenol (PCP).[60,61] The reactive epoxide intermediate may spontaneously convert to PCP or alternatively conjugate with glutathione. Studies to determine the storage, metabolism, and elimination of HCB have been conducted that suggest that PCP and pentachlorobenzenethiol (PCBT) are the major metabolites of HCB processing by hepatic cytochrome p450 pathways in humans. In one study, high levels of HCB (as high as 3025 ng/g) in feces when compared with undetectable urine HCB levels indicate elimination by feces to be the primary removal route for the parent chemical. Conversely, both PCP and PCBT have been detected in 100% of urine samples examined, but detected in only 51% and 55% of fecal matched samples, respectively. However, it should also be noted that removal by the above mechanisms only accounts for a small fraction of the estimated concentration of HCB within the lipophilic body burden of the test population.[61] In rats, it has been demonstrated that PCP formed from HCB metabolism in hepatic microsomes may undergo further transformation to tetrachlorohydroquinone (TCHQ).[62] Further, TCHQ has been found to conjugate to protein within the hepatic microsomes. This suggests that TCHQ formed from HCB metabolism may be responsible for producing reactive oxygen, which can subsequently bind to protein macromolecules to produce cellular damage. Among other metabolites, tetrachlorophenol, pentachlorobenzene, and 3 isomers of tetrachlorobenzene have been identified.[62]

The ability of HCB to directly modulate endocrine functioning has not been well documented. HCB has been tentatively classified as a non-estrogenic xenobiotic.[63] Interestingly, however, it has been reported that HCB can disrupt gene transcription by interference with the thyroid response element.[64] It is not yet clear what the mechanism of binding and action may be. PCP, one of the hydroxylated metabolites of HCB detoxification, is regarded as an endocrine-disrupting chemical. PCP appears to interfere with the metabolism of steroid hormones, resulting in an imbalance of steroid concentration and regulation in aquatic invertebrates.[65] PCP has also been shown to compete with estrogen for binding to the estrogen receptor.[66] Similarly, PCP binds to the thyroid receptor and, therefore, may compete or interfere with these nuclear signaling pathways as well.[67] PCP has also been shown to cause a reduction in circulating thyroxine and other thyroid hormones such as triiodothyronine (T_3) in rats, presumably by competing with these hormones at pituitary or hypothalamic binding sites.[68] In a related study of eight pesticides tested, PCP was the strongest competitor of circulating thyroxine hormone proteins for binding to T_3 in human plasma. This binding assay showed that PCP decreased the binding of T_3 by 48% as compared to control levels. PCP was equally effective in disrupting T_3 binding in chicken, bullfrog, and salmon plasma as well.[69]

PCP's potential effect on the human female reproduction system has been indicated through a cohort study in which 65 women with PCP exposure levels exceeding 20 µg/liter of serum were matched with a control group of 106 women.[70] All women in the study had similar gynecological conditions, such as decreased fertility and menstrual dysfunction. Several hormone levels were significantly different between the PCP-exposed group as compared to the control group. Specifically, follicle-stimulating hormone (FSH) and T_3 were statistically higher in the control group. This *in vivo* T_3 study supports the above *in vitro* binding assays, in that a decrease in circulating T_3 could be related to the lack of thyroxine hormone-binding sites caused by competition with PCP. Differences in adrenal hormone levels between the two groups of women were measured as well. Testosterone, dehydrotestosterone (DHT), dehydroepiandrosterone (DHEA), hydroxypregnenolone, and hydroxyprogesterone were lower in PCP-exposed women when compared with controls. Although the above studies strongly support the likelihood that PCP interferes with thyroid function, the potential effects of HCB or its metabolites on the endocrine system overall are not yet well understood.

The carcinogenic potential and mechanisms of action of HCB in humans is currently in debate. Similar to DDT, IARC includes HCB in Group 2B: possibly carcinogenic to humans. This designation is also based primarily on animal studies. Evidence for the carcinogenic potential of HCB surfaced in the late 1970s through studies of mice and hamsters. Mice, fed a diet of 50, 100, or 200 ppm of HCB, developed hepatomas in a dose-dependent manner. Similarly, a dose-dependent yield of thyroid adenomas, liver hepatomas, and liver haemangioendotheliomas occurred in Syrian golden hamsters in a study using a comparable dosing regime.[71] Rats administered HCB in the diet also exhibited increased neoplastic nodules in the liver and parathyroid adenomas.[72-74] At the cellular level, HCB promotes glutathione S-transferase (GSTP1-1) positive foci within the liver, induces cell division-related transcription factors *c-fos* and *c-jun,* and increases reduced-glutathione.[75,76] Further, HCB may play a specific role in the alteration of gap junction communications during tumor promotion. A significant decrease in *connexin26* and *-32* mRNA levels, as well as gap junctional communication, was observed in the livers of female HCB-treated rats but not male HCB-treated rats.[77] In another study, gap junctional plaques containing connexin32 were significantly decreased in the livers of female rats treated with HCB.[78] Specific metabolites of HCB (PCP and tetrachlorohydroquinone) have also been investigated to determine potential effects on gap junctional communication. Similar to HCB, PCP has an inhibitory effect on gap junctional communication in rat liver epithelial cells, which is reversible by removal of the PCP.[79]

The direct genotoxic effects of HCB and its metabolites warrant further investigation. There is limited evidence of the ability of these chemicals to initiate cancer, but genotoxic damage has been demonstrated in human and other mammalian cell systems. Exposure of rats to PCP has resulted in increased oxidative stress-related damage, such as 8-hydroxy-2′-deoxyguanosine (8OHdG) and other DNA adducts, in liver and kidney tissues.[80] As well, formation of 8OHdG was significantly increased in mice administered PCP and was found to be dose dependent.[81] DNA single-strand breaks in hamster lung fibroblasts were demonstrated to occur after exposure to the HCB metabolite, TCHQ.[82] Exposure of primary human fetal cells to environmental concentrations of HCB results in both cytotoxic and genotoxic damage (as discussed in more detail below).[49] Moreover, HeLa cells exposed to 300 μM TCHQ resulted in oxidative DNA damage, as well as apurinic/apyrimidinic sites.[80] This effect was also observed in a calf thymus DNA assay, in the presence of Cu(II) and NADPH, strongly suggesting that redox cycling is involved in magnifying single strand DNA breaks and formation of 8OHdG in the presence of TCHQ.[83]

A direct link between exposure to HCB and human cancer has not been firmly established. However, a significantly high chronic environmental exposure to HCB by a human population in Flix, Spain, is possibly linked to increased incidence of soft tissue sarcoma and thyroid cancer.[84] Recently, testicular cancer in men has been correlated to maternal lipid body burden of a mixture of persistent organic pollutants, including HCB.[85]

The above epidemiological reports and additional studies using rodent models have indicated an association of HCB to the carcinogenic process, specifically thyroid adenomas, renal cell adenomas, and liver cancers, as well as bile-duct hyperplasia. The classical rodent initiation-promotion model demonstrating that HCB can act as a promotor during the carcinogenic process is well documented. There is evidence, however, to suggest that cellular DNA damage by exposure to HCB or the metabolites, PCP and TCHQ, may be sufficient to initiate the carcinogenic process.

4.3.1 EFFECTS OF HCB ON FETAL AND EMBRYONIC MAMMALIAN CELLS AT LOW ENVIRONMENTAL CONCENTRATIONS

In defining the concentrations of HCB for the research described below, the mean concentration measured in the same human newborn cord blood samples as previously discussed for DDE (1.2.1) was used.[49] Because this geographical area and population group has not been directly exposed to HCB, the relatively low concentrations (but consistently measurable) within the newborn cord blood most likely derive from a combination of biotransformation and bioaccumulation through the worldwide food chain.[49] Each table or figure within this section containing the term "1X HCB" is the arithmetic mean of actual cord blood concentrations and is equal to 0.1 µg HCB per liter of media, "10X HCB" is equal to 1.0 µg HCB per liter of media, etc.[49]

Following the same reasoning as discussed above, the short-term and long-term direct toxic effects of HCB exposure upon the same two immature mammalian cell types in culture, NIH 3T3 and WS1, were investigated.

4.3.2 SHORT-TERM EFFECTS OF HCB TOXICITY ON IMMATURE MAMMALIAN CELLS

Table 4.4 is a demonstration of both the percentage of viable and total number of NIH 3T3 and WS1 cells, between 2 to 24 hours after exposure to 1X or 10X HCB, when compared with control cells receiving the ethanol vehicle alone. Overall,

TABLE 4.4
HCB: SHORT-TERM CELL VIABILITY and % TOTAL CELLS[a]

Cell Type	Treatment	% Viable[b] (% Total)[c]			
		2h	6h	12h	24h
NIH 3T3	1X HCB	100 (99)	100 (83)[c]	93[b] (87)[c]	100 (104)
	10X HCB	99 (93)[c]	98 (79)[c]	92[b] (84)[c]	99 (84)[c]
WS1	1X HCB	100 (95)	100 (99)	100 (99)	104 (92)[c]
	10X HCB	101 (83)[c]	100 (82)[c]	97 (83)[c]	101 (88)[c]

[a] Viable cells at 2, 6, 12, and 24 hours of treatment, as compared to controls, were identified by differential permeability to DNA-binding dyes in the ViaCount Reagent. Cell total was determined by combination of all viable and nonviable cells per plate. Both total viabilities and total cells were determined by flow cytometry and converted to percentage of control values (Guava Technology Inc.).
[b] Significant decrease ($p < 0.05$) in viable cells as compared to NIH 3T3 control cells, as determined by one-way ANOVA and Schiffe's comparisons.
[c] Significant decrease ($p < 0.05$) in total cell number as compared to NIH 3T3 or WS1 control cells, as determined by one-way ANOVA and Schiffe's comparisons.
(Modified from Salmon, M.L., Madanagopal, S.G., Blando, R., Berner, J. and Williams, K., *Toxicology in Vitro*, 16, 539, 2002. With permission.)

statistical analysis revealed a slightly significant decreased viability of NIH 3T3 cells only at the 12-hour time point at both 1X and 10X HCB exposure groups. Table 4.4, however, reveals more significant decreases in NIH 3T3 cell numbers at 6 and 12 hours after exposure to 1X HCB and at all time periods tested (2, 6, 12, 24 hours) within the 10X HCB-exposed NIH 3T3 cells as compared to the number of control cells. WS1 cells, in contrast, did not exhibit decreased cell viability after exposure to 1X or 10X HCB at any time up to 24 hours. However, WS1 cells did have a significant decrease in cell number by 24 hours after 1X HCB exposure and at all time periods tested (2, 6, 12, 24 hours) after the 10X HCB exposure, similar to the effect on NIH 3T3 cells after exposure to 10X HCB. Table 4.4, in comparison to Table 4.1, demonstrates that HCB appears to have a similar cytotoxic effect as DDE on NIH 3T3 cells, but HCB has a much stronger cytotoxic effect than DDE on WS1 cells at these low environmental concentrations. This cytotoxic effect of HCB, as compared to DDE, is intriguing in that the average environmental concentration of HCB used in this investigation is approximately one third the average molar concentration of DDE (1 M:3.13M, respectively).

To determine if chromosomal damage occurs after HCB exposure to either of these two types of immature cells, the comet assay was performed (as described previously). Table 4.5 contains the average nuclear chromosomal lengths of individual NIH 3T3 and WS1 cells exposed to ethanol alone (control), 1X or 10X HCB. Similar to DDE results (Table 4.2), there was a significant increase in NIH 3T3 total DNA length after 4 hours exposure to both 1X and 10X HCB. Interestingly, WS1 cells also exhibited a significant increase in the total DNA length in the 1X HCB-exposed cells and an even greater increase in the 10X HCB-exposed cells (Table 4.5). These results are unlike DDE exposure to WS1 cells, which did not appear to cause any genotoxicity to these cells (Table 4.2).[45,49]

This significantly increased chromosomal damage to both immature cell types after exposure to both 1X and 10X HCB might, therefore, contribute to the overall decrease in cell number of both cell types, as well as decreased viability to NIH 3T3 cells (Table 4.4). Flow cytometric analyses of the growth fraction of each cell population at specific time points was performed to determine if the observed decreases in cell viability and total cell numbers within Table 4.4 might be attributed to cell cycle arrest of either cell type. Figure 4.2A is the flow cytometric analysis of NIH 3T3 cells exposed to 1X and 10X HCB as compared to control cells. Similar to the DDE flow cytometric experiments, the NIH 3T3 cell cycle does not appear to be significantly affected by HCB treatments at the concentrations used in these studies. Figure 4.2B is the flow cytometric analysis of WS1 cells exposed to 1X and 10X HCB as compared to control cells. In contrast to NIH 3T3 cells, but similar to effects of DDE exposure, WS1 cells, after HCB exposure, do appear to undergo a decrease in the growth fraction. The percentage of dividing WS1 cells decreases considerably up to 24 hours after initial exposure to 10X HCB. Interestingly, DDE (Figure 4.1B) appeared to have a stronger effect on the cell cycle of WS1 cells than HCB (Figure 4.2B). Perhaps the stronger effect on the WS1 cell cycle by DDE, as compared to HCB, is indicative of a protective effect by the cell. In agreement with this hypothesis, all other short- and long-term experimental responses to DDE exposure did not demonstrate significant toxicity to WS1 cells, with the exception

TABLE 4.5
HCB: CHROMOSOMAL DAMAGE[a]

Cell Type	Treatment 4h	Total DNA Length Average
NIH 3T3	Control	11.14 mm
	1X HCB	31.74 mm[b]
	10X HCB	31.84 mm[b]
WS 1	Control	8.6 mm
	1X HCB	26.2 mm[b]
	10X HCB	32.9 mm[b,c]

[a] The comet assay was performed to determine if a 4-hour exposure to 1X or 10X HCB resulted in DNA damage. Single- and double-strand chromosomal breaks within chromosomal DNA of individual cells results in an increased ability of the DNA to migrate through agarose during electophoresis and is observed as an increase in total DNA length. The total DNA length (the displacement between the leading edge of the chromosomal DNA and the end of the tail) of a minimum of 50 cells per treatment was measured and the average length calculated.

[b] Significant increase ($p < 0.01$) in DNA migration, indicating increased strand breakage, as compared to NIH 3T3 or WS1 control cells, as determined by one-way ANOVA and Schiffe's comparisons.

[c] Significant increase ($p < 0.01$) in DNA migration, indicating increased strand breakage, as compared to WS1 1X HCB-treated cells, as determined by one-way ANOVA and Schiffe's comparisons. (From Salmon, M.L., Madanagopal, S.G., Blando, R., Berner, J. and Williams, K., *Toxicology in Vitro*, 16, 539, 2002. With permission.)

of wide fluctuations over time of cellular GSH concentration, indicating cellular protective response to oxidative damage.

WS1 GSH and GSSG ratios were determined to measure potential alterations in the intracellular redox state after exposure to HCB.[49] As illustrated in Figure 4.3, the molar ratio of reduced to oxidized glutathione (2GSH/GSSG) is significantly decreased as compared to controls for up to 6 hours after exposure to all HCB concentration tested (1X, 10X, and 50X), indicating consistent increased oxidation of GSH, or decreased reduction of GSSG, in the presence of HCB. As predicted,

HCB: CELL CYCLE KINETICS

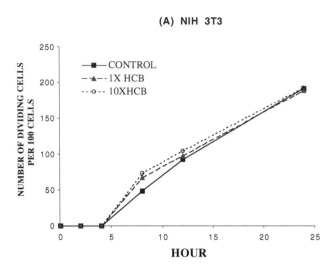

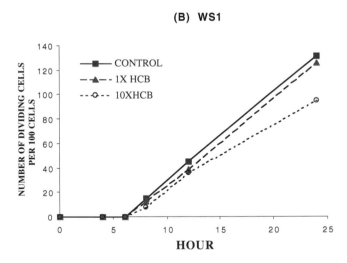

FIGURE 4.2 NIH 3T3 (A) and WS1 (B) cells were exposed to media containing BrdU, deoxycytidine, and either ethanol alone (control), 1X, or 10X HCB. Samples(in duplicate) were harvested by trypsinization at the indicated time points and underwent BrdU–Hoescht flow cytometric analysis for number of dividing cells per 100 living cells. (From Salmon, M.L., Madanagopal, S.G., Blando, R., Berner, J., and Williams, K., *Toxicology in Vitro*, 16, 539, 2002. With permission.)

HCB: GLUTATHIONE RATIOS *

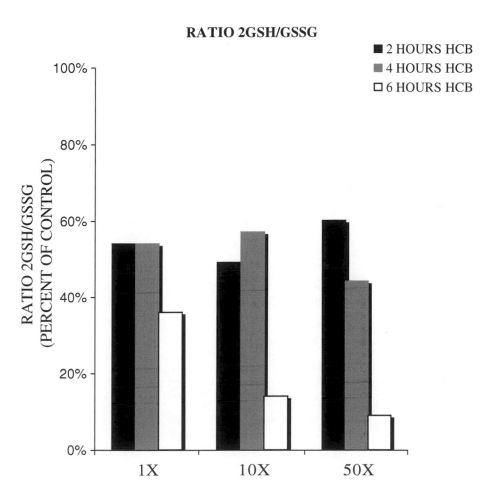

RATIO 2GSH/GSSG

FIGURE 4.3 WS1 cells were assayed for reduced glutathione (GSH) and total glutathione for subsequent determination of 2GSH/GSSG ratios. Intracellular GSH and total glutathione were measured after WS1 cells were plated and exposed to ethanol alone (control), 1X, 10X, or 50X HCB at the indicated time points.

* All HCB concentrations at all time points were significantly different from controls by one-way ANOVA ($p < 0.05$). (Modified from Salmon, M.L., Madanagopal, S.G., Blando, R., Berner, J., and Williams, K., *Toxicology in Vitro*, 16, 539, 2002. With permission.)

NIH 3T3 glutathione concentrations did not exhibit alterations at any time point after HCB exposure, for reasons discussed previously (results not shown).[49] This again indicates the possibility that this redox pathway is contributing to the protection of WS1 cells from cytotoxic events resulting from exposure to HCB.

4.3.3 LONG-TERM EFFECTS OF HCB TOXICITY ON IMMATURE MAMMALIAN CELLS

We initially examined the long-term toxicity of chronic HCB treatment by measuring colony-forming ability by individual cells. The size and number of colonies was determined after 10 days of exposure to either 1X, 10X, or 50X HCB. As illustrated in Table 4.6, NIH 3T3 cells display a significant decrease in percentage of colonies after chronic exposure to both 10X and 50X HCB but not after exposure to 1X HCB, as compared to controls. The percentage of WS1 colonies was significantly decreased only after exposure to 50X HCB. Although these results are potentially similar to the effect of DDE on WS1 colony survival, in which only 1X and 10X DDE concentrations were tested, further experiments need to be conducted to examine this possibiltiy (Table 4.3).

NIH 3T3 cell transformation during chronic exposure to HCB was examined by counting the number of foci formed after 3 to 4 weeks of contact with media containing ethanol alone (control) or HCB at 1X, 10X, or 50X concentrations (Table 4.7). There was a significant and almost linear increase in the number of foci formed at all HCB concentrations, culminating in a 2.2-fold increase in number of

TABLE 4.6
HCB: COLONY-FORMING ABILITY

Cell Type	Treatment	Percent (%) of Controls
NIH 3T3	1X HCB	96%
	10X HCB	91%*
	50X HCB	84%*
WS1	1X HCB	109%
	10X HCB	100%
	50X HCB	84%*

Long-term survival of NIH 3T3 and WS1 cells chronically exposed to HCB was determined by the total number of subsequent colonies successfully formed after 10 days. Cell survival per treatment is expressed as a percentage (%) of the number of surviving colonies on the control plates. Percentages represent the average percentage survival from three independent experiments. Asterisk (*) indicates a significant difference from ethanol alone (control) cells by one-way ANOVA ($p < 0.05$).

TABLE 4.7
HCB: NIH 3T3 TRANSFORMATION ASSAY[a]

Treatment	Total Number of Foci Counted	Fold Increase Above Control
Control	40	1
1X HCB	71	1.76
10X HCB	77	1.93
50X HCB	88	2.20
UV @ 10 J/m^2	91	2.3

[a] The NIH 3T3 transformation assay was performed to determine if exposure to 1X, 10X, or 50X HCB resulted in an increase in the number of foci. The number of foci was determined by fixing each plate of cells with 97% methanol and subsequently staining with 95% crystal violet. The foci were counted under a dissecting microscope and the results reported are a sum of five experiments. (From Salmon, M.L., Madanagopal, S.G., Blando, R., Berner, J. and Williams, K., *Toxicology in Vitro*, 16, 539, 2002. With permission.)

foci above background at 50X HCB concentration. This fold increase was almost equivalent to the positive control of NIH 3T3 exposure to 10 J/m^2 ultraviolet radiation (Table 4.7). These results are in agreement with the literature, which indicates HCB to be a potential direct carcinogen in rodents.

4.4 EFFECTS OF HCB+DDE MIXTURES ON FETAL AND EMBRYONIC MAMMALIAN CELLS AT LOW ENVIRONMENTAL CCONCENTRATIONS

For the experiments described below, concentrations of DDE (1.2.1) and HCB (1.3.1) were prepared as before,[45,49] and subsequently mixed together. The results of the experiments described in this section allow us to compare toxic effects of this environmentally relevant mixture of both chemicals on NIH 3T3 and WS1 cells in culture, to the toxic effects of DDE or HCB individually. Although the experiments described below are still an ongoing process, the importance of determining mechanisms of toxic effects of persistent organic pollutant mixtures on immature mammalian cells cannot be overestimated, as actual embryos or fetuses are seldom, if ever, exposed only to individual organic pollutants. The likelihood of different chemicals, at environmentally relevant concentrations, to interact with each other at the same, or on different, cellular targets to produce a significantly stronger cytotoxic or genotoxic response of immature human cells during embryogenesis or subsequent fetal development is of utmost importance to investigate.

4.4.1 Short-Term Effects of HCB+DDE Toxicity on Immature Human Cells

Two different methods were used to determine total cells per plate up to 24 hours after exposure to HCB+DDE. Both NIH 3T3 and WS1 cells exposed to either 1X or 10X HCB+DDE exhibited decreased cells per plate (as measured by μg DNA per plate) up to ~4 hours, when compared with controls (Figure 4.4). NIH 3T3 cells exposed to 1X HCB+DDE regained control cell numbers by 24 hours, but not NIH 3T3 cells exposed to 10X HCB+DDE, as measured both by μg DNA per plate (Figure 4.4A), and by cell count using flow cytometry (Table 4.8). WS1 cells exposed to either 1X or 10X HCB+DDE did not regain control cell numbers by 24 hours (Figure 4.4B; Table 4.8). Therefore, this environmentally relevant mix of chemicals has a significant toxic effect on WS1 cell numbers, even at 1X HCB+DDE, in direct contrast to either chemical alone (Table 4.1 and Table 4.4).

The percentage of each cell type specifically undergoing apoptosis within each treatment group was then determined. Consistent with previous cell viability and cell cycle kinetic results from exposure to either HCB or DDE individually, only NIH 3T3 cells exhibited increased apoptosis at 24 hours, which was evident at both the 1X and 10X HCB+DDE exposure concentrations (Table 4.9). Although flow cytometry to determine cell cycle kinetics has not yet been accomplished with the HCB+DDE mix, it is predictable that results will be similar to those previously reported in the presence of each chemical individually, in that NIH 3T3 cells will not have an altered cell cycle, but WS1 cells will have an increased cell cycle time indicating temporary or permanent arrest of these primary human cells.

4.4.2 Long-Term Effects of HCB+DDE Mixture Toxicity on Immature Mammalian Cells

The long-term colony-forming ability of individual cells of both NIH 3T3 and WS1 cell types was significantly decreased; at both the 1X and 10X HCB+DDE concentrations for NIH 3T3 cells, but only at the 10X HCB+DDE concentration for WS1 cells (Table 4.10). Interestingly, exposure to each chemical alone resulted in decreased colony-forming ability of WS1 cells only after exposure to 50X HCB, a concentration of HCB 5 times higher than the 10X HCB+DDE resulting in an equally decreased colony-forming efficiency for these cells (Table 4.6 and 4.10). Overall, however, NIH 3T3 cells are consistently more sensitive than WS1 cells to long-term cytotoxic effects of each chemical individually, as well as to the HCB+DDE mix (Tables 4.3, 4.6, 4.10).

The NIH 3T3 transformation assay, to determine if exposure to the HCB+DDE mix increases the number of transformed foci above background, was performed differently from the previously described assays.[45,49] The primary modes of entry and actual intracellular concentrations of these lipophilic chemicals within cell culture experiments, such as described here, have remained in question. Therefore, we sought a more physiologically relevant delivery system. First, rather than dissolving HCB and DDE separately into ethanol or acetone and subsequently combining these solutions and diluting with media, HCB and DDE were added together

HCB+DDE MIX

A.

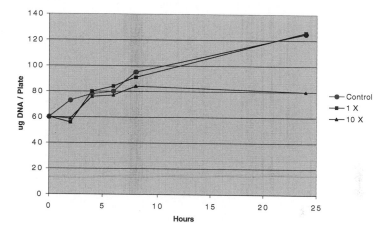

B.

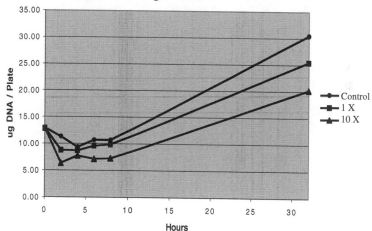

FIGURE 4.4 Assay for changes in cell number. Effect of acetone and ethanol alone (control), 1X, or 10X HCB+DDE and duration of exposure on total μg DNA per plate of two cell types. NIH 3T3 (A) and WS1 (B) cell cultures were harvested in duplicate at the indicated time points. The total DNA from each plate was determined using the diaminobenzoic acid assay. The graphs represent the average μg of DNA per duplicate sample per time point of harvest ± SD. Data points without error bars represent those duplicate samples in which the SD was too small to be represented on the graph.

TABLE 4.8
HCB+DDE: SHORT-TERM TOTAL CELLS PER PLATE[a]

		6h % Cells	12h % Cells	24h % Cells
NIH 3T3	10X HCB+DDE	91[b]	83[b]	71[b]
WS1	10X HCB+DDE	88[b]	94[b]	85[b]

[a] Total number of cells in each duplicate plate at 6, 12, and 24 hours were counted by flow cytometry, averaged and converted to percentage of average control values (% Cells) (Guava Technology Inc.).
[b] Significant decrease ($p < 0.05$) in total cell number as compared to NIH 3T3 or WS1 control cells.

TABLE 4.9
HCB+DDE: CELL APOPTOSIS AT 24 HOURS[a]

Cell Type	Treatment	Percent (%) Apoptotic
NIH 3T3	Control	6%
	1X HCB+DDE	13%
	10X HCB+DDE	17%
WS1	Control	7%
	1X HCB+DDE	8%
	10X HCB+DDE	7%

[a] Percentage (%) apoptotic cells at 24 hours after HCB+DDE treatment were identified by Guava Nexin™ kit and flow cytometry to determine apoptotic cells by detection of cells staining positive for annexin V and/or 7-AAD (Guava Technology Inc.).

into 20 ml of a lipid-rich bovine serum (Sigma) at a 1000X stock concentration of each chemical. Second, we included plates of NIH 3T3 cells that were simultaneously transfected with an activated oncogene (H-*ras,* codon 12 activating mutation G → T). Third, we mixed the lipid-rich serum containing the two organic pollutants with different commercial liposome solutions. This alternate approach was taken to determine the extent and type of toxic cellular effects when cells are exposed to a mixture of organic pollutants contained within a lipid-rich environment, similar to mammalian concentrations of persistent organic pollutants in lipid-rich areas of the body.

TABLE 4.10
HCB+DDE: COLONY-FORMING
ABILITY

Cell Type	Treatment	Percent (%) of Controls
NIH 3T3	1X	82%*
	10X	67%*
WS1	1X	100%
	10X	82%*

Long-term survival of NIH 3T3 and WS1 cells chronically exposed to HCB+DDE was determined by the total number of subsequent colonies successfully formed after 10 days. Cell survival per treatment is expressed as a percentage (%) of the number of surviving colonies on the control plates. Percentages represent the average percentage survival from three independent experiments. Asterisk (*) indicates a significant difference from ethanol alone (control) cells by one-way ANOVA ($p < 0.05$).

TABLE 4.11
HCB+DDE: NIH 3T3 TRANSFORMATION ASSAY[a]

Treatment	Fold Increase Above Control
Negative Control	1
Activated H-*ras* alone (Positive control)	3.0 – 3.8
Activated H-*ras* + 10X HCB+DDE	3.3 – 4.3
Activated H-*ras* + 100X HCB+DDE	3.1 – 6.0
10X HCB+DDE	1.5 – 2.1
100X HCB+DDE	0.95 – 1.7

[a] The NIH 3T3 transformation assay was performed to determine if exposure to activated H-*ras* and either 1X or 10X HCB resulted in an increase in the number of foci. The number of foci was determined by fixing each plate of cells with 97% methanol and subsequently staining with 95% crystal violet.

Although this approach is still developing in our laboratory, we have obtained intriguing preliminary results that indicate this altered method of introducing organic pollutants to cells in culture is at least as efficient as our previous conventional methods and is possibly significantly more relevant. As demonstrated within Table 4.11, the exposure of NIH 3T3 cells to both the HCB+DDE mix and to the activated

H-*ras* results in a higher number of foci above background than either chemical alone, or activated H-*ras* alone, regardless of the commercial liposome used (the large ranges indicate a decreased or increased transformed foci response, depending on the type of liposome used). We interpret this to indicate that cells transformed by activated H-*ras* in the presence of HCB+DDE in the lipid-rich serum and liposome solution were "driven" even more toward neoplastic transformation than toward a cytotoxic response that would result in cell death. In addition, although 10X HCB+DDE produced a range of foci somewhat above background, with the highest fold increase of 2.1 similar to previous results by exposure to HCB alone (Table 4.7), the 100X HCB+DDE exposed cells resulted in a lower response range, even falling slightly below the negative control of 1 (Table 4.11). We suspect, based on our previous results using the HCB+DDE mix, that this may indicate a sufficiently high rate of cytotoxicity such that the remaining cell population from which trans-formed foci could emerge has been severely depleted. We are currently examining cell viability and other short-term experiments, using this HCB+DDE mixture pro-tocol, to determine if this is, in fact, the case.

4.5   CONCLUDING REMARKS

Overall, each individual chemical at low environmental concentrations has demon-strated several different toxic effects on each immature cell type, each of which have the potential for long-term deleterious consequences. As a simple two-component mixture, the toxic effects to WS1 cells appear to be either potentiated or synergistic, as compared to HCB or DDE individually. This normal human fibroblast appears to be an extremely sensitive model for further mechanistic studies to determine the extent and type of direct toxic interference upon different metabolic pathways and systems within immature human cells by exposure to mixtures of persistent organic pollutants.

The results of our studies agree with rodent cancer models and human epide-miological data, as reviewed above. In rodents, these persistent organic pollutants appears to have direct acting cytotoxic effects, and neoplastic transformation is well documented, as well. Human epidemiological studies also support the hypothesis that exposure to a mixture of organic pollutants contributes to increased cancer incidence, as well as other congenital and long-term effects.

ACKNOWLEDGMENTS

This research was supported by a NOAA/NSF OPP-0002239 grant to KJW.

REFERENCES

1. *AMAP assessment report: Arctic pollution issues* Arctic Monitoring and Assessment Programme, Oslo, Norway, 1998.
2. *Toxicology: The Basic Science of Poisons*, 6th ed. McGraw-Hill, New York, 2001.

3. Toxicological Profile for DDT, DDE, DDD, *Agency for Toxic Substances and Disease Registry,* 2002.
4. Howard, P.H. et al. *Handbook of Environmental Degradation Rates,* Lewis, Chelsea, MI, 1991.
5. Jaga, K. and Dharmani, C., Global surveillance of DDT and DDE levels in human tissues, *Int. J. Occup. Med. Environ. Health* 16 (1), 7, 2003.
6. ATSDR Toxicological Profiles, *Agency for Toxic Substances and Disease Registry,* 1999.
7. Covaci, A. et al. Distribution of PCBs and organochlorine pesticides in umbilical cord and maternal serum, *The Science of the Total Environment* 298, 45, 2002.
8. Longnecker, M.P. et al. Association between maternal serum concentrations of the DDT metabolite DDE and preterm and small-for-gestational-age babies at birth, *Lancet* 358, 110, 2001.
9. Lordo, R.A., Dinh, K.T., and Schwemberger, J.G., Semivolatile organic compounds in adipose tissue: estimated averages for the US population and selected subpopulations, *Am. J. Pub. Health* 86 (9), 1253, 1996.
10. You, L. et al. Transplacental and lactational transfer of p,p'-DDE in Sprague-Dawley rats, *Toxicol. Appl. Pharmacol.* 157 (2), 134, 1999.
11. LaKind, J.S. et al. Methodology for characterizing distributions of incremental body burdens of 2,3,7,8-TCDD and DDE from breast milk in North American nursing infants, *J. Toxicol. Environ. Health, Part A* 59, 605, 2000.
12. Kelce, W.R. et al. Persistent DDT metabolite p,p'-DDE is a potent androgen receptor antagonist, *Nature* 375, 581, 1995.
13. You, L. et al. Impaired male sexual development in perinatal Sprague-Dawley and Long-Evans hooded rats exposed *in utero* and lactationally to p,p'-DDE, *Toxicol. Sci.* 45, 162, 1998.
14. Gray, L.E., Xenoendocrine disrupters: laboratory studies on male reproductive effects, *Toxicol. Lett.* 102-103, 331, 1998.
15. Kelce, W.R. et al. Vinclozolin and p,p'-DDE alter androgen-dependent gene expression: *in vivo* confirmation of an androgen receptor-mediated mechanism, *Toxicol. Appl. Pharmacol.* 142 (1), 192, 1997.
16. Sunami, O. et al. Evaluation of a 5-day Hershberger assay using young mature male rats: methyltestosterone and p,p'-DDE, but not fenitrothion, exhibited androgenic or antiandrogenic activity *in vivo.*, *J. Toxicol. Sci.* 25 (5), 403, 2000.
17. Gold, B. and Brunck, G., A mechanistic study of the metabolism of 1,1-dichloro-2,2-*bis*(p-chlorophenyl)ethane (DDD) to 2,2-*bis*(p-chlorophenyl)acetic acid (DDA), *Biochem. Pharmacol.* 33 (7), 979, 1984.
18. Gold, B. and Brunck, G., Metabolism of 1,1,1-trichloro-2,2-*bis*(p-chlorophenyl)ethane (DDT), 1,1-dichloro-*bis*(p-chlorophenyl)ethane, and 1-chloro-2,2-*bis*(p-chlorophenyl)ethene in the hamster, *Cancer Res.* 43, 2644, 1983.
19. Kitamura, S. et al. Reductive metabolism of p,p'-DDT and o,p'-DDT by rat liver cytochrome p450, *Drug Metabolism and Disposition* 30 (2), 113, 2002.
20. Noren, K. et al. Methylsulfonyl metabolites of PCBs and DDE in human milk in Sweden, 1927-1992, *Environ. Health Perspect.,* 104, 766, 1996.
21. Noren, K., Welstrand, C., and Karpe, F., Distribution of PCB congeners, DDE, hexachlorobenzene, and methylsulfonyl metabolites of PCB and DDE among various fractions of human blood plasma, *Arch. Environ. Contam. Toxicol.* 37 (3), 408, 1999.
22. Bergman, A. et al. PCB and DDE methyl sulfones in mammals from Canada and Sweden, *Environ. Toxicol. Chem.* 13, 121, 1994.

23. Jonsson, C.J. et al. Adrenocortical toxicity of 3-methylsulfonyl-DDE in mice. II. Mitochondrial changes following ecological relevant doses, *Fundam. Appl. Toxicol.* 16 (2), 365, 1991.

24. Jonsson, C.J. et al. Adrenocortical toxicity of 3-methylsulphonyl-DDE 3:studies in fetal and suckling mice, *Reprod. Toxicol.* 6 (3), 233, 1992.

25. Jonsson, C.J., Rodriguez-Martinez, H., and Brandt, I., Transplacental toxicity of 3-methylsulphonyl-DDE in the developing adrenal cortex in mice, *Reprod. Toxicol.* 9 (3), 257, 1995.

26. Lindhe, O., Skogseid, B., and Brandt, I., Cytochrome P450-catalyzed binding of 3-methylsulfonyl-DDE and o,p'-DDD in human adrenal zona fasciculata/reticularis, *Clin. Endocrinol. Metab.* 87 (3), 1319, 2002.

27. Johansson, M., Nilsson, S., and Lund, B.O., Interactions between methylsulphonyl PCBs and the glucocorticoid receptor, *Environ. Health Perspect.*, 106 (12), 769, 1998.

28. Kitchin, K.T. and Brown, J.L., Biochemical effects of DDT and DDE in rat and mouse liver, *Environ. Res.* 46 (1), 39, 1988.

29. Nims, R.W. et al. Comparative pharmacodynamics of CYP2B induction by DDT, DDE, and DDD in male rat liver and cultured rat hepatocytes, *J. Toxicol. Environ. Health A* 53 (6), 455, 1998.

30. Sierra-Santoyo, A. et al. Sex-dependent regulation of hepatic cytochrome P-450 by DDT, *Toxicol. Sci.* 54, 81, 2000.

31. Tomatis, L., Turusov, V., and Charles, R.T., Effect of long-term exposure to 1,1-dichloro-2,2-bis(p-chlorophenyl)ethylene, to 1,1-dichloro-2,2-*bis*(p-chlorophenyl)ethane and to the two chemicals combined on cf.-1 mice, *J. Natl. Cancer Inst.* 52, 883, 1974.

32. Bioassays of DDT, TDE, and *p,p'*-DDE for possible carcinogenicity, Report No. 131, 1978.

33. Rossi, L. et al. Carcinogenicity study with technical-grade dichlorodiphenyltrichloroethane and 1,1-dichloro-2,2-*bis*(p-chlorophenyl)ethylene in hamsters, *Cancer Res.* 43, 776, 1983.

34. Desaulniers, D. et al. Modulatory effects of neonatal exposure to TCDD, or a mixture of PCBs, p,p'-DDT, p,p'-DDE, on methylnitrosourea-induced mammary tumor development in the rat, *Environ. Health Perspect.*, 109 (7), 739, 2001.

35. Ruch, R.J. et al. Loss of gap junctions from DDT-treated rat liver epithelial cells, *Carcinogenesis* 15 (2), 301, 1994.

36. Mahr, U. and Miltenburger, H.G., The effect of insecticides on Chinese Hamster cell cultures, *Mutation Res.* 40, 107, 1976.

37. Zheng, T. et al. DDE and DDT in breast adipose tissue and risk of female breast cancer, *Am. J. Epidemiol.* 150 (5), 453, 1999.

38. Gammon, M.D. et al. Environmental toxins and breast cancer on Long Island. II. Organochlorine compound levels in blood, *Cancer Epidemiol., Biomarkers & Prevention* 11, 686, 2002.

39. Laden, F. et al. 1,1-Dichloro-2,2-*bis*(p-chlorophenyl)ethylene and polychlorinated biphenyls and breast cancer: Combined analysis of five U.S. studies, *J. Natl. Cancer Inst.* 93 (10), 768, 2001.

40. Demers, A. et al. Risk and aggressiveness of breast cancer in relation to plasma organochlorine concentrations, *Cancer Epidemiol., Biomarkers & Prevention* 9, 161, 2000.

41. Wolff, M.S. et al. Blood levels of organochlorine residues and the risk of breast cancer, *J. Natl. Cancer Inst.* 85 (8), 648, 1993.

42. Charlier, C. et al. Breast cancer and serum organochlorine residues, *Occup. Environ. Med.* 60 (5), 348, 2003.

43. Kupfer, D. and Bulger, W.H., Interaction of o,p'-DDT with the estrogen-binding protein (EBP) of human mammary and uterine tumors, *Res. Commun. Chem. Pathol. Pharmacol.* 16, 451, 1977.
44. Liljegren, G. et al. Case-control study on breast cancer and adipose tissue concentrations of cogener specific polychlorinated biphenyls, DDE and hexachlorobenzene, *Eur. J. Cancer Prevention* 7 (2), 135, 1998.
45. Simonetti, J., Berner, J., and Williams, K., Effects of *p, p'*- DDE on immature cells in culture at concentrations relevant to the Alaskan environment, *Toxicol. in Vitro* 15, 169, 2001.
46. Singh, N.P. et al. A simple technique for quantitation of low levels of DNA damage in individual cells, *Exp. Cell. Res.* 175 (1), 184, 1988.
47. Gocmen, A. et al. Hexachlorobenzene episode in Turkey, *Biomed. Environ. Sci.* 2, 36, 1989.
48. Toxicological profile for hexachlorobenzene, 1996.
49. Salmon, M.L. et al. Effects of hexachlorobenzene on embryonic mammalian cells, *Toxicol. in Vitro* 16, 539, 2002.
50. van Birgelen, A.P.J.M., Hexachlorobenzene as a possible major contributor to the dioxin activity of human milk, *Environ. Health Perspect.* 106 (11), 683, 1998.
51. Newhook, R. and Dormer, W., *Environ. Health Criteria* 195, 1997.
52. Polder, A. et al. Geographic variation of chlorinated pesticides, toxaphenes and PCBs in human milk from sub-arctic and arctic locations in Russia, *Sci. Total Environ.* 306, 179, 2003.
53. Sala, M. et al. Levels of hexachlorobenzene and other organochlorine compounds in cord blood: exposure across placenta, *Chemosphere* 43, 895, 2001.
54. Koopman-Esseboom, C. et al. PCB and dioxin levels in plasma and human milk of 418 Dutch women and their infants. Predictive value of PCB congener levels in maternal plasma for fetal and infant's exposure to PCBs and dioxins, *Chemosphere* 28, 1721, 1994.
55. Courtney, K.D., Andrews, J.E., and Grady, M.A., Placental transfer and fetal deposition of hexachlorobenzene in the hamster and guinea pig, *Environ. Res.* 37 (1), 239, 1985.
56. Ribas-Fito, N. et al. Association of hexachlorobenzene and other organochlorine compounds with anthropometric measures at birth, *Ped. Res.* 52 (2), 163, 2002.
57. Goldey, E.S. and Taylor, D.H., Developmental neurotoxicity following premating maternal exposure to hexachlorobenzene in rats, *Neurotoxicol. and Teratol.* 14, 15, 1992.
58. Lilienthal, H. et al. Impairment of schedule-controlled behavior by pre-and postnatal exposure to hexachlorobenzene in rats, *Arch. Toxicol.*, 174, 1996.
59. Whitlock, J.P., Genetic and molecular aspects of 2,3,7,8-tetrachlorodibenzo-*p*-dioxin action, *Annu. Rev. Pharmacol. Toxicol.* 30 (251–257), 1990.
60. den Besten, C., Peters, M.M.C.G., and van Bladeran, P.J., The metabolism of pentachlorobenzene by rat liver microsomes: the nature of the reactive intermediates formed, *Biochem. Biophys. Res. Commun.* 163, 1275, 1989.
61. To-Figueras, J. et al. Excretion of hexachlorobenzene and metabolites in feces in a highly exposed human population, *Environ. Health Perspect.*, 108 (7), 595, 2000.
62. van Ommen, B. et al. Formation of pentachlorophenol as the major product of microsomal oxidation of hexachlorobenzene, *Biochem. Biophys. Res. Commun.* 126 (1), 25, 1985.
63. Sonnenschein, C. and Soto, A.M., An updated review of environmental estrogen and androgen mimics and antagonists, *Steroid Biochem. Molec. Biol.* 65, 143, 1998.

64. Loaiza-Perez, A.I. et al. Hexachlorobenzene, a dioxin-type compound, increases malic enzyme gene transcription through a mechanism involving the thyroid hormone response element, *Endocrinology* 140 (9), 4142, 1999.

65. Parks, L.G. and LeBlanc, G.A., Reductions in steroid hormone biotransformation/elimination as a biomarker of pentachlorophenol chronic toxicity, *Aquatic Toxicol.* 34, 291, 1996.

66. Danzo, B.J., Environmental xenobiotics may disrupt normal endocrine function by interfering with the binding of physiological ligands to steroid receptors and binding proteins, *Environ. Health Perspect.,* 105, 294, 1997.

67. Brucker-Davis, F., Effects of environmental synthetic chemicals on thyroid function, *Thyroid* 8 (827-856), 1998.

68. Jekat, F.W. et al. Effects of pentachlorophenol (PCP) on the pituitary and thyroidal hormone regulation in the rat, *Toxicol. Lett.* 71, 9, 1994.

69. Ishihara, A., Sawatsuashi, S., and Yamauchi, K., Endocrine disrupting chemicals: interference of thyroid hormone binding to transthyretins and to thyroid hormone receptors, *Mol. Cell. Endocrinol.* 199, 105, 2003.

70. Gerhard, I. et al. Pentachlorophenol exposure in women with gynecological and endocrine dysfuntion, *Environ. Res. Section A* 80 (383-388), 1999.

71. Cabral, J.R. and Shubik, P., *Carcinogenic activity of hexachlorobenzene in mice and hamsters,* Oxford University Press, Lyon, France, 1986.

72. Arnold, D.L. et al. Long-term toxicity of hexachlorobenzene in the rat and the effect of dietary vitamin A., *Food Chem. Toxicol.,* 23, 779, 1985.

73. Cabral, R. et al. Medium-term bioassay for the hepatocarcinogenicity of hexachlorobenzene, *Cancer Letters* 100, 223, 1996.

74. Smith, A.G. and Cabral, R., Liver-cell tumors in rats fed hexachlorobenzene, *Cancer Letters* 11, 169, 1980.

75. Gustafson, D.L. et al. Comparative hepatocarcinogenicity of hexachlorobenzene, pentachlorobenzene, 1,2,4,5-tetrachlorobenzene, and 1,4-dichlorobenzene: application of a medium-term liver focus bioassay and molecular and cellular indices, *Toxicol. Sci.* 53, 245, 2000.

76. Ou, Y.C. et al. Stochastic simulation of hepatic preneoplastic foci development for four chlorobenzene congeners in a medium-term bioassay, *Toxicol. Sci.* 73, 301, 2003.

77. Plante, I., Charbonneau, M., and Cyr, D.G., Decreased gap junctional intercellular communication in hexachlorobenzene-induced gender-specific hepatic tumor formation in the rat, *Carcinogenesis* 23, 1243, 2002.

78. Mally, A. and Chipman, J.K., Non-genotoxic carcinogens: early effects on gap junctions, cell proliferation and apoptosis in the rat, *Toxicology* 180, 233, 2002.

79. Sai, K. et al. Inhibitory effect of pentachlorophenol on gap junctional intercellular communication in rat liver epithelial cells *in vitro, Cancer Letters* 130, 9, 1998.

80. Lin, P.-H. et al. Induction of direct adducts, apurinic/apyrimidinic sites and oxidized bases in nuclear DNA of human HeLa S3 tumor cells by tetrachlorohydroquinone, *Carcinogenesis* 22, 635, 2001.

81. Umemura, T. et al. Pentachlorophenol (PCP) produces liver oxidative stress and promotes but does not initiate hepatocarcinogenesis in B6C3F[1] mice, *Carcinogenesis* 20, 1115, 1999.

82. Dahlhaus, M. et al. Induction of 8-hydroxy-2-deoxyguanosine and single-strand breaks in DNA of V79 cells by tetrachloro-*p*-hydroquinone, *Mut. Res.* 329, 29, 1995.

83. Lin, P.-H. et al. Oxidative damage and direct adducts in calf thymus DNA induced by the pentachlorophenol metabolites, tetrachlorohydroquinone and tetrachloro-1,4-benzoquinone, *Carcinogenesis* 22, 627, 2002.

84. To-Figueras, J. et al. Accumulation of hexachlorobenzene in humans: a long standing risk., *Hum. Exp. Toxicol.* 14, 20, 1995.
85. Hardell, L. et al. Increased concentration of polychlorinated biphenyls, hexachlorobenzene, and chlordanes in mothers of men with testicular cancer, *Environ. Health Perspect.,* 111 (7), 930, 2003.

5 Dietary Phytoestrogens

Heather B. Patisaul and Patricia L. Whitten

CONTENTS

5.1 INTRODUCTION

In general, compounds classified as "endocrine disruptors" are regarded as adverse substances and presumed to have deleterious effects on mammalian systems. Human exposure to these compounds is thus recommended to be as limited as possible and great effort is being undertaken to reduce or eliminate these compounds in the environment. But one group of compounds contained within this classification is not presumed to have deleterious effects on mammalian systems but rather, quite the opposite. While most endocrine disruptors are associated with dire predictions regarding declining fertility, and increase cancer risk, this one intriguing group is touted to provide an array of beneficial effects that could provide preventative or

0-8493-2281-2/05/$0.00+$1.50
© 2005 by CRC Press

therapeutic actions in carcinogenesis, atherosclerosis, and osteoporosis. For that reason, these compounds have gained considerable notoriety in the popular literature and in October of 1999, the U.S. Food and Drug Administration (FDA) approved the health claim that daily consumption of these compounds is effective in reducing the risk of coronary artery disease in Americans.

These compounds are phytoestrogens, a group of nonsteroidal compounds found in plants, particularly soybeans and other legumes. Phytoestrogens are classically defined as any plant compound that is functionally or structurally similar to estrogen, or that produces estrogenic effects.[1] This definition includes compounds that bind to estrogen receptors, induce estrogen-responsive gene products, stimulate breast cancer cells *in vitro*, and stimulate growth of the female genital tract.[2] Although they were originally described as weak estrogens, with potencies rather similar to the *in vivo* and *in vitro* ranges reported for synthetic endocrine disruptors, many phytoestrogens are capable of acting as both estrogen agonists and antagonists depending on the target tissue.

The phytoestrogens are divided into two major classes: lignans and isoflavonoids. The latter group is the more intensely studied of the two and is further divided into the isoflavones, isoflavans, and coumestans. Mycoestrogens, or mycotoxins, are a similar group of compounds that can have potent estrogenic effects, but are not intrinsic components of plants. They are mold metabolites of the fungal genus *Fusarium,* which frequently infects pasture grasses and legumes including alfalfa and clover. Although they have received little attention in recent years compared to other phytoestrogens, they are the compounds that initially generated interest in the topic of naturally occurring estrogens, and their effects on health and reproduction. A hierarchy of phytoestrogens is presented in Figure 5.1.

Phytoestrogens occur at high levels in variety of foods, particularly those that are soy-based, such as soy infant formula, tofu, and soy flour. Numerous dietary supplements are also available that contain a wide range of phytoestrogens, particularly the isoflavones. Although they behave similarly to other endocrine-disrupting compounds on numerous molecular and cellular targets, the attitude regarding these effects by phytoestrogens is generally positive, while similar action by their synthetic counterparts often generates great concern. Much of this somewhat paradoxical position is based on the presumption that because phytoestrogens are natural, and consumed in large quantities by populations with low cancer rates such as the Japanese[3], they must be beneficial, while synthetic compounds, by virtue of their inorganic origins, must be detrimental. However, the rapidly expanding literature on phytoestrogens may in fact suggest that the highly celebrated health benefits of soy are not entirely merited, and their regular consumption should be approached with some caution. Thus, the phytoestrogens both expand our view of environmental substances with endocrine action and demonstrate that the source of the compound in question often influences the interpretation of the data.

Flavonoids
    Flavanones
        4',7-Dihydroxyflavanone
        Naringenin
    Flavones
        Apigenin
        4',5-Dihydroxyflavone
        4',6-Dihydroxyflavone
    Flavonols
        Kaempferol
    Hydroxychalcones
        Phloretin
        Isoliquirtigenin
        4,4'-Dihydroxychalcone
    Isoflavonoids
        Isoflavones
            Daidzein
            Formononetin
            Genistein
            Biochanin A
        Isoflavanones
            O-Desmethylangolensin
        Isoflavans
            Equol
        Coumestans
            Coumestrol
Lignans
    Enterlactone
    Enterodiol
Mycoestrogens
    Zearalenone
    Zearalenol
    Zearalanol (zeranol)

FIGURE 5.1 Hierarchy and classification of phytoestrogens

5.2 DIETARY SOURCES OF PHYTOESTROGENS

5.2.1 LIGNANS

Lignans are a minor component of plant cell walls. The plant lignans matairesinol and secoisolariciresinol are converted to the mammalian lignans enterlactone and enterodiol, respectively (Figure 5.2), by the resident bacterial flora of the gut.[4,5] The highest concentrations of mammalian lignans are produced from oilseeds, particularly flaxseed, which produces 50 to 100 times that of nearly every other plant studied.[6,7] Mammalian lignans are also produced from whole grains, cereal brans, legumes, and vegetables.[8,9] The *in vitro* production of lignans from some common foods is listed in Table 5.1.

TABLE 5.1
Human Lignan Production from Various Foods*

Food	Enterodiol (μg produced by fecal flora/100g sample)	Enterlactone (mg/100g)
Flaxseed meal	59,024	8,517
Flaxseed flour	40,861	11,818
Soybeans	170	693
Rapeseed	155	975
Oat bran	386	265
Wheat bran	298	269
Barley	74	41
Brown rice	128	169
Garlic	326	81
Asparagus	238	136
Broccoli	65	161
Potatoes	50	33
Pears	69	112
Bananas	14	55

* Adapted from data presented by Thompson et al. [8]

The values in the table are expressed in mg produced by human fecal flora from 100 g of nondessicated sample.

5.2.2 ISOFLAVONOIDS

The isoflavonoids are divided into three major classes: isoflavones, isoflavans, and coumestans, of which the isoflavones are the most widely studied group. The major mammalian isoflavones are genistein and daidzein, which are formed from the plant precursors formononetin and biochanin A, respectively. The most significant isoflavan is equol, a metabolite of daidzein. Coumestrol is the major coumestan. Very little is known about the coumestans compared to the other isoflavonoids. Coumestrol is the most potent phytoestrogen, with a binding affinity similar to 17β-estradiol for ERα and an affinity nearly twice that of 17β-estradiol for ERβ.[10]

Phytoestrogenic isoflavonoids are less prevalent than lignans. Legumes are the richest source of isoflavones with the highest concentrations found in soybeans and soybean-based products.[2] Soybeans can contain anywhere from 560 to 3810 mg isoflavones/kg, depending on variety and growing conditions,[9] and the isoflavone content of soy-derived foods such as tempeh, tofu, soy milk, soy protein supplements, and soy infant formula can vary considerably between brands and even between lots within the same brands.[9,11,12] Alfalfa produces only small amounts of isoflavones, but clover can contain up to 5% dry weight of various isoflavones, including genistein, formononetin, and biochanin A.[13] It is this legume that caused sterility in pasture-grazing sheep in the 1940s, hence the name "clover disease" for the affliction.[14] All of the legumes are susceptible to infection by *Fusarium* fungus, which produces high levels of

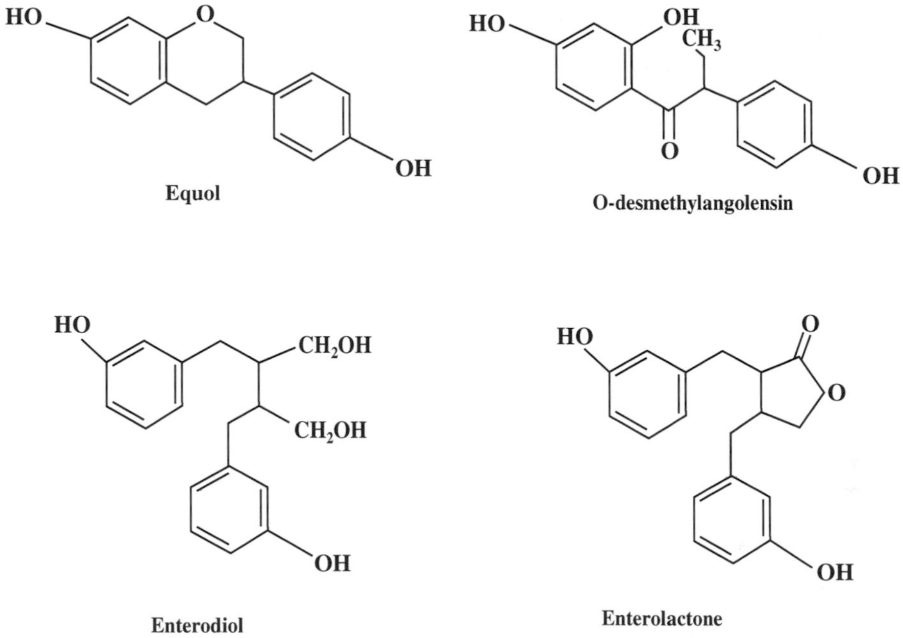

FIGURE 5.2 Mammalian metabolites of isoflavones (equol, o-desmethylangolensis) and lignans (enterodiol, enterolactone).

mycoestrogens such as zearalenone. Once infected, many legumes elevate their own phytoestrogen production, further increasing the exogenous estrogen exposure for any animal grazing on infected pasture. Whole grain products, potatoes, fruits, and vegetables also contain detectable levels of isoflavonoids.[3,9] The isoflavone content of a variety of soy-based foods is summarized in Table 5.2.

5.2.3 METABOLISM

In plants, phytoestrogens are most frequently found conjugated with glucose in their glycosidic form. Once ingested, these biologically inactive glycosides are metabolized into the active aglycone forms as well as other conjugated forms. The exact metabolic processes and pharmacokinetics of how each individual compound is converted are not completely characterized and vary between species, but in all mammals gut flora are essential for the initial hydrolysis and metabolism of these compounds. Only after this has occurred can the metabolites be absorbed by the animal, where they may undergo further conjugation and degradation by liver enzymes. Complete metabolism in most species involves several intermediate compounds, some of which have a higher binding affinity for the estrogen receptors than the end products.

In humans, the two most common bioactive aglycone isoflavones, genistein and daidzein, are produced through the hydrolysis of their glucoside conjugates (genistin and daidzin) or though metabolism of biochanin A and formononetin, respectively.

TABLE 5.2
Isoflavone Content of Various Foods

Food	Daidzein (μg/g)	Genistein (μg/g)	Coumestrol (μg/g)	Method	Ref
Soy beans — dry, whole	700	200	None detected	HPLC	235
Soybean seeds, dry	846.25	1106.75	None detected	HPLC	236†
Soybean seeds, roasted	848.1	1105.5	None detected	HPLC	236
Soybean seeds, boiled	68.5	69.4	None detected	HPLC	236
Green soybeans	54.6	72.9	None detected	HPLC	236
Soy flour	523.5	854.1	None detected	HPLC, GC-MS	3,235,236*
Soy protein — textured	523.25	636.25	None detected	HPLC	235‡
Soy nuts	575	935	None detected	HPLC	235
Soybean sprouts	138	230	7	HPLC	235
Soy hot dogs	49	139	N/A	HPLC	235
Soy cheese	14	20	N/A	HPLC	235
Tempeh	190	320	N/A	HPLC	235
Tofu	76	166	None detected	HPLC	235
Soy sauce	8	5	None detected	HPLC	235
Poppy seeds	17.9	16.7	N/A	GC-MS	3
Green split peas	72.6	None detected	None detected	HPLC	236
Kala chana seeds — dry	None detected	6.4	61.3	HPLC	236
Alfalfa sprouts	None detected	None detected	46.8	HPLC	236
Clover sprouts	None detected	3.5	280.6	HPLC	236
Garlic	2.08	1.45	N/A	GC-MS	3
Carrots	1.6	1.7	N/A	GC-MS	3

† Table values are averages of the values from all reported trials in the referenced paper.
* Table values are averages of the values reported in all three papers.
‡ Table values are averages of the values listed in the referenced paper.

Genistein ultimately metabolizes to 6'-hydroxy-*O*-demethlangolensin (6'-OH-*O*-DMA), which has unknown effects.[15] Daidzein is further metabolized into dihydro-daidzein, then equol, and *O*-demethylangolensin (*O*-DMA) in humans. Of particular interest in this pathway is equol, a superior antioxidant with a relatively high affinity for both estrogen receptors, particularly ERβ. Several studies have now demonstrated that many individuals apparently lack the ability to metabolize daidzein to equol, or can only produce it in negligible quantities. In fact, only about 35% of the population excretes appreciable levels of equol, and even among equol-producers, levels of equol in urine can vary up to 800-fold.[16-20] The factors governing equol production remain largely elusive, but the specific population of microflora present in the intestine combined with a diet low in fat and rich in carbohydrates may play an important role.[21,22]

Interestingly, the ability to metabolize daidzein to equol may increase with prolonged soy ingestion in women, but not men,[23] suggesting a sex difference in the way daidzein is metabolized. Sex differences may exist for other phytoestrogens as well. Men have been shown to excrete more of the mammalian lignan enterolactone and less enterodiol than women,[24] and both adult and adolescent women excrete more daidzein than men.[23]

Human metabolism and excretion of phytoestrogens in general varies substantially between populations as well as among individuals. Numerous studies in several countries have all revealed that vegetarians excrete the highest levels of lignans while breast cancer patients excrete the lowest. Japanese men and women have among the highest levels of urinary isoflavones, but low values of lignans.[3,25-27] Most of these differences are due to dietary variation. Asian diets are particularly high in soy, while vegetarian diets are high in whole grains, vegetables, legumes, and other sources of lignans.[28]

This variation might be due to interindividual differences in the quantity and composition of intestinal microflora. A portion of this variation can also be attributed to specific dietary intake because the phytoestrogen content of soy and other foods varies widely due to differences in processing and preparation. Soy processing also appears to influence isoflavone bioavailability. Urinary recovery of daidzein and genistein in men was higher for subjects consuming tempeh than for those consuming unfermented soy, suggesting that the aglycone conjugate of isoflavones found in fermented food may be more bioavailable than the glucoside conjugates that predominate in unfermented soy.[17] The phytoestrogenic content of edible plants also changes from season to season and year to year, depending on the growing conditions.[29] What has not been considered to date when attempting to account for individual variability is the effect of body size and body composition, which may play a critical role in the metabolism of these compounds.

Metabolism of phytoestrogens is also species specific. Cows produce significantly more equol than sheep, and clear it from their systems far more slowly.[13,30] As a result, small amounts of equol are present in meat and dairy products derived from cows. In ruminants, many isoflavones including genistein and biochanin A are broken down to non-estrogenic p-ethyl phenol and organic acids in the rumen, resulting in poor absorption. Humans, on the other hand, absorb considerable amounts, and conjugates of the isoflavones are found in all bodily fluids.[30,31]

Although the literature regarding the species-specific metabolism of numerous phytoestrogens is growing rapidly, relatively little work has been done on the most commonly used species for phytoestrogen research: rodents. Very few studies have examined the pharmacokinetics of phytoestrogen metabolism in rodents, but the current literature suggests that it shares many characteristics with the human system. For example, rodents generate appreciable levels of equol 24 to 48 hours after a meal,[32,33] and daidzein appears to be more bioavailable than genistein.[32,34] However, a more recent study using a different strain of rats found that daidzein was only poorly absorbed and thus only minimally bioavailable.[35] Overall, nearly all rodents generate equol, a characteristic shared with only around 35% of the human population. This critical difference may make it difficult to extrapolate experimental results from rodent models to humans. Without a more complete description of the pharmacokinetics of phytoestrogens in rodents, it will be difficult to accurately translate results gained from rodent experiments to human health concerns.

5.4 ACTIVITY

5.4.1 ESTROGEN RECEPTOR BINDING

Phytoestrogens get their name from their ability to mimic the actions of endogenous estrogens. Structurally, the isoflavonoid phytoestrogens and endogenous estrogens are markedly similar, as shown in Figure 5.2. For both groups of compounds, the A-ring is aromatic. There is a hydroxyl group at the C3 position in steroidal estrogens and in the equivalent position in phytoestrogens (7 in ring A and 4 in ring B). The D-ring of natural estrogens is a cyclopentano ring, but the terminal ring is aromatic in the isoflavonoids.[36] The lignans show less structural similarity to natural estrogens. All are diphenols but have a strikingly different conformation.

Because of their structural similarity to endogenous estrogens, isoflavonoid phytoestrogens can bind to estrogen receptors (ERs). ER belongs to a large family of nuclear receptor transcription factors defined by five distinct domains associated with ligand binding, DNA binding, and transactivation. There are two distinct isoforms of the estrogen receptor, ERα and ERβ, which both act as ligand-activated transcriptional regulators. The DNA-binding domain is highly conserved between the two isoforms (96% homology) but only a moderate level of conservation exists in the ligand-binding domain (58% homology).[37,38] The appreciable difference in the amino acid sequence of the ligand-binding domain drove the hypothesis that phytoestrogens bind with different affinities to ERβ than to ERα. Numerous studies have now clearly demonstrated that the majority of phytoestrogens have a far lower binding affinity for either ERα or ERβ than 17β-estradiol, but have a higher overall affinity for ERβ than ERα.[29,39-41] The one notable exception to this observation is coumestrol, which may have an affinity for ERα comparable to that of 17β-estradiol, and an even higher affinity for ERβ than any endogenous estrogen.[10]

The two ER isoforms exhibit distinct but overlapping patterns of tissue distribution [42,43] and are present in nearly all mammalian organs including the ovaries, prostate, spleen, bone, thymus, vasculature, and the brain.[37,38,44-46] In contrast, a number of studies have now shown that ERβ may be the dominant isoform in the fetus, indicating that it may play a significant role in the growth and development of the fetus.[47-49]

There is intense interest in the differential roles of each isoform but to date very little is known about their relationship to each other. Numerous studies using ER knockout mice suggest that each isoform has a distinct biological role. Both male and female ERα-knockout mice display numerous physiological and behavioral defects, including sterility, while male ERβ-knockout mice remain fertile but have prostate and bladder hyperplasia and females show ovulatory disfunction.[50-53] The degree to which the phytoestrogens can affect estrogen-dependent processes depends heavily on their ability to function as ligands through both ER isomers, and the relative roles each isomer plays in mammalian systems.

Successful binding to the estrogen receptors occurs though two distinct steps: receptor recognition and stabilization of the receptor-ligand complex.[54] For endogenous estrogens, receptor recognition is achieved by hydrogen bonding between the C3 hydroxyl group on the estrogen, and amino acid side chain in the binding domain of the ER. Stabilization is achieved through hydrogen binding to the D-ring, but does not require a hydroxyl group.[54,55]

Biological potencies of phytoestrogens relative to 17β-estradiol through both ERα and ERβ appear to be largely determined by the orientation of the AF-2 region of the ligand binding domain of the receptor upon binding with the phytoestrogen. Crystal analysis of the tertiary structure of the ligand-binding domain revealed that this region is made up of 12 highly conserved helices, of which the last one (H12) makes up the critical core of the AF-2 region.[56] The recruitment surface for a number of nuclear coactivators required for transcriptional activation is partially defined by H12, suggesting that the optimal efficiency of the ER-ligand complex is at least partially dependent on the orientation of this helix.[57-59] Whether or not a compound acts as an estrogen agonist or antagonist is well correlated to the position of H12 relative to the ligand-binding cavity in both isoforms of ligand-bound ER. Genistein binds to the ligand-binding domain of ERβ in an orientation similar to that of 17β-estradiol, but H12 lies in an orientation similar to that seen with estrogen antagonists.[60] This orientation is similar to selective estrogen receptor modulators, such as raloxifene, which are defined by their mixed agonist/antagonist effects through both ERα and ERβ.[57]

Once formed, the ligand-receptor complex is taken into the cell and functions as a nuclear transcription factor by binding to an estrogen response element (ERE) and facilitating assembly of a functional transcription complex. Many attempts have been made to quantify the relative binding affinities and potencies of phytoestrogens compared to estradiol. Depending on which assay is used, widely different values have been obtained, creating discrepancies about which phytoestrogens are the most estrogenic. Given the large number of coactivator and corepressor molecules needed for optimal ER action, these assays are likely only of limited value given that they cannot completely replicate the complex and tissue-specific cellular environment seen *in vivo*. With these limitations in mind, these assays suggest that the mycoestrogens and coumestrol are nearly as potent as 17β-estradiol,[39-41] while genistein and equol are only moderately potent.[40,61] Biochanin A, formononetin, and genistein are the least potent and may have only minimal biological activity.[29,40] Although the exact order in which these phytoestrogens should be placed in relation to estrogenic potency is not clear, these studies and others comparing them to each other and to other related compounds reveal that the 4′-hydroxy position on the B ring and its spatial orientation in relation to the 7-position hydroxy group on the A ring are primarily responsible for the estrogenicity of flavonoids.[62] This is illustrated by the reduced potency of biochanin A compared with genistein. Biochanin A has a methyl group in this position but is otherwise structurally identical to genistein, and has a much lower potency. This structural difference is depicted in Figure 5.2.

The discovery of a second estrogen receptor introduced a whole new level of complexity to the actions and activity of phytoestrogens in animals. It appears that some tissues, which contain little or no ERα, contain relatively high levels of ERβ, particularly during development. Because the isoflavonoids preferentially bind to ERβ over ERα, these compounds may have a profound impact on developmental processes, particularly in the brain, where hormones are critical for sexual differentiation and determination.

5.4.2 Mechanisms of Action not Mediated by Estrogen Receptors

Phytoestrogens also have many ER-independent effects. Enterolactone, genistein, and daidzein have been shown *in vitro* to stimulate hormone-binding globulin (SHBG) synthesis in liver cells,[63] and several phytoestrogens are capable of competitively displacing both 17β-estradiol and testosterone from SHBG in plasma.[64] Only the unbound fraction of endogenous hormone is bioactive. Thus, by altering either the total amount or availability of SHBG, phytoestrogens could affect the free fraction of endogenous hormones in circulation. However, studies in both Western and Asian women evaluating SHBG levels after a dietary soy challenge providing between 32 and 68 mg of isoflavones per day have only demonstrated nonsignificant decreases in SHBG serum levels averaging less than 2%.[65-67] This modest decrease was coupled with a nonsignificant decrease in luteal phase progesterone levels,[65,67] although one other group has found that a soymilk diet delivering isoflavone levels approximately twice as high can decrease luteal phase progesterone levels by as much as 45% and follicular phase 17β-estradiol levels by 25%.[68] This result is consistent with previous studies showing minimal[66,69] decreases in follicular phase plasma 17β-estradiol levels with isoflavone consumption.

The observed decreases in circulating endogenous estrogen levels may be due to disruption of aromatase. Isoflavones and lignan phytoestrogens, including equol, genistein, and biochanin A are potent inhibitors of the ovarian aromatase enzyme, which produces estrogen from androstenedione and testosterone in humans.[70-72] Coumestrol has been shown *in vitro* to reduce the conversion of [3H]-estrone to [3H]-estradiol by inhibiting the estrogen-specific enzyme 17β-hydroxysteroid oxidoreductase Type 1, in a dose-dependent fashion beginning with concentrations as low as 0.12 μM.[73] Genistein was more weakly inhibitory but demonstrated a similar dose-dependent effect.

Genistein is a unique phytoestrogen with a variable array of physiological effects. In addition to the effects listed above, genistein is a potent inhibitor of tyrosine protein kinases (PTKs).[74,75] PTKs catalyze phosphorylation of their own tyrosine residues and those of other proteins, including growth factors involved in tumor cell proliferation. By inhibiting PTKs, genistein can potentially slow tumerogenesis. Genistein can also inhibit DNA topoisomerases I and II, enzymes essential for DNA replication.[2,76]

5.5 PHYSIOLOGICAL EFFECTS

Phytoestrogens were first discovered to have physiological effects early last century when Australian sheep grazing on legume-rich pasture began to develop unusual reproductive abnormalities. Abortion rates were extraordinarily high in several flocks and many ewes became permanently sterile. In 1946, Bennetts et al. described severe clinical abnormalities in these animals including prolapse of the uterus, dystocia in ewes, low lambing rates, enlargement of the bulbo-urethral glands, and death.[14] This syndrome came to be known as "clover disease" and is still a potential problem that must be carefully managed by farmers today.

The observed infertility was ultimately found to be caused by anatomical changes in the cervix and uterus, which compromised the transport of spermatozoa through the cervix after insemination.[13,77] In the ewe, the genes controlling sexual differentiation do not completely deactivate after birth. Exposure to high levels of estrogen for several months can continue the differentiation process, resulting in a cervix that anatomically resembles the uterus in both histological appearance and function, and prevents normal sperm transport. The discovery that certain plants could induce reproductive abnormalities, including sterility, prompted an intense investigation aimed at identifying which phytochemicals could produce physiological effects in animals and humans, and what exactly those effects were.

Phytoestrogens are classically defined as weak estrogens but are now widely recognized to act as both agonists and antagonists of estrogen in mammalian systems depending upon the dose given, the timing of exposure, and the tissue of interest. They have been found to have both beneficial and deleterious effects on numerous physiological endpoints across several species, prompting an intense public health debate regarding their regular consumption. In that discourse, the early findings demonstrating that phytoestrogens could produce severe reproductive abnormalities in farm animals was drowned out by epidemiological evidence that populations consuming high amounts of phytoestrogens had lower cancer rates and fewer cardiovascular problems than populations consuming only small amounts of phytoestrogens.[25,78,79] A number of studies have now also demonstrated that breast cancer patients have far fewer isoflavones in their urine than women with healthy breast tissue, suggesting a link between phytoestrogen consumption and breast cancer rates.[80-82] A growing literature now also suggests that phytoestrogens may lower cholesterol, prevent bone mass reduction in postmenopausal women, and alleviate the symptoms of menopause including hot flashes. All of this evidence recently prompted the FDA to recommend that Americans consume 25 mg of soy a day. Daily soy consumption in the United States is now closer to only 1 to 3 g, while in Asian populations daily soy consumption typically ranges from 10 to 50 g.[83] There are now hundreds of soy-based dietary supplements and foods available to consumers that market themselves as "heart healthy" based on that FDA guideline. With all the hype surrounding soy, it is critical to evaluate all of the physiological effects of these compounds in context, and critically evaluate the validity of all the health claims that currently surround soy phytoestrogens.

5.5.1 Hormonal and Reproductive Effects

The earliest evidence that phytoestrogens could produce significant reproductive effects came from farm animals. Heifers grazing on phytoestrogen rich red clover developed 35% longer teats on average and had an accumulation of fluid in the vagina and uterus. Uterine tone increased, as did uterine size in ovariectomized animals.[84] Although phytoestrogen-induced infertility in cattle is rare today, phytoestrogens can cause cystic ovaries, irregular estrus, and anestrus in sheep, cattle, and rodents.[13,85,86]

Of all the biological effects phytoestrogens have been affiliated with, infertility is the one that causes the most concern. First seen in sheep, phytoestrogen-related infertility has now been observed in an array of species. A 1976 study confirmed that the breeding success of California quail depend on the phytoestrogen content of forbs growing in their breeding ranges.[87] Genistein and formononetin were present in significantly higher concentrations in forbs growing in dry years than in forbs growing in wet years. Consequently, as a result of consuming a phytoestrogen-rich diet, breeding was generally unsuccessful and many birds left California as early as June for their winter roosts.

One of the most recent examples of phytoestrogen-related infertility involves captive cheetahs. In the 1980s, high mortality coupled with low fertility threatened to drastically reduce captive cheetah populations in North American zoos. The most prevalent cause of death in these animals was liver disease of unknown etiology, and nearly 60% of all North American cheetahs had venocclusive disease.[88] Additionally, only 9 to 12% of North American captive female cheetahs were producing viable cubs, compared with 60 to 80% of African captive female cheetahs. The vast majority of these animals were primarily fed a commercially prepared diet containing between 5 and 13% soy protein, exposing each cheetah to 50 mg/day of phytoestrogens including high levels of genistein and daidzein.[88] When four cheetahs at the Cincinnati Zoo were placed on a soy-free diet for three months, their liver condition improved significantly, and a few females became pregnant, implying that the soy in the commercial diet was contributing to the illness and the infertility. Estrogens are known to produce changes in blood coagulation with secondary liver involvement[89] and have cholestatic effects, which causes bile retention and alterations in the shunting of substances into the vascular compartment.[90] Phytoestrogens, by nature of their estrogenicity, may produce similar effects.

Humans may be facing a very similar situation. Infertility among young couples inexplicably tripled between 1965 and 1982,[91] and there is some evidence to suggest that mean sperm density and seminal volume has declined over the past 50 years.[92,93] The issue is contentious and the subject of intense debate,[94] but although exogenous estrogens such as DDT and PCBs are hypothesized to be one of the primary causes of declining human fertility,[95,96] dietary phytoestrogens are almost totally absent from this discussion.

Only a handful of studies have evaluated the effect of phytoestrogen consumption on reproductive health in men. A recent study found that dietary supplementation with soy scones providing 120 mg/day of isoflavones reduced serum testosterone;[97]

other studies have found that consumption of an isoflavone supplement containing 40 mg of isoflavones or flaxseeds had no effect on sperm quality or production.[98,99] However, if phytoestrogens and other endocrine disruptors can decrease sperm quality, disruption during the organizational period of Sertoli cell development rather than in adulthood would be the more likely mechanism of action. Timing, more than dose or duration of exposure, may be the most critical factor in the relationship between phytoestrogens and male fertility and warrants further investigation.

Phytoestrogens may also decrease sexual motivation and function in females. Coumestrol and soy isoflavones have been shown to disrupt estrogen-dependent gene expression in the brain,[100,101] an effect that subsequently leads to decreased sexual behavior in female rats.[102,103] Whether or not soy has a similar effect in women is completely unknown, but there is anecdotal evidence that the breast cancer drug tamoxifen, an endocrine-disrupting drug with similar molecular properties to the isoflavones, decreases sexual desire and increases sexual discomfort.[104,105] Phytoestrogens are also known to affect other reproductive endpoints in women. Several studies have attempted to examine the effects of soy on menstrual cycle length, but only a few have been conducted with true control groups in a well-powered, randomized crossover or parallel arm design. All three suggest that phytoestrogens increase cycle length but only by about 12 hours, not a biologically or statistically significant extension.[66,69,106] Only one study has found a significant association with soy consumption and decreased cycle length (1.2 days), an effect the authors hypothesize would ultimately result in 2 fewer years of menstruation and thus a lower risk of breast cancer.[107] However, the results were drawn from interviewing a nonrepresentative sample of 200 Singapore Chinese women, thus the results are highly dependent on the accuracy of those self-reports.

Phytoestrogen consumption may also influence the metabolism of endogenous estrogen. There are many estrogen metabolites but two have generated a lot of interest because the ratio between the relatively inert

2-hydroxylated estrogens to the more genotoxic 4- and 16 α -hydroxylated forms are believed to be correlated with breast cancer risk.[108,109] 16α-Hydroxyestrogen (16α-OHE) induces DNA synthesis[110] while 4-hydroxyestradiol (4-OHE$_2$) and 4-hydroxyestrogen (4-OHE$_1$) have been shown to generate mutations that initiate cancer.[111] There is good evidence that isoflavones may significantly increase the ratio of 2-OH to both 16α-OHE and 4-OHE. Consumption of a dietary supplement containing at least 65 mg of isoflavones per day improved the 2- to 4-(OHE) ratio by 33% and the 2-to-16αOHE ratio by 67%, compared to a supplement containing only 10 mg of isoflavones.[112] Other studies using isolated soy protein or soy milk have found similarly compelling effects,[68,113] while at least one study using isolated soy protein delivering only 38 mg of isoflavones per day found only modest 7% increase in the 2-16αOHE ratio.[69] Interestingly, urinary levels of 16α-OHE are only positively associated with urinary levels of isoflavones in equol-producing women, and within that group, the ratio of 16α-OHE to 2-OHE is significantly positively correlated to equol excretion, suggesting that this daidzein metabolite may be critical for this effect.[114]

5.5.2 DEVELOPMENTAL EFFECTS

Estrogens and androgens play a critical role in development and influence growth and differentiation in tissues including the gonads and the brain. Because of their ability to produce estrogenic effects, phytoestrogens may influence fetal development and ultimately affect reproductive physiology and behavior in adulthood. As a fetus develops, there are specific, critical periods when it is particularly sensitive to hormones. In rats, this critical period lasts through the final third of gestation and into the first 10 days of life.[115] This suggests that timing of exposure may be as or even more important than the level of exposure. When examining the effects of phytoestrogens on fetal development, it is important to consider the stage of development along with the level of phytoestrogen exposure.

The developmental effects of phytoestrogens have been studied mostly in rats and interpreted to have implications for human health. The results of some of these studies are presented in Table 5.3. Rats exposed to coumestrol, lignans, or genistein during the perinatal period have severe reproductive tract abnormalities as well as altered neuroendocrine function and abnormal reproductive behaviors as adults.[116-119] Prenatal exposure to genistein at doses between 5 and 300 mg produce a variety of developmental effects including low birth weight and delayed vaginal opening in females, and shortened anogenital distances, decreased testicular size, and lower endogenous testosterone levels in males.[116,120]

Exposure to phytoestrogens during lactation also impair reproductive function and gonadotropin secretion in adulthood. Coumestrol administration (10 to 100 µg) immediately after birth significantly increased uterine weight and severely reduced ER levels in the uterus.[121] Twenty days after exposure, uterine weight was lower in coumestrol-treated animals than the controls, while ER levels were still below normal. Treatment with 40 mg of genistein per kg of body weight per day during

---

TABLE 5.3
Developmental Effects of Phytoestrogens and Mycoestrogens in Rodents

Tissue	Phytoestrogen	Effect	Reference
Uterus	Coumestrol, Zearalenone	Reduced number of glands and ER expression	121,237
Vagina	Coumestrol, Genistein	Cornification, metaplasia, delayed opening	86,120,238
Breast	Genistein	Increased duct development	181
Anogenital	Genistein	Decreased distance in males	120
Prostate	Coumestrol, Daidzein	Increased c-fos, prevention of DES lesions	239
Hypothalamus	Coumestrol	Premature anovulation, abnormal sexual behavior in males	86,240
Pituitary	Coumestrol, Genistein, Zearalenone	Altered LH response, decreased basal LH	125,241
SDN-POA	Coumestrol, Genistein	Enlarged in females	125,241

lactation (PND 1 to 21) advanced vaginal opening, increased uterine weight, and induced a permanent estrus state.[122] Daily treatment with 1 mg genistein or daidzein (approximately 100 mg/kg body weight) for PND 1 to 5 resulted in earlier vaginal opening and prolonged or persistent estrus in genistein- but not daidzein-treated females.[123] Ovaries were smaller in both genistein- and daidzein-treated females at 60 days of age and lacked corpora lutea in the genistein-treated females. Persistent exposure to coumestrol through lactation after the first 10 post-natal days resulted in acyclicity in early adulthood due to a deficit in the regulation of gonadotropin secretion and suppressed early growth, resulting in lower than average weight at vaginal opening.[117] Genistein also suppressed LH in a dose-dependent fashion[124] when administered during the first 10 days of life.

Perinatal phytoestrogen exposure also effects sexual differentiation in the rodent brain. The sexually dimorphic nucleus in the preoptic area of the hypothalamus (SND-POA) is normally 2 to 5 times larger in male than female rats, and this estrogen-dependent sexual differentiation occurs between gestation day 16 and post-natal day 5.[115] Perinatal exposure of female rats to DES, or high doses (500 µg or 1000 µg) of either zearalenone or genistein during the critical period, results in significantly larger SDN-POA volumes than female controls.[124,125] Interestingly, this effect of genistein is only significant in ovariectomized but not intact rat neonates,[125] suggesting that the endogenous hormone status of the animal is an important determinant in the biological activity of phytoestrogens on SND-POA volume.

Early exposure to phytoestrogens may influence not only reproductive physiology in adulthood, but also behavior. Neonatal treatments with genistein, but not daidzein, lowered lordotic activity in female rats,[123] and male rats exposed to either genistein or coumestrol through lactation exhibit a number of deficits in sexual behavior as adults. Exposed males have a lower ejaculation rate, a longer latency to first mount interval, and fewer overall mount attempts than unexposed males.[116,117] Very few studies have examined the influence of phytoestrogens on sexual behavior, and more research in this area is badly needed.

5.5.2.1 Phytoestrogen Exposure in Infants

In light of these developmental actions, concern has been raised over human infant exposure to phytoestrogens. Although they were initially introduced as an alternative to bovine milk formulas for babies with a milk allergy, soy infant formula has grown in popularity, largely because of numerous articles in the popular media celebrating the beneficial effects of soy, and now makes up approximately 25% of the formula market in the United States. Total isoflavone content in soy infant formula varies widely largely due to the influence of environmental and genetic differences between batches and sources but in general is quite high with as much as 122 µg genistein and 77 µg daidzein per gram of formula.[126-129] This translates to a daily intake of approximately 6 to 9 mg/kg body weight per day, an amount, when adjusted for body weight, which is 4 to 7 times higher than the amounts regularly consumed by adults meeting the FDA guidelines for soy consumption or Asians consuming a traditional soy-based diet (0.3 to 1.2 mg/kg per day).[130] Infants fed soy formula have circulating phytoestrogen concentrations of approximately 1 µg/ml, 13,000 to 22,000 times higher than endogenous estrogens, which range from 40 to 80 pg/ml in infancy.[131] These are levels high enough to produce many of the physiological effects already discussed in this chapter. In fact, a recent study in marmoset monkeys using a co-twin design demonstrated that a soy formula providing 1.6 to 3.5 mg isoflavone/kg/day suppressed the neonatal testosterone surge and increased Leydig cell number in comparison to a cow milk formula.[132]

Milk-based formulas contain significantly lower levels of phytoestrogens, with equol being the only isoflavone present in significant concentrations in the plasma of infants fed bovine milk-based formulas. This result is consistent with data showing that cows produce and excrete more equol than any other phytoestrogen.[13] Similar to the adult population, only about 30% of all infants examined to date had detectable levels of equol in their plasma, suggesting that the ability to produce equol varies in infants as well as adults. Infants do not have a full complement of gut flora at birth, and food consumption during the first year of life may ultimately dictate the nature of their colonic population, providing a mechanism for examining the emergence and regulation of equol production in humans.

Composition of human breastmilk is even more variable than either soy or bovine formula, not only between different women, but also within the same woman over the course of a day. Isoflavones enter breastmilk in a dose-dependent fashion in a biphasic pattern with maximum levels at 10 to 12 hours post-consumption and resumption of baseline values in as much as 2 to 4 days, depending on the isoflavone dose.[126,133] Peak genistein and daizein levels in breastmilk range from 10 nmol/L after consumption of only 5 g of roasted soybeans to 70 nmol/L after consumption of 20 to 25 g of roasted soybeans.

Although circulating isoflavone levels are highest among infants consuming soy formula, the fraction of bioavailable isoflavones may be higher in breast-fed infants with mothers who regularly consume soy.[126,128] Very few studies to date have examined the pharmacokinetics of phytoestrogens in infants, particularly those other than the isoflavones, but given the high levels of genistein and daizein seen in both breast-fed and soy formula-fed infants, it is an area that certainly warrants further investigation.

The considerable evidence in animal studies suggesting that perinatal exposure to phytoestrogens, particularly the isoflavones, can disrupt gonadotropin secretion,

TABLE 5.4
Isoflavone Content of Commercial Soy Infant Formulas

Soy Product (dry)	Daidzein (μg/g)	Genistein (μg/g)	Method	Reference
Prosobee	17	22	HPLC	127
Isomil	19	23	HPLC	127
Isomil	15	19	GC-MS	242
Jevity Isotonic	0.3	3.1	GC-MS	3

alter reproductive physiology, and compromise reproductive behavior in adulthood had generated great concern that soy-rich formulas may disrupt hormone-dependent development in human infants. However, to date there has only been one epidemiologic study comparing reproductive endpoints in adults fed soy- or milk-based formula as infants. This well-publicized study found modest increases in menstrual cycle length (0.37 days) and discomfort among the soy-fed women but no other appreciable effects.[134] Although it gained much attention when it was published, it has since been criticized for being underpowered and was conducted using retrospective surveys as a follow-up to a previous study undertaken when the subjects were infants, requiring the respondents to accurately recall events (such as age at first menarche) that took place as much as 20 years earlier. Clearly more evidence is needed to make any kind of conclusive determination about the safety of soy consumption by infants.

5.5.3 MENOPAUSAL SYMPTOMS

Menopause produces a wide range of hypoestrogenic symptoms in women including hot flashes, mood swings, and decreased sexual interest. In the United States, the hot flash is the hallmark of menopausal symptoms. Asian populations have a much lower incidence of both hot flashes and osteoporosis than American populations,[135,136] suggesting that phytoestrogens may reduce the incidence of these symptoms. Many women now believe that soy and soy-based supplements help relieve the symptoms of menopause, largely because of the overwhelming amount of advertisements and articles and popular media articles celebrating this supposed benefit.

Given all hype surrounding the association of soy to menopause relief, surprisingly few studies have actually attempted to validate this claim, and the results are mixed and largely discouraging.[137] The first, and most widely cited, study was conducted nearly a decade ago.[138] Women were given either soy or wheat flour for 12 weeks in a randomized, double-blind trial. Although hot flash frequency and intensity decreased by 40% over the 12-week trial in the group given soy flour, the same effect was seen in the wheat flour group, and by the end of the study, there were no statistically significant differences between the two groups. This large placebo effect has been seen in numerous subsequent studies, with some women reporting as much as a 60% reduction in hot flashes with placebo. As with this first study, although a measurable reduction in hot flash frequency and intensity is sometimes detected, these improvements are minimal and rarely reach statistical significance.[139-142] A recent analysis of the published studies found that the treatment efficacy of these trials is largely determined by the initial hot flash frequency of the subjects, with those patients with the more intense symptoms reporting the greatest benefits.[143] Although more studies are necessary, on the basis of these studies it appears unlikely that soy will have any appreciable benefit on hot flash intensity or frequency in women and that the anecdotal reports of symptom relief with soy supplements may be little more than a reflection of the placebo effect found with using "natural" therapies to treat menopausal symptoms.

5.6 OSTEOPOROSIS

Osteoporosis affects more than 10 million adults and although not exclusively a disease of women, estrogen deficiency is strongly associated with increased risk. Hormone replacement therapy (HRT) has proved an invaluable option for the prevention and treatment of this disorder, by preventing bone loss and minimizing the risk of fractures.[144] Unfortunately, a series of studies suggesting that long-term use of HRT may increase the risk of breast and endometrial cancers[145,146] and that it may not provide measurable cardioprotective effects as hoped[145] has discouraged many women and sparked an interest in alternative therapies. There is strong epidemiologic evidence demonstrating that Asians consuming a soy-rich diet have a significantly lower risk of suffering a hip fracture, despite the low calcium content of this diet.[147-149] Although diet may at least partially account for this difference, numerous other factors including body weight; skeletal mass; excretion rates of minerals such as potassium, phosphorus and calcium; and anatomical differences in hip structure are likely to also have a consequential role. The epidemiological association of a phytoestrogen-rich diet and higher bone density, particularly after menopause, has made this one of the fastest-growing areas of phytoestrogen research. Although most of the experimental evidence of an osteoprotective effect remains circumstantial, it is beginning to appear that soy isoflavones may offer measurable protection from the development of osteoporosis.

Studies on the actions of phytoestrogens on both osteoblasts, responsible for bone formation, and osteoclasts, responsible for bone resorption, *in vitro* have been very encouraging. For example, coumestrol has been shown to both inhibit bone resorption and stimulate bone mineralization *in vitro*,[150] and these findings have been replicated in at least one *in vivo* study, which demonstrated that daily injections of 1.5 µmol coumestrol twice weekly for six weeks significantly reduced bone loss in the spine and femur of ovariectomized rats.[151] These effects were accompanied by reduced urine calcium levels and excretion rates of the bone resorption markers pyridinoline and deoxypyridinoline. The soy isoflavones genistein and daidzein have been found to stimulate bone formation while simultaneously decreasing bone resorption *in vitro* through multiple mechanisms, including induction of apoptosis, activation of protein tyrosine phosphatase in osteoclasts, and stimulation of protein synthesis and alkaline phosphatase release in osteoblasts.[152-158] These studies and numerous others specifically examining the mechanism by which phytoesrogens may have osteoprotective effects have demonstrated that although both ERα and ERβ are abundant in human osteoblasts,[159-161] activity through estrogen receptors is likely only one of multiple and complex mechanisms by which the isoflavones may preserve bone density.

The *in vitro* studies in animals have produced similarly encouraging results. Most use ovariectomized animals, and both the dietary concentration of isoflavones and the observed effects vary considerably, but surprisingly nearly all of the studies using ovariectomized rodents have found that isoflavones have bone-sparing effects on both trabecular and cortical bone.[158] Genistein and daidzein have biphasic, dose-dependent effects on bone mineral density, with lower doses being more effective than higher doses.[162,163] This *in vivo* evidence combined with the compelling *in vitro* literature has sparked a wave of clinical trials examining the effects of a number of isoflavone-rich foods and supplements on bone mineral density in women.

One particularly interesting phytoestrogen in the discussion of phytoestrogens and bone density is the synthetic isoflavone ipriflavone. Ipriflavone has been shown to reduce osteoclast recruitment and differentiation, thereby inhibiting bone resorption, perhaps by the direct inhibition of parathyroid hormone on bone.[164] An early long-term study in postmenopausal women found that women taking 200 mg of ipriflavone daily (2.5 mg/kg) over a 2-year period along with a 1 g calcium supplement showed significantly lower bone loss than women given a placebo treatment along with the calcium supplement.[165] Nearly 10% of all ipriflavone consumed in a day will be metabolized into daidzein, suggesting that daidzein, taken at higher doses (e.g., > 1.8 mg/kg), may produce similar effects. Women given GnRH agonists to treat a variety of severe estrogen-dependent conditions including endometriosis and uterine fibroids enter a hypoestrogenic state, which alleviates the symptoms of the condition, but produces a variety of menopausal side effects including hot flashes and decreased bone density. Women given 600 mg of ipriflavone along with 500 mg calcium every day for 6 months showed no bone loss compared to women given the calcium supplements alone.[166] The results of these studies and others led to the approval of the drug for the treatment of osteoporosis in a number of countries but a recent, 3-year multicenter clinical study found it to be no better than placebo and associated it with an increased risk of developing lymphocytopenia, generating concerns about its long-term use.[167]

5.7 THE CANCER CONNECTION

The association between a soy-rich diet and cancer rates is one of the most well-studied and controversial areas of phytoestrogen research. The epidemiologic observation that Asian populations have much lower incidences of breast and prostate cancer than Western populations[3] has prompted great interest in the preventive and therapeutic effects of diet on these and other hormone-dependent cancers.[168,169] The case for a dietary rather than genetic role in this disparity was strengthened by the observation that when individuals of Chinese or Japanese descent move to North America and then assume a more typical Western diet, their risk of both breast and prostate cancer increases rapidly to at least half that of the indigenous population.[65,78,170] Dietary surveys from as far back as the 1960s indicate that Japanese populations consume considerably more soy-based food than individuals in the United States, which translates to higher isoflavone levels in blood, urine, feces, and prostatic fluid.[3,27,79,171] Urinary and plasma levels of phytoestrogens correlate negatively with rates of breast and prostate cancer risk.[25,80,172] All of this evidence is circumstantial, but suggests that consumption of phytoestrogens, particularly soy isoflavones, are protective against hormone-dependent cancers. It is also important to note that besides being rich in soy, the traditional Asian diet is low in fat and red meat and contains a lot of fish, which are rich in fatty acids. This overall diet pattern, even without the soy, is believed to be associated with decreased cancer risk. The experimental data linking soy to a decreased risk of cancer is not nearly as clear-cut.

Numerous *in vitro* studies have examined the effects of isoflavones, particularly genistein, on the proliferation of dozens of tumor cell lines with mixed effects.[3,173] Part of the conflict has arisen because of the different doses used to test for antiproliferative effects of phytoestrogens. Studies that use low concentrations (< 1 to 10 μM) have discovered that some phytoestrogens including genistein, daidzein, biochanin A, enterolactone, and coumestrol actually stimulate tumor proliferation, while other studies using higher concentrations of the same compounds have found antiproliferative effects.[174-176] This biphasic dose response is likely due to the mixed agonistic/antagonistic effects of isoflavones and is particularly significant given that human plasma levels are most often in the lower dose range. This would seem to suggest that phytoestrogen consumption would result in an increased cancer risk, but this is in direct conflict with the extensive epidemiological data. This apparent paradox would be resolved if organs such as the breasts and prostate have the ability to concentrate phytoestrogens. One study has already revealed that the prostate has this ability,[171] and the concentration of endogenous estrogens in normal breast ductal fluid is as much as 40-fold higher than that in serum, indicating that the breast may have the ability to concentrate phytoestrogens as well.[62] This observation makes understanding the effects of phytoestrogens on cancer cell growth at both high and low doses critical and emphasizes the need to pay particular attention to the concentration of phytochemicals in human tissues, not just plasma levels.

There is also some controversy surrounding the doses required *in vivo* to produce effects seen *in vitro* and how to normalize data gathered from different *in vitro* assays. Yeast estrogen screening assays are sensitive enough to produce results at much lower concentrations than those required for mammalian cell cultures,[41] but there are a multitude of assays developed by different labs, and not all of them are capable of adequately testing for antiestrogenic effects.[40] Because phytoestrogens can interact with SHBG and other proteins, the concentrations needed to produce biological effects in an animal or human will necessarily be much higher than the concentrations needed in an *in vitro* assay or cell culture.[177] Estrogen action occurs through multiple pathways, each with their own set of transcriptional cofactors and corepressors, the presence of which varies between tissues and cell types, thus making the *in vivo* environment difficult to replicate *in vitro*. To date there is no reliable way reconcile the results gathered from the multitude of available *in vitro* assays into a relevant and predictive model of *in vivo* effects making it difficult to draw any definitive conclusions from the data obtained from them.

5.7.1 Breast Cancer

A multitude of epidemiological studies have shown that subjects with breast cancer excrete lower amounts of lignans and isoflavonoids than healthy women, and that women living in low-risk countries have higher amounts of these compounds in their plasma and urine than women living in high-risk countries.[5,78,80,135,168,169,178] The mechanism behind this protection may come from reduced exposure to endogenous estrogens. Asian women have much lower levels of circulating estrogens than Western women.[26,179] It is unclear if these lower levels are attributable to diet or genetics. Numerous *in vitro* studies using breast cancer cell lines have found that in general, phytoestrogens inhibit tumor growth at super-physiological concentrations but stimulate growth at low concentrations. Rodent studies have yielded similarly conflicting results and, when considered as a whole, do not find a preventive effect of any phytoestrogen[173] except when phyoestrogen exposure occurs during development.[180] Early exposure to isoflavones, particularly genistein, may be critical for reducing the risk of breast cancer in adulthood. Female rats injected with 5 mg of genistein on post-natal days 2, 4, and 6 developed fewer dimethylbenz[a]anthracene (DMBA)-adenocarcinomas and had an increased mean-time to tumor development compared to control rats. The treated rats, however, had significantly reduced circulating progesterone, earlier vaginal opening, and follicular abnormalities including atretic antral follicles and fewer corpora lutea.[181] A second study found that female rats injected with 500 µg of genistein per gram of body weight on post-natal days 16, 18, and 20 also developed nearly half as many DMBA-induced mammary tumors as controls, but showed none of the reproductive side effects documented in the earlier study.[182] In both studies, genistein caused immediate and significant proliferation in the mammary glands, resulting in the creation of more differentiated terminal ductal structures. (lobules II). Premenarchal women have many undifferentiated terminal ductal structures that progress to more differentiated lobules during pregnancy. The earlier pregnancy is achieved, the lower the risk of breast cancer, indicating the protective effect of differentiation. More recent studies have found that physiological levels of genistein enhance ductal cell differentiation without any observable effects on the reproductive tract.[183]

Genistein is the most widely studied phytoestrogen in the cancer literature because it has numerous biochemical actions unrelated to its estrogenic activity. In addition to being an estrogen agonist/antagonist, it is the most powerful antioxident of all the phytoestrogens and has the ability to both increase the activities of antioxidant enzymes as well as directly inhibit hydrogen peroxide production. Female rats fed 250 ppm of genistein daily for 30 days showed a 10 to 30% increase in the activities of glutathione peroxidase, glutathione reductase, catalase, and superoxide dismutase.[184] Genistein is also a potent inhibitor of protein kinases, an effect that may be one of the most important and significant mechanisms for the hypothesized cancer-protective effects of genistein.[75] Several *in vitro* studies have also demonstrated that genistein can inhibit both topoisomerase I and II,[185] along with 5α-reductase, phenol sulfatase, aromatase, and 3β-hydroxysteroid dehydorgenase.[83,186] Genistein may also suppress angiogenesis and promote apoptosis in malignant tumors.[3,187] However, given that these effects are seen *in vivo* and the rodent *in vivo* literature has not found a preventative effect of genistein, it is not clear whether these mechanisms are physiologically relevant.

5.7.2 HUMAN DATA

The epidemiological studies assessing the relationship between dietary soy intake and cancer risk has been comprehensively reviewed[188] and suggest that soy consumption is not significantly associated with cancer protection. Three have found that frequent soy consumption is protective in premenopausal women[189-191] but only consider subjects of Asian descent, a population where soy consumption is likely to have been life-long. One case control study only found protective effects of soy in non-U.S.-born Asian Americans, leading the authors to propose that soy consumption is only protective when consumed at younger ages, a hypothesis consistent with the rodent literature.[180,192] A more recent study has also associated an increase in cancer protection by soy with early exposure, but again the findings were made using an Asian population.[193] Although these results are encouraging, it is likely that the results cannot be directly extrapolated to a Western population, where phytoestrogen intake is universally low and circulating endogenous estrogen levels are markedly higher.

Although they have received far less attention in the popular media, lignans may also have a protective effect against breast cancer. A comprehensive analysis of eight prospective studies found a measurable, but non-significant effect of lignans at the highest consumption levels.[194] It is important to note that these studies based their finding on urine or plasma levels of enterolactone rather than controlled dietary intake, making it impossible to accurately determine consumption levels in any of these studies. Although these findings are far from conclusive, they are encouraging given that lignans are more prevalent in the Western diet than isoflavones and are thus more likely to be consumed regularly over the lifespan.

5.8   CHOLESTEROL AND HEART DISEASE

It has long been known that a diet high in soluble fiber helps protect against heart disease. A recent study in middle-aged, Finnish, male smokers found that supplementing a normal diet with only 10 g of fiber reduces that risk of coronary death by 18%.[195] A second study found that a similar increase in fiber intake reduces the risk of coronary heart disease by as much as 20% in women.[196] Soluble dietary fiber is packed with bioactive compounds suggested to reduce the risk of heart disease including pectin, psyllium, and lignans. It is unclear what role, if any, lignans alone play in this reduction. Lignans, indigestible starch, antioxidants, trace minerals, and phenolic compounds are all found in fiber-rich whole grains and could reduce the risk of heart disease.[197]

There is an even larger body of literature indicating that soy products can effectively lower total blood cholesterol levels in animals and humans, particularly LDL and VLDL cholesterol.[198-200] Research from as early as 1940 demonstrated that animal protein (casein) is more atherogenic than soy protein.[201] More recent studies in both animals and humans have drawn similar conclusions.[202-204] Plasma LDL cholesterol reductions ranging from 8 to 16% have been reported for human patients with moderate to severe type II hypercholesterolemia after consuming soy protein, with HDL levels rising an average of 2% in most patients.[199,200,205] The exact mechanism of how soy products can lower blood cholesterol is unknown, but there are several theories, most of which center around the bioactivity of soy isoflavones, particularly genistein and daidzein. Soy protein-containing isoflavones significantly reduce total and LDL cholesterol in hyperocholesterolemic subjects,[206,207] an effect that is lost if the isoflavones are stripped from the soy protein by ethanol extraction.[208]

Several animal studies have also demonstrated the importance of isoflavones in cholesterol reduction.[202,209,210] However, a growing body of evidence has now demonstrated that isoflavone extracts alone do not appreciably lower LDL cholesterol levels, suggesting that the composition and context of the isoflavone source is critical.[211,212] These findings culminated in the U.S. Food and Drug Administration's approval of a health claim in 1999 that "25 g of soy protein a day, as part of a diet low in saturated fat and cholesterol, may reduce the risk of heart disease."[213]

The mechanism by which soy lowers serum cholesterol levels is largely unknown but could be related to an increase in thyroxine (T4) levels [214,215] or a direct effect on hepatic metabolism of cholesterol. 3-Hydroxy-3-methylglutaryl coenzyme A (HMG CoA) reductase activity increased in rats fed soy in addition to their normal diets.[216] This theory has not received as much attention and has only been studied in a limited range of animals. There is good evidence, however, that soy foods increase fecal excretion of bile acids. This depletes the body's store of bile and results in the recruitment of circulating cholesterol for increased bile production. This mechanism for the hypocholesterolemic effect of soy has been well documented in rabbits and rats,[216] but reports in other species, especially humans, are less consistent and thus less conclusive.[217]

Soy has other cardioprotective effects, in addition to its lipid lowering properties. Soy isoflavones have been found to decrease thrombin formation[218] and improve systemic arterial compliance[211,219] and may reduce LDL oxidative susceptibility.[220-222] There is also growing but conflicting evidence that soy may affect endothelium-mediated vasodilation in both humans and monkeys.[200]

Although the beneficial effects of soy on numerous markers of cardiovascular health are encouraging, the real test of their usefulness is whether or not these effects actually translate to a measurable decrease the risk of cardiac disease. Artherosclerosis is a common disease in older Americans and results from the formation of plaques on the inner layers of the arteries. The development and proliferation of these plaques is regulated by a long list of cytokines and growth factors. PTKs phosphorylate many of the proteins that regulate cell function, and many growth factors depend on PTK activity to bind properly to their receptor. As discussed earlier, genistein is a potent inhibitor of PTKs. Genistein has also been shown to inhibit vascular permeability factor-induced relaxation in canine coronary arteries, suppress lipopolysaccharide induction of cytokines and NF-κB, and inhibit fibronectin EIIIA mRNA induction in rat aortic rings at levels at or below 37μmol/l.[223] At higher levels genistein has been shown to inhibit chemotaxis and smooth muscle growth,[224] alter nitric oxide formation, and inhibit platelet aggregation[225] in vitro. Atherosclerotic female macaques had enhanced arterial dilator response to acetylcholine after consuming a diet high in isoflavones for 6 months,[226] and the same group has now linked long-term soy isoflavone consumption by postmenopausal monkeys to decreased, but not statistically significant, levels of coronary artery atherosclerosis.[227] Whether or not these effects will translate to humans remains to be seen and several clinical studies are currently underway to examine that possibility.

5.9 EQUOL: THE KEY TO THE BENEFITS OF SOY?

A tremendous hurdle in comprehensively interpreting the data from studies attempting to evaluate the health benefits of isoflavones is that much of the data is incongruent and inconsistent, especially in the human studies. No matter what endpoint is being considered, there is a wide range of interindividual variation, and this necessitates the acquisition of enormous sample sizes to generate sufficient power necessary to produce statistically meaningful results. There are likely many reasons for the observed variability but because phytoestrogen metabolism and absorption is critically dependent on bacterial degradation, interindividual differences in colonic bacterial populations are perhaps the biggest factor. More specifically, the observed benefits of soy may hinge upon the ability to convert daidzein to equol, an ability that only 30% of Western individuals have. Urinary excretion varies up to 800-fold among individuals and is far higher in Asian populations that Western populations.[228,229] Equol has a high affinity for both ERα and ERβ and is superior to all other isoflavones in its antioxidant activity.[230]

A recent study has found that premenopausal women who excrete equol have a plasma hormone profile associated with lowered risk of breast cancer.[81] Although the study is small and only contains data from 14 women, it suggests that the ability to convert genistein to equol may be the key for many of the observed effects of soy. Very few studies have examined the clinical effects of equol, but urinary equol excretion has been linked with follicular phase length in cycling women[67,231] and preserved bone mineral density in postmenopausal women.[230,232] Retrospective analysis of the data from at least one previously published report on the effects of soy foods on plasma lipid levels found that appreciable changes in cholesterol levels were only seen in subjects with high plasma levels of equol.[230] Many other published human studies examining the effects of soy on bone density, and cardiovascular protection had marginal but non-significant effects. It is possible that these effects would become more pronounced if the subjects were sorted by their ability to excrete appreciable levels of equol.

5.10 CONCLUSION

Phytoestrogens are a unique group of endocrine-disrupting compounds that have gained widespread attention because of their supposed health benefits, even though they have been found to produce some of the same reproductive abnormalities as their more vilified synthetic brethren. Most estrogen-disrupting industrial chemicals and pesticides, including polychlorinated biphenyls and, most notably, DDT and its metabolites, have lower binding affinities for estrogen receptors than isoflavones or coumestans,[10] and their negative effects are seen at far higher doses.[94,233] However, although there is widespread concern surrounding the long-term effects of these compounds, there is an enthusiastic push for phytoestrogen consumption. This biased presumption that "natural" endocrine disruptors are beneficial, while synthetic endocrine disruptors are deleterious has driven the research on these two types of compounds in totally opposite directions. For example, phytoestrogens were hypothesized to be anti-carcinogenic in the breast while synthetic compounds such as DDT and PCBs were presumed to increase the risk of breast cancer. Despite the hype, neither of those hypotheses have proven to be true.[188,234]

Both phytoestrogens and synthetic endocrine disruptors have been found to impair similar reproductive and neuroendocrine endpoints, including sexual differentiation and maturation, fertility, malformation of the genital tract, and sexual behavior, suggesting that they have similar mechanisms of action. Indeed, both can act as either estrogen agonists or antagonists depending upon dose, timing of exposure, tissue type, gender, and species. Still, "natural" is presumed to be good and "synthetic" is presumed to be deleterious. One of these presumptions is wrong. Either the phytoestrogens are not as good for us as they are advertised be, or their synthetic brethren are not as toxic as generally believed.

If the epidemiological data are a true indication of the biological activity of phytoestrogens, then increased consumption of these compounds could greatly reduce the risk of cancer and provide other benefits as well, including lower cholesterol and reduce the risk of osteoporosis. However, there are few data available on the most effective or optimal dose range for any of these compounds, and some animal studies have indicated that they can have severe reproductive consequences if consumed at high levels for a long period of time. Like other estrogens, these natural substances appear to have the capacity to produce both beneficial and adverse effects. The potential reproductive impact for humans is unclear. Further studies in this area must be made before any definite dietary recommendations can be made. Once again the epidemiological data indicates that populations consuming significant quantities of phytoestrogens, including vegetarians and many Asian cultures, suffer no adverse effects and live long, healthy lives. This may be an indication that lignans and soy foods should be part of the Western diet.

REFERENCES

1. Knight, D. C. and Eden, J. A., A review of the clinical effects of phytoestrogens, *Obstetrics and Gynecology* 87 (5 pt.2), 897–, 1996.
2. Kurzer, M. S. and Xia, X., Dietary Phytoestrogens, *Annual Review of Nutrition* 17, 353–381, 1997.
3. Adlercreutz, H. and Mazur, W., Phyto-oestrogens and western diseases, *Ann. Med.* 29, 95–120, 1997.
4. Borriello, S., Setchell, K., Axelson, M., and Lawson, A., Production and metabolism of lignans by the human fecal flora, *J. Appl. Bacteriol.* 58, 37–43, 1985.
5. Adlercreutz, H., Phytoestrogens: epidemiology and a possible role in cancer protection, *Environ. Health Persp.* 130 (suppl 7), 103–112, 1995.
6. Axelson, M., Sjovall, J., Gustafsson, B., and KD, S., Origin of lignans in mammals and identification of a precursor from plants, *Nature* 298, 659–660, 1982.
7. Nesbitt, P. and Thompson, L., Lignans in homemade and commercial products containing flaxseed, *Nutr. Cancer* 29, 222–227, 1997.
8. Thompson, L. U., Robb, P., Serraino, M., and Cheung, F., Mammalian lignan production from various foods, *Nutr. Cancer* 16 (1), 43–52, 1991.
9. Fletcher, R., Food sources of phyto-estrogens and their precursors in Europe, *Br. J. Nutr.* 89 (Suppl 1), S39–43, 2003.

10. Kuiper, G. G. J. M., Lemmen, J. G., Carlsson, B., Corton, J. C., Safe, S. H., Van Der Saag, P. T., Van Der Berg, B., and Gustafsson, J.-Å. Interaction of estrogenic chemicals and phytoestrogens with estrogen receptor β, *Endocrinology* 139, 4252–4263, 1998.

11. Setchell, K. D., Brown, N. M., Desai, P., Zimmer-Nechemias, L., Wolfe, B. E., Brashear, W. T., Kirschner, A. S., Cassidy, A., and Heubi, J. E., Bioavailability of pure isoflavones in healthy humans and analysis of commercial soy isoflavone supplements, *J. Nutr.* 131 (4 Suppl), 1362S–75S, 2001.

12. Setchell, K. D. and Cole, S. J., Variations in isoflavone levels in soy foods and soy protein isolates and issues related to isoflavone databases and food labeling, *J. Agric. Food Chem.* 51 (14), 4146–55, 2003.

13. Adams, N. R., Detection of the effects of phytoestrogens on sheep and cattle, *J. Anim. Sci.* 73, 1509–1515, 1995.

14. Bennetts, H. W., Underwood, E. J., and Shier, F. L., A specific breeding problem of sheep on subterranean clover pastures. in Western Australia, *Austral. Vet. J.* 22, 2, 1946.

15. Joannou, G. E., Kelley, G. E., Reeder, A. Y., Waring, M., and Nelson, C., A urinary profile study of dietary phytoestrogens. The identification and mode of metabolism of new isoflavonoids, *J. Steroid Biochem.* 54 (3/4), 167–184, 1995.

16. Setchell, K. D., Borriello, S. P., Hulme, P., Kirk, D. N., and Axelson, M., Nonsteroidal estrogens of dietary origin: possible roles in hormone-dependent disease, *Am. J. Clin. Nutr.* 40 (3), 569–78, 1984.

17. Hutchins, A. M., Slavin, J. L., and Lampe, J. W., Urinary isoflavonoid phytoestrogen and lignan excretion after consumption of fermented and unfermented soy products, *J. Am. Diet. Assoc.* 95 (5), 545–551, 1995.

18. Kelly, G. E., Joannou, G. E., Reeder, A. Y., Nelson, C., and Waring, M. A., The variable metabolic response to dietary isoflavones in humans, *Proc. Soc. Exp. Biol. Med.* 208, 40–43, 1995.

19. Morton, M. S., Wilcox, G., Wahlqvist, M. L., and Griffiths, K., Determination of lignans and isoflavonoids in human female plasma following dietary supplementation., *J. Endocrinol.* 142, 251–259, 1994.

20. Lampe, J., Karr, S., Hutchins, A., and Slavin, J., Urinary equol excretion with a soy challenge: influence of habitual diet, *PSEBM* 217, 335–339, 1998.

21. Bowey, E., Adlercreutz, H., and Rowland, I., Metabolism of isoflavones and lignans by the gut microflora: a study in germ-free and human flora associated rats, *Food Chem. Toxicol.* 41 (5), 631–6, 2003.

22. Rowland, I. R., Wiseman, H., Sanders, T. A., Adlercreutz, H., and Bowey, E. A., Interindividual variation in metabolism of soy isoflavones and lignans: influence of habitual diet on equol production by the gut microflora, *Nutr. Cancer* 36 (1), 27–32, 2000.

23. Lu, L. J. and Anderson, K. E., Sex and long-term soy diets affect the metabolism and excretion of soy isoflavones in humans, *Am. J. Clin. Nutr.* 68 (6 Suppl), 1500S–1504S, 1998.

24. Kirkman, L. M., Lampe, J. W., Campbell, D. R., Martini, M. C., and Slavin, J. L., Urinary lignan and isoflavonoid excretion in men and women consuming vegetable and soy diets, *Nutr. Cancer* 24, 1–12, 1995.

25. Adlercreutz, H., Goldin, B. R., Gorbach, S. L., Höckerstedt, K. A. V., Watanabe, S., Hamalainen, E. K., Markkanen, M. H., Mäkela, T. H., and Wähälä, K. T., Soybean phytoestrogen intake and cancer risk, *J. Nutr.* 125, 757–770S, 1995.

26. Shimizu, H., Ross, R. K., Pike, M. C., and Henderson, B. E., Serum oestrogen levels in postmenopausal women: comparison of American whites and Japanese in Japan, *Br. J. Cancer* 62, 451–453, 1990.

27. Morton, M. S., Arisaka, O., Miyake, N., Morgan, L. D., and Evans, B. A., Phytoestrogen concentrations in serum from Japanese men and women over forty years of age, *J. Nutr.* 132 (10), 3168–71, 2002.

28. Lampe, J. W., Gustafson, D. R., Hutchins, A. M., Martini, M. C., Li, S., Wahala, K., Grandits, G. A., Potter, J. D., and Slavin, J. L., Urinary isoflavonoid and lignan excretion on a Western diet: relation to soy, vegetable, and fruit intake, *Cancer Epidemiol. Biomarkers Prev.* 8 (8), 699–707, 1999.

29. Markiewicz, L., Garey, J., Adlercreutz, H., and Gurpide, E., *In vitro* bioassays of non-steroidal phytoestrogens, *J. Steroid Biochem. Mol. Biol.* 45 (5), 399–405, 1993.

30. Lundh, T., Metabolism of estrogenic isoflavones in domestic animals, *Pro. Soc. Exp. Biol. Med.* 208 (1), 33–39, 1995.

31. Adlercreutz, H., van der Wildt, J., Kinzel, J., Attalla, H., Wähälä, K., Mäkelä, T., Hase, T., and Fotsis, T., Lignan and isoflavonoid conjugates in human urine, *J. Steroid Biochem. Mol. Biol.* 52 (1), 97–103, 1995.

32. King, R. A., Broadbent, J. L., and Head, R. J., Absorption and excretion of the soy isoflavone genistein in rats, *J. Nutr.* 126 (1), 176–82, 1996.

33. Axelson, M., Sjovall, J., Gustafsson, B. E., and Setchell, K. D., Soya—a dietary source of the non-steroidal oestrogen equol in man and animals, *J. Endocrinol.* 102 (1), 49–56, 1984.

34. King, R. A., Daidzein conjugates are more bioavailable than genistein conjugates in rats, *Am. J. Clin. Nutr.* 68 (6 Suppl), 1496S–1499S, 1998.

35. Bayer, T., Colnot, T., and Dekant, W., Disposition and biotransformation of the estrogenic isoflavone daidzein in rats, *Toxicol. Sci.* 62 (2), 205–11, 2001.

36. Clarke, R., Hilakivi-Clarke, L., Cho, E., James, M. R., and Leonessa, F., Estrogens, phytoestrogens and breast cancer, in *Dietary Phytochem. Cancer Prevention Treatment*, *Res.*, A. I. f. C. Plenum Press, New York, 1996, pp. 63–85.

37. Kuiper, G. G. J. M., Enmark, E., Pelto-Huikko, M., Nilsson, S., and Gustafsson, J.-Å. Cloning of a novel estrogen receptor expressed in rat prostate and ovary, *Proc. Nat. Acad. Sci. U.S.* 93, 5925–5930, 1996.

38. Mosselman, S., Polman, J., and Dijkema, R., ERβ: identification and characterization of a novel human estrogen receptor, *FEBS Lett.* 392, 49–53, 1996.

39. Miksicek, R. J., Interaction of naturally occurring nonsteroidal estrogens with expressed recombinant human estrogen receptor, *J. Steroid Biochem. Mol. Biol.* 47, 39–48, 1994.

40. Coldham, N. G., Dave, M., Sivapathasundaram, S., McDonnell, D. P., Connor, C., and Sauer, M. J., Evaluation of a recombinant yeast cell estrogen screening assay, *Environ. Health Persp.* 105, 734–742, 1997.

41. Collins, B. M., McLachlan, J. A., and Arnold, S. F., The estrogenic and antiestrogenic activities of phytochemicals with the human estrogen receptor expressed in yeast, *Steroids* 62, 365–372, 1997.

42. Kuiper, G. G. J. M., Carlsson, B., Grandien, K., Enmark, E., Häggblad, J., Hilsson, S., and Gustafsson, J.-Å. Comparison of the ligand binding specificity and transcript tissue distribution of estrogen receptors α and β, *Endocrinology* 138 (3), 863–870, 1997.

43. Barkhem, T., Carlsson, B., Nilsson, Y., Enmark, E., Gustafsson, J., and Nilsson, S., Differential response of estrogen receptor α and estrogen receptor β to partial estrogen agonists/antagonists, *Mol. Pharmacol.* 54, 105–112, 1998.

44. Iafrati, M. D., Karas, R. H., Aronovitz, M., Kim, S., Sullivan, T. R. J., Lubahn, D. B., O'Donnell, T. F. J., Korach, K. S., and Mendelsohn, M. E., Estrogen inhibits the vascular injury response in estrogen receptor α-deficient mice, *Nat. Med.* 3 (5), 545–548, 1997.

45. Shughrue, P. J., Komm, B., and Merchenthaler, I., The distribution of estrogen receptor-β mRNA in the rat hypothalamus, *Steroids* 61, 678–681, 1996.

46. Shughrue, P. L., Scrimo, P., Lane, M. V., and Merchenthaler, I., The distribution of estrogen receptor-β mRNA in forebrain regions of the estrogen receptor-α knockout mouse, *Endocrinology* 138, 5649–5652, 1997.

47. Brandenberger, A. W., Tee, M. K., Lee, J. Y., Chao, V., and Jaffe, R. B., Tissue distribution of estrogen receptors and alpha (ER-α) and beta (ER-β) in the midgestational human fetus, *J. Clin. Endocrinol. Metab.* 82 (10), 3509–3512, 1997.

48. Gaskell, T. L., Robinson, L. L., Groome, N. P., Anderson, R. A., and Saunders, P. T., Differential expression of two estrogen receptor beta isoforms in the human fetal testis during the second trimester of pregnancy, *J. Clin. Endocrinol. Metab.* 88 (1), 424–32, 2003.

49. Takeyama, J., Suzuki, T., Inoue, S., Kaneko, C., Nagura, H., Harada, N., and Sasano, H., Expression and cellular localization of estrogen receptors alpha and beta in the human fetus, *J. Clin. Endocrinol. Metab.* 86 (5), 2258–62, 2001.

50. Hewitt, S. C. and Korach, K. S., Oestrogen receptor knockout mice: roles for oestrogen receptors alpha and beta in reproductive tissues, *Reproduction* 125 (2), 143–9, 2003.

51. Ogawa, S., Chan, J., Chester, A., Gustafsson, J., Korach, K., and Pfaff, D., Survival of reproductive behaviors in estrogen receptor β gene-deficient (βERKO) male and female mice, *Proc. Nat. Acad. Sci. U.S.* 96 (22), 12887–12892, 1999.

52. Couse, J. F. and Korach, K. S., Exploring the role of sex steroids through studies of receptor deficient mice, *J. Mol. Med.* 76 (7), 497–511, 1998.

53. Krege, J. H., Hodgin, J. B., Couse, J. F., Enmark, E., Warner, M., Mahler, J. F., Sar, M., Korach, K. S., Gustafsson, J.-A., and Smithies, O., Generation and reproductive phenotypes of mice lacking estrogen receptor β, *Proc. Natl. Acad. Sci. U.S.* 95, 15677–15682, 1998.

54. Raynaud, J. P., Ojasco, T., Bouton, M. M., Bignon, E., Pons, M., and Crastes de Paulet, A., Structure-activity relationships of steroid estrogens, in *Estrogens in the Environment*, McLachlan, J. A. Elsevier Science Publishing Company, New York, 1985, pp. 24–41.

55. Anstead, G. M. and Kym, P. R., Benz(a)anthracene diols: predicted carcinogenicity and structure-estrogen receptor binding affinity relationships, *Steroids* 60, 383–394, 1995.

56. Henttu, P. M., Kalkhoven, E., and Parker, M. G., AF-2 activity and recruitment of steroid receptor coactivator 1 to the estrogen receptor depend on a lysine residue conserved in nuclear receptors, *Mol. Cell Biol.* 17 (4), 1832–9, 1997.

57. Pike, A. C., Brzozowski, A. M., and Hubbard, R. E., A structural biologist's view of the oestrogen receptor, *J. Steroid Biochem. Mol. Biol.* 74, 261–268, 2000.

58. Feng, W., Ribeiro, R. C., Wagner, R. L., Nguyen, H., Apriletti, J. W., Fletterick, R. J., Baxter, J. D., Kushner, P. J., and West, B. L., Hormone-dependent coactivator binding to a hydrophobic cleft on nuclear receptors, *Science* 280 (5370), 1747–9, 1998.

59. Brzozowski, A., Pike, A., Dauter, Z., Hubbard, R., Bonn, T., Engstrom, O., Ohman, L., Greene, G., Gustafsson, J., and Carlquist, M., Molecular basis of agonism and antagonism in the oestrogen receptor, *Nature* 389, 753–758, 1997.

60. Pike, A. C., Brzozowski, A. M., Hubbard, R. E., Bonn, T., Thorsell, A. G., Engstrom, O., Ljunggren, J., Gustafsson, J. A., and Carlquist, M., Structure of the ligand-binding domain of oestrogen receptor beta in the presence of a partial agonist and a full antagonist, *Embo. J.* 18 (17), 4608–18, 1999.

61. Arts, C. J. M. and Van Den Berg, H., Multi-residue screening of bovine urine on xenobiotic oestrogens with an oestrogen radioreceptor assay, *J. Chromatogr.* 489, 225–234, 1989.

62. Zava, D. T. and Duwe, G., Estrogenic and antiproliferative properties of genistein and other flavonoids in human breast cancer cells *in vitro*, *Nutr. Cancer* 27 (1), 31–40, 1997.

63. Adlercreutz, H., Mousavi, Y., Clark, J., Höckersted, K., Hämäläinen, E. K., Wähälä, K., Mäkelä, T., and Hase, T., Dietary phytoestrogens and cancer: *in vitro* and *in vivo* studies, *J. Steroid Biochem. Mol. Biol.* 41, 331–337, 1992.

64. Dechaud, H., Ravard, C., Claustrat, F., and Brac de la Perriere, A., Xenoestrogen interaction with human sex hormone-binding globulin (hSHBG), *Steroids* 64, 328–334, 1999.

65. Wu, A. H., Stanczyk, F. Z., Hendrich, S., Murphy, P. A., Zhang, C., Wan, P., and Pike, M. C., Effects of soy foods on ovarian function in premenopausal women, *Br. J. Cancer* 82 (11), 1879–86, 2000.

66. Nagata, C., Takatsuka, N., Inaba, S., Kawakami, N., and Shimizu, H., Effect of soymilk consumption on serum estrogen concentrations in premenopausal Japanese women, *J. Natl. Cancer Inst.* 90 (23), 1830–5, 1998.

67. Cassidy, A., Bingham, S., and Setchell, K. D. R., Biological effects of a diet of soy protein rich in isoflavones on the menstrual cycle of premenopausal women, *Am. J. Clin. Nutr.* 60, 333–340, 1994.

68. Lu, L. J., Cree, M., Josyula, S., Nagamani, M., Grady, J. J., and Anderson, K. E., Increased urinary excretion of 2-hydroxyestrone but not 16alpha-hydroxyestrone in premenopausal women during a soya diet containing isoflavones, *Cancer Res.* 60 (5), 1299–305, 2000.

69. Martini, M. C., Dancisak, B. B., Haggans, C. J., Thomas, W., and Slavin, J. L., Effects of soy intake on sex hormone metabolism in premenopausal women, *Nutr. Cancer* 34 (2), 133–9, 1999.

70. Wang, C., Makela, T., Hase, T. A., Adlercreutz, C. H. T., and Kurzer, M. S., Lignans and isoflavonoids inhibit aromatase enzyme in human preadipocytes, *J. Steroid Biochem. Mol. Biol.* 50, 205–212, 1994.

71. Pelissero, C., Lenczowski, M., Chinzi, D., Davail-Cuisset, B., Sumpter, J., and Fostier, A., Effects of flavonoids on aromatase activity, and *in vitro* study, *J. Steroid Biochem. Mol. Biol.* 57 (3–4), 215–223, 1996.

72. Chen, S., Kao, Y. C., and Laughton, C. A., Binding characteristics of aromatase inhibitors and phytoestrogens to human aromatase, *J. Steroid Biochem. Mol. Biol.* 61 (3–6), 107–15., 1997.

73. Franke, A. A. and Custer, L. J., High-performance liquid chromatographic assay of isoflavonoids and coumestrol from human urine, *J. Chromatogr. B: Biomed. Appl.* 662, 47–60, 1994.

74. Piontek, M., Hangels, K. J., Porschen, R., and Strohmeyer, G., Anti-proliferative effect of tyrosine kinase inhibitors in epidermal growth factor-stimulated growth of human gastric cancer cells, *Anticancer Res.* 13, 2119–2123, 1993.

75. Boutin, J. A., Minireview - Tyrosine protein kinase inhibition and cancer, *Int. J. Biochem. Cell Biol.* 26, 1203–1226, 1994.

76. Okura, A., Arakawa, H., Oka, H., Yoshinari, T., and Monden, Y., Effect of genistein on topoisomerase activity and on the growth of [Val 12] Ha-ras-transformed NIH 3T3 cells, *Biochem. Biophys. Res. Commun.* 157, 183–189, 1988.

77. Adams, N. R., Organizational and activational effects of phytoestrogens on the reproductive tract of the ewe, *Proc. Soc. Exp. Biol. Med.* 208 (1), 87–91, 1995.

78. Stanford, J. L., Herrinton, L. J., Schwartz, S. M., and Weiss, N. S., Breast cancer incidence in Asian migrants to the United States and their descendants, *Epidemiology* 6, 181–183, 1995.

79. Uehar, M., Arai, Y., Watanabe, S., and Adlercreutz, H., Comparison of plasma and urinary phytoestrogens in Japanese and Finnish women by time-resolved fluoroimmunoassay, *Biofactors* 12 (1–4), 217–25, 2000.

80. Ingram, D., Sanders, K., Kolybaba, M., and Lopez, D., Case-control study of phyto-oestrogens and breast cancer, *Lancet* 350, 990–994, 1997.

81. Duncan, A. M., Merz-Demlow, B. E., Xu, X., Phipps, W. R., and Kurzer, M. S., Premenopausal equol excretors show plasma hormone profiles associated with lowered risk of breast cancer, *Cancer Epidemiol. Biomarkers Prev.* 9 (6), 581–6, 2000.

82. Murkies, A., Dalais, F. S., Briganti, E. M., Burger, H. G., Healy, D. L., Wahlqvist, M. L., and Davis, S. R., Phytoestrogens and breast cancer in postmenopausal women: a case control study [In Process Citation], *Menopause* 7 (5), 289–96, 2000.

83. Messina, M. J., Persky, V., Setchell, K. D., and Barnes, S., Soy intake and cancer risk: a review of the *in vitro* and *in vivo* data, *Nutr. Cancer* 21 (2), 113–31, 1994.

84. Nwannenna, A. I., Madej, A., Lundh, T. J.-O., and Fredriksson, G., Effects of oestrogenic silage on some clinical and endocrinological parameters in ovariectomized heifers, *Acta Veterinaria Scandinavia* 35 (2), 173–183, 1994.

85. Whitten, P. L., Russell, E., and Naftolin, F., Effects of a normal, human-concentration, phytoestrogen diet on rat uterine growth, *Steroids* 57, 98–106, 1992.

86. Whitten, P. L., Lewis, C., and Naftolin, F., A phytoestrogen diet induces the premature anovulatory syndrome in lactationally exposed female rats, *Biol. Reprod.* 49, 1117–1121, 1993.

87. Leopold, A., Erwin, M., Oh, J., and Browning, B., Phytoestrogens: adverse effects on reproduction in California quail, *Science* 191 (4222), 98–100, 1976.

88. Setchell, K. D. R., Gosselin, S. J., Welsh, M. B., Johnston, J. O., Balistreri, W. F., Kramer, L. W., Dresser, B. L., and Tarr, M. J., Dietary estrogens — a probable cause of infertility and liver disease in captive cheetahs, *Gastroenterology* 93, 225–233, 1987.

89. Almen, T., Hartel, M., Nylander, G., and Olivercrona, H., The effect of estrogen on the vascular endothelium and its possible relation to thrombosis, *Surg. Gyn. Obstet.* 140, 938–40, 1975.

90. Adlercreutz, H. and Tenhunen, R., Some aspects of the interaction between natural and synthetic female hormones and the liver, *Am. J. Med.* 49, 630–648, 1970.

91. Mosher, W. D. and Pratt, R. F., Fecundity and infertility in the United States, 1965–1982, in *Advance Data from Vital and Health Statistics,* Public Health Service, New York, 1985.

92. Carlsen, E., Giwercman, A., Keiding, N., and Skakkebaek, N., Evidence for decreasing quality of semes during past 50 years, *Br. Med. J.* 305, 609–613, 1992.

93. Feichtinger, W., Environmental factors and fertility, *Hum. Reprod.* 6, 1170–1175, 1991.

94. Safe, S. H., Endocrine disruptors and human health—is there a problem? An update, *Environ. Health Perspect.* 108 (6), 487–93, 2000.

95. Koifman, S., Koifman, R. J., and Meyer, A., Human reproductive system disturbances and pesticide exposure in Brazil, *Cad. Saude Publica.* 18 (2), 435–45, 2002.

96. Sharpe, R. and Skakkebaek, N., Are oestrogens involved in falling sperm counts and disorders of the male reproductive tract, *The Lancet* 341, 1292–1395, 1993.

97. Gardner-Thorpe, D., O'Hagen, C., Young, I., and Lewis, S. J., Dietary supplements of soya flour lower serum testosterone concentrations and improve markers of oxidative stress in men, *Eur. J. Clin. Nutr.* 57 (1), 100–6, 2003.

98. Mitchell, J. H., Cawood, E., Kinniburgh, D., Provan, A., Collins, A. R., and Irvine, D. S., Effect of a phytoestrogen food supplement on reproductive health in normal males, *Clin. Sci. (Lond.)* 100 (6), 613–8, 2001.

99. Shultz, T. D., Bonorden, W. R., and Seaman, W. R., Effect of short-term flaxseed consumption on lignan and sex hormone metabolism in men, *Nutr. Res.* 11, 1089–1100, 1991.

100. Patisaul, H., Whitten, P., and Young, L., Regulation of estrogen receptor beta mRNA in the brain: opposite effects of 17β-estradiol and the phytoestrogen, coumestrol., *Brain Res. Mol. Brain Res.* 67, 165–171, 1999.

101. Patisaul, H. B., Melby, M., Whitten, P. L., and Young, L. J., Genistein affects ERβ- but not ERα-dependent gene expression in the hypothalamus, *Endocrinology* 143, 2189–2197, 2002.

102. Patisaul, H. B., Dindo, M., Whitten, P. L., and Young, L. J., Soy isoflavone supplements antagonize reproductive behavior and ERα- and ERβ-dependent gene expression in the brain, *Endocrinology* 142, 2001.

103. Patisaul, H. B., Luskin, J. R., and Wilson, M. E., A soy supplement and tamoxifen inhibit sexual behavior in female rats, *Hormones Behav.*, Submitted.

104. Mourits, M. J., De Vries, E.G., Willemse, P. H., Ten Hoor, K. A., Hollema, H., and Van der Zee, A. G., Tamoxifen treatment and gynecologic side effects: a review, *Obstet. Gynecol.* 97 (5 Pt 2), 855–66, 2001.

105. Day, R., Quality of life and tamoxifen in a breast cancer prevention trial: a summary of findings from the NSABP P-1 study. National Surgical Adjuvant Breast and Bowel Project, *Ann. N. Y. Acad. Sci.* 949, 143–50, 2001.

106. Daniels, D. and Flanagan-Cato, L. M., Functionally-defined compartments of the lordosis neural circuit in the ventromedial hypothalamus in female rats, *J. Neurobiol.* 45 (1), 1–13, 2000.

107. Jakes, R. W., Alexander, L., Duffy, S. W., Leong, J., Chen, L. H., and Lee, W. H., Dietary intake of soybean protein and menstrual cycle length in pre-menopausal Singapore Chinese women, *Public Health Nutr.* 4 (2), 191–6, 2001.

108. Gupta, M., McDougal, A., and Safe, S., Estrogenic and antiestrogenic activities of 16alpha- and 2-hydroxy metabolites of 17beta-estradiol in MCF-7 and T47D human breast cancer cells, *J. Steroid Biochem. Mol. Biol.* 67 (5–6), 413–9, 1998.

109. Lord, R. S., Bongiovanni, B., and Bralley, J. A., Estrogen metabolism and the diet-cancer connection: rationale for assessing the ratio of urinary hydroxylated estrogen metabolites, *Altern. Med. Rev.* 7 (2), 112–29, 2002.

110. Telang, N. T., Suto, A., Wong, G. Y., Osborne, M. P., and Bradlow, H. L., Induction by estrogen metabolite 16 alpha-hydroxyestrone of genotoxic damage and aberrant proliferation in mouse mammary epithelial cells, *J. Natl. Cancer Inst.* 84 (8), 634–8, 1992.

111. Cavalieri, E. L., Stack, D. E., Devanesan, P. D., Todorovic, R., Dwivedy, I., Higginbotham, S., Johansson, S. L., Patil, K. D., Gross, M. L., Gooden, J. K., Ramanathan, R., Cerny, R. L., and Rogan, E.G., Molecular origin of cancer: catechol estrogen-3,4-quinones as endogenous tumor initiators, *Proc. Natl. Acad. Sci. U. S. A.* 94 (20), 10937–42, 1997.

112. Xu, X., Duncan, A. M., Merz, B. E., and Kurzer, M. S., Effects of soy isoflavones on estrogen and phytoestrogen metabolism in premenopausal women, *Cancer Epidemiol. Biomarkers Prev.* 7 (12), 1101–8, 1998.

113. Xu, X., Duncan, A. M., Wangen, K. E., and Kurzer, M. S., Soy consumption alters endogenous estrogen metabolism in postmenopausal women, *Cancer Epidemiol. Biomarkers Prev.* 9 (8), 781–6, 2000.

114. Atkinson, C., Skor, H. E., Dawn Fitzgibbons, E., Scholes, D., Chen, C., Wahala, K., Schwartz, S. M., and Lampe, J. W., Urinary equol excretion in relation to 2-hydroxyestrone and 16alpha-hydroxyestrone concentrations: an observational study of young to middle-aged women, *J. Steroid Biochem. Mol. Biol.* 86 (1), 71–7, 2003.

115. Preslock, J. P. and McCann, S., Lesions of the sexually dimorphic nucleus of the preoptic area: effects upon LH, FSH, and prolactin in rats, *Brain Res. Bull.* 18, 127–134, 1987.

116. Wisniewski, A. B., Klein, S. L., Lakshmanan, Y., and Gearhart, J. P., Exposure to genistein during gestation and lactation demasculinizes the reproductive system in rats, *J. Urol.* 169 (4), 1582–6, 2003.

117. Whitten, P. L., Lewis, C., Russell, E., and Naftolin, F., Phytoestrogen influences on the development of behavior and gonadotropin function, *Proc. Soc. Exp. Biol. Med.* 208 (1), 82–86, 1995.

118. Strauss, L., Makela, S., Joshi, S., Huhtaniemi, I., and Santti, R., Genistein exerts estrogen-like effects in male mouse reproductive tract, *Mol. Cell Endocrinol.* 144 (1–2), 83–93, 1998.

119. Tou, J. C., Chen, J., and Thompson, L. U., Dose, timing, and duration of flaxseed exposure affect reproductive indices and sex hormone levels in rats, *J. Toxicol. Environ. Health A* 56 (8), 555–70, 1999.

120. Levy, J. R., Faber, K. A., Ayyash, L., and Hughes, C. L., Jr., The effect of prenatal exposure to the phytoestrogen genistein on sexual differentiation in rats, *Proc. Soc. Exp. Biol. Med.* 208 (1), 60–66, 1995.

121. Medlock, K. L., Branham, W. S., and Sheehan, D. M., Effects of coumestrol and equol on the developing reproductive tract of the rat, *Proc. Soc. Exp. Biol. Med.* 208 (1), 67–71, 1995.

122. Lewis, R. W., Brooks, N., Milburn, G. M., Soames, A., Stone, S., Hall, M., and Ashby, J., The effects of the phytoestrogen genistein on the postnatal development of the rat, *Toxicol. Sci.* 71 (1), 74–83, 2003.

123. Kouki, T., Kishitake, M., Okamoto, M., Oosuka, I., Takebe, M., and Yamanouchi, K., Effects of neonatal treatment with phytoestrogens, genistein and daidzein, on sex difference in female rat brain function: estrous cycle and lordosis, *Horm. Behav.* 44 (2), 140–5, 2003.

124. Faber, K. A. and Hughes, C. L., Jr., Dose-response characteristics of neonatal exposure to genistein on pituitary responsiveness to gonadotropin releasing hormone and volume of the sexually dimorphic nucleus of the preoptic area (SDN-POA) in postpubertal castrated female rats, *Reprod. Toxicol.* 7 (1), 35–9, 1993.

125. Faber, K. A. and Hughes, C. L. J., The effect of neonatal exposure to diethylstilbestrol, genistein, and zearalenone on pituitary responsiveness and sexually dimorphic nucleus volume in the castrated adult rat, *Biol. Reprod.* 45, 649–653, 1991.

126. Franke, A. A., Custer, L. J., and Tanaka, Y., Isoflavones in human breast milk and other biological fluids, *Am. J. Clin. Nutr.* 68 (6 Suppl), 1466S–1473S, 1998.

127. Setchell, K. D. R. and Welsh, M. B., High-performance liquid chromatographic analysis of phytoestrogens in soy protein preparations with ultraviolet electrochemical and thermospray mass spectrometric detection, *J. Chromatog. A* 386, 315–323, 1987.

128. Setchell, K. D. R., Zimmer-Nechemias, L., Cai, J., and Heubi, J. E., Exposure of infants to phyto-oestrogens from soy-based infant formula, *Lancet* 350, 23–27, 1997.

129. Johns, P., Dowlati, L., and Wargo, W., Determination of isoflavones in ready-to-feed soy-based infant formula, *J. AOAC Int* 86 (1), 72–8, 2003.

130. Barnes, S., Effect of genistein on *in vitro* and *in vivo* models of cancer, *J. Nutr.* 125 (Suppl 3), S777–783, 1995.

131. Winter, J. S. D., Hughes, I. A., Reyes, F. I., and Faiman, C., Pituitary-gonadal relations in infancy: patterns of serum gonadal steroid concentrations in man from birth to two years of age, *J. Clin. Endocrinol. Metab.* 42, 679–686, 1976.

132. Sharpe, R. M., Martin, B., Morris, K., Greig, I., McKinnell, C., McNeilly, A. S., and Walker, M., Infant feeding with soy formula milk: effects on the testis and on blood testosterone levels in marmoset monkeys during the period of neonatal testicular activity, *Hum. Reprod.* 17 (7), 1692–703, 2002.

133. Franke, A. A. and Custer, L. J., Daidzein and genistein concentrations in human milk after soy consumption, *Clin. Chem.* 42 (6), 955–964, 1996.

134. Strom, B. L., Schinnar, R., Ziegler, E. E., Barnhart, K. T., Sammel, M. D., Macones, G. A., Stallings, V. A., Drulis, J. M., Nelson, S. E., and Hanson, S. A., Exposure to soy-based formula in infancy and endocrinological and reproductive outcomes in young adulthood, *JAMA* 286 (7), 807–14, 2001.

135. Tang, G., The climacteric of Chinese factory workers, *Maturitas* 19, 177–182, 1994.

136. Nagata, C., Shimizu, H., Takami, R., Hayashi, M., Takeda, N., and Yasuda, K., Hot flushes and other menopausal symptoms in relation to soy product intake in Japanese women, *Climacteric* 2, 6–12, 1999.

137. The role of isoflavones in menopausal health: consensus opinion of The North American Menopause Society, *Menopause* 7 (4), 215–29, 2000.

138. Murkies, A., Lombard, C., Strauss, B., Wilcox, G., Burger, H., and Morton, M., Dietary flour supplementation decreases post-menopausal hot flushes: effect of soy and wheat, *Maturitas* 21, 189–195, 1995.

139. Tice, J. A., Ettinger, B., Ensrud, K., Wallace, R., Blackwell, T., and Cummings, S. R., Phytoestrogen supplements for the treatment of hot flashes: the Isoflavone Clover Extract (ICE) Study: a randomized controlled trial, *JAMA* 290 (2), 207–14, 2003.

140. Burke, G. L., Legault, C., Anthony, M., Bland, D. R., Morgan, T. M., Naughton, M. J., Leggett, K., Washburn, S. A., and Vitolins, M. Z., Soy protein and isoflavone effects on vasomotor symptoms in peri- and postmenopausal women: the Soy Estrogen Alternative Study, *Menopause* 10 (2), 147–53, 2003.

141. St Germain, A., Peterson, C. T., Robinson, J. G., and Alekel, D. L., Isoflavone-rich or isoflavone-poor soy protein does not reduce menopausal symptoms during 24 weeks of treatment, *Menopause* 8 (1), 17–26, 2001.

142. Kronenberg, F. and Fugh-Berman, A., Complementary and alternative medicine for menopausal symptoms: a review of randomized, controlled trials, *Ann. Intern. Med.* 137 (10), 805–13, 2002.

143. Messina, M. and Hughes, C., Efficacy of soyfoods and soybean isoflavone supplements for alleviating menopausal symptoms is positively related to initial hot flush frequency, *J. Med. Food* 6 (1), 1–11, 2003.

144. Blank, R. D. and Bockman, R. S., A review of clinical trials of therapies for osteoporosis using fracture as an end point, *J. Clin. Densitom.* 2 (4), 435–52, 1999.

145. Investigators, W. G. f. t. W. s. H. I., Risks and benefits of estrogen plus progestin in healthy postmenopausal women: principal results from the Women's Health Initiative randomized controlled trial, *JAMA* 288 (3), 321–33, 2002.

146. Lacey, J. V., Jr., Mink, P. J., Lubin, J. H., Sherman, M. E., Troisi, R., Hartge, P., Schatzkin, A., and Schairer, C., Menopausal hormone replacement therapy and risk of ovarian cancer, *JAMA* 288 (3), 334–41, 2002.

147. Lau, E. M., Lee, J. K., Suriwongpaisal, P., Saw, S. M., Das De, S., Khir, A., and Sambrook, P., The incidence of hip fracture in four Asian countries: the Asian Osteoporosis Study (AOS), *Osteoporos. Int.* 12 (3), 239–43, 2001.

148. Lau, E. M. and Cooper, C., The epidemiology of osteoporosis. The oriental perspective in a world context, *Clin. Orthop.* (323), 65–74, 1996.

149. Lauderdale, D. S., Thisted, R. A., and Goldberg, J., Is geographic variation in hip fracture rates related to current or former region of residence?, *Epidemiology* 9 (5), 574–7, 1998.

150. Tustsumi, N., Effect of coumestrol on bone metabolism in organ culture, *Biol. Pharm. Bull.* 18, 1012–1015, 1995.

151. Draper, C. R., Edel, M. J., Dick, I. M., Randall, A. G., Martin, G. G., and Prince, R. L., Phytoestrogens reduce bone loss and bone resorption in oophorectomized rats, *J. Nutr.* 127, 1795–1799, 1997.

152. Blair, H. C., Jordan, S. E., Peterson, T. G., and Barnes, S., Variable effects of tyrosine kinase inhibitors on avian osteoclastic activity and reduction of bone loss in ovariectomized rats, *J. Cell Biochem.* 61 (4), 629–37, 1996.

153. Gao, Y. H. and Yamaguchi, M., Suppressive effect of genistein on rat bone osteoclasts: apoptosis is induced through Ca2+ signaling, *Biol. Pharm. Bull.* 22 (8), 805–9, 1999.

154. Gao, Y. H. and Yamaguchi, M., Suppressive effect of genistein on rat bone osteoclasts: involvement of protein kinase inhibition and protein tyrosine phosphatase activation, *Int. J. Mol. Med.* 5 (3), 261–7, 2000.

155. Rassi, C. M., Lieberherr, M., Chaumaz, G., Pointillart, A., and Cournot, G., Downregulation of osteoclast differentiation by daidzein via caspase 3, *J. Bone Miner. Res.* 17 (4), 630–8, 2002.

156. Li, B. and Yu, S., Genistein prevents bone resorption diseases by inhibiting bone resorption and stimulating bone formation, *Biol. Pharm. Bull.* 26 (6), 780–6, 2003.

157. Viereck, V., Grundker, C., Blaschke, S., Siggelkow, H., Emons, G., and Hofbauer, L. C., Phytoestrogen genistein stimulates the production of osteoprotegerin by human trabecular osteoblasts, *J. Cell Biochem.* 84 (4), 725–35, 2002.

158. Setchell, K. D. and Lydeking-Olsen, E., Dietary phytoestrogens and their effect on bone: evidence from *in vitro* and *in vivo*, human observational, and dietary intervention studies, *Am. J. Clin. Nutr.* 78 (3 Suppl), 593S–609S, 2003.

159. Wiren, K. M., Chapman Evans, A., and Zhang, X. W., Osteoblast differentiation influences androgen and estrogen receptor-alpha and -beta expression, *J. Endocrinol.* 175 (3), 683–94, 2002.

160. Bodine, P. V., Henderson, R. A., Green, J., Aronow, M., Owen, T., Stein, G. S., Lian, J. B., and Komm, B. S., Estrogen receptor-alpha is developmentally regulated during osteoblast differentiation and contributes to selective responsiveness of gene expression, *Endocrinology* 139 (4), 2048–57, 1998.

161. Arts, J., Kuiper, G., Janssen, J., Gustafsson, J.-A., Lowik, C., Pols, H., and van Leeuwen, J., Differential expression of estrogen receptors α and β mRNA during differentiation of human osteoblast SV-HFO cells, *Endocrinology* 138 (11), 5067–5070, 1997.

162. Anderson, J. J., Ambrose, W. W., and Garner, S. C., Biphasic effects of genistein on bone tissue in the ovariectomized, lactating rat model, *Proc. Soc. Exp. Biol. Med.* 217 (3), 345–50, 1998.

163. Ishimi, Y., Arai, N., Wang, X., Wu, J., Umegaki, K., Miyaura, C., Takeda, A., and Ikegami, S., Difference in effective dosage of genistein on bone and uterus in ovariectomized mice, *Biochem. Biophys. Res. Commun.* 274 (3), 697–701, 2000.

164. Valente, M., Bufalino, L., Castiglione, G., D'Angelo, R., Mancuso, A., Galoppi, P., and Zichella, L., Effects of 1-year treatment with ipriflavone on bone in postmenopausal women with low bone mass, *Calcified Tissue Int.* 54 (5), 377–380, 1994.

165. Adami, S., Bufalino, L., Cervetti, R., Di Marco, C., Di Munno, O., Fantasia, L., Isaia, G., Serni, U., Vecchiet, L., and Passeri, M., Ipriflavone prevents radial bone loss in postmenopausal women with low bone mass over 2 years, *Osteoporosis Int.* 7 (2), 119–125, 1997.

166. Gambacciani, M., Spinetti, A., Piaggesi, L., Cappagli, B., Taponeco, F., Manetti, P., Weiss, C., Teti, G. C., Commare, P. I., and Facchini, V., Ipriflavone prevents the bone mass reduction in premenopausal women treated with gonadotropin hormone-releasing hormone agonists, *Bone and Mineral* 26, 19–26, 1994.

167. Alexandersen, P., Toussaint, A., Christiansen, C., Devogelaer, J. P., Roux, C., Fechtenbaum, J., Gennari, C., and Reginster, J. Y., Ipriflavone in the treatment of postmenopausal osteoporosis: a randomized controlled trial, *JAMA* 285 (11), 1482–8, 2001.

168. Rose, D. P., Boyar, A. P., and Wynder, E. L., International comparison of mortality rates for cancer of the breast, ovary, prostate, and colon, and per capita food consumption, *Cancer* 58, 2363–2371, 1986.

169. Armstrong, B. E. and Doll, R., Environmental factors and cancer incidence and mortality in different countries with special reference to dietary practices, *Int. J. Cancer* 15, 617–631, 1975.

170. Shimizu, H., Ross, R. K., Bernstein, L., Yatani, R., Henderson, B. E., and Mack, T. M., Cancers of the prostate and breast among Japanese and white immigrants in Los Angeles County, *Br. J. Cancer* 63 (6), 963–6, 1991.

171. Morton, M. S., Chan, P. S. F., Cheng, C., Blacklock, N., Matos-Ferreira, A., Abranches-Monteiro, L., Correia, R., Lloyd, S., and Griffiths, K., Lignans and isoflavonoids in plasma and prostatic fluid in men: samples from Portugal, Hong Kong, and the United States, *Prostate* 32, 122–128, 1997.

172. Carter, B. S., Cater, H. B., and Isaacs, J. T., Epidemiologic evidence regarding predisposing factors to prostate cancer, *Prostate* 16, 187–197, 1996.

173. Anderson, J., Anthony, M., Messina, M., and Garner, S., Effects of phyto-oestrogens on tissues, *Nutr. Res. Rev.* 12, 75–116, 1999.

174. Wang, C. and Kurzer, M. S., Phytoestrogen concentration determines effects on DNA synthesis in human breast cancer cells, *Nutr. Cancer* 28 (3), 236–247, 1997.

175. Dees, C., S, F. J., Ahamed, S., and Wimalasena, J., Dietary estrogens stimulate human breast cancer cells to enter the cell cycle, *Environ. Health Persp.* 105 (Suppl 3), 633–636, 1997.

176. Mousavi, Y. and Adlercreutz, H., Enterolactone and estradiol inhibit each other's proliferative effect on MCF-7 breast cancer cells in culture, *J. Steroid Biochem. Mol. Biol.* 14 (3–8), 615–619, 1992.

177. Arnold, S. F., Collins, B. M., Robinson, M. K., Guillette, L. J., Jr., and McLachlan, J. A., Differential interaction of natural and synthetic estrogens with extracellular binding proteins in a yeast estrogen screen, *Steroids* 61, 642–646, 1996.

178. Adlercreutz, H., Fotsis, T., Lampe, J., Wähälä, K., Mäkelä, T., Brunow, G., and Hase, T., Quantitative determination of lignans and isoflavonoids in plasma of ominvorous and vegetarian women by isotope dilution gas chromatography-mass spectrometry, *Scand. J. Clin. Lab. Invest.* 215 (Suppl), 5–18, 1993.

179. Bernstein, L., Ross, R. K., Pike, M. C., Brown, J. B., and Henderson, B. E., Hormone levels in older women: a study of postmenopausal breast cancer and healthy population controls, *Br. J. Cancer* 61, 298–302, 1990.

180. Lamartiniere, C. A., Protection against breast cancer with genistein: a component of soy, *Am. J. Clin. Nutr.* 71 (6 Suppl), 1705S–7S; discussion 1708S–9S, 2000.

181. Lamartiniere, C. A., Moore, J. B., Brown, N. M., Thompson, R., Hardin, M. J., and Barnes, S., Genistein supresses mammary cancer in rats, *Carcinogenesis* 16 (11), 2833–2840, 1995.

182. Murrill, W. B., Brown, N. M., Zhang, J., Manzolillo, P. A., Barnes, S., and Lamartiniere, C. A., Prepubertal genistein exposure suppresses mammary cancer and enhances gland differentiation in rats, *Carcinogenesis* 17 (7), 1451–1457, 1997.

183. Brown, N. M., Wang, J., Cotroneo, M. S., Zhao, Y. X., and Lamartiniere, C. A., Prepubertal genistein treatment modulates TGF-alpha, EGF and EGF-receptor mRNAs and proteins in the rat mammary gland, *Mol. Cell Endocrinol.* 144 (1–2), 149–65, 1998.

184. Wei, H., Bowen, R., Cai, Q., Barnes, S., and Wang, Y., Antioxidant and antipromotional effects of the soybean isoflavone genistein, *Proc. Soc. Exp. Biol. Med.* 208 (1), 124–130, 1995.

185. Constantinou, A., Kiguchi, K., and Huberman, E., Induction of differentiation and DNA strand breakage in human HL-60 and D-562 leukemia cells by genistein, *Cancer Research* 50, 2618–2624, 1990.

186. Adlercreutz, H., Phytoestrogens and breast cancer, *J. Steroid Biochem. Mol. Biol.* 83 (1–5), 113–8, 2002.

187. Bylund, A., Zhang, J. X., Bergh, A., Damber, J. E., Widmark, A., Johansson, A., Adlercreutz, H., Aman, P., Shepherd, M. J., and Hallmans, G., Rye bran and soy protein delay growth and increase apoptosis of human LNCaP prostate adenocarcinoma in nude mice, *Prostate* 42 (4), 304–14, 2000.

188. Peeters, P. H., Keinan-Boker, L., van der Schouw, Y. T., and Grobbee, D. E., Phytoestrogens and breast cancer risk. Review of the epidemiological evidence, *Breast Cancer Res. Treat.* 77 (2), 171–83, 2003.

189. Lee, H. P., Gourley, L., Duffy, S. W., Esteve, J., Lee, J., and Day, N. E., Risk factors for breast cancer by age and menopausal status: a case-control study in Singapore, *Cancer Causes Control* 3 (4), 313–22, 1992.

190. Lee, H. P., Gourley, L., Duffy, S. W., Esteve, J., Lee, J., and Day, N. E., Dietary effects on breast-cancer risk in Singapore, *Lancet* 337 (8751), 1197–200, 1991.

191. Hirose, K., Tajima, K., Hamajima, N., Inoue, M., Takezaki, T., Kuroishi, T., Yoshida, M., and Tokudome, S., A large-scale, hospital-based case-control study of risk factors of breast cancer according to menopausal status, *Jpn J. Cancer Res.* 86 (2), 146–54, 1995.

192. Wu, A. H., Ziegler, R. G., Horn-Ross, P. L., Nomura, A. M., West, D. W., Kolonel, L. N., Rosenthal, J. F., Hoover, R. N., and Pike, M. C., Tofu and risk of breast cancer in Asian-Americans, *Cancer Epidemiol. Biomarkers Prev.* 5 (11), 901–6, 1996.

193. Shu, X. O., Jin, F., Dai, Q., Wen, W., Potter, J. D., Kushi, L. H., Ruan, Z., Gao, Y. T., and Zheng, W., Soyfood intake during adolescence and subsequent risk of breast cancer among Chinese women, *Cancer Epidemiol. Biomarkers Prev.* 10 (5), 483–8, 2001.

194. Smith-Warner, S. A., Spiegelman, D., Yaun, S. S., Adami, H. O., Beeson, W. L., van den Brandt, P. A., Folsom, A. R., Fraser, G. E., Freudenheim, J. L., Goldbohm, R. A., Graham, S., Miller, A. B., Potter, J. D., Rohan, T. E., Speizer, F. E., Toniolo, P., Willett, W. C., Wolk, A., Zeleniuch-Jacquotte, A., and Hunter, D. J., Intake of fruits and vegetables and risk of breast cancer: a pooled analysis of cohort studies, *JAMA* 285 (6), 769–76, 2001.

195. Pietinen, P., Rimm, E., and Korhonen, P., Intake of dietery fiber and risk of coronary heart disease in a cohort of Finnish men: the ATBC study, *Circulation* 94, 2720–2727, 1996.

196. Wolk, A., Manson, J. E., Stampfer, M. J., Colditz, G. A., Hu, F. B., Speizer, F. E., Hennekens, C. H., and Willett, W. C., Long-term intake of dietary fiber and decreased risk of coronary heart disease among women, *JAMA* 281 (21), 1998–2004, 1999.

197. Slavin, J., Jacobs, D., and Marquart, L., Whole-grain consumption and chronic disease: protective mechanisms, *Nutr. Cancer* 27 (1), 14–21, 1997.

198. Carrol, K. K. and Kurowska, E. M., Soy consumption and cholesterol reduction: review of animal and human studies, *J. Nutr.* 125 (Suppl 3), 594–597s, 1995.

199. Sirtori, C. R., Lovati, M. R., Manzoni, C., Monetti, M., Pazzucconi, F., and Gatti, E., Soy and cholesterol reduction: clinical experience, *J. Nutr.* 125 (Suppl 3), 598–605s, 1995.

200. Clarkson, T. B., Soy, soy phytoestrogens and cardiovascular disease, *J. Nutr.* 132 (3), 566S–569S, 2002.

201. Kritchevsky, D., Dietary protein, cholesterol and artherosclerosis: a review of the early history, *J. Nutr.* 125 (Suppl 3), 589–593s., 1995.

202. Anthony, M. S., Clarkson, T. B., Hughes, C. L., Jr., Morgan, T. M., and Burke, G. L., Soybean isoflavones improve cardiovascular risk factors without affecting the reproductive system of peripubertal rhesus monkeys, *J. Nutr.* 126, 43–50, 1996.

203. Hung, L. M., Chen, J. K., Huang, S. S., Lee, R. S., and Su, M. J., Cardioprotective effect of resveratrol, a natural antioxidant derived from grapes, *Cardiovasc Res.* 47 (3), 549–55, 2000.

204. Kris-Etherton, P. M., Hecker, K. D., Bonanome, A., Coval, S. M., Binkoski, A. E., Hilpert, K. F., Griel, A. E., and Etherton, T. D., Bioactive compounds in foods: their role in the prevention of cardiovascular disease and cancer, *Am. J. Med.* 113 Suppl 9B, 71S–88S, 2002.

205. Anderson, J. W., Johnstone, B. M., and Cook-Newell, M. E., Meta-analysis of the effects of soy protein intake on serum lipids, *N. Engl. J. Med.* 333 (5), 276–82, 1995.

206. Merz-Demlow, B. E., Duncan, A. M., Wangen, K. E., Xu, X., Carr, T. P., Phipps, W. R., and Kurzer, M. S., Soy isoflavones improve plasma lipids in normocholesterolemic, premenopausal women, *Am. J. Clin. Nutr.* 71 (6), 1462–9, 2000.

207. Wangen, K. E., Duncan, A. M., Xu, X., and Kurzer, M. S., Soy isoflavones improve plasma lipids in normocholesterolemic and mildly hypercholesterolemic postmenopausal women, *Am. J. Clin. Nutr.* 73 (2), 225–31, 2001.

208. Crouse, J. R., 3rd, Morgan, T., Terry, J. G., Ellis, J., Vitolins, M., and Burke, G. L., A randomized trial comparing the effect of casein with that of soy protein containing varying amounts of isoflavones on plasma concentrations of lipids and lipoproteins, *Arch. Intern. Med.* 159 (17), 2070–6, 1999.

209. Anthony, M. S., Clarkson, T. B., Bullock, B. C., and Wagner, J. D., Soy protein versus soy phytoestrogens in the prevention of diet-induced coronary artery atherosclerosis of male cynomolgus monkeys, *Arterioscler. Thromb. Vasc. Biol.* 17 (11), 2524–31, 1997.

210. Balmir, F., Staack, R., Jeffrey, E., Jimenez, M. D., Wang, L., and Potter, S. M., An extract of soy flour influences serum cholesterol and thyroid hormones in rats and hamsters, *J. Nutr.* 126 (12), 3046–53, 1996.

211. Nestel, P. J., Yamashita, T., Sasahara, T., Pomeroy, S., Dart, A., Komesaroff, P., Owen, A., and Abbey, M., Soy isoflavones improve systemic arterial compliance but not plasma lipids in menopausal and perimenopausal women, *Arterioscler. Thromb. Vasc. Biol.* 17 (12), 3392–8, 1997.

212. Simons, L. A., von Konigsmark, M., Simons, J., and Celermajer, D. S., Phytoestrogens do not influence lipoprotein levels or endothelial function in healthy, postmenopausal women, *Am. J. Cardiol.* 85 (11), 1297–301, 2000.

213. Food labeling: health claims; soy protein and coronary heart disease. Food and Drug Administration, HHS. Final rule, *Fed. Regist.* 64 (206), 57700–33, 1999.

214. Forsythe, W. A., III, Soy protein, thyroid regulation and cholesterol metabolism, *J. Nutr.* 125 (Suppl 3), 619–623s, 1995.

215. Ham, J. O., Chapman, K. M., Esses-Sorlie, D., Bakhit, R. M., Prabhudesai, M., Winter, L., Erdman, J. W., and Potter, S. M., Endocrinological response to soy protein and fiber in mildly hypercholesterolemic men, *Nutr. Res.* 13, 873–884, 1993.

216. Potter, S. M., Overview of proposed mechanisms for the hypocholesterolemic effect of soy, *J. Nutr.* 125 (Suppl 3), 606–611s, 1995.

217. Fumagalli, R., Soleri, L., Farini, R., Musanti, R., Mantero, O., Noseda, G., Gatti, E., and Sirtori, C. R., Fecal cholesterol excretion studies in type II hypercholesterolemic patients treated with soybean protein diet, *Atherosclerosis* 43, 341–353, 1982.

218. Sargeant, P., Farndale, R. W., and Sage, S. O., The tyrosine kinase inhibitors methyl 2,5-dihydroxycinnamate and genistein reduce thrombin-evoked tyrosine phosphorylation and Ca2+ entry in human platelets, *FEBS Lett* 315 (3), 242–6, 1993.

219. Teede, H. J., Dalais, F. S., Kotsopoulos, D., Liang, Y. L., Davis, S., and McGrath, B. P., Dietary soy has both beneficial and potentially adverse cardiovascular effects: a placebo-controlled study in men and postmenopausal women, *J. Clin. Endocrinol. Metab.* 86 (7), 3053–60, 2001.

220. Tikkanen, M. J., Wahala, K., Ojala, S., Vihma, V., and Adlercreutz, H., Effect of soybean phytoestrogen intake on low density lipoprotein oxidation resistance, *Proc. Natl. Acad. Sci. USA* 95 (6), 3106–10, 1998.

221. Meng, Q. H., Lewis, P., Wahala, K., Adlercreutz, H., and Tikkanen, M. J., Incorporation of esterified soybean isoflavones with antioxidant activity into low density lipoprotein, *Biochim. Biophys. Acta* 1438 (3), 369–76, 1999.

222. Wiseman, H., O'Reilly, J. D., Adlercreutz, H., Mallet, A. I., Bowey, E. A., Rowland, I. R., and Sanders, T. A., Isoflavone phytoestrogens consumed in soy decrease F(2)-isoprostane concentrations and increase resistance of low-density lipoprotein to oxidation in humans, *Am. J. Clin. Nutr.* 72 (2), 395–400, 2000.

223. Raines, E. W. and Ross, R., Biology of atherosclerotic plaque formation: possible role of growth factors in lesion development and the potential impact of soy, *J. Nutr.* 125 (Suppl 3), 624–630s, 1995.

224. Shimokado, K., Umezawa, K., and Ogata, J., Tyrosine kinase inhibitors inhibit multiple steps of the cell cycle of vascular smooth muscle cells, *Exp. Cell Res.* 220, 266–273, 1995.

225. Gaudette, D. C. and Holub, B. J., Effect of genistein, a tyrosine kinase inhibitor, on U46619-induced phosphoinositide phosphorylation in human platelets, *Biochem. Biophys. Res. Commun.* 170, 238–242, 1990.

226. Honore, E. K., Williams, J. K., Anthony, M. S., and Clarkson, T. B., Soy isoflavones inhance coronary vascular reactivity in atherosclerotic female macaques, *Fertility and Sterility* 67 (1), 148–154, 1997.

227. Clarkson, T. B., Anthony, M. S., and Morgan, T. M., Inhibition of postmenopausal atherosclerosis progression: a comparison of the effects of conjugated equine estrogens and soy phytoestrogens, *J. Clin. Endocrinol. Metab.* 86 (1), 41–7, 2001.

228. Arai, Y., Uehara, M., Sato, Y., Kimira, M., Eboshida, A., Adlercreutz, H., and Watanabe, S., Comparison of isoflavones among dietary intake, plasma concentration and urinary excretion for accurate estimation of phytoestrogen intake, *J. Epidemiol.* 10, 127–135, 2000.

229. Setchell, K. D., Brown, N. M., Desai, P. B., Zimmer-Nechimias, L., Wolfe, B., Jakate, A. S., Creutzinger, V., and Heubi, J. E., Bioavailability, disposition, and dose-response effects of soy isoflavones when consumed by healthy women at physiologically typical dietary intakes, *J. Nutr.* 133 (4), 1027–35, 2003.

230. Setchell, K. D., Brown, N. M., and Lydeking-Olsen, E., The clinical importance of the metabolite equol-a clue to the effectiveness of soy and its isoflavones, *J. Nutr.* 132 (12), 3577–84, 2002.

231. Cassidy, A., Bingham, S., and Setchell, K., Biological effects of isoflavones in young women: importance of the chemical composition of soyabean products, *Br. J. Nutr.* 74 (4), 587–601, 1995.

232. Lydeking-Olsen, E., Jensen, J.-B. E., Setchell, K. D. R., Daamhus, M., and Jensen, T. H., Isoflavone-rich soymilk prevents bone-loss in the lumbar spine of postmeno-pasual women. A 2 year study, *J. Nutr.* 132, 581S (abs), 2002.

233. Daston, G. P., Gooch, J. W., Breslin, W. J., Shuey, D. L., Nikiforov, A. I., Fico, T. A., and Gorsuch, J. W., Environmental estrogens and reproductive health: a discussion of the human and environmental data, *Reprod. Toxicol.* 11 (4), 465–81, 1997.

234. Snedeker, S. M., Pesticides and breast cancer risk: a review of DDT, DDE, and dieldrin, *Environ. Health Perspect.* 109 Suppl 1, 35–47, 2001.

235. Reinli, K. and Block, G., Phytoestrogen content of foods — a compendium of literature values, *Nutrition and Cancer* 26, 123–148, 1996.

236. Franke, A. A., Custer, L. J., Cerna, C. M., and Narala, K., Rapid HPLC analysis of dietary phytoestrogens from legumes and from human urine, *Proc. Soc. Exp. Biol. Med.* 208 (1), 18–26, 1995.

237. Sheehan, D. M., Branham, W. S., Medlock, K. L., and Shamugasundaram, E. R. B., Estrogenic activity of zearalenone and zearalanol in the neonatal rat uterus, *Teratology* 29, 383–392, 1984.

238. Burroughs, C. D., Long-term reproductive tract alterations in female mice treated neotanally with coumestrol, *Proc. Soc. Exp. Biol. Med.* 208 (1), 78–81, 1995.

239. Mäkelä, S., Chemoprevention of prostate cancer. Role of plant estrogens in normal and estrogen-related growth of rodent prostate, *Turun Yliopiston Julkaisuja Annales Universitatis Turkuensis* Ser. D, 170, 1995.

240. Leavitt, W. W. and Meismer, D. M., Sexual development altered by neonatal oestrogens, *Nature* 218, 181–182, 1968.

241. Register, B., Bethel, M. A., Thompson, N., Walmer, D., Blohm, P., Ayyash, L., and Hughes, C., Jr., The effect of neonatal exposure to diethylstilbestrol, coumestrol, and β-sitosterol on pituitary responsiveness and sexually dimorphic nucleus volume in the castrated adult rat, *Proc. Soc. Exp. Biol. Med.* 208 (1), 72–77, 1995.

242. Lu, L. J. W., Broemeling, L. D., Marshall, M. V., and Ramanujam, V. M. S., A simplified method to quantify isoflavones in commercial soybean diets and human urine after legume consumption, *Cancer Epidemiol. Biomarkers and Prevention* 4, 497–503, 1995.

6 Estrogens, Xenoestrogens, and the Development of Neoplasms

A.M. Soto and C. Sonnenschein

CONTENTS

0-8493-2281-2/05/$0.00+$1.50

6.1 INTRODUCTION

Sharpe and Skakkebaek postulated that environmental, hormone-like chemicals may be the underlying cause of increased incidences of testicular cancer, undescended testis, and malformations of the male genital tract during the last half of this century.[1] Davis extended this correlation to the increase in breast cancer incidence during the same time interval.[2] Epidemiological studies and experimental carcinogenesis in animal models reveal a strong link between hormonal exposure and neoplasia and are the basis for both hypotheses.

Endogenous estrogens are considered the main risk factor for of breast cancer. Also, estrogen-replacement therapy has been shown to increase the incidence of endometrial cancer. Exposure to diethylstilbestrol (DES) *in utero* resulted in the development of clear cell adenocarcinoma of the vagina that appeared after exposed girls reached puberty. The recent discovery of hormonally active compounds in the environment— as well as in materials such as food packaging, food additives, cosmetics, and toiletries— suggested that in addition to exposure to exogenous hormones for medical purposes, humans are exposed to many synthetic chemicals that have hormonal activity.

While the role of natural estrogens in carcinogenesis is well documented, the role of other sex steroids such as androgens is less compelling. Androgens are a main factor in the development of prostate cancer; however, there is no evidence at present of environmental contaminants that act as androgen mimics. Some environmental contaminants do, however, possess antiandrogenic properties. Although these compounds may disrupt the development of the male genital tract, it is not yet known whether they play a role in carcinogenesis.

An aspect seldom considered when dealing with carcinogenic properties of environmental endocrine disruptors (EEDs) is defining the targets of these chemicals that lead to deleterious effects. Research on chemical carcinogenesis has been based so far on the premise that— in addition to its intoxicating effects that somehow are overcome by the host— these chemicals generate mutations in the DNA of somatic cells that, as they accumulate, will generate a tumor. Research based on these notions has led to the two-stage model of carcinogenesis whereby an "initiating" agent causes permanent DNA damage and an unspecific "promoting" agent induces proliferation of the genetically altered cells.[3] Although this view is somewhat consistent with some experiments on skin carcinogenesis, there is a substantial body of experimental evidence that contradicts this simplistic interpretation of the data.[4,5] We discuss below alternative interpretations of the data and incorporate novel observations that offer a significantly different perspective on how and on which targets these endocrine disruptors may act to increase the incidence of cancers in exposed populations.

6.2 XENOESTROGENS

Xenobiotics of widely diverse chemical structures have estrogenic properties.[6,7,8] This diversity makes it difficult to predict the estrogenicity of chemicals solely on a structural basis. Hence, their identification as estrogens has relied on bioassays using diverse end points on which estrogens play a direct or indirect role (e.g., cell proliferation, uterine growth, induction of specific genes). Hertz argued convincingly that the proliferative effect of natural estrogens on the female genital tract is the hallmark of estrogen action; thus, this property was adopted to determine whether or not a chemical is an estrogen in animal or cell culture models.[9] This requires measuring increases of proliferative activity in tissues of the female genital tract after estrogen administration. We developed an equally reliable, easy, and rapid method using estrogen-target, serum-sensitive breast cancer MCF7 cells. The E-SCREEN bioassay measures cell proliferation as a specific marker of estrogenicity.[10,11] Other *in vitro* assays rely on the induction of endogenous genes, such as PS2 and PgR, or transfected reporter genes.[12,13] The record shows, however, that the E-SCREEN appears to be the most sensitive and reliable bioassay available to identify xenoestrogens.[14,15]

6.2.1 CUMULATIVE EFFECT OF XENOESTROGENS

Humans and wildlife are exposed to a variety of chemicals simultaneously.[16,17] Residues of diverse estrogenic xenobiotics coexist in the fat and body fluids of exposed individuals.[17] Thus, it is likely that they may become bioavailable, for example, during fasting or nursing. At such time, they may act cumulatively. That is, when present at individual levels lower than those needed to express overt estrogenicity, their activity may add up to a level sufficient to trigger a full estrogenic response.[18,19,20] We explored this concept and found that xenoestrogens indeed act cumulatively in the E-SCREEN assay.[18,19] Silva et al. showed significant additive effects of low doses of xenoestrogens.[21] Hence, we surmise that measuring the total estrogenic burden due to environmental contaminants present in plasma/tissue samples may be more meaningful than measuring the levels of each of the known xenoestrogens individually. This is significant when one considers the implications of evaluating human conditions suspected to be caused by xenoestrogens, such as undescended testis (cryptorchidism), testicular and breast cancer, and the decline in sperm counts and quality seen during the last 50 years.[1,22,23]

6.2.2 NOVEL XENOESTROGENS

Novel xenoestrogens have been found among antioxidants (alkylphenols, butylhydroxyanisole), plasticizers (bisphenol-A [BPA], dibutylphthalate, butylbenzylphthalate), PCB congeners, disinfectants (o-phenylphenol), pesticides (toxaphene, dieldrin, endosulfan, lindane), and sunscreens.[24,25,26,27] The newly identified estrogens not only induce cell proliferation but also increase the expression of pS2 and progesterone receptor (PgR). These xenoestrogens compete with estradiol for binding to the estrogen receptors (ERs) α and β. Their relative binding affinities to the ERs correlate well with their potency to induce both cell proliferation and the expression of marker gene products such as pS2 and PgR.[25] Thus, binding to the "conventional" or nuclear ER present in epithelial cells appears as a likely pathway to explain the mode of action of xenoestrogens at the cellular level of hierarchical complexity. Recently, ERs located in the plasma membrane have been characterized; they have been proposed to mediate nongenomic effects as well as cell proliferation.[28,29] The binding of xenoestrogens to these receptors has yet to be explored in depth. Another issue that awaits exploration is whether these chemicals exert additional effects on tissues as units of biological complexity (see below) through stroma-epithelium interactions. There is evidence of these stroma-mediated effects for natural estrogens[30] during the development of the genital tract and in mammary gland morphogenesis.

No qualitative differences could be found when comparing animal assays and MCF7-based assays. That is, the estrogenic properties of compounds characterized using animal bioassays was also ascertained by measuring cell proliferation or gene induction in cell culture bioassays. From a pharmacokinetic perspective, these *in vitro* assays measure estrogenicity at the target cellular level under conditions where estrogen concentrations are mostly constant, much like the ones achieved when animals are treated with estrogen-filled silastic implants. This approach is more relevant to chronic environmental exposure than that of measuring acute effects after a single dose. Estrogen-target cells in culture have a limited metabolic repertory. For example, it is likely that the estrogenic activity of nonylphenol diethoxylate, a compound that does not bind to estrogen receptor, results from metabolism to the free phenol.[31] Similarly, methoxychlor was believed to be inactive until metabolized to free phenols, presumably in the liver. Methoxychlor tested positive when assayed by the E-SCREEN test. Therefore, even though the putative proestrogens tested so far were estrogenic when assayed by the E-SCREEN test, an added step in the quest for identifying all xenoestrogens may include their metabolic activation by liver microsome extracts prior to their testing by the E-SCREEN assay.

Regarding quantitative effects, while kepone is 100,000 to 1,000,000 times less potent than estradiol according to the E-SCREEN assay, an increase of the rat uterine wet weight comparable to that of estradiol occurred with a 1000- to 5000-fold higher dose of chlordecone than that of estradiol.[6] This discrepancy may be due to rapid metabolism of estradiol and persistence and bioaccumulation of chlordecone in animals. BPA, the only novel xenoestrogen tested so far for endocrine disruption upon exposure *in utero,* was found to produce effects at doses lower than expected from its potency measured in adult animals and *in vitro.*[32,33] Moreover, when BPA was given to adult animals, it was also found to be more potent than what was expected from *in vitro* data.[34,35]

6.2.3 Developmental Effects

Significant progress has been made in establishing that perinatal exposure to low, environmentally relevant doses of xenoestrogens induces morphological and functional alterations in the male[32] and female genital tract[36,37,38] and the mammary gland.[39] The *homeobox* (Hox) and *wingless* (Wnt) families of genes have recently been identified as hormone-sensitive candidates that relay information on tissue patterning within the developing uterus, vagina, and mammary gland, particularly regarding the relationship between the epithelial and stromal compartments, which is critical to normal development. Hoxa-9, hoxa-10, hoxa-11, and hoxa-13 are all expressed along the paramesonephric duct in the embryonic mouse; by birth and into adulthood, these genes establish a spatial co-linearity such that they are expressed in the Fallopian tubes, uterus, uterus and uterine cervix, and upper vagina, respectively. In late gestation, hoxd-10 and 11, hoxd-12, and hoxd-13 are also expressed in the oviduct, uterus, and posterior uterus/vagina, respectively.[40] Wnt 4, Wnt 5a, and Wnt 7a are expressed in specific mesenchymo-epithelial patterns during perinatal development of the uterus,[41] while Msx 1, Msx 2, and Wnt 10b are expressed during prenatal mammary gland morphogenesis.[42]

Recently, the expression of some of these developmental genes was shown to oscillate in response to changes in circulating levels of steroid hormones during the murine estrous cycle, or down-regulate following ovariectomy. Therefore, the subsequent findings that prenatal exposure to the potent estrogen DES altered the expression of Wnt 7a and Hoxa-10 during uterine morphogenesis in the mouse established an important correlation between chemical exposure and the ensuing developmental abnormalities associated with endocrine disruption.[43,44,45] This link was made even more credible when the phenotype of mice carrying specific Hox and Wnt null mutations was observed to be strikingly similar to that of human and mouse "DES daughters." The Wnt genes are associated with cellular responses such as cell proliferation, apoptosis, and cell-cell communication (through the β-catenin/E-cadherin complex). Changing patterns of expression due to environmental chemical exposure can thus provide insight into how these chemicals influence cell fate determination and tissue morphogenesis in hormone-sensitive organs.

6.3 NEOPLASIA

An accurate definition for cancer has been difficult to come by. No single, comprehensive definition satisfies all aspects of this disease. This shortcoming is an acknowledgment of our limited understanding of cancer pathogenesis.

Cancer is both a biological problem and a medical one. Each property of neoplasias is also expressed in normal cells (e.g., invasiveness, ability to proliferate, etc.) From an evolutionary perspective, neoplasias appear with the advent of multicellular organisms. Their purview spans several hierarchical levels of organization from the cellular to the population one.[46,47]

The process by which neoplasias are generated is called carcinogenesis. In epithelia, precursor lesions are called hyperplasia (increased cell proliferation), metaplasia (the ectopic appearance of otherwise normal epithelium), dysplasia (the epithelium shows altered organization and signs of increased proliferative activity), and carcinoma *in situ* (the epithelium resembles a neoplasia that had not yet invaded normal adjacent tissue). Whether these epithelial changes are an expression of the direct or indirect effect of the carcinogen on these cells is the subject of heated controversy (see below).

Definitions of neoplasias and even of their precursor lesions are fraught with unwarranted assumptions about the carcinogenetic process.[48] They are usually circular, and they are additionally contradicted by either the behavior of a particular neoplasm or by that of a normal cell type. For example, Willis states that "a tumor is an abnormal mass of tissue, the growth of which exceeds and is uncoordinated with that of the normal tissues, and persists in the same excessive manner after cessation of the stimuli which evoked the change."[49] This definition (1) fails to distinguish a simple hyperplasia from a neoplasia, (2) does not establish in which regard this "abnormal mass of tissue" differs from other anomalies that are not neoplastic, (3) invokes stimuli that are presently unknown, and (4) does not take into consideration the phenomenon of regression that may occur during carcinogenesis or even neoplasia. True and complete spontaneous regressions of early stage melanomas[50] and some neuroblastomas[51] have been well documented. Regression often occurs in hormonal carcinogenesis after hormone withdrawal. Another drawback of Willis' definition is that it does not take into consideration the tissue organization defects that allow the diagnosis of neoplasia at the histological level.[52] For all these reasons, we will leave neoplasia undefined, and we will paraphrase the pronouncement of U.S. Supreme Court Justice Potter Stewart about pornography: While it is difficult to define, we recognize it when we see it.

Neoplasias are viewed in three contexts: (1) as an aberration of development, (2) as a problem of tissue organization, and (3) as an aberration of the control of cell proliferation.

6.4 THEORIES ON THE MECHANISMS OF CARCINOGENESIS

6.4.1 GENETIC ORIGIN AND THE SOMATIC MUTATION THEORY OF CARCINOGENESIS

The somatic mutation theory (SMT) of cancer has survived practically unchallenged as dogma for almost a century. Since first articulated by Boveri in 1914, it has been updated from time to time to accommodate new findings; however, it has never predicted outcomes that would validate or falsify it. In other words, a theory that can accommodate all outcomes can be hardly verified or falsified. In its latest incarnation it postulates that cancer arises through mutations in putative *oncogenes* (positive mediators) and in *tumor-suppressor genes* (negative mediators) that have been proposed to regulate cell proliferation.[53] Methodologically— and consistent with the notion that carcinogenesis is a cellular or intracellular-based phenomenon— those who favored the SMT used a two-dimensional experimental model (cells in glass or plastic culture flasks) to define the genes responsible for the cancer phenotype.

Research on chemical carcinogenesis has been based on the premise that, in addition to any toxic effects, these chemicals generate somatic mutations. This research led to the above-mentioned two-stage model whereby an "initiating" agent causes permanent DNA damage and an unspecific "promoting" agent induces proliferation of the genetically altered cells.[3]. Although this view is somewhat consistent with some experiments on skin carcinogenesis, there is a substantial body of experimental evidence that contradicts this simplistic interpretation of the data both in these experimental cancers as well as those induced in other organs.[4,5] Despite claims by supporters of the SMT, an unequivocal identification of the candidate mutated genes responsible for tumor formation in sporadic cancers has been elusive. This has been acknowledged by both Varmus[54] and Bishop,[55] the original proponents of a crucial role for oncogenes in carcinogenesis. Other cancer researchers have recently concurred on this evaluation.[56]

A major reason to invoke a genetic origin for sporadic cancers has been the existence of familial cancers inherited through the germ line. However, this fact by itself does not provide an explanation of how carcinogenesis takes place. The lethal giant larvae mutant [l(2)gl] in *Drosophila* is the best studied model. Homozygosity of this mutant gene results in the appearance of neuroblastomas in the third instar larvae.[57] The wild-type gene codes for an intracellular, cytoskeleton-associated protein that is expressed in the early embryo, long before the morphogenesis of the nervous system takes place. Replacement of the mutated sequence in early homozygous embryos with the *wild* allele results in normal flies, indicating that expression of this gene at this embryonal stage, not later, is required for the development of normal neuroblasts.[58] The difficulty remains in trying to understand how the affected gene resulted in a neoplasia, since this protein does not appear to have a direct role on the control of neuroblast proliferation. We have interpreted the presence of syndromes whereby mutated genes transmitted through the germ line are linked to the appearance of tumors in several organs as "inborn errors of development."

Analogous to inborn errors of metabolism that were extensively described during the second half of the 20th century,[59] these cancers represent syndromes that involve the appearing of uni- or multilocular tumors at different times during development. For instance, these syndromes may appear shortly after birth as in retinoblastoma,[60] after puberty or early adulthood like in multiple endocrine cancers,[61] or prior to the age of incidence for the non-familial form in breast cancers due to BRCA1 and BRCA2 gene mutations,[62] and in colorectal cancers due to APC mutations. The distinction between hereditary and sporadic cancers is intended to separate two sets of tumors that have a distinct etiology (genetic versus epigenetic, respectively) but share a common pathogenesis (tissue architecture disruption).

6.4.2 Epigenetic Origin: Development and Neoplasia

The epigenetic origin of sporadic cancers is invoked on the basis of data that appear to be incompatible with DNA mutational events as the ultimate cause of carcinogenesis. Most of this evidence has been collected from models generated in animal experiments. One example is represented by the development of embryonal carcinomas when embryonal tissues are implanted in the testis of certain strains of mice. When a few of these tumor cells were in turn injected into normal blastocysts, they contributed to different tissues of these "mosaic" mice. These tissues included oocytes and spermatozoa that generated normal, fertile progeny.[63] A second experimental example that argues against the SMT is the development of normal tadpoles when nuclei of triploid frog renal carcinoma cells were transplanted into enucleated diploid eggs.[64] In addition, certain tumors arising during development from fetal tissue appear in association with developmental anomalies (nephroblastoma with horse-shoe kidney, hypospadias, cryptorchidism), suggesting that these neoplasias may develop when normal development is affected.[65] The frequent regression of neuroblastomas in infants suggests that cancer cells may revert to normalcy when placed in a permissive environment. Thus, the dictum "once a cancer cell, always a cancer cell" is unsupported by data.[66]

6.4.3 Control of Cell Proliferation and Neoplasia

A significant shortcoming in establishing a successful research program in carcinogenesis has been the lack of resolution of the fundamental controversy regarding the default proliferative state of cells in metazoa.

Self-replication is the *sine qua non* of life. It is generally accepted that proliferation is a built-in property of the cells of unicellular organisms and metaphyta. Unicellular organisms and metaphyta cells dissociated from tissues and placed in culture proliferate maximally as long as they are exposed to nutrients. The state of proliferative quiescence appeared with the advent of multicellularity. There are only two possible choices: The default state of cells in metazoa is either *quiescence* or *proliferation*. Most researchers studying metazoa assume that the quiescent state observed *in situ* is their default state. This means that cells will not proliferate unless stimulated. However, from an evolutionary perspective, this argument is not compelling since multicellular organisms evolved from unicellular ones. Every organism starts as a single cell, the egg. It is highly unlikely for that single cell to forgo the property of self-replication. An almost complete homology between the machinery to replicate yeast cells and human cells suggests that the machinery for cell replication has remained constant throughout evolution.[67]

The prevailing idea that *quiescence* appeared as a new default state in metazoans has never been adequately supported by either argument or data.[68] As mentioned above, multicellular organisms do have quiescent cells. However, it is unlikely that this quiescent state is a newly acquired default state for metazoan cells, rather than the consequence of a regulatory event imposed by the organism on specific cell types, always within the constrains of evolutionary strategies during development. Why would organisms relinquish the fundamental property of self-replication? If one would consider *quiescence* as a newly acquired default state, important incompatibilities would surface. For instance, all cells of the organism have a similar genome, and in experimental conditions, somatic cell nuclei may generate whole individuals when placed in enucleated oocytes. Segregated germ cells, like their somatic counterparts, also undergo control of cell proliferation, as evidenced by the "dormancy" of oogenesis and spermatogenesis at certain developmental stages in metazoa. If the built-in capacity to proliferate within these cells were not curtailed by organismal control, their exponential proliferation would destroy the soma and threaten the viability of the organism.[69]

The choice made by cancer researchers about the default state in metazoan cells subsequently shaped their research program. Those accepting *quiescence* as the default state searched for growth factors and other possible endogenous stimulators of cell proliferation (oncogenes), while those accepting *proliferation* as the default state searched for inhibitory factors.[67]

6.4.3.1 Control of Cell Proliferation by Sex Steroids

Sex hormones (androgens and estrogens) regulate the proliferative activity of their target cells. Studies in animal models have shown that estrogens and androgens control epithelial cell numbers in their target organs by (1) inhibiting cell death,[70] (2) indirectly inducing cell proliferation (Step 1), and later 3) directly inhibiting cell proliferation (proliferative shutoff effect, Step 2).[71,72] These three effects have been shown to segregate in different experimental models, suggesting that they are controlled by discrete, separate mechanisms.

6.4.3.2 Control of Initiation of Cell Proliferation by Estrogens (Step 1)

Three hypotheses aim at explaining the role of estrogens on the induction of cell proliferation: (1) The direct positive hypothesis proposes that estrogens trigger *per se* (without an intermediary step) the proliferation of their target cells.[73] (2) The indirect positive hypothesis proposes that estrogens induce the synthesis of growth factors that, in turn, cause proliferation of estrogen-sensitive cells via stroma-epithelium, paracrine,[74] or autocrine[75] interactions. (3) The indirect negative hypothesis posits that estrogens cancel the effect of plasma-borne inhibitory molecules (estrocolyone-I).[76,77,75] The first two hypotheses are based on the premise that proliferation is an inducible function (that is, the default state of cells is *quiescence*). On the contrary, the third hypothesis assumes that *proliferation* is a constitutive property of cells.

Either a falsification of one of the two premises or a synthesis has yet to emerge. This implies that important evidence needed to fully understand estrogen control of cell proliferation is either still missing or remains unacknowledged. A brief reference to data collected using a variety of models follows, and a resolution of the controversy will be proposed.

(1) Whole animal models: After estradiol administration to ovariectomized or prepubescent rodents, the expression of cellular oncogenes,[78] growth factors,[79] and their receptors[80] are increased in a temporal pattern consistent with their involvement in the proliferative process. To explain these data, it was proposed that estrogens act by inducing epidermal growth factor (EGF) receptors and EGF synthesis in uterine epithelium *in situ*.[79] EGF implants induced both cell proliferation and estrogen-regulated genes in uterine and vaginal epithelia in mice.[81] However, EGF does not induce uterotropic effects in estrogen receptor-knockout mice.[82] These contradictory results leave unresolved the identity of the ultimate causal agent responsible for entry of cells into the reproductive cycle.

(2) Primary culture experiments: Rodent uterine epithelial cells are fully responsive to estrogens for the induction of specific genes; however, estradiol does not increase their proliferative rate.[83,84] In fact, these cells proliferate both in estrogenless and serumless defined medium, suggesting that estrogens may act indirectly in order to induce cell proliferation.[83,85,86] Lack of a proliferative effect by estrogens in primary cultures is inconsistent with the autocrine hypothesis. Moreover, proliferation occurs even in the absence of growth factors.[85] Also, mice mammary luminal epithelial cells are estrogen-sensitive for gene expression but not for cell proliferation.[87] Epithelial cells in vaginal explants undergo rapid proliferation in basal medium devoid of growth factors, regardless of the presence of estrogens. Inferred paracrine mechanisms involving stromal cells are inconsistent with data obtained using explants from ovariectomized mice.[88] This suggests that the intact stroma in the explant fails to mediate estrogen-induced epithelial cell proliferation and that these cells are instead released from inhibitory signals operating in the animal.[88]

(3) Established estrogen-target cell lines: Estrogen-mediated proliferation in culture conditions occurs only when the medium contains serum made estrogenless by charcoal-dextran stripping (CD). Contradictory data were reported on the proliferative effect of estrogens in serumless medium. They varied from a much reduced[89] to a null effect.[90,91,92] These discrepancies may have been due to 1) the presence of a proliferation inhibitor in serum,[76,77,91,92] 2) a permissive effect of serum growth factors,[93] or 3) a synergism between these growth factors and estrogens.[94] Human breast MCF7 cells become quiescent in culture when growth medium is supplemented with CD serum and estrogens specifically release them from this proliferative quiescence.[75] A subline of MCF7 cells (MCF7-SF9) has been propagated in defined medium without growth factors for several thousand generations.[95] These cells proliferate at comparable rates in defined medium regardless of the presence of estrogens. Still, CD serum inhibits their proliferation while estrogens cancel the CD serum-mediated inhibition. The very existence of these cell lines challenges the notion of synergism between growth factors and estrogen and strongly supports the existence of a negative control mechanism involving a serum-borne inhibitor, albumin (estrocolyone-I).[75,76,77] Remarkably, these human breast cells form tumors only in estrogen-treated athymic mice.[96]

(4) The role of serum inhibitors: Serum fractionation protocols resulted in the coelution of the inhibitory activity with serum albumin. Removal of human albumin (HA) from CD serum resulted in a preparation lacking the inhibitory effect. HA inhibition was cell type and protein specific. Only estrogens cancelled HA inhibition; recombinant growth factors and other hormones were ineffective. Recombinant HA and a truncated peptide spanning Domains I and II inhibited cell proliferation. Domain I was also inhibitory, albeit less potent than HA.[76] Domain III lacked inhibitory activity. These results suggest that (1) albumin or a portion of it (most likely within Domains I and II) is the specific inhibitory signal for the proliferation of human breast estrogen-target, serum-sensitive cells, (2) estrogens specifically cancel this inhibition, (3) inhibitory signals prevail over putative growth factors, and (4) the default state in these cells is *proliferation*.

(5) Role of ERs on induction of cell proliferation by estrogens: Stable expression of transfected ERα gene constructs in previously ERα-negative cells renders these cells able to evoke an estrogen-induced proliferative shutoff (Step 2, see above). However, no induction of estrogen-sensitive cell proliferation has been observed.[97] This suggests that ERα expression is necessary, but not sufficient, for conferring estrogen-sensitivity for induction of cell proliferation. We have presented evidence involving a plasma membrane-bound ER complex where an albumin-binding protein plays a role in the mechanism, whereby these estrogen-target cells are allowed to express their proliferative capabilities.[28,29] ER is not present in all serum-sensitive, estrogen-target cells, and most likely, it does not play a role on the control of the proliferation of these cells.[98]

6.4.3.3 Control of the Expression of the Proliferative Shutoff by Estrogens (Step-2) in Normalcy, Carcinogenesis, and Tumor Regression

Stormshak et al. found that estrogens not only induced the proliferation of their target cells in rats, but that their chronic administration resulted in a proliferative shutoff.[71] Later, Gorski's and Stancel's groups demonstrated that this inhibitory effect is a physiological response to estrogens,[99,100] while Bruchovsky et al. showed a comparable response of rat prostate cells to androgens.[101] Mukku et al. found that a second injection of estradiol, given 18 hours after the first one, reduced the peak of mitosis normally observed in the endometrium 24 hours after a single hormone dose.[100] Wiklund et al. explored the difference in responses of the anterior pituitary in Holtzman and Fischer rats: estrogen implants induced a proliferative response that lasted only 5 to 6 days in female Holtzman rats, while it continued in Fisher rats that eventually went on to develop pituitary tumors. Wiklund et al. concluded that "the quantitative relationships of estrogen doses to 'refractoriness' suggest to us that estrogens induce the accumulation of some product that limits the ability of the cells to respond to additional estrogen."[102]

High doses of estrogens induce regression of clinical breast cancer at rates similar to those obtained with antiestrogens. In fact, the usefulness of tamoxifen was tested in comparison with DES. Both were equally effective, but tamoxifen was adopted because of its less-severe side effects.[103] As mentioned above, transfection of ER into mammary breast cells, fibroblasts, HeLa cells, etc., resulted in a phenotype expressing Step 2 only. In 7,12-dimethylbenzanthracene (DMBA)-induced tumors, high doses of estrogen inhibited the development of mammary tumors.[104] The development of variants of the MCF7 cell line that express Step 1, Step 2, both, or neither suggest that these two effects are controlled through independent pathways.[105,106] The existence of an estrogen-induced shutoff effect indicates that the proliferative effect does not follow a linear dose-response curve.[106,107] We have postulated that Step 2 (shutoff) is mediated by estrogen-induced intracellular effectors. A comparable pattern was described in the human prostate cancer cell line LNCaP,[108,109] and the gene product mediating this inhibitory effect has been identified.[110,111]

6.4.4 EPIGENETIC ORIGIN: TISSUE MAINTENANCE AND NEOPLASIA

We have postulated that the process of carcinogenesis in adulthood, that is, the development of sporadic cancers, takes place at the tissue level of hierarchical organization. This, together with the premise that *proliferation* is the default state of all cells, constitute the *tissue organization field theory of carcinogenesis* (TOFT).[47,46] We posit that there are discrete *units of tissue maintenance or organization* in normal, adult, multicellular organisms. They comprise the parenchyma and the stroma of organs. We are proposing to use the name *tissulon* to abbreviate this concept. Like morphogenetic fields, which act during embryogenesis to instruct the formation of tissues and organs, tissulons operating during postnatal life are tridimensional entities that carry positional information. They maintain the normal architecture of all organs and guide tissue turnover, remodeling, and healing through a dynamic process. During embryogenesis, the stroma exerts instructive and permissive influences on the overlying epithelium, dictating its phenotypic characteristics. According to data collected by J.W. Orr and his colleagues almost half a century ago, these properties are maintained by the stroma during adulthood,[112] and carcinogen-exposed stroma was able to evoke a neoplastic phenotype in adjacently grafted epithelia never exposed to the carcinogen. In our view, *tissulons,* present within all organs, are the ultimate targets of carcinogenic agents. There are likely *tissulons* that are more susceptible to carcinogenesis than others (breast, prostate, colon, uterus, etc.), and this susceptibility is probably linked to the extent of remodeling activity in these organs.

Developmental biology is now tackling the problems of pattern formation and morphogenesis, thereby providing the basis for the study of interactions among cells and tissues. It is hoped that the application of these principles in the context of the TOFT will shed light into the study of carcinogenesis.

The exploration of an epigenetic paradigm such as the one proposed by the TOFT would require experimental models where the level of biological complexity at which carcinogenesis takes place is defined. For over two decades, a few laboratories favored the use of tridimensional tissue culture models to test the role of the microenvironment in the expression of the neoplastic phenotype.[113,114] These data show that the neoplastic phenotype is not fixed in the interior of neoplastic cells, but rather it can be "normalized" by altering the composition of the extracellular matrix.[115] Further efforts in this direction will require the recreation of stroma-epithelium interactions in a tri-dimensional setting.

A complementary approach is the study of stroma-epithelium recombinants *in vivo*. Using this approach Barcellos-Hoff and Ravani showed that radiation-induced changes in the stromal microenvironment contributed to the neoplastic progression of non-irradiated, quasi-normal, established COMMA-1 mammary epithelial cells.[116] Maffini et al. observed that exposure of the mammary gland stroma to a carcinogen results in the neoplastic transformation of epithelial mammary cells, regardless of whether or not the epithelial cells were exposed to the carcinogen. These observations suggest that the stroma, rather than the epithelium, is the target of physical and chemical carcinogens.[117] These results challenge the value of the mutational origin of neoplasias, while buttressing the epigenetic hypothesis.[117]

6.5   HORMONAL CARCINOGENESIS

At present, it is difficult to unambiguously establish the role played by hormones in the development of neoplasias. However, it is evident that estrogens represent a significant risk factor in human breast cancer. It is important to accurately define how exposure to estrogens at large influences the incidence of this cancer and, when possible, to recommend measures that may reduce its incidence. We will next attempt to place the role of natural and synthetic xenoestrogenic hormones on carcinogenesis under the context of the *competing theories of carcinogenesis*.

Within the SMT, two roles have been postulated for hormones: (1) that they induce mutations and (2) that they act as promoters. For proponents of the epigenetic perspective, extemporaneous exposure to hormones is considered teratogenic. Hence, according to the TOFT, neoplasias are the result of altered development. Finally, some think that the genetic and epigenetic options are not mutually exclusive. In this case, sex hormones would contribute to the development of neoplasia by acting on all three end points: mutation, control of cell proliferation, and organogenesis-tissue maintenance.

6.5.1   HORMONES AS MUTAGENS

Supporters of the genetic causation hypothesis (two-step model of carcinogenesis) propose that certain estrogens are able to form DNA adducts. This would lead to mutations in yet-to-be-identified genes that, in turn, would result in neoplasms through yet-to-be-defined pathways.[118,119] These inferential pathways involve entities such as oncogenes and tumor-suppressor genes.

The main research program in this endeavor has been to elucidate metabolic pathways leading to the formation of estrogen metabolites that form DNA adducts in estrogen-target tissues. When misrepaired, these DNA adducts would originate mutations. One prediction of the mutagenic hypothesis is that not all estrogenic compounds are carcinogenic. In other words, only those that are mutagenic are expected to induce tumor formation. For example, 2-fluoroestradiol, a compound with an estrogenic potency similar to estradiol, does not induce tumorigenesis in the Syrian hamster model, while estradiol does. This is explained by the fact that estradiol is metabolized to 2-hydroxy metabolites while 2-fluoroestradiol is not metabolized.[120] From a similar perspective, DES is metabolized to an unstable semiquinone that can react with DNA.[121,122] Others have postulated that DES may interact with spindle formation, causing aneuploidy.[123] Bradlow et al. suggested that estradiol is metabolized through two mutually exclusive pathways resulting in a 2-OH estrone and 16"-estrone; they propose that the genotoxic activity is entirely due to 16"-estrone.[124,2] From this perspective, carcinogenesis may be induced by chemicals that affect the metabolism of natural estrogens, enhancing the formation of 16"-estrone. Estrogens have also been implicated in the development of prostate cancer in rats,[125] and mutational mechanisms were invoked.[126] The link between estrogens, mutations, and neoplasia remains circumstantial, and a demonstration of causality is still missing.

6.5.1.1 Xenoestrogens and the Mutational Hypothesis

Xenoestrogen exposure appears to be a risk factor for neoplasms of the female genital tract, breast, and prostate. If mutations are the first step in carcinogenesis, how are xenoestrogens thought to act? Accumulation in a target cell would be proportional to the binding affinity for the xenoestrogens by estrogen receptors. Therefore, a linear dose-response curve may be assumed when associating exposure to effects. However, once xenoestrogens are accumulated in the target tissue, the rate of conversion to the metabolites able to produce DNA adducts must be dependent on their affinity for the enzymes involved in this pathway. If xenoestrogens act by altering the metabolism of endogenous estrogens, the mutagenic activity would be disassociated from their estrogenic activity and instead linked with their ability to induce or activate enzymes that regulate the metabolism of endogenous estrogens. Therefore, a linear dose-response curve would be expected. However, mutagenic potency may not be directly related to estrogenic potency. In conclusion, while the estrogenic potency of xenoestrogens may be important, it does not seem to be the main determinant for their potential mutagenicity.

6.5.2 Hormones as Promoters

Animal models and observational data in humans indicate that tumors in estrogen and androgen-target organs are rare in individuals that had been gonadectomized before or during early adulthood. It is postulated that the role of sex steroids in this context is to sustain cell proliferation in genetically susceptible individuals (i.e., only certain strains develop tumors upon sustained hormone exposure).

In normal sex hormone-target tissues, cell number is tightly regulated, and sex steroids both induce cell proliferation (Step 1) and later inhibit it (Step 2). The "initiated" cells must overcome the restraining mechanisms of Step 2 in order to proliferate selectively and become a hyperplasia and, later on, a tumor. Once the tumor develops, it may or may not require hormones to propagate further (hormone-sensitive or -insensitive, respectively). In this view, a cell "mutated" in its ability to proliferate would acquire a selective advantage to multiply over those impervious to the carcinogen-mutagen. This is a rarely analyzed paradox. The paradox could be reconciled if those mutations are shown to be only in suppressor genes or colyogenes. Proponents of oncogenes state that cancer cells have lost the ability to respond to organismal signals that inhibit cell proliferation.[127] However, none of these hypotheses take into consideration that the precursor lesions that appear during carcinogenesis show altered tissue organization.

Hormones are not only necessary during the process of carcinogenesis, but may also play a role in the propagation of these tumors. Thus, breast and prostate cancers in humans regress after estrogens or androgens, respectively, are withdrawn or suppressed. In animal models, regression may "cure" the tumor, whereas in humans, clinical regressions are temporary due to the selection of "hormone-insensitive" phenotypes. This process is called tumor progression; this recurrence has been attributed to genetic (further mutations) or epigenetic (adaptive) mechanisms due to short-lived therapeutic regimes.[106,109,128,129]

6.5.2.1 Xenoestrogens and the Promotional Hypothesis

As explained above, the issue regarding how estrogen levels may affect proliferation and carcinogenesis remains unsolved. To assess whether or not xenoestrogens significantly increase normal adult women's exposure to estrogen, one first has to ask how ovarian estrogen levels affect proliferation in their target organs. For example, ductal cell proliferation in the breast is maximal from late follicular phase and throughout the luteal phase (i.e., when endogenous estrogen levels are high).[130] Further increases in the estrogen levels may not affect cell proliferation, since the endogenous levels of estrogen at this point are already triggering a full proliferative response followed by a proliferative shutoff. The ubiquitous presence of xenoestrogens in foods, their persistence in the environment, the fact that they are not bound by the plasma carrier protein sex hormone binding globulin, and their cumulative action[18,19,25,131,132] may increase the "basal" levels of estrogens during the early follicular phase of the menstrual cycle. This may result in an early onset of proliferative activity of the organs of the female genital tract and breast, consequently prolonging the period of proliferative activity during each cycle, leading to a higher incidence of breast tumors in later years. Hence, the assumption of a linear dose-response curve is not appropriate when evaluating the role of xenoestrogens as promoters.

6.5.3 Hormones as Teratogens According to the TOFT

According to developmental biologists, extemporaneous hormonal activity is being essentially teratogenic. These untimely exposures would favor the persistence of cell populations past the point at which they should disappear during normal development.[133,134,135] Steroid hormone-target organs undergo morphogenetic changes during postnatal life, and hormones play a main role in these morphogenetic processes. Hence, their role in carcinogenesis may be attributed to disturbance of these processes when hormone levels are excessive or exposures occur extemporaneously.

6.5.3.1 The DES Model

Genital tract organogenesis occurs during the first trimester of gestation in humans and at gestational days 9 to 16 in mice. The role of estrogenic hormones in the normal development of the mammalian reproductive tract is not completely understood, although it is clear that ER must be present for estradiol to mediate biological activity.[136] Exposure to exogenous estrogens during early development results in several anomalies of the human genital tract, including neoplasia. Some of these effects entail the persistence of tissues that regress or express different cellular markers during development. For example, Mullerian ducts (structures that give rise to organs of the female genital tract) normally regress during development in males, but they persist in those exposed to estrogens during development. Women exposed to DES *in utero* manifested a series of anomalies of the genital tract (adenosis, ectropion, anomalies of the cervix) and an increased incidence of clear cell adenocarcinoma of the vagina (risk from birth to 34 years of age is 1:1000).[137] Exposure to DES occurred before the 13th week of *in utero* development in women that developed clear cell adenocarcinoma. The fact that 90% of the cases were diagnosed between ages 15 and 27 suggests that, in addition to *in utero* exposure, the hormonal environment present at puberty is required for the development of this lesion. Interestingly, in the mouse model, a main effect of DES exposure was that animals developed uterine adenocarcinomas after 4 months of age.[138] Before this point in development, exposed mice had exhibited hypoplastic uteri with few or no glands.[139] This suggests that the primary effect may be neither proliferative nor mutational. Instead, the primary effect may be altered tissue organization in the sense that cell populations that should have disappeared did not.

The cohort of women exposed to DES *in utero* is now reaching the age at which breast cancer is diagnosed. Consequently, it is not yet known whether prenatal DES exposure increases breast cancer risk. It is worth noting that an increased risk has been reported in the mothers that received DES during pregnancy.[140] Recently published data by Palmer et al.[141] shows an overall 40% excess breast cancer risk in women exposed *in utero* to DES; the authors of this report remarked that this result "raises a concern calling for continued investigation."[141] Bern[142,143] and Newbold and McLachlan[138] studied the effect of prenatal and early postnatal exposure to DES on the genital tract of mice and found that the most important feature of this syndrome is that some of the morphological alterations are not readily recognizable at birth, but they manifest themselves during puberty and adult life. In the uterus, cystic endometrial hyperplasia, leiomyomas, adenocarcinomas, and stromal cell sarcomas were observed. In the vagina, the proliferative lesions reported were basal cell hyperplasia combined with hyperkeratinization, epidermoid tumors, and adenocarcinomas. It should be noted that vaginal adenocarcinomas appeared when mice were exposed to relatively low doses (2.5 µg/kg/day), while uterine adenocarcinomas appeared at higher exposure levels (100 µg/kg/day) on days 9 to 16 of gestation.[144]

Ovariectomy before puberty prevented the development of these neoplasias. Prolactinomas were observed in mice exposed on days 16 to 17 of prenatal development.[145]

Another interesting consequence of neonatal exposure to DES in mice infected with murine mammary tumor viruses is a shortened latency period and an increased incidence of mammary tumors. In the CD-1 strain of mice, which has high incidence of spontaneous mammary tumors, offspring of females exposed *in utero* had a significantly higher incidence of ovarian and mammary tumors than offspring of females exposed to vehicle.[146] DES induced vaginal adenocarcinomas and squamous cell carcinomas in Wistar rats treated on days 18 to 20 of gestation.[147] More recently, it was reported that male mice exposed *in utero* to DES can transmit a carcinogenic effect to their offspring.[148] Walker and Kurth showed that female mice exposed *in utero* can transmit a carcinogenic effect to their offspring.[149] Using blastocyst transfers, it was shown that offspring of normal blastocysts, which had been transferred to mice exposed prenatally to DES, developed uterine adenocarcinomas (7%). Offspring from blastocysts from female mice exposed to DES *in utero* transferred to mice exposed to vehicle, also developed endometrial adenocarcinomas (16%). Hence, the neoplastic effects of intrauterine exposure may be due to "germ cell modification" (mutation or gene imprinting), as well as to alteration of the maternal environment.

6.5.3.2 Xenoestrogens and the Developmental Hypothesis

Time of exposure appears to be crucial for eliciting developmental mishaps. In addition, some of the developmental alterations mediated by estrogens occur at significantly lower doses than those necessary for causing estrogenic effects in adults. For example, Burroughs et al. have found that hypoplasia of uterine glands occurs after neonatal exposure to extremely low doses of coumestrol, a phytoestrogen.[150,151] In addition, vom Saal observed significant increases in the size of the prostate in adult animals exposed *in utero* to higher levels of estrogen due to a positional effect (a male between two females versus a male between two males).[152,153] Moreover, *in utero* exposure to low doses of BPA also resulted in increased prostate size in the adult[33] and to altered mammary gland development.[154,37,39] It should be noted that in vom Saal's experiments, the dose-response curve looks like an inverted U. This means that the higher doses were less effective in inducing these effects than the lower ones.[32,33] In summary, there are stages of particular vulnerability during development and the developing organism seems to be far more sensitive to minute variations of hormone levels than the adult organism.

6.5.4 Hormones as Agents of Tissue Maintenance and Remodeling

During postnatal life, the mammary gland and the endometrium undergo massive architectural changes, comparable to those usually associated with organogenesis. These changes occur in response to various physiological hormonal environments such as those of puberty and pregnancy. For example, the mammary gland ducts grow by invading the adjacent connective tissue. A similar process takes place in the prostate gland during development and maturation. Moreover, these changes can be repeatedly induced experimentally by endocrine manipulation. These organizational changes occur through interactions between the stroma and the epithelium.[155,156] We have observed that the mammary glands of mice exposed to environmentally relevant doses of the xenoestrogen BPA during prenatal development undergo changes that manifest as altered patterns of bromodeoxyuridine into DNA at 10 days of age, as decreased rates of migration of the ductal tree at puberty, and finally as excessive accumulation of ducts and alveolar structures at 6 months of age.[37,39]

6.6 ANIMAL MODELS FOR HORMONAL CARCINOGENESIS

6.6.1 "Spontaneous" Neoplasia of Estrogen-Target Organs in Animal Models

Neoplasia of endocrine and reproductive organs seldom occur in wildlife and laboratory animals subjected to a restricted diet. Long-term studies in laboratory animals revealed that mammary tumors occur spontaneously in some laboratory rat and mouse strains. For example, Sprague-Dawley and ACI aging virgin females develop mammary tumors spontaneously. Ovariectomy and multiple pregnancies during early adulthood significantly decreased the incidence of these tumors. Endometrial tumors also develop in Han:Wistar, BDII/Han, and Donryu strains.[157] Ovariectomy inhibits the development of these neoplasias.[158] Spontaneous prolactinomas develop in certain rat (Sprague-Dawley) and mouse strains (C57BL/6).[159] Adenoma and adenocarcinoma of the magnum of the oviduct and leiomyoma of the ventral ligament of the oviduct are the most frequent spontaneous neoplasias in the reproductive tract of hens,[160] which correlate with high plasma estrogen levels.[161]

6.6.2 Experimental Neoplasia as a Result of Hormonal Manipulation in Animal Models

Hormonal carcinogenesis started as a result of experiments to study the role of endocrine organs by means of organ ablation-hormone replacement experiments.[65] Ovarian hormones were found to play a role in tumor development of the mammary gland. Pituitary tumors could be obtained by estrogen treatment (rat), and were also induced by thyroidectomy in mice. Thyroid tumors in mice were induced by goitrogens, through an increase in plasma TSH levels. Ovarian tumors were induced by transplanting the ovary into the spleen in ovariectomized rats and mice (presumably gonadotropin induced). Gonadectomy induced adrenocortical tumors in guinea pigs, rats, mice, and hamsters.

6.6.3 Ovarian Hormones and Neoplasia

The search for a role for ovarian hormones in breast neoplasia can be traced to the end of the 19th century when Beatson reported that ovariectomy resulted in clinical regression of advanced breast cancer.[162] This result may be interpreted today as evidence for the trophic role of estrogens in tumor growth and cell survival, as ovariectomy drastically reduced the incidence of breast cancer. Endometrial cancer in humans is also related to estrogen exposure. Vaginal clear cell carcinoma in young women appears as a consequence of *in utero* exposure to DES. Understandably, experimentation in humans is restricted by ethical concerns. On the other hand, animal models provide valuable insights, although they are not always directly applicable to humans. Estrogens were found to induce pituitary neoplasia (rat, mouse, European hamster), mammary cancer (rat and mouse), and kidney tumors (male Syrian and European hamsters). These kidney tumors are estrogen sensitive. Although they do not seem to have an equivalent in human pathology, they are currently used to explore the role of estrogens as mutagens.

6.6.3.1 Endometrial Tumors

Endometrial tumors occur at a relatively high incidence in certain strains of rats. DES exposure throughout adult life results in a 1.7% incidence of uterine adeno-carcinoma in mice, while neonatal (day 1 to5) administration results in 90% incidence. Tumors did not develop in animals ovariectomized before puberty.[144] These tumors required estrogens for continuous growth when transplanted. Adenocarcinomas of the uterus may also be developed by administration of the carcinogen *n*-nitroso-*n*-methylurea (NMU) to intact adult mice.[163] Progestagens inhibited the development of tumors in estrogen-treated animals.[164]

In humans, endometrial adenocarcinoma rates increased in women taking estrogen-replacement therapy.[165] Simultaneous administration of estrogens and progestagens (hormone-replacement therapy) results in a much lower incidence of this type of cancer (almost similar to those of untreated women).[166,167] Recently, it has been suggested that the xenoestrogen hypothesis should be tested by focusing on endometrial rather than on breast cancer.[168] This is predicated on the rapid increase in the incidence of endometrial cancer in postmenopausal women treated with unopposed estrogens and the otherwise low incidence of this malignancy when compared with that of breast cancer. However, it is likely that xenoestrogen exposure would not increase the risk of endometrial cancer in mature, cycling women since their ovaries produce progesterone. Many postmenopausal women are taking hormone-replacement therapy to avoid osteoporosis and heart disease. Only those postmenopausal women not taking progesterone may be at risk of developing endometrial tumors.

6.6.3.2 Mammary Gland Tumors

In 1928, Murray demonstrated that mammary cancer could be induced to when ovaries were transplanted into male mice of a strain in which almost 100% of the females developed mammary cancer.[169] Lacassagne reproduced these results by treating male mice with ovarian extracts ("folliculin").[170] While it is possible to obtain a high tumor yield by prolonged treatment of susceptible rats with estrogens, this only happens in mice infected with mouse mammary tumor viruses.

Mammary tumors can be induced in the Sprague-Dawley and other rat strains by prolonged treatment with estrogens. Estrogens shorten the latency period and increase the incidence of tumors that otherwise would appear if those animals were observed for their entire life span. For example, the spontaneous incidence of mammary adenocarcinomas in female ACI rats was reported to be 7%, whereas treatment with 5-mg pellets of DES at 80 days of age increased the incidence to 52% after 200 days of observation.[171] Regardless of whether or not the resulting neoplasia behaves as a hormone-sensitive tumor, it develops only in intact, non-ovariectomized animals.[172]

Experimental estrogen-induced mammary tumors required prolonged treatment with hormones; the latency periods were extremely long and the incidence was usually low. The discovery that chemical carcinogens such as methylcholanthrene and DMBA-induced mammary carcinomas in some rat strains greatly facilitated the study of these tumors, since the latency period was shortened and the incidence was higher than that of estrogen-induced tumors. Interestingly, the tumors obtained with DMBA or nitroso-methylurea were histologically similar to human breast tumors. Several factors play a role in the induction of mammary carcinomas by these agents: genetic background, estrogen exposure, pituitary hormone exposure, and age.[173] Tumors only develop in certain strains. Over 80% of these carcinogen-treated rats from Fisher, Wistar-Furth, Sprague-Dawley, and other inbred and outbred strains present tumors after 90 days of observation. This incidence is significantly lowered, or nonexistent, with other strains, e.g., Copenhagen.

In nulliparous Sprague-Dawley rats, mammary cancer develops spontaneously. Similarly, estrogens are necessary for the development of DMBA- and NMU-induced mammary cancer in rats. Ovariectomy prior to carcinogen treatment inhibits tumor formation. Estrogen treatment of ovariectomized animals results in comparable tumor incidence rates and latency periods as those observed in intact animals. Paradoxically, high doses of estrogen increase the latency period, decrease the size of tumors, and result in a lower tumor yield per animal.[104] Hence, estrogens also have a biphasic effect on the induction of mammary carcinoma.

Hypophysectomy prevents the development of DMBA-induced tumors. Prolactin appears to stimulate the growth of DMBA-induced mammary carcinomas in ovariectomized, adrenalectomized, and hypophysectomized rats.[174] However, estrogens seem to be essential for the prolonged growth of these tumors.[175,176] This contradicts the hypothesis that estrogens act by inducing the secretion of prolactin.

In DMBA-induced mammary cancer in rats, a "window of vulnerability" was identified between the 45th and 55th day of life;[177] carcinogen administration during this period significantly increases the incidence of carcinomas and decreases the latency period. Multiparity further decreases the incidence of carcinomas. These effects are explained by the intense proliferative activity of structures called terminal end buds, from which new gland ducts are originated during this window of vulnerability.[173] Further development of the gland produces structures that become "carcinogen resistant."[177]

Prenatal exposure to DES results in increased incidence of mammary carcinomas and decreased latency period in Sprague-Dawley rats that were treated with DMBA at 50 days of age.[178,179] Mammary gland carcinogenesis can also be induced in adult

ACI females by persistent treatment with estradiol or DES. In this model, prenatal treatment with a total DES dose of 42.8 µg/kg resulted in an increased incidence of mammary tumors and a decreased latency period.[180] A significant increase in the incidence of mammary gland tumors followed if these animals were challenged with a postnatal exposure to DES from 12 to 22 weeks of age. Prenatal exposure to a total dose of 4 µg/kg DES (a standard dose to elicit a uterotropic response) also results in a significant increase in the incidence of mammary gland carcinomas when these animals were treated with a DES pellet from 12 to 22 weeks of age. These two models provide evidence that prenatal exposure to DES increases the risk of mammary gland carcinogenesis.

In humans, only a small percentage (5 to 10%) of breast cancer is attributed to genetic inheritance. Otherwise, risk factors are mostly related to cumulative lifetime exposure to endogenous ovarian hormones,[181] from early menarche and late menopause. Pregnancy also plays a role. Nulliparous women have a higher risk than those that had undergone full-term pregnancies in their early 20s, and a first pregnancy in the late 30s and 40s increases the risk of breast cancer.[181] There is also some evidence that the level of estrogen exposure during development *in utero* may influence the risk of breast cancer.[182] Exposure to radiation during adolescence and early adulthood is also a risk factor. Epidemiological studies have, for the most part, examined exposure to estrogens from the viewpoint that they act as promoters. For example, a study by Toniolo et al. showed a significant correlation between free (unbound to sex steroid binding globulin) estrogen levels in postmenopausal women and their incidence of breast cancer a few years later.[183]

6.6.3.3 Pituitary Tumors

Chronic estrogen treatment in Fischer, ACI, or Wistar-Furth rats results in the development of pituitary adenomas and transplantable neoplasms that grow as estrogen-sensitive tumors. The proliferative response to estrogens ceased after a few days, in spite of the continuous presence of estrogens in strains that did not develop adenomas (proliferative shutoff).[99,184] Rat strains in which the proliferative response was maintained as long as estrogens were administered developed neoplasms. Hence, tumors appear to develop in animals that have lost the ability to express the estrogen-induced proliferative shutoff.

6.6.3.4 Testicular Neoplasias

There are no animal models that closely parallel the human disease. Hence, we will discuss current thoughts about the genesis of this disease in humans. Germ cell tumors develop from carcinoma *in situ*.[185] The age-specific pattern of tumor incidence in males shows a small peak from birth to 4 years of age, and a second increase after puberty reaching another peak between 20 and 30 years of age for malignant teratoma, and at 30 to 40 years for seminoma.[186] While incidence has increased recently in young men, there is no clear evidence of an increase in boys.[187] Although histological examination of testicular parenchyma adjacent to tumors in adult men revealed the presence of carcinoma *in situ*, this association was not found in tissue from boys;[188] this suggests separate etiologies. The age distribution for incidence of testicular cancer suggests that exposure to risk factors occurs early in life, and that the progression from carcinoma *in situ* to clinical cancer is influenced by androgens or pituitary hormones. The risk of testicular cancer is increased in men with a history of testicular maldescent, gonadal dysgenesis, androgen insensitivity, intersex states, and infertility. Testicular maldescent is associated with a five- to tenfold relative risk increase. When undescent is unilateral, testicular cancer may arise in the contralateral testicle, or in both.[189] In addition, orchidopexy may not prevent testicular cancer.[190] This suggests that an inherent germinal defect present in germinal epithelium may be responsible for the two pathologies.[191] Testicular dysgenesis is an etiologic factor in cryptorchidism.[192] Also, dysgeneic tissue is frequently found in undescended testis.[193] In addition, approximately 20% of the cases of testicular cancer have a history of maldescent. A twofold increase in incidence of undescended testis has been reported from 1950 to 1970;[194] similar increases in hypospadias have been reported.[195,196,197] The hypothesis that high estrogen exposure *in utero* may be a risk factor for testicular cancer is supported by the increased incidence of this pathology in dizygotic twins (a condition that results in increased estrogen exposure).[198]

Mouse strains where testicular cancer arises spontaneously have been described.[186] Mice exposed *in utero* to DES offer a model for testicular maldescent.[139] This pathology is strongly correlated with testicular cancer of germinal cell origin in humans. However, the testicular cancer associated with DES exposure in mice originates in the rete testis (non-germinal origin). For the most part, hormone-induced testicular cancers in laboratory rodents are Leydig cell adenomas, and DES treatment induces these tumors in European hamsters.[199]

6.6.3.5 Prostate Cancer

The etiology of human prostate cancer is unknown. However, like other cancers of the genital tract, its incidence is practically non-existent in men who were castrated before 40 years of age.[200] In addition, most cases of clinical prostate cancer regress after castration. Several models for prostate cancer have been developed in animal systems. Most pathologists believe that rat ventral prostate tumors are not representative of the human disease, while those of the dorsolateral prostate are good models for human carcinoma.[201]

(1) Spontaneous cancer: Cribriform carcinoma of the ventral prostate develops frequently in the aging ACI rats[201] and in AXC rats.[202] Adenocarcinoma of the dorsolateral prostate develops in the Lobund-Wistar rat.[201] One interesting feature of the ACI tumors is that their incidence rate increases in animals exposed to a high-fat diet.[203] This is consistent with correlations derived from human studies.

(2) Hormone-induced cancer: Prostate cancer may be induced in rats by treatment with chemical carcinogens, androgens, carcinogens plus androgens, and androgens plus estrogens. Treatment with chemical carcinogens in otherwise normal males resulted in ventral prostate tumors in the F344 and MRC rat.[201] Lobund-Wistar rats developed spontaneous prostate cancer. Prolonged treatment with testosterone increased the tumor yield and decreased the latency period.[204] Interestingly, increasing the fat content in the diet resulted in further shortening of the latency period.

Combinations of chemical carcinogens and testosterone in various protocols increased the tumor incidence over that obtained with carcinogen alone. Moreover, carcinomas also appeared in the seminal vesicles and coagulating glands. However, the most striking results are those obtained with a combination of estradiol or ethynyl-estradiol and testosterone. Noble originally found that estradiol plus testosterone was more effective than testosterone alone.[205] These hormones induce epithelial dysplasia and, subsequently, adenocarcinoma in the dorsolateral prostate of NBL rats[205] and F344 rats treated with the carcinogen 3,2'-dimethyl-4 aminobiphenyl (DMAB).[206] An interesting feature of the DMAB model is that testosterone alone, as well as testosterone plus ethynyl-estradiol, significantly decreases the incidence of ventral prostate carcinoma below that obtained with DMAB alone, while increasing carcinoma incidence of the lateral, dorsal, and anterior prostates. Testosterone and estrogen levels increased two- to threefold during this treatment. The role of estrogens in this process is unknown. However, several studies found a cooperative effect of estrogens given together with androgens in normal prostate growth.[207,208] Others have suggested that the role of estrogens is to produce DNA damage.[126] Most interestingly, 5″-dihydrotestosterone, which is not metabolized into estrogens, failed to induce prostate cancer in Lobund-Wistar rats[209] and in the DMAB model.[206]

6.7 ENDOCRINE DISRUPTORS AND NEOPLASIA IN ANIMAL MODELS

6.7.1 DDT AND ESTROGEN-SENSITIVE TUMOR GROWTH

Estrogen-sensitive mammary MT2 cells grow as a tumor when inoculated into ovariectomized syngeneic hosts treated with estradiol. The full estrogen agonist o,p′DDT sustained tumor growth at the same rate achieved with estradiol pellets. The congener p,p′DDD, which is a partial agonist less potent than p,p′DDT, did not increase the tumor size over that found in ovariectomized controls.[210]

6.7.2 NEOPLASIAS IN ANIMALS TREATED WITH ESTROGENIC PESTICIDES

As reviewed above, natural estrogens induce neoplasias in reproductive and endocrine organs. There is no consensus on whether they do so through non-hormonal mechanisms (as mutagens) or through their hormonal activity (promotional, developmental, and tissue organization effects). In addition, carcinogens devoid of hormonal activity, such as NMU, induce mammary neoplasias that behave as estrogen-sensitive tumors. Carcinogenicity studies done by long-term exposure to maximum tolerable doses of a chemical are unsuitable to address the question of whether or not their carcinogenicity is mediated by their hormonal activity. The results of the few studies reported in the literature are summarized below. It should be noticed that, for the most part, interpretation of these long-term studies is obfuscated by high mortality due to general toxicity, sample loss, or insufficient sampling.[211,212]

6.7.2.1 Mammary Gland Neoplasias

Methoxychlor treatment resulted in a doubling of the mammary tumor incidence in Osborne-Mendel female rats.[211] In this strain endosulfan induced fibroadenomas and carcinomas.[212]

6.7.2.2 Neoplasias of the Female Genital Tract

Endosulfan increased the incidence of benign endometrial polyps, stromal cell sarcoma, and endometrial adenocarcinoma.[212]

6.7.2.3 Pituitary Neoplasias

Methoxychlor increased the percentage of pituitary adenomas and carcinomas in Osborne-Mendel female rats.[211] Lindane increased the incidence of adenomas and carcinomas both in female and male Osborne-Mendel rats.[213]

6.7.2.4 Ovary Neoplasias

DDT, methoxychlor, and lindane induced carcinomas in Osborne-Mendel rats; these tumors were not seen in the vehicle-treated controls.[211,213,214,215]

6.7.2.5 Testicular Neoplasias

Methoxychlor induced interstitial cell carcinomas in Balb/c mice; estrogens also induce this type of tumor in the Balb/c strain.[211]

6.7.2.6 Adrenal Gland Neoplasias

Methoxychlor doubled the incidence of adenomas and carcinomas in female Osborne-Mendel rats.[211] Lindane also increased the number of these tumors in females and males.[213]

6.7.2.7 Thyroid Neoplasias

Lindane exposure resulted in an increased incidence of adenomas and adenocarcinomas in both male and female Osborne-Mendel rats.[213]

6.8   PESTICIDES AND BREAST CANCER

Correlations have been found between occupational sources of exposure to organic solvents and pesticides and excess breast cancer.[216] Among the estrogenic xenobiotics, PCBs and DDT were considered suitable markers of exposure for breast cancer because they were released massively into the environment beginning approximately 50 years ago, and they are persistent. Their presence in serum may represent cumulative exposure during a lifetime. Early studies, which showed no correlation between breast cancer incidence and xenoestrogen levels, were comprised of a small number of cases and controls that were not matched for other risk factors. However, three recent studies do show a correlation between the occurrence of breast cancer and the levels of xenoestrogens. Wolff et al. found that serum DDE levels correlated with breast cancer incidence in a study of 58 breast cancer patients and 171 controls that were well-matched for risk factors and age.[23] Another study documented that estrogen-receptor-positive breast cancer correlated with higher concentrations of DDE in tissues from these patients.[217] Krieger et al. studied 150 women with breast cancer and 150 controls, where each set was comprised of 50 African-American, 50 Caucasian, and 50 Asian-American women. When the data from all ethnic groups were pooled, no significant correlation was observed between plasma levels of DDE and breast cancer.[218] However, when the cases and matching controls were evaluated separately, according to their ethnic group, high serum DDE levels were correlated to breast cancer incidence in Caucasian and African-American women; there was no significant correlation in Asian-American women. More recent studies were unable to document such a correlation.[219,220,221]

Evidence of a link between exposure to PCBs and breast cancer incidence is also equivocal.[222,221] Hoyer et al. found a significant relation between exposure to dieldrin and breast cancer incidence,[223] and an inverse relationship between levels of exposure and survival. An issue seldom taken into consideration is the relevance of time of exposure. In case-control studies, levels of exposure are measured once the cancer is diagnosed. In nested-case-control studies, exposure is measured before the cancer is diagnosed, but usually it represents exposure during adulthood. From animal studies, we know that the susceptibility of the mammary gland to carcinogenesis is different at different ages. One of these periods of vulnerability is puberty, during invasion of the stroma by the ductal tree (see above). In humans, we know that susceptibility to X-rays is also maximal during puberty and early adulthood.[224] For example, a prospective nested case-control study was performed in a population exposed to DDT during childhood and adolescence at the time of active DDT use in the U.S. Blood was drawn at the time of exposure. In this study, risk of breast cancer increased with increasing concentrations of serum DDT and was significantly stronger in women exposed before age 15 than in those exposed later in life.[225,226]

Another relevant issue is whether single pesticides such as dieldrin and DDT, their metabolites, or PCBs (either total, or individual congeners) are worthy markers of total xenoestrogen exposure. In fact, there are good reasons to think that they are not, because (1) not all the PCB congeners and pesticide metabolites are estrogenic; (2) foods are not uniformly contaminated with all these xenoestrogens, and hence, levels of exposure will be different for different xenoestrogens; (3) different xenoestrogens have dissimilar physical and chemical properties, so that one of them cannot represent the whole; and (4) xenoestrogens act additively among themselves and with ovarian estrogens.[21] In addition, the newly identified estrogens are usually less persistent than PCBs and DDT metabolites. However, these new xenoestrogens are widely used. Hence, it may be inferred that exposure occurs steadily due to their presence in foods.[25] Methods to measure the new xenoestrogens in blood plasma are yet to be developed. Nevertheless, the crux of the problem is whether or not the combined exposure to xenoestrogens correlates with breast cancer incidence. Methodology developed to measure the total xenoestrogen burden[19,227] is being used to assess this hypothesis.[228]

6.9 DISCUSSION AND CONCLUSIONS

The development of neoplasias has been a topic of intense research during the current century. However, little is known about mechanisms underlying this phenomenon. Research during the last four decades has focused on the SMT, probably due to the technological advances that allow for the study of DNA. In spite of this extensive effort, the SMT has not provided a clear understanding of carcinogenesis.

As pointed out at the beginning of this review, most of the data on carcinogenesis has been collected under the premise that the default state of cells in metazoa is *quiescence*. Instead, we have argued that the default state of all living cells is *proliferation*.[229] In the context of carcinogenesis, according to the SMT, putative carcinogens would play the role of direct or indirect stimulators of cell proliferation. In the alternative paradigm, carcinogens become disruptors of inhibitory processes by affecting genetic or epigenetic pathways of homeostasis. Their ultimate effects allow cells to ignore inhibitory signals and exercise their built-in capacity to proliferate. The adoption of *proliferation* as the default state and, consequently, the search for genuine negative signals may be more productive in harnessing the constitutive ability of cells to proliferate than strategies used so far to learn *how* cells proliferate and what may be the role of elusive stimulators of cell proliferation.

In contrast to the SMT, the epigenetic causation hypothesis has not generated a comparable research program because it has not singled out mechanisms that may result in neoplasia. In addition, epigenetic phenomena may act at several hierarchical levels, which means that they cannot be easily explored using the tools of linear thought and molecular biology, which are the traditional equipment of the genetic hypothesis. This may soon change, since the theoretical grounds have been articulated (the tissulon theory) and recent advances in developmental biology will allow researchers to explore the interactions between tissues and cells that operate in morphogenesis and tissue maintenance.[46]

Endogenous sex steroids are a major causal agent in the development of neoplasias in their target organs, and gonadectomy prevents this neoplastic development. The genetic background of animals plays a permissive role in the induction of neoplasms by sex steroids. However, the underlying mechanisms of resistance and susceptibility are presently unknown.

Experimental carcinogenesis studies in animal models and observational studies in humans have produced data consistent with the notion that sex steroids are causal agents because they control the development of their target organs and the proliferation of their target cells. In addition, estrogens induce the formation of DNA adducts, which may result in DNA mutations.

Models for hormone-induced carcinogenesis were developed to obtain high tumor yields with short latency periods by administering supraphysiological levels of hormones alone or in combination with chemical carcinogens. However, this conflicted with the normal plasma levels of hormones implicated in carcinogenesis that were found in susceptible strains that developed these hormone-sensitive tumors. Genome mutations in the epithelial cells of these susceptible strains were considered to be ultimate causes of this susceptibility. Although they may indeed play a role, these genetic factors are not a sufficient cause. Estrogens are still required for the development of a neoplasia

The apparently normal levels of hormones represent a static measure of a time point, which falls within normal ranges. For females, "normal ranges" comprise the wide fluctuations of the estrual and menstrual cycles. Minute increases in estrogen concentration at the beginning of the cycle, when the estrogen level is at its minimum, may be sufficient to produce an effect that does not occur at lower doses. In contrast, an increase in the concentration of estrogens at the point of the cycle where they naturally peak may not produce further effects. In addition, hormones are released in pulses, and this pulsatile pattern of hormone secretion has been shown to be important in determining qualitative aspects of the response. These considerations point to areas of research that has not been explored in relation to carcinogenesis.

The incidence of hormone-induced tumors may be enhanced in animals fed high-fat diets without apparent changes in the plasma levels of hormones. Epidemiological studies also suggest that diet plays an important role in the development of these neoplasias in humans.

It has been observed that extemporaneous administration of sex hormones during development leads to permanent lesions in the genital tract. In turn, this teratogenic effect results in tissues predisposed to neoplasia. Remarkably, developmental effects occur at doses lower than those needed to trigger responses in adult animals. On the other hand, neoplasias of the genital tract in animals exposed *in utero* or neonatally to DES occurred at pharmacological doses. However, recent experiments indicate that females exposed to DES *in utero* transmit a neoplastic phenotype to blastocysts from normal animals.[149] These data indicate that alterations of the maternal environment may lead to neoplasia.

Whether environmental hormonally active agents have a causal role in the development of malignancies of estrogen-and androgen-target organs has not been exhaustively explored. Consequently, it is premature to draw definitive conclusions regarding their contribution to the increase of breast, testicular, and prostate cancer incidence. The plausibility of this hypothesis is based on evidence that exposure to natural estrogens is a main risk factor for endometrial and breast cancers, that exposure to androgens is a risk factor for prostate cancer, and that estrogenic pesticides induce endocrine and reproductive tumors in some rodent strains. As explained above, our understanding of mechanisms of carcinogenesis in general, and of the role of hormones in this process, is still rudimentary.

The main criticism raised against the xenoestrogen hypothesis is that these chemicals are generally less potent than natural estrogens and that current exposure levels are supposedly insignificant when compared to the levels of endogenous hormones. This criticism is based on a slanted reading of biological phenomena. The few epidemiological studies addressing this problem dealt mostly with exposure to DDT metabolites and organochlorines that are not estrogenic. DDT is just one of the many xenoestrogens to which humans are exposed, and evidence of exposure to newly identified xenoestrogens has yet to be gathered. The relatively low potency of xenoestrogens, when compared to ovarian estrogens, is magnified in binding assays and studies done in tissue culture because these studies do not address metabolic rates or bioavailability. These assays may underestimate the potency of xenoestrogens in whole organisms.

A second criticism is based on the assumption of linearity in dose-responses for these chemicals. In this regard, there is evidence that the dose-response to estrogens is not linear, but biphasic. It induces cell proliferation at low doses and inhibits it at high doses. From this perspective, the pattern of exposure may be relevant since estrogen levels are low in the early follicular phase of the menstrual cycle. Steady exposure to xenoestrogens may result in significant increases of the estrogen levels early in the menstrual cycle and, consequently, result in the early onset of proliferative activity in the breast. In contrast, xenoestrogen levels may not affect cell proliferation in the luteal phase, since the endogenous levels of estrogens are already triggering a full proliferative response. Additionally, developmental effects seem to occur at lower doses than those effective in adult animals. The scant dose-response data on developmental effects show an inverted U shape. Moreover, xenoestrogens act cumulatively, and until data on exposure to all known xenoestrogens becomes available, the possibility that their cumulative level is relevant in carcinogenesis cannot be ruled out. The relevance of cumulative effects is heightened by recent evidence indicating that xenoestrogens act additively.[18,19,21]

Finally, given the many uncertainties about basic mechanisms on the control of cell proliferation and carcinogenesis, the shape of the dose-response curve, levels of xenoestrogen exposure, and timing of exposure, what should be done from the perspective of public and environmental health? Exploring these basic questions will take years, even decades, of intense research. Should we wait for the basic science to be done, or should we adopt a preventive approach, diminishing exposures to endocrine disruptors now? The answer is that the enactment of an aggressive preventive approach is not incompatible with a meticulous reappraisal of the implicit premises in this field.

ACKNOWLEDGMENTS

This work was partially supported by grants from the NIH-ES08314, NIH-CA13410, and NIH-CA 55574. We thank Cheryl Michaelson, Janine Calabro, and April Flynn for their editorial assistance.

REFERENCES

1. Sharpe, R. M. and Skakkebaek, N. E., Are oestrogens involved in falling sperm count and disorders of the male reproductive tract? *Lancet*, 341, 1392–1395, 1993.
2. Davis, D. L., Bradlow, H. L., Wolff, M., Woodruff, T., Hoel, D. G., and Anton-Culver, H., Medical hypothesis: xenoestrogens as preventable causes of breast cancer. *Environ. Health Perspect.*, 101, 372–377, 1993.
3. Berenblum, I. and Shubik, P., A new quantative approach to the study of the stages of chemical carcinogenesis in the mouse's skin. *Br. J. Cancer*, 1346, 383–391, 1947.
4. Iversen, O. H., The reverse experiment in two-stage skin carcinogenesis. *APMIS*, 101, 1–96, 1993.

5. Rubin, H., Epigenetic nature of neoplastic transformation, in *Developmental Biology and Cancer*, Hodges, G. M. and Rowlatt, C., Eds., CRC Press, Boca Raton, FL, 1993, 61–84.

6. Hammond, B., Katzenellenbogen, B. S., Kranthammer, N., and McConnell, J., Estrogenic activity of the insecticide chlordecone (kepone) and interaction with uterine estrogen receptors. *Proc. Nat. Acad. Sci. USA*, 76, 6641–6645, 1979.

7. Meyers, C. Y., Matthews, W. S., Ho, L. L., Kolb, V. M., and Parady, T. E., Carboxylic acid formation from kepone, in *Catalysis in Organic Synthesis*, Smith, G. W., Ed., Academic Press, New York, 1977, 213–255.

8. Soto, A. M., Michaelson, C. L., Prechtl, N. V., Weill, B. C., Sonnenschein, C., Olea-Serrano, M. F., and Olea, N., Assay to measure estrogen and androgen agonists and antagonists, in *in vitro Germ Cell Developmental Toxicology: From Science to Social and Industrial Demand.*, del Mazo, J., Ed., Plenum Press Publishing Co., New York, 1998.

9. Hertz, R., The estrogen problem—-retrospect and prospect, in *Estrogens in the Environment II- Influences on Developement*, McLachlan, J. A., Ed., Elsevier, New York, 1985, 1–11.

10. Soto, A. M., Justicia, H., Wray, J. W., and Sonnenschein, C., p-Nonyl-phenol: an estrogenic xenobiotic released from "modified" polystyrene. *Environ. Health Perspect.*, 92, 167–173, 1991.

11. Soto, A. M., Lin, T.-M., Justicia, H., Silvia, R. M., and Sonnenschein, C., An "in culture" bioassay to assess the estrogenicity of xenobiotics, in *Chemically Induced Alterations in Sexual and Functional Development: The Wildlife/Human Connection*, Colborn, T. and Clement, C., Eds., Princeton Scientific Publishing, Princeton, NJ, 1992, 295–309.

12. Routledge, E. J. and Sumpter, J. P., Structural features of alkylphenolic chemicals associated with estrogenic activity. *J. Biol. Chem.*, 272, 3280–3288, 1997.

13. Collins, B. M., McLachlan, J. A., and Arnold, S. F., The estrogenic and antiestrogenic activities of phytochemicals with the human estrogen receptor expressed in yeast. *Steroids*, 62, 365–372, 1997.

14. Andersen, H. R., Andersson, A. M., Arnold, S. F., Autrup, H., Barfoed, M., Beresford, N. A., Bjerregaard, P., Christiansen, L. B., Gissel, B., Hummel, R., Jorgensen, E. B., Korsgaard, B., Le Guevel, R., Leffers, H., McLachlan, J., Moller, A., Nielsen, J. B., Olea, N., Oles-Karasko, A., Pakdel, F., Pedersen, K. L., Perez, P., Skakkebaek, N. E., Sonnenschein, C., Soto, A. M., Sumpter, J. P., Thorpe, S. M., and Grandjean, P., Comparison of short-term estrogenicity tests for identification of hormone-disrupting chemicals. *Environ. Health Perspect.*, 107(Supple 1), 89–108, 1999.

15. Fang, H., Tong, W., Perkins, R., Soto, A. M., Prechtl, N. V., and Sheehan, D. M., Quantitative comparisons of *in vitro* assays for estrogenic activities. *Environ. Health Perspect.*, 108, 723–729, 2000.

16. Fox, G. A., Epidemiological and pathobiological evidence of contaminant-induced alterations in sexual development in free-living wildlife, in *Chemically Induced Alterations in Sexual and Functional Development: The Wildlife/Human Connection*, Colborn, T. and Clement, C., Eds., Princeton Scientific Publishing, Princeton, NJ, 1992, 147–158.

17. Thomas, K. B. and Colborn, T., Organochlorine endocrine dispruptors in human tissue, in *Chemically Induced Alterations in Sexual Development: The Wildlife/Human Connection*, Colborn, T. and Clement, C., Eds., Princeton Scientific Publishing Co., Princeton, NJ, 1992, 365–394.

18. Soto, A. M., Chung, K. L., and Sonnenschein, C., The pesticides endosulfan, toxaphene, and dieldrin have estrogenic effects on human estrogen sensitive cells. *Environ. Health Perspect.*, 102, 380–383, 1994.

19. Soto, A. M., Fernandez, M. F., Luizzi, M. F., Oles Karasko, A. S., and Sonnenschein, C., Developing a marker of exposure to xenoestrogen mixtures in human serum. *Environ. Health Perspect.*, 105, 647–654, 1997.

20. Arnold, S. F., Bergeron, J. M., Tran, D. Q., Collins, B. M., Vonier, P. M., Crews, D., Jr., and McLachlan, J. A., Synergistic responses of steroidal estrogens *in vitro* (yeast) and *in vivo* (turtles). *Biochem. Biophys. Res. Commun.*, 235, 336–342, 1997.

21. Silva, E., Rajapakse, N., and Kortenkamp, A., Something from "nothing" — eight weak estrogenic chemicals combined at concentrations below NOECs produce significant mixture effects. *Environ. Sci. Technol.*, 36, 1751–1756, 2002.

22. Giwercman, A., Carlsen, E., Keiding, N., and Skakkebaek, N. E., Evidence for increasing incidence of abnormalities of the human testis: a review. *Environ. Health Perspect.*, 101, 65–71, 1993.

23. Wolff, M. S., Toniolo, P. G., Lee, E. W., Rivera, M., and Dubin, N., Blood levels of organochlorine residues and risk of breast cancer. *J. Nat. Cancer Inst.*, 85, 648–652, 1993.

24. Soto, A. M. and Sonnenschein, C., Environmental sex hormone agonists and antagonists. *Comment. Tox.*, 5, 329–346, 1996.

25. Soto, A. M., Sonnenschein, C., Chung, K. L., Fernandez, M. F., Olea, N., and Olea-Serrano, M. F., The E-SCREEN assay as a tool to identify estrogens: an update on estrogenic environmental pollutants. *Environ. Health Perspect.*, 103, 113–122, 1995.

26. Ma, R., Cotton, B., Lichtensteiger, W., and Schlumpf, M., UV filters with antagonistic action at androgen receptors in the MDA-kb2 cell transcriptional-activational assay. *Toxicol. Sci.*, 74, 43–50, 2003.

27. Schlumpf, M., Cotton, B., Conscience, M., Haller, V., Steinmann, B., and Lichtensteiger, W., *In vitro* and *in vivo* estrogenicity of UV screens. *Environ. Health Perspect.*, 109, 239–244, 2001.

28. Powell, C. E., Soto, A. M., Michaelson, C. L., Diba, F., Mounier, F., Verroust, P. J., and Sonnenschein, C., Plasma membrane-resident albumin binding protein associated with the proliferation of MCF7 serum-sensitive cells. *Steroids*, 68, 487–496, 2003.

29. Powell, C. E., Soto, A. M., and Sonnenschein, C., Identification and characterization of membrane estrogen receptor from MCF7 estrogen-target cells. *J. Steroid Biochem. Molec. Biol.*, 77, 97–108, 2001.

30. Buchanan, D. L., Setiawan, T., Lubahn, D., Taylor J.A., Kurita, T., Cunha, G., and Cooke, P. S., Tissue compartment-specific estrogen receptor-a participation in the mouse uterine epithelial secretory response. *Endocrinology*, 140, 484–491, 1999.

31. White, R., Jobling, S., Hoare, S. A., Sumpter, J. P., and Parker, M. G., Environmentally persistent alkylphenolic compounds are estrogenic. *Endocrinology*, 135, 175–182, 1994.

32. vom Saal, F. S., Timms, B. G., Montano, M. M., Palanza, P., Thayer, K. A., Nagel, S. C., Ganjam, V. K., Parmigiani, S., and Welshons, W. V., Prostate enlargement in mice due to fetal exposure to low doses of estradiol or diethylstilbestrol and opposite effects at high doses. *Proc. Nat. Acad. Sci. USA*, 94, 2056–2061, 1997.

33. Nagel, S. C., vom Saal, F. S., Thayer, K. A., Dhar, M. G., Boechler, M., and Welshons, W. V., Relative binding affinity-serum modified access (RBA-SMA) assay predicts the relative *in vivo* bioactivity of the xenoestrogens bisphenol A and octylphenol. *Environ. Health Perspect.*, 105, 70–76, 1997.

34. Steinmetz, R., Brown, N. G., Allen, D. L., Bigsby, R. M., and Ben-Jonathan, N., The environmental estrogen bisphenol A stimulates prolactin release *in vitro* and *in vivo*. *Endocrinology*, 138, 1780–1786, 1997.

35. Colerangle, J. B. and Roy, D., Profound effects of the weak environmental estrogen-like chemical bisphenol A on the growth of the mammary gland of Noble rats. *J. Steroid Biochem. Molec. Biol.*, 60, 153–160, 1997.

36. Howdeshell, K. L., Hotchkiss, A. K., Thayer, K. A., Vandenbergh, J. G., and vom Saal, F. S., Exposure to bisphenol A advances puberty. *Nature*, 401, 763–764, 1999.

37. Markey, C. M., Coombs, M. A., Sonnenschein, C., and Soto, A. M., Mammalian development in a changing environment: exposure to endocrine disruptors reveals the developmental plasticity of steroid-hormone target organs. *Evolution and Development*, 5, 1–9, 2003.

38. Rubin, B. S., Murray, M. K., Damassa, D. A., King, J. C., and Soto, A. M., Perinatal exposure to low doses of bisphenol-A affects body weight, patterns of estrous cyclicity and plasma LH levels. *Environ. Health Perspect.*, 109, 675–680, 2001.

39. Markey, C. M., Luque, E. H., Munoz de Toro, M. M., Sonnenschein, C., and Soto, A. M., *In utero* exposure to bisphenol A alters the development and tissue organization of the mouse mammary gland. *Biol. Reprod.*, 65, 1215–1223, 2001.

40. Taylor, H. S., Heuvel, G. B. V., and Igarash, P., A conserved Hox axis in the mouse and human female reproductive system:late establishment and persistent adult expression of the *Hoxa* cluster genes. *Biol. Reprod.*, 57, 1338–1345, 1997.

41. Miller, C., Pavlova, A., and Sassoon, D. A., Differential expression patterns of Wnt genes in the murine female reproductive tract during development and the estrous cycle. *Mechanisms of Development*, 76, 91–99, 1998.

42. Phippard, D. J., Weber-Hall, S. J., Sharpe, P. T., Naylor, M. S., Jayatalake, H., Maas, R., Woo, I., Roberts-Clark, D., Francis-West, P. H., Liu, Y., Maxson, R., Hill, R. E., and Dale, T. C., Regulation of Msx-1, Msx-2, Bmp-2 and Bmp-4 during foetal and postnatal mammary gland development. *Development*, 122, 2729–2737, 1996.

43. Kitajewski, J. and Sassoon, D. A., The emergence of molecular gynecology: homeobox and Wnt genes in the female reproductive tract. *Bioessays*, 22, 902–910, 2000.

44. Miller, C., Degenhardt, K., and Sassoon, D. A., Fetal exposure to DES results in de-regulation of Wnt7a during uterine morphogenesis. *Nature Genet.*, 20, 228–230, 1998.

45. Sassoon, D. A., Wnt genes and endocrine disruption of the female reproductive tract: a genetic approach. *Mol. Cell. Endocrinol.*, 158, 1–5, 2001.

46. Sonnenschein, C. and Soto, A. M., Epilogue: moving toward the integration of cell proliferation, carcinogenesis, and neoplasia into biology, in *The Society of Cells: Cancer and Control of Cell Proliferation*, Springer Verlag, New York, 1999, 134–143.

47. Sonnenschein, C. and Soto, A. M., The somatic mutation theory of carcinogenesis: Why it should be dropped and replaced. *Mol. Carcinog.*, 29, 1–7, 2000.

48. Peng, A. and Ackerman, A. B., Neoplasm? *Dermatopathology*, 4, 41–45, 1998.

49. Willis, R. A., *Pathology of Tumors*, Butterworths, London, 1967.

50. Clark, W. H., Tumour progression and the nature of cancer. *Br. J. Cancer*, 64, 631–644, 1991.

51. Turkel, S. B. and Itabashi, H. H., The natural history of neuroblastic cells in the fetal adrenal gland. *Am.J.Pathol.*, 76(2), 225–236, 1974.

52. Rowlatt, C., Some consequences of defining the neoplasm as focal self-perpetuating tissue disorganization., in *New Frontiers in Cancer Causation*, Iversen, O. H., Ed., Taylor & Francis, Washington, D.C., 1994, 45–58.

53. Varmus, H. E. and Weinberg, R. A., *Genes and the Biology of Cancer*, Scientific American Library, New York, 1992, 123.

54. Varmus, H. E., The molecular genetics of cellular oncogenes. *Annu. Rev. Genet.*, 18, 553–612, 1984.

55. Bishop, J. M., Cellular oncogenes and retroviruses. *Annu. Rev. Biochem.*, 52, 301–354, 1983.

56. Hahn, W. C. and Weinberg, R. A., Modeling the molecular circuitry of cancer. *Nat.Rev.Cancer*, 2, 331–342, 2002.

57. Gateff, E. and Schneiderman, H. A., Neoplasms in mutant and cultured wild-type of Drosophila. *National Cancer Institute Monographs*, 31, 365–397, 1969.

58. Mechler, B. M., Strand, D., Kalmes, A., Merz, R., Schmidt, M., and Torok, I., Drosophila as a model system for molecular analysis of tumorogenesis. *Environ. Health Perspect.*, 93, 63–71, 1991.

59. Schaub, J., *Inborn Errors of Metabolism*, Lippincott, Williams & Wilkins, Philadelphia, 1991.

60. Knudson, A. G., Jr., Pediatric molecular oncology: Past as prologue to the future. *Cancer*, 71, 3320–3324, 1993.

61. Poisson, A., Zablewska, B., and Gaudray, P., Menin interacting proteins as clues toward the understanding of multiple endocrine neoplasia type 1. *Cancer Lett.*, 189, 1–10, 2003.

62. Iau, P. T., Macmillian, R. D., and Blamey, R. W., Germ line mutations associated with breast cancer susceptibility. *Eur. J. Cancer*, 37, 300–321, 2001.

63. Mintz, B. and Ilmensee, K., Normal genetically mosaic mice produced from malignant teratocarcinoma cells. *Proc. Nat. Acad. Sci. USA*, 72, 3585–3589, 1975.

64. McKinnell, R. G., Deggins, B. A., and Labbat, D. D., Transplantation of pluripotent nuclei from triploid frog tumors. *Science*, 165, 394–396, 1969.

65. Foulds, L., *Neoplastic Development,* Academic Press, New York, 1969/

66. Pierce, G. B. and Cox, W. F. Jr., Neoplasms as tissue caricatures of tissue renewal, in *Cell Differentiation and Neoplasia*, Saunders, G. F., Ed., Raven Press, New York, 1978, 57–66.

67. Sonnenschein, C. and Soto, A. M., Cell proliferation: the background and the premesis; Cell proliferation, call nutrition and evolution, in *The Society of Cells: Cancer and Control of Cell Proliferation*, Springer Verlag, New York, 1999, 1–30.

68. Alberts, B., Johnson, A., Lewis, J. G., Raff, M., Roberts, K., and Walter, P., Default state defined, in *Molecular Biology of the Cell*, Garland Publishing Inc., New York, 2002, 1015.

69. Soto, A. M. and Sonnenschein, C., Estrogens, xenoestrogens and the development of neoplasms, in *Endocrine disruptors: effects on the male and female reproductive systems.*, Naz, R. K., Ed., CRC Press, Boca Raton, FL, 1999, 125–163.

70. Martin, L., Estrogens, antiestrogens and the regulation of cell proliferation in the female reproductive tract *in vivo*, in *Estrogens in the Environment*, McLachlan, J. A., Ed., Elsevier/North-Holland, New York, 1980, 103–130.

71. Stormshak, F., Leake, R., Wertz, N., and Gorski, J., Stimulatory and inhibitory effects of estrogen on uterine DNA synthesis. *Endocrinology*, 99, 1501–1511, 1976.

72. Mukku, V. R., Kirkland, J. L., Hardy, M., and Stancel, G. M., Hormonal control of uterine growth: temporal relationships between estrogen administration and deoxyribonucleic acid synthesis. *Endocrinology*, 111, 480–487, 1982.

73. Stack, G. and Gorski, J., Direct mitogenic effect of estrogen on the prepubertal rat uterus: studies on isolated nuclei. *Endocrinology*, 115, 1141–1150, 1984.

74. Cooke, P. S., Uchima, F. D. A., Fujii, D. K., Bern, H. A., and Cunha, G. R., Restoration of normal morphology & estrogen responsiveness in cultured vaginal & uterine epithelia transplanted with stroma. *Proc. Nat. Acad. Sci. USA*, 83, 2109–2113, 1986.

75. Soto, A. M. and Sonnenschein, C., The role of estrogens on the proliferation of human breast tumor cells (MCF-7). *J. Steroid Biochem.*, 23, 87–94, 1985.

76. Sonnenschein, C., Soto, A. M., and Michaelson, C. L., Human serum albumin shares the properties of estrocolyone-I, the inhibitor of the proliferation of estrogen-target cells. *J. Steroid Biochem. Molec. Biol.*, 59, 147–154, 1996.

77. Soto, A. M., Silvia, R. M., and Sonnenschein, C., A plasma-borne specific inhibitor of the proliferation of human estrogen-sensitive breast tumor cells (estrocolyone-I). *J. Steroid Biochem. Molec. Biol.*, 43, 703–712, 1992.

78. Chiappetta, C., Kirkland, J. L., Loose-Mitchell, D. S., Murthy, L., and Stancel, G. M., Estrogen regulates expression of the jun family of protooncogenes in the uterus. *J. Steroid Biochem. Molec. Biol.*, 41, 113–123, 1992.

79. Huet-Hudson, Y. M., Chakraborty, C., De, S. K., Suzuki, Y., Andrews, G. K., and Dey, S. K., Estrogen regulates the synthesis of epidermal growth factor in mouse uterine epithelial cells. *Mol. Endocrinol.*, 4, 510–523, 1990.

80. Stancel, G. M., Chiappetta, C., Gardner, R. M., Kirkland, J. L., Lin, T. H., Lingham, R. B., Loose-Mitchell, D. S., Mukku, V. R., and Orengo, C. A., Regulation of the uterine epidermal growth factor receptor by estrogen. *Prog. Clin. Biol. Res.*, 322, 213–226, 1990.

81. Nelson, K. G., Takahashi, T., Bossert, N. L., Walmer, D. K., and McLachlan, J. A., Epidermal growth factor replaces estrogen in the stimulation of female genital-tract growth & differentiation. *Proc. Nat. Acad. Sci. USA*, 88, 21–25, 1991.

82. Curtis, S. W., Washburn, T., Sewall, C., Diaugustine, R., Lindzey, J., Couse, J. F., and Korach, K. S., Physiological coupling of growth factor and steroid receptor signaling pathways: Estrogen receptor knockout mice lack estrogen-like response to epidermal growth factor. *Proc. Nat. Acad. Sci. USA*, 93, 12626–12630, 1996.

83. Uchima, F. D. A., Edery, M., Iguchi, T., and Bern, H. A., Growth of mouse endometrial luminal epithelia cells *in vitro*: functional integrity of the oestrogen receptor system and failure of oestrogen to induce proliferation. *J. Endocrinol.*, 128, 115–120, 1991.

84. Uchima, F. D. A., Edery, M., Iguchi, T., Larson, L., and Bern, H. A., Growth of mouse vaginal epithelial cells in culture: functional integrity of the estrogen receptor system and failure of estrogen to induce proliferation. *Cancer Lett.*, 35, 227–235, 1987.

85. Fukamachi, H. and McLachlan, J. A., Proliferation and differentiation of mouse uterine epithelial cells in primary serum-free culture: Estradiol-17b suppresses uterine epithelial proliferation cultured on a basement membrane-like substratum. *in vitro Cell. Dev. Biol.*, 27A, 907–913, 1991.

86. Julian, J., Carson, D. D., and Glasser, S. R., Polarized rat uterine epithelium *in vitro* constitutive expression of estrogen "induced" proteins. *Endocrinology*, 130, 79–87, 1992.

87. Yang, J., Richards, J., Guzman, R., Imagawa, W., and Nandi, S., Sustained growth in primary culture of normal mammary epithelial cells embedded in collagen gels. *Proc. Nat. Acad. Sci. USA*, 77(4), 2088–2092, 1980.

88. Tsai, P. S. and Bern, H. A., Estrogen-independent growth of mouse vaginal epithelium in organ culture. *J. Exp. Zool.*, 259, 238–245, 1991.

89. Darbre, P. D., Curtis, S., and King, R. J., Effects of estradiol and tamoxifen on human breast cancer cells in serum-free culture. *Cancer Res.*, 44, 2790–2793, 1984.

90. Butler, W., Kirkland, W. L., Gargala, T., Goran, N., Kelsey, W. H., and Berlinski, P., Steroid stimulation of plasminogen activator production in a human breast cancer cell line (MCF-7). *Cancer Res.*, 43, 1637–1641, 1983.

91. Soto, A. M. and Sonnenschein, C., Mechanism of estrogen action on cellular proliferation: evidence for indirect and negative control on cloned breast tumor cells. *Biochem. Biophys. Res. Commun.*, 122, 1097–1103, 1984.

92. Lykkesfeldt, A. E. and Briand, P., Indirect mechanism of oestradiol stimulation of cell proliferation of human breast cancer cell lines. *Br. J. Cancer*, 53, 29–35, 1986.

93. van der Burg, B., Rutteman, G. R., Blankenstein, M. A., De Laat, S. W., and van Zoelen, E. J., Mitogenic stimulation of human breast cancer cells in a growth factor-defined medium: synergistic action of insulin and estrogen. *J. Cell Physiol.*, 134, 101–108, 1988.

94. van der Burg, B., De Groot, R. P., Isbrucker, L., Kruijer, W., and De Laat, S. W., Direct stimulation by estrogen of growth factor signal transduction pathways in human breast cancer cells. *J. Steroid Biochem. Molec. Biol.*, 43, 111–115, 1992.

95. Briand, P. and Lykkesfeldt, A. E., Long-term cultivation of a human breast cancer cell line, MCF7, in chemically defined medium. *Anticancer Res.*, 6, 85–90, 1986.

96. Soule, H. D. and McGrath, C. M., Estrogen responsive proliferation of clonal human breast carcinoma cells in athymic mice. *Cancer Lett.*, 10, 177–189, 1980.

97. Jiang, S.-Y. and Jordan, V. C., Growth regulation of estrogen-receptor negative breast cancer cells transfected with cDNAs for estrogen receptor. *J. Nat. Cancer Inst.*, 84, 580–591, 1992.

98. Krege, J. H., Hodgin, J. B., Couse, J. F., Enmark, E., Warner, M., Mahler, J. F., Sar, M., Korach, K. S., Gustafsson, J. A., and Smithies, O., Generation and reproductive phenotypes of mice lacking estrogen receptor beta. *Proc .Nat. Acad. Sci. USA*, 95, 15677–15682, 1998.

99. Wiklund, J., Rutledge, J., and Gorski, J., A genetic model for the inheritance of pituitary tumor susceptibility in F344 rats. *Endocrinology*, 109, 1708–1714, 1981.

100. Mukku, V. R., Kirkland, J. L., Hardy, M., and Stancel, G. M., Stimulatory and inhibitory effects of estrogen and antiestrogen on uterine cell division. *Endocrinology*, 109, 1005–1010, 1981.

101. Bruchovsky, N. and Lesser, B., Control of proliferative growth in androgen responsive organs and neoplasms. *Advances in Sex Hormone Research*, 2, 1–55, 1976.

102. Wiklund, J. A. and Gorski, J., Genetic differences in estrogen-induced deoxyribonucleic acid synthesis in the rat pituitary: correlations with pituitary tumor susceptibility. *Endocrinology*, 111, 1140–1149, 1982.

103. Ingle, J. N., Ahman, D. L., and Green, S. J., Randomized clinical trial of DES versus tamoxifen in post-menopausal women with advanced breast cancer. *New Engl. J. Med.*, 304, 16–21, 1981.

104. Meites, J., The relation of estrogen and prolactin to mammary tumorigenesis in the rat, in *Estrogen target tissues and neoplasia*, Dao, T. L., Ed., Univ. of Chicago Press, Chicago, 1972, 275–286.

105. Soto, A. M. and Sonnenschein, C., Cell proliferation of estrogen-sensitive cells: the case for negative control. *Endocr. Rev.*, 8, 44–52, 1987.

106. Sonnenschein, C., Szelei, J., Nye, T. L., and Soto, A. M., Control of cell proliferation of human breast MCF7 cells; serum and estrogen resistant variants. *Oncology Res.*, 6, 373–381, 1994.

107. Amara, J. F. and Dannies, P. S., 17 b-Estradiol has a biphasic effect on gh cell growth. *Endocrinology*, 112, 1141–1143, 1983.

108. Sonnenschein, C., Olea, N., Pasanen, M. E., and Soto, A. M., Negative controls of cell proliferation: human prostate cancer cells and androgens. *Cancer Res.*, 49, 3474–3481, 1989.

109. Soto, A. M., Lin, T. M., Sakabe, K., Olea, N., Damassa, D. A., and Sonnenschein, C., Variants of the human prostate LNCaP cell line as a tool to study discrete components of the androgen-mediated proliferative response. *Oncology Res.*, 7, 545–558, 1995.

110. Maffini, M. V., Geck, P., Powell, C. E., Sonnenschein, C., and Soto, A. M., Mechanism of androgen action on cell proliferation AS3 protein as a mediator of proliferative arrest in the rat prostate. *Endocrinology*, 143, 2708–2714, 2002.

111. Geck, P., Maffini, M. V., Szelei, J., Sonnenschein, C., and Soto, A. M., Androgen-induced proliferative quiescence in prostate cancer: the role of AS3 as its mediator. *Proc. Nat. Acad. Sci. USA*, 97, 10185–10190, 2000.

112. Orr, J. W., The mechanism of chemical carcinogenesis. *Br. Med. Bull.*, 14, 99–101, 1958.

113. Bissell, M. J. and Radisky, D., Putting tumours in context. *Nat. Rev. Cancer*, 1, 46–54, 2001.

114. Park, C. C., Bissell, M. J., and Barcellos-Hoff, M. H., The influence of the microenvironment on the malignant phenotype. *Molecular Medicine Today*, 6, 324–329, 2000.

115. Weaver, V. M., Petersen, O. W., Wang, F., Larabell, C. A., Briand, P., Damsky, C., and Bissell, M. J., Reversion of the malignant phenotype of human breast cells in three-dimensional culture and *in vivo* integrin blocking antibody. *J .Cell Biol.*, 137, 231–245, 1997.

116. Barcellos-Hoff, M. H. and Ravani, S. A., Irradiated mammary gland stroma promotes the expression of tumorigenic potential by unirradiated epithelial cells. *Cancer Res.*, 60, 1254–1260, 2000.

117. Maffini, M. V., Soto, A. M., Calabro, J. M., Ucci, A. A., and Sonnenschein, C., Rat mammary gland chemical carcinogenesis: the stroma as a crucial target. *J. Cell Sci.*, 2004.

118. Liehr, J. G., Genotoxicity of the steroidal oestrogens oestrone and oestradiol: possible mechanism of uterine and mammary cancer development. *Human Reproduction Update*, 7, 273–281, 2001.

119. Yue, W., Santen, R. J., Wang, J. P., Li, Y., Verderame, M. F., Bocchinfuso, W. P., Korach, K. S., Devanesan, P., Todorovic, R., Rogan, e.g., and Cavalieri, E. L., Genotoxic metabolites of estradiol in breast: potenital mechanism ofestradiol induced carcinogenesis. *J. Steroid Biochem. Molec. Biol.*, 86, 477–486, 2003.

120. Liehr, J. G., Stancel, G. M., Chorich, L. P., Bousfield, G. R., and Ulubelen, A. A., Hormonal carcinogenesis; separation of estrogenicity from carcinogenicity. *Chem. Biol. Interactions*, 59, 173–184, 1986.

121. Bhat, H. K., Han, X., Gladek, A., and Liehr, J. G., Regulation of the formation of the major diethylstilbestrol-DNA adduct and some evidence of its structure. *Carcinogenesis*, 15, 2137–2142, 1994.

122. Roy, D., Bernhardt, A., Strobel, H. W., and Liehr, J. G., Catalysis of the oxidation of steroid and stilbene estrogens to estrogen quinone metabolites by the beta-naphthoflavone-inducible cytochrome P450 IA family. *Arch. Biochem. Biophys.*, 296, 450–456, 1992.

123. Barrett, J. C., Wong, A., and McLachlan, J. A., Diethylstilbestrol induces neoplastic transformation of cells in culture without measurable somatic mutation at two loci. *Science*, 212, 1402–1404, 1981.

124. Bradlow, H. L., Davis, D. L., Lin, G., Sepkovic, D., and Tiwari, R., Effects of pesticides on the ratio of 16 alpha/2-hydroxyestrone: a biologic marker of breast cancer risk. *Environ. Health Perspect.*, 103 Suppl 7, 147–150, 1995.

125. Noble, R. L., The development of prostatic adenocarcinoma in Nb rats following prolonged sex hormone administration. *Cancer Res.*, 37, 1929–1933, 1977.

126. Han, X., Liehr, J. G., and Bosland, M. C., Induction of a DNA adduct detectable by 32P-postlabeling in the dorsolateral prostate of NBL/Cr rats treated with estradiol-17 beta and testosterone. *Carcinogenesis*, 16, 951–954, 1995.

127. Alberts, B., Bray, D., Lewis, J. G., Raff, M., Roberts, K., and Watson, J. D., *<[13] Book Title>*, Garland Publishing Inc., New York, 1994, 1280–1281.

128. Szelei, J., Jimenez, J., Soto, A. M., Luizzi, M. F., and Sonnenschein, C., Androgen-induced inhibition of proliferation in human breast cancer MCF7 cells transfected with androgen receptor. *Endocrinology*, 138, 1406–1412, 1997.

129. Sonnenschein, C. and Soto, A. M., Cell proliferation in metazoans: negative control mechanisms, in *Regulatory Mechanisms in Breast Cancer.*, Lippman, M. E. and Dickson, R. B., Eds., Kluwer, Boston, 1991, 171–194.

130. Meyer, J. S., Cell proliferation in normal human breast ducts, fibroadenomas, and other ductal hyperplasias measured by nuclear labeling with tritiated thymidine. *Hum. Pathol.*, 8, 67–81, 1977.

131. Brotons, J. A., Olea-Serrano, M. F., Villalobos, M., and Olea, N., Xenoestrogens released from lacquer coating in food cans. *Environ. Health Perspect.*, 103, 608–612, 1994.

132. Olea, N., Pulgar, R., Perez, P., Olea-Serrano, F., Rivas, A., Novillo-Fertrell, A., Pedraza, V., Soto, A. M., and Sonnenschein, C., Estrogenicity of resin-based composites and sealants used in dentistry. *Environ. Health Perspect.*, 104(3), 298–305, 1996.

133. Ozawa, S., Iguchi, T., Sawada, K., Ohta, Y., Takasugi, N., and Bern, H. A., Postnatal vaginal nodules induced by prenatal diethylstilbestrolof ovary-independent vaginal and uterine changes in mice. *Cancer Lett.*, 58, 167–175, 1991.

134. Takasugi, N., Cytological basis for permanent vaginal changes on mice treated neonatally with steroid hormones. *Int. Rev. Cytol.*, 44, 193–224, 1976.

135. Bern, H. A., *<[13] Book Title>*, Li, J., Nandi, S., and Li, S. A., Eds. Springer Verlag, New York, 1992.

136. Lubahn, D. B., Moyer, J. S., Golding, T. S., Couse, J. F., Korach, K. S., and Smithies, O., Alteration of reproductive function but not prenatal sexual development after insertional disruption of the mouse estrogen receptor gene. *Proc. Nat. Acad. Sci. USA*, 90, 11162–11166, 1993.

137. Mittendorf, R., Teratogen update: carcinogenesis and teratogenesis associated with exposure to diethylstilbestrol (DES) *in utero. Teratology*, 51, 435–445, 1995.

138. Newbold, R. R. and McLachlan, J. A., Diethylstilbestrol associated defects in murine genital tract development., in *Estrogens in the Environment II: Influences on Development*, McLachlan, J. A., Ed., Elsevier Science Publishing Co.,Inc., New York, 1985, 288–318.

139. Newbold, R. R., Cellular and molecular effects of developmental exposure to diethylstilbestrol: Implications for other environmental estrogens. *Environ. Health Perspect.*, 103 (Suppl 7), 83–87, 1995.

140. Giusti, R. M., Iwamoto, K., and Hatch, E. E., Diethylstilbestrol revisited: a review of the long-term health effects. *Ann. Intern. Med.*, 122, 778–788, 1995.

141. Palmer, J. R., Hatch, E. E., Rosenberg, C. L., Hartge, P., Kaufman, R. H., Titus-Ernstoff, L., Noller, K. L., Herbst, A. L., Rao, R. S., Troisi, R., Colton, T., and Hoover, R. N., Risk of breast cancer in women exposed to diethylstilbestrol *in utero*: preliminary results (United States). *CCC*, 13, 753–758, 2002.

142. Bern, H. A., The fragile fetus, in *Chemically-Induced Alterations in Sexual and Functional Development: The Wildlife/Human Connection.*, Colburn, T. and Clement, C., Eds., Princeton Scientific Publishing Co., Inc., Princeton, NJ, 1992, 9–15.

143. Bern, H. A., Jones, L. A., and Mills, K. T., Use of the neonatal mouse in studying long-term effects of early exposure to hormones and other agents. *J. Toxicol. Environ. Health – Suppl.*, 1, 103–116, 1976.

144. Newbold, R. R., Bullock, B. C., and McLachlan, J. A., Uterine adenocarcinoma in mice following developmental treatment with estrogens: a model for hormonal carcinogenesis. *Cancer Res.*, 50, 7677–7681, 1990.

145. Walker, B. E. and Kurth, L. A., Pituitary tumors in mice exposed prenatally to diethylstilbestrol. *Cancer Res.*, 53, 1546–1549, 1993.

146. Walker, B. E., Tumors in female offspring of control and diethylstilbestrol- exposed mice fed high-fat diets. *J. Nat. Cancer Inst.*, 82, 50–54, 1990.

147. Baggs, R. B., Miller, R. K., and Odoroff, C. L., Carcinogenicity of diethylstilbestrol in the Wistar rat: effect of postnatal oral contraceptive steroids. *Cancer Res.*, 51, 3311–3315, 1991.

148. Turusov, V. S., Trukhanova, L. S., Parfenov, Y. D., and Tomatis, L., Occurance of tumours on the descendants of CBA male mice prenatally treated with diethylstilbestrol. *Int. J. Cancer*, 50, 131–135, 1992.

149. Walker, B. E. and Kurth, L. A., Multi-generational carcinogenesis from diethylstilbestrol investigated by blastocyst transfers in mice. *Int. J. Cancer*, 61, 249–252, 1995.

150. Burroughs, C. D., Bern, H. A., and Stokstad, E. L., Prolonged vaginal cornification and other changes in mice treated neonatally with coumestrol, a plant estrogen. *J. Toxicol. Environ. Health*, 15, 51–61, 1985.

151. Burroughs, C. D., Mills, K. T., and Bern, H. A., Long-term genital tract changes in female mice treated neonatally with coumestrol. *Reproductive Toxicology*, 4, 127–135, 1990.

152. vom Saal, F. S., Montano, M. M., and Wang, M. H., Sexual differentiation in mammals, in *Chemically-Induced Alterations in Sexual and Functional Development: the Wildlife/Human Connection.*, Colborn, T. and Clement, C., Eds., Princeton Scientific Publishing Co.,Inc., Princeton, NJ, 1992, 17–83.

153. Nonneman, D. J., Ganjam, V. K., Welshons, W. V., and vom Saal, F. S., Intrauterine position effects on steroid metabolism and steroid receptors of reproductive organs in male mice. *Biol. Reprod.*, 47, 723–729, 1992.

154. Markey, C. M., Rubin, B. S., Soto, A. M., and Sonnenschein, C., Endocrine disruptors from Wingspread to environmental developmental biology. *J. Steroid Biochem. Molec. Biol.*, 83, 235–244, 2003.

155. Cunha, G. R., Bigsby, R. M., Cooke, P. S., and Sugimura, Y., Stromal-epithelial interactions in adult organs. *Cell Different.*, 17, 137–148, 1985.

156. Hayward, S. W., Rosen, M. A., and Cunha, G. R., Stromal-epithelial interactions in the normal and neoplastic prostate. *Brit. J. Urol.*, 79 Suppl 2, 18–26, 1997.

157. Nagaoka, T., Onodera, H., Matsushima, Y., Todate, A., Shibutani, M., Ogasawara, H., and Maekawa, A., Spontaneous uterine adenocarcinomas in aged rats and their relation to endocrine imbalance. *J .Cancer Res. Clin. Oncol.*, 116, 623–628, 1990.

158. Deerberg, F. and Kaspareit, J., Endometrical carcinoma in BD II/Han rats: model of a spontaneous hormone-dependent tumor. *J. Nat. Cancer Inst.*, 78, 1245–1251, 1987.

159. Greenman, D. L., Highman, B., Chen, J., Sheldon, W., and Gass, G., Estrogen-induced thyroid follicular cell adenomas in C57BL/6 mice. *J. Toxicol. Environ. Health*, 29, 269–278, 1990.

160. Anjum, A. D. and Payne, L. N., Spontaneous occurence and experimental induction of leiomyoma of the ventral ligament of the oviduct of the hen. *Research in Veterinary Science*, 45, 341–348, 1988.

161. Anjum, A. D. and Payne, L. N., Concentration of steroid sex hormones in the plasma of hens in relation to oviduct tumours. *Brit. Poultry Sci.*, 29, 729–734, 1988.

162. Beatson, G. T., On the treatment of inoperable cases of carcinoma of the mamma: Suggestions for a new method of treatment with illustrative cases. *Lancet*, 2, 104–106, 1896.

163. Niwa, K., Murase, T., Furui, T., Morishita, S., Mori, H., and Tanaka, T., Enhancing effects of estrogens on endometrial carcinogenesis initiated by N-methyl-N-nitrosourea in ICR mice. *Jpn. J. Cancer Res.*, 84, 951–955, 1993.

164. Niwa, K., Morishita, S., Murase, T., Itoh, N., Tanaka, T., Mori, H., and Tamaya, T., Inhibitory effects of medroxyprogesterone acetate on mouse endometrial carcinogenesis. *Jpn. J. Cancer Res.*, 86, 724–729, 1995.

165. Ziel, H. K., Estrogen's role in endometrial cancer. *Obstet. Gynecol.*, 60, 509–515, 1982.

166. Brinton, L. A. and Schairer, C., Estrogen replacement therapy and breast cancer risk. *Epidemiologic Reviews*, 15, 66–79, 1993.

167. Hulka, B. S., Kaufman, D. G., Fowler, W. C., Jr., Grimson, R. C., and Greenberg, B. G., Predominance of early endometrial cancers after long-term estrogen use. *J. Am. Med. Assoc.*, 244, 2419–2422, 1980.

168. Adami, H. O., Lipworth, L., Titus-Ernstoff, L., Hsieh, C. C., Hanberg, A., Ahlborg, U., Baron, J., and Trichopoulos, D., Organochlorine compounds and estrogen-related cancers in women. *CCC*, 6, 551–566, 1995.

169. Murray, W. S., Ovarian secretion and tumor incidence. *J. Cancer Res.*, 12, 18–25, 1928.

170. Lacasagne, A., Aparition de cancers de la mammelle chez la souris male, soumise a des injections de folliculine. *C.R. Hebd. Seances Acad. Sci.*, 195, 630–632, 1932.

171. Shellabarger, C. J., Stone, J. P., and Holtzman, S., Rat differences in mammary tumor induction with estrogen and neutron radiation. *J .Nat. Cancer Inst.*, 61, 1505–1508, 1978.

172. Nandi, S., Guzman, R., and Yang, J., Hormones and mammary carcinogenesis in mice, rats, and humans: a unifying hypothesis. *Proc. Nat. Acad. Sci. USA*, 92, 3650–3657, 1995.

173. Russo, J. and Russo, I. H., Biological and molecular bases of mammary carcinogenesis. *Lab. Invest.*, 57, 112–137, 1987.

174. Talwalker, P. K. and Meites, J., Mammary lobulo-alveolar growth induced by anterior pituitary hormones in adreno-ovariectomized and adreno-ovariectomized-hypophysectomized rats. *Proc. Soc. Exp. Biol. Med.*, 107, 880–883, 1961.

175. Leung, B. S. and Sasaki, G. H., On the mechanism of prolactin and estrogen action in 7,12-dimethylbenzanthracene-induced mammary carcinoma in the rat. II. *In vivo* tumor responses and estrogen receptor. *Endocrinology*, 97, 564–572, 1975.

176. Welsch, C. W., Host factors affecting the growth of carcinogen-induced rat mammary carcinomas: a review and tribute to Charles Brenton Huggins. *Cancer Res.*, 45, 3415–3443, 1985.

177. Russo, J. and Russo, I. H., DNA labeling index and structure of the rat mammary gland as determinants of its susceptibility to carcinogenesis. *J. Nat. Cancer Inst.*, 61, 1451–1459, 1978.

178. Boylan, E. S. and Calhoon, R. E., Transplacental action of diethylstilbestrol on mammary carcinogenesis in female rats given one or two doses of 7,12-dimethyl-benz(a)anthracene. *Cancer Res.*, 43, 4879–4884, 1983.

179. Boylan, E. S. and Calhoon, R. E., Prenatal exposure to diethylstilbestrol: ovarian-independent growth of mammary tumors induced by 7,12-dimethyl-benz[a]anthracene. *J. Nat. Cancer Inst.*, 66, 649–652, 1981.

180. Rothschild, T. C., Boylan, E. S., Calhoon, R. E., and Vonderhaar, B. K., Transplacental effects of diethylstilbestrol on mammary development and tumorigenesis in female ACI rats. *Cancer Res.*, 47, 4508–4516, 1987.

181. Hulka, B. S. and Stark, A. T., Breast cancer: cause and prevention. *Lancet*, 346, 883–887, 1995.

182. Ekbom, A., Trichopoulos, D., Adami, H. O., Hsieh, C. C., and Lan, S. J., Evidence of prenatal influences on breast cancer risk. *Lancet*, 340, 1015–1018, 1992.

183. Toniolo, P. G., Levitz, M., Zeleniuch-Jacquotte, A., Banerjee, S., Koenig, K. L., Shore, R. E., Strax, P., and Pasternack, B. S., A prospective study of endogenous estrogens and breast cancer in postmenopausal women. *J. Nat. Cancer Inst.*, 87, 190–197, 1995.

184. Wiklund, J. A., Wertz, N., and Gorski, J., A comparison of estrogen effects on uterine and pituitary growth and prolactin synthesis in F344 and Holtzman rats. *Endocrinology*, 109, 1700–1707, 1981.

185. Skakkebaek, N. E., Bethelsen, J. G., Giwercman, A., and Muller, J., Carcinoma in situ of the testis: possible origin from gonocytes and precursor of all types of germ cell tumors except spermatocytoma. *Int. J. Androl.*, 10, 19–28, 1987.

186. Horwich, A., Mason, M. D., and Hendry, W. F., Urological cancer, in *Oxford Textbook of Oncology.*, Peckham, M., Pinedo, H., and Veronesi, U., Eds., Oxford University Press, New York, 1995, 1407–1530.

187. Moller, H., Jorgensen, N., and Forman, D., Trends in incidence of testicular cancer in boys and adolescent men. *Int. J. Cancer*, 61, 761–764, 1995.

188. Jorgensen, N., Muller, J., Giwercman, A., Visfeldt, J., Moller, H., and Skakkebaek, N. E., DNA content and expression of tumour markers in germ cells adjacent to germ cell tumours in childhood: probably a different origin for infantile and adolescent germ cell tumours. *J. Pathol.*, 176, 269–278, 1995.

189. Johnson, D. E., Woodhead, D. M., Pohl, D. R., and Robison, J. R., Cryptorchidism and testicular tumorigenesis. *Surgery*, 63, 919–922, 1968.

190. Senturia, Y. D., The epidemiology of testicular cancer. *Brit. J. Urol.*, 60, 285–291, 1987.

191. Sohval, A. R., Testicular dysgenesis in relation to neoplasm of the testicle. *J. Urol.*, 75, 285–291, 1956.

192. Sohval, A. R., Testicular dysgenesis as an etiologic factor in cryptorchidism. *J. Urol.*, 72, 693–702, 1953.

193. Paulson, D. F., Einhorn, L. H., Peckham, M. J., and Williams, S. D., Cancer of the testis, in *Cancer principles & practice of oncology*, DeVita, V. T., Hellman, S., and Rosenberg, S. A., Eds., J.B.Lippincott Company, Philadelphia, 1982, 786–822.

194. Chilivers, C., Pike, M. C., Forman, D., Fogelman, K., and Wadsworth, M. E. J., Apparent doubling of frequency of undescended testis in England and Wales in 1962–81. *Lancet*, 330–332, 1984.

195. Kallen, B., Case control study of hypospadias, based on registry information. *Teratology*, 38, 45–50, 1988.

196. Kallen, B., Castilla, E. E., Robert, E., Lancaster, P. A., Kringelbach, M., Martinez-Frias, M. L., and Mastroiacovo, P., An international case-control study on hypospadias. The problem with variability and the beauty of diversity. *European Journal of Epidemiology*, 8, 256–263, 1992.

197. Paulozzi, L. J., Erickson, J. D., and Jackson, R. J., Hypospadias trends in two US surveillance systems. *Pediatrics*, 100, 831–834, 1997.

198. Braun, M. M., Ahlbom, A., Floderus, B., Brinton, L. A., and Hoover, R. N., Effect of twinship on incidence of cancer of the testis, breast, and other sites (Sweden). *CCC*, 6, 519–524, 1995.

199. Reznik-Schuller, H., Carcinogenic effects of diethylstilbestrol in male Syrian golden hamsters and European hamsters. *J. Nat .Cancer Inst.*, 62, 1083–1088, 1979.

200. Moore, R. A., Benign hypertrophy and carcinoma of the prostate. *Surgery*, 16, 152–167, 1944.

201. Bosland, M. C., Animal models for the study of prostate carcinogenesis. *J. Cell. Biochem.–Supplement*, 16H, 89–98, 1992.

202. Shain, S. A., McCullough, B., Nitchuk, M., and Boesel, R. W., Prostate carcinogenesis in the AXC rat. *Oncology*, 34, 114–122, 1977.

203. Iizumi, T., Yazaki, T., Kanoh, S., Kondo, I., and Koiso, K., Establishment of a new prostatic carcinoma cell line (TSU-Pr1). *J. Urol.*, 137, 1304–1306, 1987.

204. Pollard, M. and Luckert, P. H., Tumorigenic effects of direct- and indirect-acting chemical carcinogens in rats on a restricted diet. *J. Nat. Cancer Inst.*, 74, 1347–1349, 1985.

205. Noble, R. L., Prostate carcinoma of the Nb rat in relation to hormones. *International Review of Experimental Pathology*, 23, 113–159, 1982.

206. Shirai, T., Imaida, K., Masui, T., Iwasaki, S., Mori, T., Kato, T., and Ito, N., Effects of testosterone, dihydrotestosterone and estrogen on 2′-dimethyl-4-aminobiphenyl-induced rat prostate carcinogenesis. *Int. J .Cancer*, 57, 224–228, 1994.

207. Walsh, P. C. and Wilson, J. D., The induction of prostatic hypertrophy in the dog with androstanediol. *J. Clin. Invest.*, 57, 1093–1097, 1976.

208. Ofner, P., Bosland, M. C., and Vena, R. L., Differential effects of diethylstilbestrol and estradiol-17 beta in combination with testosterone on rat prostate lobes. *Toxicology and Applied Pharmacology*, 112, 300–309, 1992.

209. Pollard, M., Snyder, D. L., and Luckert, P. H., Dihydrotestosterone does not induce prostate adenocarcinoma in L- W rats. *Prostate*, 10, 325–331, 1987.

210. Robison, A. K., Sirbasku, D. A., and Stancel, G. M., DDT supports the growth of an estrogen-responsive tumor. *Toxicol. Lett. (Amst)*, 27, 109–113, 1985.

211. Reuber, M. D., Carcinogenicity and toxicity of methoxychlor. *Environ. Health Perspect.*, 36, 205–219, 1980.

212. Reuber, M. D., The role of toxicity in the carcinogenicity of endosulfan. *Sci. Total Environ.*, 20, 23–47, 1981.

213. Reuber, M. D., Carcinogenicity of lindane. *Environmental Research*, 19, 460–481, 1979.

214. Reuber, M. D., Carcinomas of the liver in Osborne-Mendel rats ingesting DDT. *Tumori*, 64(6), 571–577, 1978.

215. Reuber, M. D., Carcinomas of the liver in Osborne-Mendel rats ingesting methoxychlor. *Life Sci.*, 24, 1367–1371, 1979.

216. Band, P. R., Le, N. D., Fang, R., Deschamps, M., Gallagher, R. P., and Yang, P., Identification of occupational cancer risks in British Columbia. A population-based case-control study of 995 incident breast cancer cases by menopausal status, controlling for confounding factors. *Journal of Occupational & Environmental Medicine*, 42, 284–310, 2000.

217. Dewailly, E., Dodin, S., Verreault, R., Ayotte, P., Sauve, L., Morin, J., and Brisson, J., High organochlorine body burden in women with estrogen receptor positive breast cancer. *J. Nat. Cancer Inst.*, 86, 232–234, 1994.

218. Krieger, N., Wolff, M. S., Hiatt, R. A., Rivera, M., Vogelman, J., and Orentreich, N., Breast cancer and serum organochlorines:a prospective study among white, black, and Asian women. *J. Nat. Cancer Inst.*, 86, 589–599, 1994.

219. Romieu, I., Hernandez-Avila, M., Lazcano-Ponce, E., Weber, J. P., and Dewailly, E., Breast cancer, lactation history, and serum organochlorines. *Am. J. Epidemiol.*, 152, 363–370, 2000.

220. Wolff, M. S., Zeleniuch-Jacquotte, A., Dubin, N., and Toniolo, P., Risk of breast cancer and organochlorine exposure. *Cancer Epidem. Biomar.*, 9, 271–277, 2004.

221. Stellman, S. D., Djordjevic, M. V., Britton, J. A., Muscat, J. E., Citron, M. L., Kementy, M., Busch, E., and Gong, L., Breast cancer risk in relation to adipose concentrations of organochlorine pesticides and polychlorinated biphenyls in Long Island, New York. *Cancer Epidem. Biomar.*, 9, 1241–1249, 2000.

222. Wolff, M. S. and Toniolo, P. G., Environmental organochlorine exposure as a potential etiologic factor in breast cancer. *Environ. Health Perspect.*, 103, 141–145, 1995.

223. Hoyer, A. P., Grandjean, P., Jorgensen, T., Brock, J. W., and Hartvig, H. B., Organochloride exposure and risk of breast cancer. *Lancet*, 352, 1816–1820, 1998.

224. Carmichael, A., Sami, A. S., and Dixon, J. M., Breast cancer risk among the survivors of atomic bomb and patriets exposed to therapeutic iosising radiation. *European Journal of Surgical Oncology*, 29, 475–479, 2003.

225. Cohn, B., Wolff, M., Cirillo, P., Sholtz, R., Christianson, R., van den Berg, B., and Siiteri, K., Timing of DDT exposure and breast cancer before age 50. Proceedings of the International Society for Environmental Epidemiology. *Epidemiology*, 13, S197, 2002.

226. Hoyer, A. P., Jorgensen, T., Brock, J. W., and Grandjean, P., Organochloride exposure and breast cancer survival. *J. Clin. Epidemiol.*, 53, 323–330, 2000.

227. Sonnenschein, C., Soto, A. M., Fernandez, M. F., Olea, N., Olea-Serrano, M. F., and Ruiz-Lopez, M. D., Development of a marker of estrogenic exposure in human serum. *Clin. Chem.*, 41, 1888–1895, 1995.

228. Pazos, P., Perez, P., Rivas, A., Nieto, R., Botella, B., Crespo, S., Olea-Serrano, F., Fernandez, M. F., Esposito, J., Olea, N., and Pedraza, V., Development of a marker of estrogen exposure in breast cancer patients. *Adv. Exp. Med. Biol.*, 444, 29–40, 1998.

229. Soto, A. M. and Sonnenschein, C., Regulation of cell proliferation: the negative control perspective. *Ann. NY Acad. Sci.*, 628, 412–418, 1991.

7 Molecular Mechanisms of Endocrine Disruption in Estrogen Dependent Processes

Robert M. Bigsby, Minerva Mercado-Feliciano, and Josephine Mubiru

CONTENTS

7.1 INTRODUCTION

Estrogens are normally produced in cyclic fashion in adult females and induce transient effects in reproductive organs, brain, and pituitary, allowing for cyclic reproductive activity. In addition, the natural pattern of estrogen secretion at puberty is responsible for changes in the body known as secondary sexual characteristics, such as hairless facial skin, breast development, and body fat distribution. Estrogens also program developmental processes resulting in permanent morphological changes such as sexually dimorphic areas of the brain or short stature in women

0-8493-2281-2/05/$0.00+$1.50
© 2005 by CRC Press

due to closure of the epiphyseal plates of long bones. Thus, estrogens or environmental mimics of estrogen can produce permanent, heritable changes in cells and tissues, either as a natural course of gender differences or as pathological manifestations of inappropriate exposure from exogenous sources. It is because of the irreversible nature of developmental effects that special attention must be paid to the actions of environmental estrogens during embryonic and fetal stages.[1]

The first description of an environmental estrogen arose from observations of sheep herds in Australia that had reduced fertility after extended grazing on pastures containing a particular clover.[2] It was found that the clover produced estrogenic effects that either temporarily or permanently reduced fertility in the ewes. Individual females from herds left on pastures containing estrogenic clover were permanently infertile; that is, they did not regain reproductive capacity when moved from the estrogenic clover-laden pasture to another that was free of the clover. Examination of the reproductive tracts of the permanently affected animals revealed altered morphogenesis of the cervix leading to a deficiency in sperm transport. Experimental evidence showed that this type of permanent morphological change could be achieved by treating ewes repeatedly with estradiol for several months.[3]

The next environmental estrogen to be recognized was a manmade compound. In the early 1960s, wildlife researchers noted a dramatic decline in the numbers of birds of prey.[4] The problem was traced to a diet of fish contaminated by the pesticide dichlorodiphenyltrichloroethane (DDT) that had entered streams, lakes, and oceans through agricultural runoff.[5,6–8] The birds had a deficiency in their oviducts that resulted in production of eggs with shells too thin to sustain the weight of the nesting adult. With the discovery that one of the congeners of DDT present in the technical mixture, o,p'-DDT, was estrogenic,[9] the estrogen-receptor interaction hypothesis was put forward to explain the altered reproductive capacity in these bird populations. However, we now know that p,p'-DDE, not o,p'-DDT, was responsible for eggshell thinning, and that the mechanism does not involve estrogen receptor but rather is the result of inhibition of prostaglandin synthesis in the eggshell gland mucosa.[10]

The seminal observations derived from animal husbandry and wildlife management became connected to human health concerns in 1971 with the appearance of a rare form of gynecologic cancer, clear cell carcinoma of the vagina, in young adult women whose mothers had been treated during pregnancy with the potent estrogen, diethylstilbestrol (DES).[11,12] Early experimental animal work, particularly that performed on rhesus monkeys, had indicated that DES posed no concern of toxicity or carcinogenicity (see Hertz, 1985).[13] With this assurance, DES was administered to pregnant women in an attempt to reduce preterm delivery. Although there was never any clinical data supporting the use of DES for this purpose, it was administered to millions of women during the period of 1948 to 1971.[14] In addition to an increased risk of developing vaginal cancer, female offspring of DES-treated mothers were at a higher risk of suffering from a dysfunctional cervix, leading to reduced fertility.[15]

Experimental work with mice has since shown that DES administered during crucial developmental periods leads to adult anomalies in the female reproductive tract, such as persistent, estrogen-independent hyperplasia of the vaginal epithelium and adenomyosis in the uterus.[16,17] Male offspring can also be affected by inappropriate exposure to estrogen during organogenesis. A clinical study showed that men who were exposed to DES *in utero* had a threefold increase in genital malformations, but there was no decrease in fertility among these individuals, with or without the malformations.[18] Although experimental evidence in mice indicates that perinatal exposure to DES increases susceptibility of males to testicular tumors, even in the "grandchildren" of the exposed mother,[19] to date, men exposed to DES *in utero* do not appear to be at a higher risk for developing cancer of any type.[20]

Epidemiological studies also link estrogens to cancers of the endometrium and breast.[21,22,23] Both types of cancer are associated with conditions of excess estrogen, such as obesity due to conversion of circulating androgens to estrogens by the aromatase enzyme present in adipose cell or estrogen treatment in post-menopausal women, but the latter relationship remains controversial.[24] The molecular mechanisms through which an estrogen can permanently transform a cell have not been definitively determined, but recent evidence reviewed below suggests several possibilities.

The experimental evidence that has accumulated over the past 3 decades indicates a role for estrogen in regulating sexually dimorphic developmental processes and carcinogenesis. During the same period, we have become increasingly aware that numerous environmental chemicals, both natural and manmade, are capable of exerting estrogenic effects. These chemicals come from a variety of sources and exhibit a variety of structures. Figure 7.1 lists some environmental chemicals known either to act as estrogens (xenoestrogens) or to disrupt endocrine processes related to estrogen action. Compounds such as ethinyl estradiol (EE2) and diethylstilbestrol were synthesized as pharmaceuticals. EE2, a component of some oral contraceptive formulations, has been found in the effluent of sewage treatment plants and thereby contaminates freshwater streams.[25,26,27] DES was used in humans as a means of preventing premature labor and has been used extensively in animal husbandry as a growth promoter.[14,28] Although banned in most of the industrialized world, organochlorines, such as the pesticides DDT and hexachlorocyclohexane (HCH) and the electronic insulating chemical polychlorinated biphenyls (PCB), persist in the environment and have accumulated in the food chain.[29] The plasticizer bisphenol A (BPA) leaches into foods from plastic-lined containers.[30] Genistein is representative of estrogenic compounds found in many plants and vegetables.[31] Dioxin is a product of combustion of waste, particularly plastics or chlorine-containing organic materials,[32] and, although it is not estrogenic itself, it impinges on estrogen action in a variety of ways (see below). We are exposed to these chemicals mainly through a dietary route, either as a natural component of foodstuffs or as contaminants in our food. Should we be concerned with the presence of these compounds in our environment? Which compounds might be harmful? Which of them might be beneficial? Answers to these questions require an understanding of the mechanisms through which these chemicals affect biochemical and cellular processes. This review focuses on the current knowledge of the molecular mechanisms of action of environmental endocrine disruptor chemicals that affect estrogenic processes.

For the most part, knowledge of the mechanisms of action of xenoestrogens follows progress in our understanding of how natural estrogens exert their effects

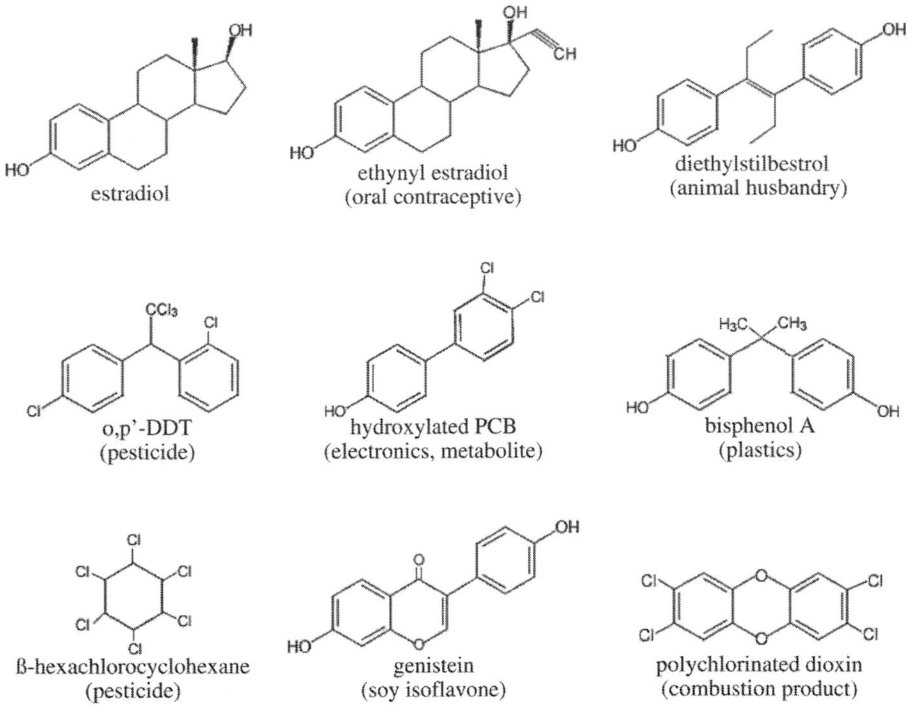

FIGURE 7.1 Structures of representative endocrine disruptor chemicals.

at the cellular and molecular levels. Since the discovery of the estrogen receptor (ER) in the late 1950s, there has been an appreciation of how this ligand-activated transcription factor functions. Research in this area has led to an understanding of mechanisms not only at the molecular level but, indeed, down to the intramolecular level. Also, mechanisms for cross-talk between growth factor stimulated pathways and nuclear estrogen receptor have been discovered, and extra-nuclear actions of estrogens and estrogen receptors have been elucidated. It appears that these newly discovered mechanisms account for hitherto unexplained rapid, nongenomic actions of estrogen. In addition to these direct cellular pathways, xenobiotics can disrupt normal estrogen physiology by altering metabolism, leading to decreased levels of the endogenous hormone. Metabolism also plays a role in transforming weak xenoestrogens into ones that are more potent. Furthermore, metabolic products of natural hormones and xenoestrogens can be mutagenic. Thus, this review covers three areas of research on xenoestrogens: genomic action through ligand activation of ER; nongenomic mechanisms of action that is either ER-dependent or ER-independent; and the role of metabolism. Throughout, we attempt to link molecular mechanisms with toxicities associated with environmental endocrine disruptor chemicals.

7.2 GENOMIC ACTION

7.2.1 TRANSCRIPTIONAL ACTIVATION BY ESTROGEN RECEPTOR

Two estrogen receptors have been identified in mammals to date, ERα and ERβ. These proteins belong to a large family of ligand-activated transcription factors. Some members of this family have no known natural ligand and are referred to as "orphan receptors." An explosive body of research over the past 30 years has led to an understanding of the mechanisms through which ligands alter the conformation of ER, thereby leading to its activation, binding to specific sites on DNA in the promoter regions of target genes, and recruiting other proteins that in turn interact with the chromatin and transcriptional machinery to enhance gene transcription. The reader is referred to excellent reviews on these topics.[33-37] The molecular and intramolecular mechanisms of ER action will be described briefly here to allow discussion of how xenoestrogens act.

Structurally, the two ERs are very similar. The receptors contain a ligand binding domain (LBD), a DNA binding domain (DBD), and two regions important to transcriptional activation, activation function-1 (AF-1) and activation function-2 (AF-2) in the N-terminal and C-terminal portions of the protein, respectively. There is a high degree of homology between the two receptors at the LBD, AF-2, and DBD, but they deviate from each other in the N-terminal regions. The receptors exist as globular proteins made of alpha helices and turns in the AF-1 and LBD/AF-2 regions and a zinc-finger structure in the DBD. Ligand activation of the receptor leads to its interaction with a specific DNA sequence, the estrogen response element (ERE), in the promoter region of target genes. It has been shown that ligand activation also leads to protein–protein interactions in the AF-2. If the ligand is an agonist the receptor recruits one of many coactivator proteins, most of which either have histone acetylase transferase (HAT) activity or will recruit other proteins with HAT activity.

If the ligand is an antagonist, the receptor recruits a corepressor protein having histone deacetylase (HDAC) activity. The LBD/AF-2 region has been crystallized and its structure determined in the presence of various ligands. The crystallography shows that the position of a particular alpha-helix, helix 12, plays a key role in determining whether coactivator protein can or cannot bind to the receptor, and the position of this helix is determined by the ligand present in the ligand binding pocket. In addition to these inter-protein interactions at the C-terminal portion of the receptor protein there also is an important, but yet to be fully defined, intramolecular interaction between AF-1 and AF-2 that enhances the transcriptional activation function of the receptor. Likewise, certain coactivator proteins are known to bind to the AF-1 region, but the precise nature of this interaction is unknown. Thus, as shown in Figure 7.2A, once activated, the estrogen receptor binds to the ERE and recruits associated proteins, and this complex in turn interacts with the chromatin and the general transcription machinery in the promoter region to enhance gene activation.

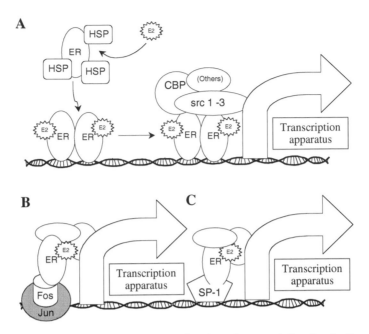

FIGURE 7.2 Models of estrogen receptor action through transcriptional activation.

Certain ER ligands, such as 4-transhydroxytamoxifen (TOT), can behave as either an antagonist, blocking gene transcription through the ERE, or as an agonist, activating transcription of genes that do not include an ERE in the promoter region. The latter effect is achieved by tethering the receptor to the promoter DNA sequences in an indirect manner. The AP-1 cis element in promoters binds the protein dimer complex, c-Jun/c-Fos (Figure 7.2B). ERα that has been activated by binding of TOT will bind to the c-Jun/c-Fos complex and thereby recruit its associated coactivator proteins to the gene promoter.[38] Similarly, E2 can activate genes containing a serum response element (SRE) in the promoter region by inducing a dimerization of ER with the transcription factor SP1[39] (see Figure 7-2C).

In addition to activation by ligand binding, estrogen receptors are also the targets of cellular kinases, which specifically phosphorylate the receptor on several serine or tyrosine sites. Growth factor-activated intracellular pathways lead to phosphorylation of receptor in the absence of estrogen ligand; this topic will be discussed in greater detail below. Estradiol-17β (E2) also has been shown to induce phosphorylation of ERα through hormone-induced tyrosine kinase and casein kinase II and other, yet-to-be-identified kinases.[35]

A fourth mode of action of ER at the genomic level has been suggested recently by studies with the environmental contaminant dioxin. Although dioxins generally exert an antiestrogenic effect through activation of the aryl hydrocarbon receptor (AhR),[40] dioxins can be associated with induction of endometriosis and estrogen-dependent tumors. The mechanism of such a stimulatory activity may be through dioxin-induced heterodimerization of the AhR and the unliganded ER, thereby recruiting the co-activator p300 to estrogen-responsive promoters.[41]

Of course, the key to setting these processes in motion is the ligand-receptor interaction. The natural hormones are bound to the receptor by fitting into a well-defined hydrophobic pocket in the globular protein. The affinity of the ligand-receptor interaction is governed by the degree of fit and the extent of the intermolecular interactions made between the ligand and the amino acid residues in the pocket.[36,37,42] The sensitivity of gene transcription driven by ER is dependent on the affinity of the ligand-receptor interaction. Accordingly, the relative binding affinity (RBA) of a putative estrogen receptor ligand is often used to predict its ability to act as a receptor agonist or antagonist. The RBAs of select compounds believed to act as environmental estrogens are listed in Table 7.1. More extensive listings of the physico-chemical characteristics and RBA of potentially estrogenic compounds have been reported.[43,56,57] It can be seen that many of these compounds, even those with proven environmental relevance, have very low RBAs. For example, the prototypical environmental estrogen, o,p′-DDT, has an RBA of as little as 0.01% for ERα, indicating that 50% saturation of ERα binding would require a concentration of o,p′-DDT 10,000-fold higher than the concentration of E2 that produces the same receptor saturation. Such a large discrepancy between the binding affinity of the natural hormone and the xenobiotic would suggest that there might be little risk associated with the compound through its estrogenic action. However, as discussed below, biological evidence suggests that such simple stoichimetric considerations may be misleading.

As predicted from their RBA, most xenoestrogens are very weak agonist of the receptors. Accordingly, most of these compounds only affect estrogen target genes if they are present in culture medium at high concentrations or if they are administered to animals at high doses. However, the route and means of administration of these chemicals suggest that pharmacokinetics plays a large role in their efficacy. For example, when administered in bolus injections, BPA induces gene expression or cell proliferation in the uterus of ovariectomized rats only at approximately 40 mg/kg body weight or higher; however, if BPA is delivered by a continuous, slow-release capsule, then it is effective at a dose that is approximately 40 µg/kg/day.[58–60] The difference between these observations may be that environmental compounds can be converted to more active compounds through metabolic hydroxylation reactions. The pesticide methoxychlor was originally designed to replace DDT in the anticipation that it would be less estrogenic. However, methoxychlor is metabolized to its mono- and di-hydroxy metabolites by liver enzymes and these compounds are 10 to 100 times more potent than the parent compound[61,62] due to a corresponding increase in RBA to ERα (see Table 7.1). Similarly, experimental work in the developing prostate has shown BPA to be much more potent than would be predicted by its RBA or by its ability to induce gene transcription *in vivo*.[63] Recent work by Yoshihara and co-workers has identified a metabolite of BPA in rodents that is at least 100 times more potent than the parent compound.[64,65]

Most xeonestrogens have been shown to work through activation of ER, either ERα or ERβ, in a manner similar to natural ligands. Xenoestogens enhance ERα binding to DNA and induce ERα-coactivator interactions.[66,67] As expected, studies have shown that xenoestrogens stimulate expression of individual estrogen-responsive genes.[54,59,60] More recent work utilizing cDNA arrays shows that xenoestrogens

TABLE 7.1
Relative Binding Affinities of Endocrine Disruptor Chemicals for ERα and ERβ

Chemical	ERα[a]	ERβ[a]	References
17β-estradiol	100	100	
Pharmaceuticals			
Ethynyl estradiol	85 – 220	2 – 24	1, 6, 14
DES	118 – 580	220 – 295	1, 3, 6, 14, 15
4-OH-tamoxifen	175 – 257	232 – 339	1, 2, 7
Tamoxifen	0.6 – 7	3 – 6	1, 2, 3, 6, 7, 15
ICI 164384	15 – 85	166	1, 2
Diphenyl alkanes (plasticizers)			
Bisphenol A	0.008 – 0.056	0.002 – 0.33	1–3, 5, 8, 15
Bisphenol B	0.086		1
Bisphenol F	0.15		5
MM6	0.25		5
Organochlorine pesticides			
4-chlorophenol	0.004		1
o,p'-DDT	0.01 – 0.4	0.02	1, 3, 6, 7
p,p'-DDT	0 – 0.09		1, 3, 7
methoxychlor	0 – 0.02	0.0005 – 0.13	1, 2, 3, 6, 7, 15
Di-OH-methoxychlor (HPTE)	0.253 – 1.7		1, 3
Mono-OH-methoxychlor	0.130		1
β-HCH	0		16, 17
Emulsifiers			
4-nonylphenol	0.01 – 0.05	0.09 – 0.11	1, 3, 6, 7, 15
4-tert-octylphenol	0.01 – 0.2	0.011 – 0.03	1, 3, 7, 15
Polychlorinated biphenyls			
3,4-BP	0		4
4'-OH-3,4-BP	0.3		4
2,5-BP	0		4
4'OH-2,5-BP	0.033 – 0.036		1, 4
4'OH-2,3,4,5-BP	0.228 – 7.2		1, 7
Phytochemicals			
Coumestrol	11 – 94	93 – 185	2, 7, 14
Genistein	0.59 – 5	2 – 87	2, 7, 14, 15
β-Zearalanol	16	14	2
Zearalenone	2.4 – 10	4.8 – 18	7, 14
Daidzein	0.1 – 0.2	0.5 – 1	7, 14, 15
Apigenin	0.19 – 0.3	0.1 – 6	7, 14, 15
Quercetin	0.01 – 0.074	0.002 – 0.124	7, 13, 15
Kaempferol	0.07 – 0.144	0.002 – 3.9	7, 13, 14; 15
Isorhamnetin	0.032	0.19	13
Naringenin	0.01	0.11 – 0.2	7, 14
Phloretin	0.2	0.01 – 0.7	7, 14
Lupinalbin A	9.3	150	14

TABLE 7.1 (CONTINUED)
Relative Binding Affinities of Endocrine Disruptor Chemicals for ERα and ERβ

Chemical	ERα[a]	ERβ[a]	References
Metals[b]			
Cobalt	29		10
Nickel	100		10
Lead	27		10
Mercury	27		10

[a] Relative binding affinity (RBA) was based on the IC50 for estradiol and the test compound in receptor binding assays and is expressed as a percentage. The sources of receptor included tissue or cell extract (ERα) or recombinant protein (ERα and ERβ) from human, mouse, and rat. [b] Estimated RBAs based on relative potency in a bioassay.

regulate expression of numerous genes that are also responsive to E2, but, interestingly, some xenoestrogens can also stimulate genes that are not E2-regulated.[68–71] This latter observation suggests that xenoestrogens not only work through ER-mediated pathways but also exert genomic effects through other, distinct molecular pathways.

Blood levels of environmental chemicals are generally very low, on the order of 0.1 to 20 ng/ml or lower,[72–75] suggesting that at most the xenoestrogen may only activate a very small fraction of the ER in a target cell. Can such scant ER activation have a significant effect on cell physiology? In an experimental system using cultured rat pituitary cells, Chun and co-workers[76] found that the extent of E2-induced gene transcription closely paralleled the predicted level of saturation of ERα but that E2-induced cell proliferation required only a very small fraction, less than 1%, of the receptors to be occupied. In an *in vivo* experimental model we have found that an o,p′-DDT blood concentration of 42 ng/ml (approximately 0.1 μM) was associated with significant increases in vaginal epithelial proliferation in the ovariectomized mouse.[77] Such results suggest that a complex cellular response, such as cell proliferation, occurs through a system of amplification that is set in motion by only very small increments in gene activation. Moreover, with the advent of gene array technology, it is now appreciated that estrogens induce a broad spectrum of genes,[68–71] and it is likely that the cellular response to the hormone is not due to the induction of one or several genes, but to the induction of a battery of genes, the products of which act in concert to produce the physiological effect.

Phyto- and mycoestrogens are naturally occurring non-steroidal plant and fungal compounds, respectively, with estrogen-like biological activity.[31,78] Phytoestrogens are loosely classified into major phenolic subgroups, that is, isoflavonoids, flavonoids, stilbenes, lignins and non-phenolic compounds, terpenoids, and saponins.[78] Phytoestrogens are structurally similar to E2 (Figure 7.1), and binding assays have shown that phytoestrogens are bound by both ERα and ERβ, but with wide-ranging binding affinities (Table 7.1). Of note is the observation that genistein has a higher

RBA for ERβ, suggesting that it may preferentially activate that form of receptor in cells that exhibit both ERα and ERβ.[35] Thus, in accordance with their ability to act as ER ligands, phytoestrogens stimulate transcription of estrogen-responsive genes[49,79,80] and proliferation of estrogen-responsive breast cancer cells in culture.[80,81] Early work pointed to an association between low prevalence of estrogen-mediated diseases, such as breast and prostate cancer, and diets rich in flavonoids, suggesting that these compounds have protective anti-estrogenic properties;[31,82] however, continued epidemiological study does not support this contention.[83]

It is worthwhile to note that some polyphenolic phytochemicals that are structurally similar to estradiol are antiestrogenic. Although largely unstudied, glyceollins have been shown to weakly inhibit estrogen-induced activity in ER-positive MCF-7 and Ishikawa cells at 10 nM to 1 μM, concentrations associated with ER agonist action of many phytoestrogens.[84] In addition, the glyceollins essentially lacked the ER agonist capacity to induce cell proliferation.[84] Furthermore, the glyceollins displayed greater affinity to, and preferential suppression of, ERα compared to ERβ. The inability of the antiestrogen ICI 182,780 to suppress this effect suggested an ER-independent mechanism.

As discussed above, ERs are members of a family of nuclear transcription factors. Some members of this family do not bind natural hormones, and their ligands, if they have any, have not been identified.[85] Three of these "orphan receptors" are referred to as estrogen-related receptors (ERRα, β, and γ). It has recently been demonstrated that the estrogenic flavones and isoflavones can bind to and thereby activate the ERRs.[86] In an experimental cell system, phytoestrogen-activated ERRs induced transcription through a consensus ERE. These observations suggest yet another way in which environmental estrogens can affect cellular physiology.

Divalent metals are another source of natural endocrine disruptor chemicals that act through the ER (see Martin et al.[51] and references therein). Exposure to metals has been linked to infertility, miscarriage, menstrual cycle disturbances, precancerous lesions of the cervix, and carcinoma of the breast. Experimental work with breast cancer cells shows that copper, cobalt, nickel, lead, mercury, tin, chromium, or vandadate induced cell proliferation and gene expression in an ER-dependent manner. Furthermore, the ability to stimulate ER-mediated effects was lost when the ligand-binding domain of the ER was mutated. The metals were able to compete with E2 for ERα binding, and radioisotopes of cobalt and nickel were found to bind to ERα with high affinity. These observations suggest that interaction with ER plays an important role in the reproductive toxicity of metal ions.

Man-made environmental contaminants that do not interact with ER may also exert antiestrogenic effects through genomic mechanisms. Dioxins and other halogenated hydrocarbons, such as PCB, activate the AhR, which in turn is recognized by the dioxin response element (DRE) in the promoter region of specific genes; this typically enhances expression of those genes involved in the response to dioxin. However, in some estrogen responsive genes there are inhibitory DREs (iDRE) that mediate a suppressive effect on gene transcription.[40] In addition, dioxins induce proteasomal degradation of the ER through an undefined mechanism.[87] Both of these mechanisms are likely to be involved in the reduction of estrogen-induced gene expression and cell proliferation in breast cancer cells by dioxins and PCB.[88–92]

7.2.2 CHANGES IN GENE EXPRESSION ASSOCIATED WITH DES EXPOSURE

The inadvertent but tragic experiment represented by the DES story served as a warning that environmental estrogens can have long-lasting effects. The mouse has proven to be an important research model for studying the mechanisms through which DES exerts these effects. Recent evidence from the mouse has led to an understanding of the role of homeobox genes in development and physiology of the female reproductive tract. Homeobox genes produce transcription factors that are involved in developmental regulation of tissue patterning in organ systems. It was found that several homeobox genes are expressed in the female reproductive tract in specific spatial and temporal patterns that are associated with key developmental, morphogenetic events.[93] Many of the defects seen in the reproductive tract of adult mice that had been treated with DES perinatally are also present in animals in which the hoxa-10 and hoxa-11 genes have been mutated.[94,95] Indeed, maternal DES treatment results in a disrupted spatial patterning of hox gene expression in the reproductive tracts of female offspring.[96] The role of ERα in these effects was demonstrated by the lack of altered gene expression or tissue morphogenesis in ERαKO offspring.[97] It has not been determined whether the hox genes in the reproductive tissues were permanently altered by estrogen or whether altered expression of these genes at a critical point in development led to permanently altered tissue differentiation.

The Wnt genes produce another family of proteins that are involved in developmental regulation of tissue growth and differentiation. Wnt proteins are secreted factors that play a role in tissue-tissue interactions important to organogenesis. Expression of Wnt4, Wnt5a, and Wnt7a is hormonally regulated in the uterus.[98] Mutation of Wnt7a leads to many of the malformations displayed in the female reproductive tract of the DES-treated animal,[99] and exposure to DES leads to a transient decrease in Wnt7a expression during a critical period of postnatal development of the lower reproductive tract in mice.[98] It may be that once the tissue differentiation has been determined in the absence of the normal amount of Wnt7a, the altered morphogenesis becomes permanent.

7.2.3 EPIGENETIC EFFECTS

Can DES or other estrogens induce a permanent change in a gene or genes thereby affecting tissue differentiation and function? It is well established that CpG island methylation is one mechanism through which genes are permanently regulated during tissue differentiation in development. Generally, genes with a high degree of cytosine methylation in the promoter region are silenced, while hypomethylation may lead to constitutive gene expression.[100] Li and coworkers found that perinatal treatment of mice induced a constitutive expression of the normally estrogen-regulated gene lactoferrin and that this was associated with a decrease in CpG island methylation in the promoter region of that gene.[101] On the other hand, perinatal DES treatment results in suppressed hoxa-10 expression in the female reproductive tract of mice, but this does not involve altered methylation of the gene promoter sequence.[102] It may be that genes regulating hoxa-10 were permanently silenced.

Gene activity can also be altered through mutation. Metabolic pathways that act on E2, DES, or other xenoestrogens are known to produce reactive intermediate metabolites that can form DNA adducts.[103–106] This topic will be discussed in further detail in Section 7.4.

7.3 INTRACELLULAR SIGNALING MECHANISMS

Several observations suggest that E2 and some environmental estrogens act through mechanisms that either do not involve the ER or act on the receptor indirectly. Kepone, E2, and 4-OH-E2 induced gene expression in ERαKO mouse uterus, and this effect was not blocked by the antiestrogen ICI182,780, suggesting the presence of a distinct estrogen signaling pathway doesn't rely on ER.[107,108] Crude preparations of the pesticide/pediculicide lindane contain the beta-isomer of hexachlorocyclohexane (β-HCH). Although ERα doesn't bind β-HCH, it induces transcription of estrogen-responsive genes in culture systems,[54] and this effect requires the presence of estrogen receptor.[109] Vaginal and uterine epithelia of ovariectomized mice are stimulated by β-HCH at blood concentrations that are relevant to human exposure levels.[77] These effects may be mediated by cellular mechanisms working through growth factor signaling pathways.

Actions of phytoestrogen may also involve pathways other than the classical ER-mediated events. Dose-response studies of phytoestrogen activity in cell culture systems often show a biphasic effect; i.e., the compounds are stimulatory at low concentrations but are inhibitory at high concentrations. Generally, phytoestrogens at concentrations 10 μM or greater cause cell death,[80] but antiestrogenic effects can be achieved through high concentratinons without inducing cytotoxicity.[110] Evidently, phytoestrogen-induced cell cytotoxicity was not mediated through direct antagonism of ER since the cytotoxic effect could not be reversed by addition of E2, and it also occurred in ER-negative HeLa cells.[80] Quercetin and resveratrol were shown to inhibit proliferation of Ishikawa cells, an endometrial cancer cell line, through suppression of EGF expression, but it was not determined whether this effect was mediated by the ER.[111,112]

It was suggested nearly 30 years ago that estrogen acted not only at the nuclear receptor level but also through a membrane-bound receptor to induce rapid intracellular changes in second messenger molecules such as Ca^{2+} and cAMP.[113,114] More recently, several potential molecular mechanisms have been described for estrogen action at the membrane or through pathways involving growth factor receptors (see reviews).[115–118] These pathways are depicted in Figure 7.3. Accordingly, estrogens have been shown to interact directly with G-protein coupled receptors (GPCR) to stimulate activation of membrane-associated proteases, such as matrix metalloprotease, that cause release of membrane-bound growth factor peptides, which in turn activate members of the erbB family of growth factor receptors. Activation of the GPCR also has the effect of increasing adenylate cyclase activity, increasing cAMP, and activating protein kinase A (PKA). Alternatively, estrogen may interact directly with erbB proteins, thereby activating the intracellular signaling mechanisms. Other research has shown that ligand activated ERα can interact with non-receptor tyrosine kinase, c-Src, to stimulate changes in cell shape and motility. The mitogen-activated

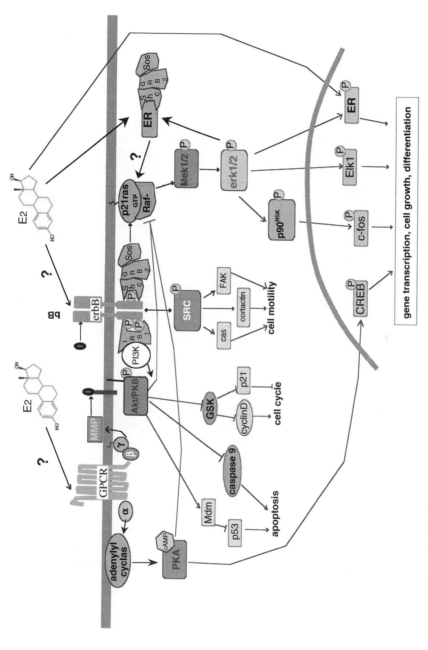

FIGURE 7.3 Intracellular molecular signaling pathways affected by estrogens.

protein kinases (MAPK) ERK-1 and ERK-2 can phosphorylate ERα, thereby enhancing its transactivation function. Phosphorylated ERα also interacts with the intermediary protein, Shc, allowing it to form a complex with Grb-2 and Sos; this complex may bind and activate the Ras/Raf complex. Each of these pathways leads to physiological changes within the cell and to transcriptional activation through activation of ER and other transcription factors such as Elk1, AP-1 (Jun/Fos), and CREB. These pathways are known to impinge on cellular proliferation, apoptosis, and differentiation.

Although these intracellular pathways may explain some actions of environmental estrogens, to date, only a few studies have explored this possibility. The estrogen-like activity of β-HCH and o,p'-DDT has been ascribed to a direct activation of an erbB protein, thereby activating the mechanisms leading to phosphorylation of MAPK.[119–121] Likewise, Burow and coworkers have shown that estrogenic flavonoids and DDT can activate MAPK, either ERK-1/-2 or p38, and thereby induce estrogen-like activity.[122,123] The antiestrogenic action of flavonoids and isoflavanoids may be related to their ability to inhibit tyrosine kinases[124] or phosphoinositide-3 kinase.[125]

7.4 METABOLIC MECHANISMS

Aside from conversion of a proestrogenic compound to an estrogenic metabolite, as discussed above, metabolic pathways may be involved in endocrine disruption by altering hormone synthesis or metabolic clearance of endogenous hormone, or through production of reactive metabolic intermediates from endogenous estrogens or xenoestrogens.

7.4.1 ESTROGEN SYNTHESIS

The biosynthetic pathways leading to production of estrogens are well documented (Figure 7.4). In the ovaries, granulosa cells synthesize estrogens from androgens secreted by surrounding thecal cells. The testes mostly secrete androgens, but the Leydig cells also convert some of the androgen to estrogen. In peripheral tissues, such as fat cells and the mammary epithelial cells, estrogens are synthesized from circulating androgens that originate from gonadal or adrenal secretions. Thus, two key enzymes in estrogen biosynthesis are 17alpha-hydroxylase/17,20-lyase (CYP17), which converts pregnanes to androgens, and aromatase (CYP19arom), which aromatizes androgens to estrogens. Substances that inhibit these enzymes reduce estrogen levels, either in circulation or at local tissue levels.

Xenobiotic interference with steroid synthesis has received increasing attention. A single dose of 2,3,7,8-tetrachlorodibenzo-p-dioxin (TCDD) induced abortion in laboratory macaques, and this was accompanied by a decrease in serum estradiol (E2) concentration.[126] This observation suggested that perhaps TCDD inhibited CYP19arom. Drenth and coworkers[127] found that TCDD and other organochlorine mixtures decreased aromatase activity in cultured human choriocarcinoma cells, but later research showed that this was most likely associated with cellular toxicity rather

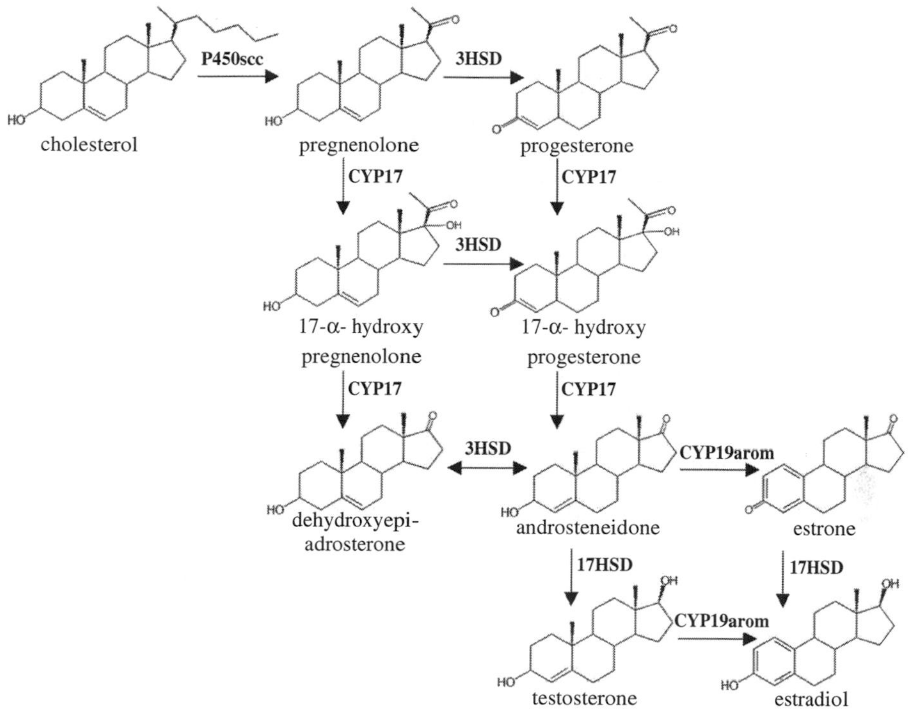

FIGURE 7.4 Estrogen synthetic pathways. P450scc = cholesterol side chain cleavage complex; 3HSD = 3β-hydroxysteroid dehydrogenase; CYP17 = 17α-hydroxylase/17,20-lyase; CYP19arom = aromatase; 17HSD = 17α-hydroxysteroid dehydrogenase.

than direct inhibition of the enzyme.[128] Using a cell line that is apparently less sensitive to the cytotoxic effects of TCDD, it was shown that TCDD-induced inhibition of estrogen secretion was due to decreased expression of CYP17.[129] BPA can also inhibit steroidogenesis *in vivo*. In studies on rats, BPA inhibited testicular secretion of testosterone and E2 due to inhibition of both CYP17 and CYP19arom expression.[130] It is also interesting to note that the effect of BPA on testicular steroidogenesis exhibited a U-shaped dose response curve, both *in vivo* and *in vitro*.[129] Serum testosterone levels were decreased by BPA at a dose of 2.4 μg/kg body weight, and testosterone secretion by isolated Leydig cells was inhibited by 0.01 nM BPA; increasing the dose tenfold in either experiment removed the inhibitory effect. This is in contrast to continued inhibition of testosterone synthesis across all doses of the potent estrogen, DES.

Flavonoids, isoflavonoids, and lignans inhibit aromatase activity.[131–136] The degree of hydroxylation and the positions of the hydroxyl groups in these molecules govern their potency to competitively bind and inhibit aromatase.[131,134] Furthermore, the aromatase inhibitory activity is not related to the estrogenic character of the compound.[131,134,136]

7.4.2 Metabolic Clearance

7.4.2.1 Catechol Estrogens and Reactive Metabolites

Endogenous estrogens and xenobiotics are cleared from the blood by two enzymatic detoxification pathways: Phase I enzymes, belonging to the CYP450 family of enzymes, modify the substrate through hydroxylation. Phase II enzymes conjugate the substrate to sulfate, glucuronide, glutathione, or methyl moieties. The reader is referred to recent excellent reviews on the subjects of these pathways.[137,138] The pathways and the points at which endocrine disruptor chemicals may be effective are described in Figure 7.5.

Estrogen hydroxylation to catecholestrogens is catalyzed by several CYP450 isoenzymes.[139] While the main pathway in liver is 2-hydroxylation, 4-hydroxylation is common in other organs. In human liver, hydroxylation at the 2-position is mostly catalyzed by CYP1A2 and the CYP3A family, while the inducible CYP1A1 is responsible for most extrahepatic 2-hydroxylation. CYP1B1 is responsible for most 4-hydroxylation, although CYP1A2 also has a high catalytic activity toward 4-hydroxylation.

Catecholestrogens are themselves signaling molecules that may play a role in normal physiological processes such as blastocyst implantation[140] or regulation of catecholamine homeostasis.[141,142] Hydroxylated estrogens can be further oxidized to yield reactive quinones capable of forming direct adducts with purines in DNA or

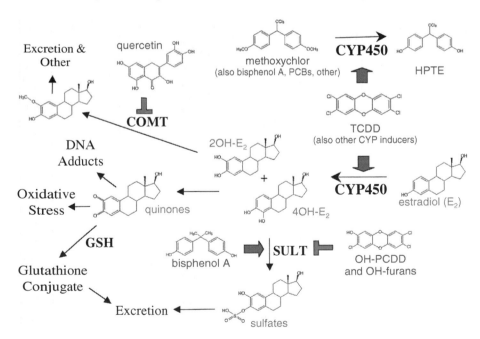

FIGURE 7.5 Metabolism of estrogens and endocrine disruptors. COMT = catechol-O-methyltransferase; SULT = sulfotransferase.

undergo redox cycling and thus produce oxidative stress.[143,144] Although both the 4-hydroxy and 2-hydroxy forms of catechol E2 (4-OHE2 and 2-OHE2, respectively) are capable of redox cycling through their quinonne intermediates, the evidence strongly suggests that it is the former that is involved in carcinogenesis. A high 4-OHE2 to 2-OHE2 concentration ratio is common in human breast cancer,[145] and 4-OHE2, but not 2-OHE2, was shown to be carcinogenic in the kidney of the Syrian golden hamster.[143,144] Furthermore, 2-OHE2 may be anticarcinogenic. There is an inverse relationship between cancer risk, and 2-hydroxylation activity in patients and induction of 2-hydroxylation by indole-3-carbinol, a component of cruciferous vegetables (e.g., broccoli, cabbage, cauliflower, and Brussels sprouts), is protective.[146]

Estrogens, their catechols, or the quinone intermediates are inactivated or detoxified by the phase II, conjugating enzymes.[137] The parent steroid or their catechols can be conjugated to glucuronide or sulfate moieties by UDP-glucuronyl transferase or sulfotransferases; the catechol estrogens can also be methylated by catechol-O-methyl transferase; the quinone intermediates can be conjugated to glutathione by glutathione-S-transferases. Each of these enzymatic steps can display large variations among individuals, thereby at least partially accounting for individual variation in susceptibility to hormone-induced carcinogenesis.[147,148]

Endocrine disruptor compounds are subject to the same metabolic clearance pathways, including production of similar intermediates. The hydroxylation of exogenous estrogens like DES and hexestrol can also lead to adduct formation *in vitro* and *in vivo* and cancer initiation in experimental mammals.[104,149–151] Metabolism of BPA may also lead to production of reactive quinones.[152,153] Final clearance of xenobiotics occurs mainly through glucuronide and sulfate conjugation.[154–156]

7.4.2.2 CYP450 and the Aryl Hydrocarbon Receptor Pathway

Induction of CYP450 isozyme expression by environmental compounds is believed to play a role in their endocrine disruptive activity through altered metabolic clearance of hormone. Environmental chemicals can induce expression of CYP450 isozymes through the aryl hydrocarbon receptor, a transcription factor that is activated by xenobiotics. TCDD is a particularly strong ligand for AhR but the receptor is activated by numerous halogenated and non-halogenated aryl hydrocarbons and phytochemicals.[157] Activated AhR binds to a specific response element known as the XRE (for xenobiotic response element) or DRE (for dioxin response element). TCDD-activated AhR enhances expression of CYP1A1 and CYP1B1 in several tissues including liver, breast cancer cells, placenta, and normal fibroblasts, and the relative responses of these two isozymes is tissue and species dependent.[158–164]

Treatment with AhR ligands is likely to reduce the levels of active hormone in blood, but it also is likely to increase the availability of reactive intermediates and therefore increase DNA adduct formation. Thus, TCDD treatment increases oxidative damage differentially in intact versus ovarectomized rats, with a higher incidence of 8-oxo-deoxyguanosine found in livers of intact animals versus ovariectomized animals, suggesting a role for increased oxidative stress due to production of reactive intermediates from endogenous estrogens.[165,166]

Herbs and foods contain a variety of AhR-binding phytochemicals that may have different activities regarding CYP450 modulation, and the natural mixtures may be agonists or antagonists of AhR-dependent effects, depending on the concentration of total mixture.[167,168] The acidic condensation products of indole-3-carbinol formed in the stomach environment have a high affinity for AhR and are potent inducers of AhR-mediated gene expression.[161,169] Extracts containing a mixture of phytochemicals from several types of herbs, such as ginseng, licorice, ginkgo biloba, and black cohosh, activated AhR.[167,170] The stilbene resverastrol, found in mulberries, peanuts, grapes, red wines, and other foods, binds AhR and inhibits TCDD-induced increases in CYP1A mRNA and enzyme activity.[171,172] Several flavones and flavonols prevent CYP1A induction at lower concentrations, but are inducers at higher concentrations.[173] In addition to these AhR-mediated effects, natural phytochemical mixtures generally contain some form of phytoestrogens that are also responsible for ER-mediated effects.

7.4.2.3   PXR and CAR Regulated CYP450

Although the CYP3A isozymes have a lesser activity for estrogen hydroxylation than the CYP1A family, they constitute about 30% of the un-induced human liver CYP450[174] and therefore may account for a large portion of liver estrogen metabolism, especially when induced. Both CYP3A4 and CYP3A5 act mainly through the 2-hydroxylation pathway for estrogens.[174,175] The CYP3A family is also responsible for the metabolism of and interactions between many pharmaceuticals and phytochemicals.

Induction of CYP3A4 is mediated by at least three different nuclear receptors: constitutive androstane receptor (CAR), pregnane X receptor (PXR), and vitamin D receptor (VDR). These three receptors belong to the subfamily of nuclear receptors, which heterodimerize with the retinoid X receptor (RXR) (see reviews).[176–178] The activity of PXR and CAR is regulated by the glucocorticoid receptor, and dexamethasone is known to induce CYP3A4 activity and potentiate induction when coadministered with PXR agonists.[179–181] The activity of VDR is associated mostly with bone, intestinal, and liver tissue and may play a role in the induction of estrogen metabolism only in the liver.[182,183]

The human PXR is strongly activated by the anti-tuberculosis drug rifampicin and phenobarbital, known inducers of CYP3A4.[184,185] Many other important pharmaceutical inducers of CYP3A4 are also PXR ligands,[184] including pregnanes, glucocorticoids, topiramate,[186] statins,[187,188] troglitazone,[189] cyclophosphamide,[179,190] and paclitaxel.[191]

The known endocrine disruptors, phthalic acid and nonylphenol, were shown to activate PXR and thereby induce expression of CYP3A1.[192] The organochlorine pesticides, dieldrin and chlordane, also induced CYP3A4 expression through PXR.[193] Although not effective in mouse, BPA was able to induce CYP3A4 gene expression through PXR in a human cell model system.[194]

While PXR is a ligand-activated receptor localized in the nucleus even when inactive, CAR is constitutively active and sequestered in the cytoplasm, translocating to the nucleus only after treatment with xenobiotics like phenobarbital or

1,4-bis[2-(3,5- dichloropyridyloxy)]benzene (TCPOBOP) and chlorpromazine. Interestingly, the xenobiotic-dependent translocation of CAR to the nucleus may not require binding of the chemical by the receptor protein. CAR, PXR, and VDR have similar DNA-binding motifs and can activate each other's target genes.[195,196]

In clinical studies, ritonavir, the antiepileptic drugs topiramate and carbamezapine, and the herb St. John's wort (*Hypericum perforatum*) were shown to cause a dose-dependent increase in the clearance of ethinyl estradiol.[193,194,197,198] In the case of topiramate, while one study found significant increases in clearance of ethinyl estradiol in women taking the drug every 12 hours;[193] another study found a non-significant increase in women taking topiramate once a day.[197] St. John's wort is known to induce CYP3A4.[199] Hyperforin is the main chemical constituent in St. John's wort that binds PXR and induces CYP3A4 in primary human hepatocytes.[192]

7.4.2.4   Conjugating Enzymes

While the action of endogenous estrogens is terminated primarily by hydroxylation, the resulting catechol estrogens (as well as the parent compounds) can be further methylated or conjugated with the hydrophilic groups glucuronide and sulfate (see review).[184] The estrogen sulfotransferases are enzymes that add a sulfate group to estrogens, thus deactivating the original molecule. Xenoestrogens and many poly-halogenated aromatic hydrocarbons are also metabolized by estrogen sulfotransferases. Of the three forms of sulfotransferases, estrogen sulfotransferase (SULT1E1) shows the greatest capacity to sulfate xenoestrogens such as DES, BPA, and non-ylphenol.[200,201]

In addition to their function in estrogen clearance, sulfotransferases can regulate tissue-specific estrogen levels (see reviews).[138] A large proportion of estrone synthesized by aromatase is converted to estrone sulfate, and hydrolysis of the sulfate back to estrone by the sulfotransferases is thought to make a major contribution to the production of active estrogen within breast tumor tissues.[202,203] Therefore, changes in sulfotransferase activity can alter both systemic deactivation of estrogen and tissue-specific estrogen homeostasis.

A few xenobiotics are known to affect sulfotransferase activity. BPA induces expression of estrogen sulfotransferase isoform 3 in rat.[71] On the other hand, hydrox-ylated metabolites of polyhalogenated aromatic hydrocarbons (PCB, polybrominated diphenyl ethers, and chlorinated BPA) can be potent inhibitors of SULT1E1.[204] Monohydroxylated dioxins and furans can inhibit the recombinant enzyme at nano-molar concentrations.[204] Sulfotransferase are also inhibited by estrogenic akylphe-nols.[205] Such observations suggest another mechanism through which xenobiotics disrupt hormonal status, either at the local tissue level or systemically.

Catechol-O-methyl transferase (COMT) catalyzes the conversion of the 2-OHE2 (or 2-OHE1) to a 2-methoxy estrogen.[137] Like other conjugation steps, this serves to facilitate clearance of the hormone from the blood and it also detoxifies the catechol estrogen, removing it from the redox cycling pathway that leads to oxidative stress. The flavonoid quercetin inhibits COMT, and it may be this effect that is responsible for the enhanced tumorigenic effect of E2 in the golden hamster kidney.[206]

7.5 SUMMARY

Environmental chemicals can affect developmental, physiological, and pathological processes that are dependent upon, or sensitive to, estrogens. The most extensively studied mechanism of endocrine disruptor activity is the interaction of these compounds with the ER as a ligand-activated transcription factor. As with the endogenous estrogens, environmental estrogens stimulate or repress numerous estrogen responsive genes, and most notably, they alter developmental expression of critical genes involved in tissue differentiation. Recent evidence suggests that both endogenous estrogens and xenoestrogens can also act through intracellular pathways that utilize growth factor receptor proteins and their intermediate signaling molecules. These intracellular pathways may intersect with ER either in its classical mode of action as a transcription factor or in a membrane-associated form, as a member of protein complexes that modulate activity of intracellular signaling molecules. Environmental compounds are also capable of affecting endogenous concentrations of estrogen, either in circulation or at the local tissue level by altering steroid synthetic or catabolic pathways. Metabolic products of these endocrine disruptor chemicals can also take part in mechanisms of oxidative stress. Thus, endocrine disruptor chemicals can act at the cellular and organismal level through several interrelated mechanisms. The results of these endocrine disruptor activities are often insidious, requiring years or generations to manifest themselves. Identification of the most sensitive of the mechanisms involved in perturbation of normal development or function will allow a relevant evaluation of risks imposed by current exposure levels.

REFERENCES

1. Bigsby, R., Chapin, R.E., Daston, G.P., et al., Evaluating the effects of endocrine disruptors on endocrine function during development, *Environ. Health Perspect.*, 107, 613, 1999.
2. Adams, N.R., Permanent infertility in ewes exposed to plant oestrogens, *Aust. Vet. J.*, 67, 197, 1990.
3. Adams, N.R., and Sanders, M.R., Persistent infertility in ewes after prolonged exposure to oestradiol-17 beta, *J. Reprod. Fertil.*, 84, 373, 1988.
4. 'Hickey, J.J., *The Perigrine Falcon Populations: Their Biology and Decline*, University of Wisconsin Press, Madison, WI, 1969.
5. Wurster, C.F.J., and Wingate, D.B., DDT residues and declining reproduction in the Bermuda petrel, *Science*, 159, 979, 1968.
6. Robinson, J., Residues of organochlorine insecticides in dead birds in the United Kingdom, *Chem. Ind.*, 47, 1974, 1967.
7. Risebrough, R.W., Menzel, D.B., Martin, D.J.J., et al., DDT residues in Pacific sea birds: a persistent insecticide in marine food chains, *Nature*, 216, 589, 1967.
8. Ratcliffe, D.A., Decrease in eggshell weight in certain birds of prey, *Nature*, 215, 208, 1967.
9. Bitman, J., Cecil, H.C., Harris, S.J., et al., Estrogenic activity of o,p′-DDT in the mammalian uterus and avian oviduct, *Science*, 162, 371, 1968.

10. Lundholm, C.D., DDE-induced eggshell thinning in birds: effects of p,p'-DDE on the calcium and prostaglandin metabolism of the eggshell gland, *Comp. Biochem. Physiol. C Pharmacol. Toxicol. Endocrinol.*, 118, 113, 1997.

11. Herbst, A.L., Ulfelder, H., and Poskanzer, D.C., Adenocarcinoma of the vagina. Association of maternal stilbestrol therapy with tumor appearance in young women, *N. Engl. J. Med.*, 284, 878, 1971.

12. Melnick, S., Cole, P., Anderson, D., et al., Rates and risks of diethylstilbestrol-related clear-cell adenocarcinoma of the vagina and cervix, *N. Engl. J. Med.*, 316, 514, 1987.

13. Hertz, R., The estogen problem: Retrospect and prospect, in: *Estrogen in the Environment II*, McLachlan, J.A., Ed., Elsevier, New York, 1985, 1.

14. Shapiro, S., and Slone, D., The effects of exogenous female hormones on the fetus, *Epidemiol. Rev.*, 1, 110, 1979.

15. Kaufman, R.H., Adam, E., Binder, G.L., et al., Upper genital tract changes and pregnancy outcome in offspring exposed *in utero* to diethylstilbestrol, *Am. J. Obstet. Gynecol.*, 137, 299, 1980.

16. Newbold, R.R., Bullock, B.C., and McLachlan, J.A., Uterine adencarcinoma in mice following developmental treatment with estrogens: a model for hormonal carcinogenesis, *Cancer Res.*, 50, 7677, 1990.

17. Newbold, R.R., Banks, E.P., Bullock, B., et al., Uterine adenocarcinoma in mice treated neonatally with genistein, *Cancer Res.*, 61, 4325, 2001.

18. Wilcox, A.J., Baird, D.D., Weinberg, C.R., et al., Fertility in men exposed prenatally to diethylstilbestrol, *N. Engl. J. Med.*, 332, 1411, 1995.

19. Newbold, R.R., Hanson, R.B., Jefferson, W.N., et al., Proliferative lesions and reproductive tract tumors in male descendants of mice exposed developmentally to diethylstilbestrol, *Carcinogenesis*, 21, 1355, 2000.

20. Strohsnitter, W.C., Noller, K.L., Hoover, R.N., et al., Cancer risk in men exposed *in utero* to diethylstilbestrol, *J. Natl. Cancer Inst.*, 93, 545, 2001.

21. Hulka, B.S., Liu, E.T., and Lininger, R.A., Steroid hormones and risk of breast cancer, *Cancer*, 74, 1111, 1994.

22. Kuller, L.H., The etiology of breast cancer—from epidemiology to prevention, *Public Health Rev.*, 23, 157, 1995.

23. Persson, I., Estrogens in the causation of breast, endometrial and ovarian cancers — evidence and hypotheses from epidemiological findings, *J. Steroid Biochem. Mol. Biol.*, 74, 357, 2000.

24. Eden, J., Progestins and breast cancer, *Am. J. Obstet. Gynecol.*, 188, 1123, 2003.

25. Williams, R.J., Johnson, A.C., Smith, J.J., et al., Steroid estrogens profiles along river stretches arising from sewage treatment works discharges, *Environ. Sci. Technol.*, 37, 1744, 2003.

26. Sumpter, J.P., Xenoendorine disrupters—environmental impacts, *Toxicol. Lett.*, 102–103, 337, 1998.

27. Aherne, G.W., and Briggs, R., The relevance of the presence of certain synthetic steroids in the aquatic environment, *J. Pharm. Pharmacol.*, 41, 735, 1989.

28. McMartin, K.E., Kennedy, K.A., Greenspan, P., et al., Diethylstilbestrol: a review of its toxicity and use as a growth promotant in food-producing animals, *J. Environ. Pathol. Toxicol.*, 1, 279, 1978.

29. Clarkson, T.W., Environmental contaminants in the food chain, *Am. J. Clin. Nutr.*, 61, 682S, 1995.

30. Soto, A. M., Sonnenschein, C., Murray, M. K., et al., Estrogenic plasticizers and antioxidants. In: *Hormonally active agents in food*, Eisenbrand, G., Ed., Wiley-Vch, Weinheim, Germany, 1998, 128.

31. Kurzer, M.S., and Xu, X., Dietary phytoestrogens, *Annu. Rev. Nutr.*, 17, 353, 1997.
32. U.S.E.P.A., Draft Exposure and Human Health Reassessment of 2,3,7,8-Tetrachlorodibenzo-p-Dioxin (TCDD) and Related Compounds. Volume 2: Sources of Dioxin-like Compounds in the United States, *http://cfpub.epa.gov/ncea/cfm/part1and2.cfm? ActType=default*, 2000.
33. McKenna, N.J., Lanz, R.B., and O'Malley, B.W., Nuclear receptor coregulators: cellular and molecular biology, *Endocr. Rev.*, 20, 321, 1999.
34. Katzenellenbogen, B.S., and Katzenellenbogen, J.A., Estrogen receptor transcription and transactivation: Estrogen receptor alpha and estrogen receptor beta: regulation by selective estrogen receptor modulators and importance in breast cancer, *Breast Cancer Res.*, 2, 335, 2000.
35. Nilsson, S., Makela, S., Treuter, E., et al., Mechanisms of estrogen action, *Physiol. Rev.*, 81, 1535, 2001.
36. Shiau, A.K., Barstad, D., Loria, P.M., et al., The structural basis of estrogen receptor/coactivator recognition and the antagonism of this interaction by tamoxifen, *Cell*, 95, 927, 1998.
37. Shiau, A.K., Barstad, D., Radek, J.T., et al., Structural characterization of a subtype-selective ligand reveals a novel mode of estrogen receptor antagonism, *Nat. Struct. Biol.*, 9, 359, 2002.
38. Kushner, P.J., Agard, D.A., Greene, G.L., et al., Estrogen receptor pathways to AP-1, *J. Steroid Biochem. Mol. Biol.*, 74, 311, 2000.
39. Safe, S., Transcriptional activation of genes by 17 beta-estradiol through estrogen receptor-Sp1 interactions, *Vitam. Horm.*, 62, 231, 2001.
40. Safe, S., and McDougal, A., Mechanism of action and development of selective aryl hydrocarbon receptor modulators for treatment of hormone-dependent cancers, *Int. J. Oncol.*, 20, 1123, 2002.
41. Ohtake, F., Takeyama, K., Matsumoto, T., et al., Modulation of oestrogen receptor signalling by association with the activated dioxin receptor, *Nature*, 423, 545, 2003.
42. Anstead, G.M., Carlson, K.E., and Katzenellenbogen, J.A., The estradiol pharmacophore: ligand structure-estrogen receptor binding affinity relationships and a model for the receptor binding site, *Steroids*, 62, 268, 1997.
43. Blair, R.M., Fang, H., Branham, W.S., et al., The estrogen receptor relative binding affinities of 188 natural and xenochemicals: structural diversity of ligands, *Toxicol. Sci.*, 54, 138, 2000.
44. Kuiper, G.G., Carlsson, B., Grandien, K., et al., Comparison of the ligand binding specificity and transcript tissue distribution of estrogen receptors alpha and beta, *Endocrinology*, 138, 863, 1997.
45. Bolger, R., Wiese, T.E., Ervin, K., et al., Rapid screening of environmental chemicals for estrogen receptor binding capacity, *Environ. Health Perspect.*, 106, 551, 1998.
46. Vakharia, D.D., and Gierthy, J.F., Use of a combined human liver microsome-estrogen receptor binding assay to assess potential estrogen modulating activity of PCB metabolites, *Toxicol. Lett.*, 114, 55, 2000.
47. Perez, P., Pulgar, R., Olea-Serrano, F., et al., The estrogenicity of bisphenol A-related diphenylalkanes with various substituents at the central carbon and the hydroxy groups, *Environ. Health Perspect.*, 106, 167, 1998.
48. Andersen, H.R., Andersson, A.M., Arnold, S.F., et al., Comparison of short-term estrogenicity tests for identification of hormone-disrupting chemicals, *Environ. Health Perspect.*, 107 Suppl. 1, 89, 1999.
49. Kuiper, G.G., Lemmen, J.G., Carlsson, B., et al., Interaction of estrogenic chemicals and phytoestrogens with estrogen receptor beta, *Endocrinology*, 139, 4252, 1998.

50. Kim, H.S., Han, S.Y., Yoo, S.D., et al., Potential estrogenic effects of bisphenol-A estimated by *in vitro* and *in vivo* combination assays, *J. Toxicol. Sci.*, 26, 111, 2001.

51. Martin, M.B., Reiter, R., Pham, T., et al., Estrogen-like activity of metals in MCF-7 breast cancer cells, *Endocrinology*, 144, 2425, 2003.

52. Oh, S.M., and Chung, K.H., Estrogenic activities of Ginkgo biloba extracts, *Life Sci.*, 74, 1325, 2004.

53. Harris, H.A., Bapat, A.R., Gonder, D.S., et al., The ligand binding profiles of estrogen receptors alpha and beta are species dependent, *Steroids*, 67, 379, 2002.

54. Steinmetz, R., Young, P.C., Caperell-Grant, A., et al., Novel estrogenic action of the pesticide residue beta-hexachlorocyclohexane in human breast cancer cells, *Cancer Res.*, 56, 5403, 1996.

55. Coosen, R., and van Velsen, F.L., Effects of the β-isomer of hexachlorocyclohexane on estrogen-sensitive human mammary tumor cells, *Toxicol. Appl. Pharmacol.*, 101, 310, 1989.

56. Fang, H., Tong, W., Shi, L.M., et al., Structure-activity relationships for a large diverse set of natural, synthetic, and environmental estrogens, *Chem. Res. Toxicol.*, 14, 280, 2001.

57. Shi, L.M., Fang, H., Tong, W., et al., QSAR models using a large diverse set of estrogens, *J. Chem. Inf. Comput. Sci.*, 41, 186, 2001.

58. Steinmetz, R., Brown, N.G., Allen, D.L., et al., The environmental estrogen bisphenol A stimulates prolactin release *in vitro* and *in vivo*, *Endocrinology*, 138, 1780, 1997.

59. Steinmetz, R., Mitchner, N.A., Grant, A., et al., The xenoestrogen bisphenol A induces growth, differentiation, and c-fos gene expression in the female reproductive tract, *Endocrinology*, 139, 2741, 1998.

60. Long, X., Burke, K.A., Bigsby, R.M., et al., Effects of the xenoestrogen bisphenol A on expression of vascular endothelial growth factor (VEGF) in the rat, *Exp. Biol. Med. (Maywood)*, 226, 477, 2001.

61. Kupfer, D., and Bulger, W.H., Metabolic activation of pesticides with proestrogenic activity, *Fed. Proc.*, 46, 1864, 1987.

62. Bulger, W.H., Feil, V.J., and Kupfer, D., Role of hepatic monoxygenases in generation estrogenic metabolites from methoxychlor and from its identified contaminants, *Mol. Pharmacol.*, 27, 115, 1985.

63. Welshons, W.V., Nagel, S.C., Thayer, K.A., et al., Low-dose bioactivity of xenoestrogens in animals: fetal exposure to low doses of methoxychlor and other xenoestrogens increases adult prostate size in mice, *Toxicol. Ind. Health*, 15, 12, 1999.

64. Yoshihara, S., Makishima, M., Suzuki, N., et al., Metabolic activation of bisphenol A by rat liver S9 fraction, *Toxicol. Sci.*, 62, 221, 2001.

65. Yoshihara, S., Mizutare, T., Makishima, M., et al., Potent estrogenic metabolites of bisphenol A and bisphenol B formed by rat liver S9 fraction: their structures and estrogenic potency, *Toxicol. Sci.*, 2003.

66. Routledge, E.J., White, R., Parker, M.G., et al., Differential effects of xenoestrogens on coactivator recruitment by ERalpha and ERbeta, *J. Biol. Chem.*, 2000.

67. Hall, J.M., McDonnell, D.P., and Korach, K.S., Allosteric regulation of estrogen receptor structure, function, and coactivator recruitment by different estrogen response elements, *Mol. Endocrinol.*, 16, 469, 2002.

68. Watanabe, H., Suzuki, A., Kobayashi, M., et al., Similarities and differences in uterine gene expression patterns caused by treatment with physiological and non-physiological estrogens, *J. Mol. Endocrinol.*, 31, 487, 2003.

69. Adachi, T., Koh, K.B., Tainaka, H., et al., Toxicogenomic difference between diethylstilbestrol and 17beta-estradiol in mouse testicular gene expression by neonatal exposure, *Mol. Reprod. Dev.*, 67, 19, 2004.
70. Larkin, P., Sabo-Attwood, T., Kelso, J., et al., Gene expression analysis of largemouth bass exposed to estradiol, nonylphenol, and p,p′-DDE, *Comp. Biochem. Physiol. B. Biochem. Mol. Biol.*, 133, 543, 2002.
71. Naciff, J.M., Jump, M.L., Torontali, S.M., et al., Gene expression profile induced by 17alpha-ethynyl estradiol, bisphenol A, and genistein in the developing female reproductive system of the rat, *Toxicol. Sci.*, 68, 184, 2002.
72. Toppari, J., Larsen, J.C., Christiansen, P., et al., Male reproductive health and envrionmental xenoestrogens, *Environ. Health Perspect.*, 104, 741, 1996.
73. Brock, J.W., Melnyk, L.J., Caudill, S.P., et al., Serum levels of several organochlorine pesticides in farmers correspond with dietary exposure and local use history, *Toxicol. Ind. Health*, 14, 275, 1998.
74. Helzlsouer, K.J., Alberg, A.J., Huang, H.Y., et al., Serum concentrations of organochlorine compounds and the subsequent development of breast cancer, *Cancer Epidemiol. Biomarkers Prev.*, 8, 525, 1999.
75. Dorgan, J.F., Brock, J.W., Rothman, N., et al., Serum organochlorine pesticides and PCBs and breast cancer risk: results from a prospective analysis (USA), *Cancer Causes Control*, 10, 1, 1999.
76. Chun, T.Y., Gregg, D., Sarkar, D.K., et al., Differential regulation by estrogens of growth and prolactin synthesis in pituitary cells suggests that only a small pool of estrogen receptors is required for growth, *Proc. Natl. Acad. Sci. U.S.A.*, 95, 2325, 1998.
77. Ulrich, E.M., Caperell-Grant, A., Hites, R.A., et al., Environmentally relevant xenoestrogen tissue concentrations correlated to biological response in mice, *Environ. Health Perspect.*, 108, 973, 2000.
78. Cos, P., De, B.T., Apers, S., et al., Phytoestrogens: recent developments, *Planta Med.*, 69, 589, 2003.
79. Schmitt, E., Dekant, W., and Stopper, H., Assaying the estrogenicity of phytoestrogens in cells of different estrogen sensitive tissues, *Toxicol. in vitro*, 15, 433, 2001.
80. Maggiolini, M., Bonofiglio, D., Marsico, S., et al., Estrogen receptor alpha mediates the proliferative but not the cytotoxic dose-dependent effects of two major phytoestrogens on human breast cancer cells, *Mol. Pharmacol.*, 60, 595, 2001.
81. Rowlands, J.C., Berhow, M.A., and Badger, T.M., Estrogenic and antiproliferative properties of soy sapogenols in human breast cancer cells *in vitro*, *Food Chem. Toxicol.*, 40, 1767, 2002.
82. Messina, M.J., Persky, V., Setchell, K.D., et al., Soy intake and cancer risk: a review of the *in vitro* and *in vivo* data, *Nutr. Cancer*, 21, 113, 1994.
83. Messina, M.J., and Loprinzi, C.L., Soy for breast cancer survivors: a critical review of the literature, *J. Nutr.*, 131, 3095S, 2001.
84. Burow, M.E., Boue, S.M., Collins-Burow, B.M., et al., Phytochemical glyceollins, isolated from soy, mediate antihormonal effects through estrogen receptor alpha and beta, *J. Clin. Endocrinol. Metab.*, 86, 1750, 2001.
85. Willson, T.M., and Moore, J.T., Genomics versus orphan nuclear receptors—a half-time report, *Mol. Endocrinol.*, 16, 1135, 2002.
86. Suetsugi, M., Su, L., Karlsberg, K., et al., Flavone and isoflavone phytoestrogens are agonists of estrogen-related receptors, *Mol. Cancer. Res.*, 1, 981, 2003.

87. Wormke, M., Stoner, M., Saville, B., et al., Crosstalk between estrogen receptor alpha and the aryl hydrocarbon receptor in breast cancer cells involves unidirectional activation of proteasomes, *FEBS Lett.*, 478, 109, 2000.

88. Connor, K., Ramamoorthy, K., Moore, M., et al., Hydroxylated polychlorinated biphenyls (PCBs) as estrogens and antiestrogens: structure-activity relationships, *Toxicol. Appl. Pharmacol.*, 145, 111, 1997.

89. Fernandez, P., and Safe, S., Growth inhibitory and antimitogenic activity of 2,3,7,8-tetrachlorodibenzo-p-dioxin (TCDD) in T47D human breast cancer cells, *Toxicol. Lett.*, 61, 185, 1992.

90. Harper, N., Wang, X., Liu, H., et al., Inhibition of estrogen-induced progesterone receptor in MCF-7 human breast cancer cells by aryl hydrocarbon (Ah) receptor agonists, *Mol. Cell. Endocrinol.*, 104, 47, 1994.

91. Krishnan, V., and Safe, S., Polychlorinated biphenyls (PCBs), dibenzo-p-dioxins (PCDDs), and dibenzofurans (PCDFs) as antiestrogens in MCF-7 human breast cancer cells: quantitative structure-activity relationships, *Toxicol. Appl. Pharmacol.*, 120, 55, 1993.

92. Moore, M., Mustain, M., Daniel, K., et al., Antiestrogenic activity of hydroxylated polychlorinated biphenyl congeners identified in human serum, *Toxicol. Appl. Pharmacol.*, 142, 160, 1997.

93. Taylor, H.S., The role of HOX genes in human implantation, *Hum. Reprod. Update*, 6, 75, 2000.

94. Benson, G.V., Lim, H., Paria, B.C., et al., Mechanisms of reduced fertility in Hoxa-10 mutant mice: uterine homeosis and loss of maternal Hoxa-10 expression, *Development*, 122, 2687, 1996.

95. Gendron, R.L., Paradis, H., Hsieh-Li, H.M., et al., Abnormal uterine stromal and glandular function associated with maternal reproductive defects in Hoxa-11 null mice, *Biol. Reprod.*, 56, 1097, 1997.

96. Block, K., Kardana, A., Igarashi, P., et al., In utero diethylstilbestrol (DES) exposure alters Hox gene expression in the developing mullerian system, *FASEB J.*, 14, 1101, 2000.

97. Couse, J.F., Dixon, D., Yates, M., et al., Estrogen receptor-alpha knockout mice exhibit resistance to the developmental effects of neonatal diethylstilbestrol exposure on the female reproductive tract, *Dev. Biol.*, 238, 224, 2001.

98. Miller, C., Degenhardt, K., and Sassoon, D.A., Fetal exposure to DES results in de-regulation of Wnt7a during uterine morphogenesis, *Nat. Genet.*, 20, 228, 1998.

99. Parr, B.A., and McMahon, A.P., Sexually dimorphic development of the mammalian reproductive tract requires Wnt-7a, *Nature*, 395, 707, 1998.

100. Ehrlich, M., Expression of various genes is controlled by DNA methylation during mammalian development, *J. Cell. Biochem.*, 88, 899, 2003.

101. Li, S., Washburn, K.A., Moore, R., et al., Developmental exposure to diethylstilbestrol elicits demethylation of estrogen-responsive lactoferrin gene in mouse uterus, *Cancer Res.*, 57, 4356, 1997.

102. Li, S., Ma, L., Chiang, T., et al., Promoter CpG methylation of Hox-a10 and Hox-a11 in mouse uterus not altered upon neonatal diethylstilbestrol exposure, *Mol. Carcinog.*, 32, 213, 2001.

103. Hayashi, N., Hasegawa, K., Komine, A., et al., Estrogen-induced cell transformation and DNA adduct formation in cultured Syrian hamster embryo cells, *Mol. Carcinog.*, 16, 149, 1996.

104. Thomas, R.D., and Roy, D., Stilbene estrogen produces higher levels of mitochondrial DNA adducts than nuclear DNA adducts in the target organ of cancer (liver) of male Sprague Dawley rats, *Oncol. Rep.*, 8, 1035, 2001.

105. Atkinson, A., and Roy, D., In vivo DNA adduct formation by bisphenol A, *Environ. Mol. Mutagen.*, 26, 60, 1995.

106. Roy, D., and Liehr, J.G., Estrogen, DNA damage and mutations, *Mutat. Res.*, 424, 107, 1999.

107. Das, S.K., Taylor, J.A., Korach, K.S., et al., Estrogenic responses in estrogen receptor-alpha deficient mice reveal a distinct estrogen signaling pathway, *Proc. Natl. Acad. Sci. USA*, 94, 12786, 1997.

108. Das, S.K., Tan, J., Raja, S., et al., Estrogen targets genes involved in protein processing, calcium homeostasis, and Wnt signaling in the mouse uterus independent of estrogen receptor-alpha and -beta, *J. Biol. Chem.*, 275, 28834, 2000.

109. Bigsby, R.M., unpublished data, 2004.

110. Collins-Burow, B.M., Burow, M.E., Duong, B.N., et al., Estrogenic and antiestrogenic activities of flavonoid phytochemicals through estrogen receptor binding-dependent and -independent mechanisms, *Nutr. Cancer*, 38, 229, 2000.

111. Kaneuchi, M., Sasaki, M., Tanaka, Y., et al., Resveratrol suppresses growth of Ishikawa cells through down-regulation of EGF, *Int. J. Oncol.*, 23, 1167, 2003.

112. Kaneuchi, M., Sasaki, M., Tanaka, Y., et al., Quercetin regulates growth of Ishikawa cells through the suppression of EGF and cyclin D1, *Int. J. Oncol.*, 22, 159, 2003.

113. Pietras, R.J., and Szego, C.M., Endometrial cell calcium and oestrogen action, *Nature*, 253, 357, 1975.

114. Pietras, R.J., and Szego, C.M., Specific binding sites for oestrogen at the outer surfaces of isolated endometrial cells, *Nature*, 265, 69, 1977.

115. Pietras, R.J., Nemere, I., and Szego, C.M., Steroid hormone receptors in target cell membranes, *Endocrine*, 14, 417, 2001.

116. Filardo, E.J., Epidermal growth factor receptor (EGFR) transactivation by estrogen via the G-protein-coupled receptor, GPR30: a novel signaling pathway with potential significance for breast cancer, *J. Steroid Biochem. Mol. Biol.*, 80, 231, 2002.

117. Migliaccio, A., Castoria, G., Di, D.M., et al., Sex steroid hormones act as growth factors, *J. Steroid Biochem. Mol. Biol.*, 83, 31, 2002.

118. Migliaccio, A., Castoria, G., Di, D.M., et al., Src is an initial target of sex steroid hormone action, *Ann. NY Acad. Sci.*, 963, 185, 2002.

119. Enan, E., and Matsumura, F., Activation of c-neu tyrosine kinase by o,p'-DDT and β-HCH in cell-free and intact cell preparations from MCF-7 human breast cancer cells, *J. Biochem. Toxicol.*, 12, 83, 1998.

120. Hatakeyama, M., and Matsumura, F., Correlation between the activation of Neu tyrosine kinase and promotion of foci formation induced by selected organochlorine compounds in the MCF-7 model system, *J. Biochem. Mol. Toxicol.*, 13, 296, 1999.

121. Hatakeyama, M., Zou, E., and Matsumura, F., Comparison of the characteristic of estrogenic action patterns of beta-HCH and heregulin beta1 in MCF-7 human breast cancer cells, *J. Biochem. Mol. Toxicol.*, 16, 209, 2002.

122. Frigo, D.E., Duong, B.N., Melnik, L.I., et al., Flavonoid phytochemicals regulate activator protein-1 signal transduction pathways in endometrial and kidney stable cell lines, *J. Nutr.*, 132, 1848, 2002.

123. Frigo, D.E., Tang, Y., Beckman, B.S., et al., Mechanism of AP-1-mediated gene expression by select organochlorines through the p38 MAPK pathway, *Carcinogenesis*, 2003.

124. Akiyama, T., Ishida, J., Nakagawa, S., et al., Genistein, a specific inhibitor of tyrosine-specific protein kinases, *J. Biol. Chem.*, 262, 5592, 1987.
125. Walker, H.E., Pacold, E.M., Perisic, O., et al., Structural determinants of phosphoinositide 3-kinase inhibition by wortmannin, LY294002, quercetin, myricetin, and staurosporine, *Mol. Cell*, 6, 909, 2000.
126. Guo, Y., Hendrickx, A.G., Overstreet, J.W., et al., Endocrine biomarkers of early fetal loss in cynomolgus macaques (Macaca fascicularis) following exposure to dioxin, *Biol. Reprod.*, 60, 707, 1999.
127. Drenth, H.J., Bouwman, C.A., Seinen, W., et al., Effects of some persistent halogenated environmental contaminants on aromatase (CYP19) activity in the human choriocarcinoma cell line JEG-3, *Toxicol. Appl. Pharmacol.*, 148, 50, 1998.
128. Letcher, R.J., van, H.I., Drenth, H.J., et al., Cytotoxicity and aromatase (CYP19) activity modulation by organochlorines in human placental JEG-3 and JAR choriocarcinoma cells, *Toxicol. Appl. Pharmacol.*, 160, 10, 1999.
129. Moran, F.M., VandeVoort, C.A., Overstreet, J.W., et al., Molecular target of endocrine disruption in human luteinizing granulosa cells by 2,3,7,8-tetrachlorodibenzo-*p*-dioxin: inhibition of estradiol secretion due to decreased 17alpha-hydroxylase/17,20-lyase cytochrome P450 expression, *Endocrinology*, 144, 467, 2003.
130. Akingbemi, B.T., Sottas, C.M., Koulova, A.I., et al., Inhibition of testicular steroidogenesis by the xenoestrogen bisphenol A is associated with reduced pituitary LH secretion and decreased steroidogenic enzyme gene expression in rat Leydig cells, *Endocrinology*, 2003.
131. Adlercreutz, H., Bannwart, C., Wahala, K., et al., Inhibition of human aromatase by mammalian lignans and isoflavonoid phytoestrogens, *J. Steroid Biochem. Mol. Biol.*, 44, 147, 1993.
132. Pelissero, C., Lenczowski, M.J., Chinzi, D., et al., Effects of flavonoids on aromatase activity, an *in vitro* study, *J. Steroid Biochem. Mol. Biol.*, 57, 215, 1996.
133. Mak, P., Cruz, F.D., and Chen, S., A yeast screen system for aromatase inhibitors and ligands for androgen receptor: yeast cells transformed with aromatase and androgen receptor, *Environ. Health Perspect.*, 107, 855, 1999.
134. Le, B.J.C., Champavier, Y., Chulia, A.J., et al., Effects of phytoestrogens on aromatase, 3beta and 17beta-hydroxysteroid dehydrogenase activities and human breast cancer cells, *Life Sci*, 66, 1281, 2000.
135. Whitehead, S.A., and Lacey, M., Phytoestrogens inhibit aromatase but not 17beta-hydroxysteroid dehydrogenase (HSD) type 1 in human granulosa-luteal cells: evidence for FSH induction of 17beta-HSD, *Hum. Reprod.*, 18, 487, 2003.
136. Almstrup, K., Fernandez, M.F., Petersen, J.H., et al., Dual effects of phytoestrogens result in u-shaped dose-response curves, *Environ. Health Perspect.*, 110, 743, 2002.
137. Raftogianis, R., Creveling, C., Weinshilboum, R., et al., Estrogen metabolism by conjugation, *J. Natl. Cancer Inst. Monogr.*, 27, 113, 2000.
138. Lakhani, N.J., Venitz, J., Figg, W.D., et al., Pharmacogenetics of estrogen metabolism and transport in relation to cancer, *Curr. Drug Metab.*, 4, 505, 2003.
139. Lee, A.J., Cai, M.X., Thomas, P.E., et al., Characterization of the oxidative metabolites of 17beta-estradiol and estrone formed by 15 selectively expressed human cytochrome p450 isoforms, *Endocrinology*, 144, 3382, 2003.
140. Paria, B.C., Lim, H., Das, S.K., et al., Molecular signaling in uterine receptivity for implantation, *Semin. Cell Dev. Biol.*, 11, 67, 2000.
141. Zhu, B.T., and Conney, A.H., Functional role of estrogen metabolism in target cells: review and perspectives, *Carcinogenesis*, 19, 1, 1998.

142. Xiao, L., and Becker, J.B., Effects of estrogen agonists on amphetamine-stimulated striatal dopamine release, *Synapse*, 29, 379, 1998.

143. Yager, J.D., Endogenous estrogens as carcinogens through metabolic activation, *J. Natl. Cancer Inst. Monogr.*, 27, 67, 2000.

144. Liehr, J.G., Is estradiol a genotoxic mutagenic carcinogen?, *Endocr. Rev.*, 21, 40, 2000.

145. Rogan, E.G., Badawi, A.F., Devanesan, P.D., et al., Relative imbalances in estrogen metabolism and conjugation in breast tissue of women with carcinoma: potential biomarkers of susceptibility to cancer, *Carcinogenesis*, 24, 697, 2003.

146. Bradlow, H.L., Telang, N.T., Sepkovic, D.W., et al., 2-hydroxyestrone: the 'good' estrogen, *J. Endocrinol.*, 150, Suppl:S259, 1996.

147. Kristensen, V.N., and Borresen-Dale, A.L., Molecular epidemiology of breast cancer: genetic variation in steroid hormone metabolism, *Mutat. Res.*, 462, 323, 2000.

148. Mitrunen, K., and Hirvonen, A., Molecular epidemiology of sporadic breast cancer. The role of polymorphic genes involved in oestrogen biosynthesis and metabolism, *Mutat. Res.*, 544, 9, 2003.

149. Jan, S.T., Devanesan, P.D., Stack, D.E., et al., Metabolic activation and formation of DNA adducts of hexestrol, a synthetic nonsteroidal carcinogenic estrogen, *Chem. Res. Toxicol.*, 11, 412, 1998.

150. Carmichael, P.L., Mills, J.J., Campbell, M., et al., Mechanisms of hormonal carcinogenesis in the p53+/- hemizygous knockout mouse: studies with diethylstilbestrol, *Toxicol. Pathol.*, 29 Suppl., 155, 2001.

151. Green, M., Thomas, R., Gued, L., et al., Inhibition of DES-induced DNA adducts by diallyl sulfide: implications in liver cancer prevention, *Oncol. Rep.*, 10, 767, 2003.

152. Atkinson, A., and Roy, D., In vitro conversion of environmental estrogenic chemical bisphenol A to DNA binding metabolite(s), *Biochem. Biophys. Res. Commun.*, 210, 424, 1995.

153. Atkinson, A., and Roy, D., In vivo DNA adduct formation by bisphenol A, *Environ. Mol. Mutagen.*, 26, 60, 1995.

154. Nakagawa, Y., and Tayama, S., Metabolism and cytotoxicity of bisphenol A and other bisphenols in isolated rat hepatocytes, *Arch. Toxicol.*, 74, 99, 2000.

155. Elsby, R., Maggs, J.L., Ashby, J., et al., Comparison of the modulatory effects of human and rat liver microsomal metabolism on the estrogenicity of bisphenol A: implications for extrapolation to humans, *J. Pharmacol. Exp. Ther.*, 297, 103, 2001.

156. Kim, Y.H., Kim, C.S., Park, S., et al., Gender differences in the levels of bisphenol A metabolites in urine, *Biochem. Biophys. Res. Commun.*, 312, 441, 2003.

157. Denison, M.S., and Nagy, S.R., Activation of the aryl hydrocarbon receptor by structurally diverse exogenous and endogenous chemicals, *Annu. Rev. Pharmacol. Toxicol.*, 43, 309, 2003.

158. Hakkola, J., Pasanen, M., Pelkonen, O., et al., Expression of CYP1B1 in human adult and fetal tissues and differential inducibility of CYP1B1 and CYP1A1 by Ah receptor ligands in human placenta and cultured cells, *Carcinogenesis*, 18, 391, 1997.

159. Whitlock, J.P.J., Induction of cytochrome P4501A1, *Annu. Rev. Pharmacol. Toxicol.*, 39, 103, 1999.

160. Mimura, J., and Fujii-Kuriyama, Y., Functional role of AhR in the expression of toxic effects by TCDD, *Biochim. Biophys. Acta.*, 1619, 263, 2003.

161. Horn, T.L., Reichert, M.A., Bliss, R.L., et al., Modulations of P450 mRNA in liver and mammary gland and P450 activities and metabolism of estrogen in liver by treatment of rats with indole-3-carbinol, *Biochem. Pharmacol.*, 64, 393, 2002.

162. Wang, H.W., Chen, F.W., and Ueng, T.H., Induction of cytochromes P-450 1A1 and 1B1 by motorcycle exhaust particulate in human breast cancer MCF-7 cells, *J. Toxicol. Environ. Health A*, 65, 1401, 2002.

163. Spink, B.C., Hussain, M.M., Katz, B.H., et al., Transient induction of cytochromes P450 1A1 and 1B1 in MCF-7 human breast cancer cells by indirubin, *Biochem. Pharmacol.*, 66, 2313, 2003.

164. van, D.M.B., Sanderson, J.T., van, D.B.M., et al., Effects of several dioxin-like compounds on estrogen metabolism in the malignant MCF-7 and nontumorigenic MCF-10A human mammary epithelial cell lines, *Toxicol. Appl. Pharmacol.*, 190, 241, 2003.

165. Tritscher, A.M., Seacat, A.M., Yager, J.D., et al., Increased oxidative DNA damage in livers of 2,3,7,8-tetrachlorodibenzo-*p*-dioxin treated intact but not ovariectomized rats, *Cancer Lett.*, 98, 219, 1996.

166. Wyde, M.E., Wong, V.A., Kim, A.H., et al., Induction of hepatic 8-oxo-deoxyguanosine adducts by 2,3,7,8-tetrachlorodibenzo-p-dioxin in Sprague-Dawley rats is female-specific and estrogen-dependent, *Chem. Res. Toxicol.*, 14, 849, 2001.

167. Jeuken, A., Keser, B.J., Khan, E., et al., Activation of the Ah receptor by extracts of dietary herbal supplements, vegetables, and fruits, *J. Agric. Food. Chem.*, 51, 5478, 2003.

168. Henry, E.C., Kende, A.S., Rucci, G., et al., Flavone antagonists bind competitively with 2,3,7, 8-tetrachlorodibenzo-p-dioxin (TCDD) to the aryl hydrocarbon receptor but inhibit nuclear uptake and transformation, *Mol. Pharmacol.*, 55, 716, 1999.

169. Bjeldanes, L.F., Kim, J.Y., Grose, K.R., et al., Aromatic hydrocarbon responsiveness-receptor agonists generated from indole-3-carbinol *in vitro* and *in vivo*: comparisons with 2,3,7,8-tetrachlorodibenzo-*p*-dioxin, *Proc. Natl. Acad. Sci. USA*, 88, 9543, 1991.

170. Yang, X.F., Wang, N.P., Lu, W.H., et al., Effects of Ginkgo biloba extract and tanshinone on cytochrome P-450 isozymes and glutathione transferase in rats, *Acta Pharmacol. Sin.*, 24, 1033, 2003.

171. Ciolino, H.P., Daschner, P.J., and Yeh, G.C., Resveratrol inhibits transcription of CYP1A1 *in vitro* by preventing activation of the aryl hydrocarbon receptor, *Cancer Res.*, 58, 5707, 1998.

172. Casper, R.F., Quesne, M., Rogers, I.M., et al., Resveratrol has antagonist activity on the aryl hydrocarbon receptor: implications for prevention of dioxin toxicity, *Mol. Pharmacol.*, 56, 784, 1999.

173. Ashida, H., Fukuda, I., Yamashita, T., et al., Flavones and flavonols at dietary levels inhibit a transformation of aryl hydrocarbon receptor induced by dioxin, *FEBS Lett.*, 476, 213, 2000.

174. Shimada, T., Yamazaki, H., Mimura, M., et al., Interindividual variations in human liver cytochrome P-450 enzymes involved in the oxidation of drugs, carcinogens and toxic chemicals: studies with liver microsomes of 30 Japanese and 30 Caucasians, *J. Pharmacol. Exp. Ther.*, 270, 414, 1994.

175. Yokose, T., Doy, M., Taniguchi, T., et al., Immunohistochemical study of cytochrome P450 2C and 3A in human non-neoplastic and neoplastic tissues, *Virchows Arch.*, 434, 401, 1999.

176. Honkakoski, P., Sueyoshi, T., and Negishi, M., Drug-activated nuclear receptors CAR and PXR, *Ann. Med.*, 35, 172, 2003.

177. Kliewer, S.A., The nuclear pregnane X receptor regulates xenobiotic detoxification, *J. Nutr.*, 133, 2444S, 2003.

178. Carlberg, C., Current understanding of the function of the nuclear vitamin D receptor in response to its natural and synthetic ligands, *Recent Results Cancer Res.*, 164, 29, 2003.

179. Lindley, C., Hamilton, G., McCune, J.S., et al., The effect of cyclophosphamide with and without dexamethasone on cytochrome P450 3A4 and 2B6 in human hepatocytes, *Drug Metab. Dispos.*, 30, 814, 2002.

180. Zhang, W., Purchio, A., Chen, K., et al., In vivo activation of the human CYP3A4 promoter in mouse liver and regulation by pregnane X receptors, *Biochem. Pharmacol.*, 65, 1889, 2003.

181. Dvorak, Z., Modriansky, M., Pichard-Garcia, L., et al., Colchicine down-regulates cytochrome P450 2B6, 2C8, 2C9, and 3A4 in human hepatocytes by affecting their glucocorticoid receptor-mediated regulation, *Mol. Pharmacol.*, 64, 160, 2003.

182. Engman, H.A., Lennernas, H., Taipalensuu, J., et al., CYP3A4, CYP3A5, and MDR1 in human small and large intestinal cell lines suitable for drug transport studies, *J. Pharm. Sci.*, 90, 1736, 2001.

183. Elizondo, G., and Medina-Diaz, I.M., Induction of CYP3A4 by 1alpha,25-dyhydroxyvitamin D3 in HepG2 cells, *Life Sci.*, 73, 141, 2003.

184. Luo, G., Cunningham, M., Kim, S., et al., CYP3A4 induction by drugs: correlation between a pregnane X receptor reporter gene assay and CYP3A4 expression in human hepatocytes, *Drug Metab. Dispos.*, 30, 795, 2002.

185. Niemi, M., Backman, J.T., Fromm, M.F., et al., Pharmacokinetic interactions with rifampicin: clinical relevance, *Clin. Pharmacokinet.*, 42, 819, 2003.

186. Nallani, S.C., Glauser, T.A., Hariparsad, N., et al., Dose-dependent induction of cytochrome P450 (CYP) 3A4 and activation of pregnane X receptor by topiramate, *Epilepsia*, 44, 1521, 2003.

187. Gibson, G.G., el-Sankary, W., and Plant, N.J., Receptor-dependent regulation of the CYP3A4 gene, *Toxicology*, 181–182, 199, 2002.

188. Raucy, J., Warfe, L., Yueh, M.F., et al., A cell-based reporter gene assay for determining induction of CYP3A4 in a high-volume system, *J. Pharmacol. Exp. Ther.*, 303, 412, 2002.

189. Jones, S.A., Moore, L.B., Shenk, J.L., et al., The pregnane X receptor: a promiscuous xenobiotic receptor that has diverged during evolution, *Mol. Endocrinol.*, 14, 27, 2000.

190. Martin, H., Sarsat, J.P., de, W.I., et al., Induction of cytochrome P450 2B6 and 3A4 expression by phenobarbital and cyclophosphamide in cultured human liver slices, *Pharm. Res.*, 20, 557, 2003.

191. Nallani, S.C., Goodwin, B., Maglich, J.M., et al., Induction of cytochrome P450 3A by paclitaxel in mice: pivotal role of the nuclear xenobiotic receptor, pregnane X receptor, *Drug Metab. Dispos.*, 31, 681, 2003.

192. Masuyama, H., Hiramatsu, Y., Kunitomi, M., et al., Endocrine disrupting chemicals, phthalic acid and nonylphenol, activate pregnane X receptor-mediated transcription, *Mol. Endocrinol.*, 14, 421, 2000.

193. Rosenfeld, W.E., Doose, D.R., Walker, S.A., et al., Effect of topiramate on the pharmacokinetics of an oral contraceptive containing norethindrone and ethinyl estradiol in patients with epilepsy, *Epilepsia*, 38, 317, 1997.

194. Ouellet, D., Hsu, A., Qian, J., et al., Effect of ritonavir on the pharmacokinetics of ethinyl oestradiol in healthy female volunteers, *Br. J. Clin. Pharmacol.*, 46, 111, 1998.

195. Goodwin, B., Hodgson, E., D'Costa, D.J., et al., Transcriptional regulation of the human CYP3A4 gene by the constitutive androstane receptor, *Mol. Pharmacol.*, 62, 359, 2002.

196. Drocourt, L., Ourlin, J.C., Pascussi, J.M., et al., Expression of CYP3A4, CYP2B6, and CYP2C9 is regulated by the vitamin D receptor pathway in primary human hepatocytes, *J. Biol. Chem.*, 277, 25125, 2002.

197. Doose, D.R., Wang, S.S., Padmanabhan, M., et al., Effect of topiramate or carbamazepine on the pharmacokinetics of an oral contraceptive containing norethindrone and ethinyl estradiol in healthy obese and nonobese female subjects, *Epilepsia*, 44, 540, 2003.

198. Hall, S.D., Wang, Z., Huang, S.M., et al., The interaction between St. John's wort and an oral contraceptive, *Clin. Pharmacol. Ther.*, 74, 525, 2003.

199. Markowitz, J.S., Donovan, J.L., DeVane, C.L., et al., Effect of St. John's wort on drug metabolism by induction of cytochrome P450 3A4 enzyme, *JAMA*, 290, 1500, 2003.

200. Suiko, M., Sakakibara, Y., and Liu, M.C., Sulfation of environmental estrogen-like chemicals by human cytosolic sulfotransferases, *Biochem. Biophys. Res. Commun.*, 267, 80, 2000.

201. Shimizu, M., Ohta, K., Matsumoto, Y., et al., Sulfation of bisphenol A abolished its estrogenicity based on proliferation and gene expression in human breast cancer MCF-7 cells, *Toxicol. in vitro*, 16, 549, 2002.

202. Santen, R.J., Leszczynski, D., Tilson-Mallet, N., et al., Enzymatic control of estrogen production in human breast cancer: relative significance of aromatase versus sulfatase pathways, *Ann. N. Y. Acad. of Sci.*, 464, 126, 1986.

203. Raobaikady, B., Purohit, A., Chander, S.K., et al., Inhibition of MCF-7 breast cancer cell proliferation and *in vivo* steroid sulphatase activity by 2-methoxyoestradiol-bis-sulphamate, *J. Steroid Biochem. Mol. Biol.*, 84, 351, 2003.

204. Kester, M.H., Bulduk, S., van, T.H., et al., Potent inhibition of estrogen sulfotransferase by hydroxylated metabolites of polyhalogenated aromatic hydrocarbons reveals alternative mechanism for estrogenic activity of endocrine disrupters, *J. Clin. Endocrinol. Metab.*, 87, 1142, 2002.

205. Kirk, C.J., Bottomley, L., Minican, N., et al., Environmental endocrine disrupters dysregulate estrogen metabolism and Ca2+ homeostasis in fish and mammals via receptor-independent mechanisms, *Comp. Biochem. Physiol. A Mol. Integr. Physiol.*, 135, 1, 2003.

206. Zhu, B.T., and Liehr, J.G., Inhibition of catechol O-methyltransferase-catalyzed O-methylation of 2- and 4-hydroxyestradiol by quercetin. Possible role in estradiol-induced tumorigenesis, *J. Biol. Chem.*, 271, 1357, 1996.

8 2,3,7,8-Tetrachlorodibenzo-*p*-Dioxin (TCDD) and Related Environmental Antiestrogens: Characterization and Mechanism of Action

Stephen H. Safe

CONTENTS

0-8493-2281-2/05/$0.00+$1.50

8.1   ARYL HYDROCARBON RECEPTOR AGONISTS: BIOCHEMICAL AND TOXIC RESPONSES

8.1.1   INTRODUCTION

Organochlorine industrial chemicals have been extensively used in the production of plastics, flame retardants, dielectric fluids, pesticides, drugs, and a host of other commercial products. Some of these chemicals such as the organochlorine insecticides, which include DDT, are both highly stable and lipophilic, and trace residues have been detected as pollutants in air, water, sediments, fish, wildlife, human adipose tissue, blood, and milk.[1] Other halogenated aromatic compounds such as the polychlorinated biphenyls (PCBs), dibenzo-p-dioxins (PCDDs), and dibenzo-furans (PCDFs) exhibit comparable widespread environmental distribution profiles.[2,3] After initial identification of DDT, its metabolite DDE, and PCBs as environmental pollutants, regulatory agencies have either banned or restricted use of most persistent organochlorine compounds, and residue levels for most of these chemicals have dramatically declined over the past 20 to 30 years.[1]

Organochlorine contaminants induce multiple species-dependent effects that have been linked to reproductive and developmental failures of some wildlife populations in contaminated regions such as the Great Lakes.[4] Some of these adverse effects may be related to the endocrine-like activity of some organochlorine compounds, and there has been considerable scientific and public controversy regarding the potential wildlife and human health effects associated with exposure to endocrine disruptors, particularly those compounds that exhibit estrogenic activity (i.e., xenoestrogens).[4–6] Wolff and coworkers initially reported that adipose tissue PCB levels were higher in a cohort of women with breast cancer (in Connecticut), and in a nested case-control study in New York serum DDE levels were higher in breast patients than controls.[7,8] Their analysis showed that women with the highest levels of DDE had a fourfold increased risk for breast cancer, and it was concluded that "environmental contamination with organochlorine residues may be an important etiologic factor in breast cancer."[7] It was later hypothesized that xenoestrogens were a preventable cause of breast cancer,[9–11] and there has been considerable research on testing the validity of the reported correlational studies. Recent studies on women from the San Francisco Bay area, five European countries, the Nurses Health Study (comprising 121,700 women from 11 states), and three Mexico City hospitals have compared serum or tissue DDE and in some cases, PCB levels in breast cancer in patients and controls.[12–15] Subsequent studies in several laboratories concur that

DDE/PCBs are not elevated in breast cancer patients, and a recent report on women in Long Island stated the following: "In conclusion in the large population-based case-control study among women in Long Island, breast cancer risk was not increased in relation to serum organochlorine levels."[16]

The xenoestrogen-breast cancer hypothesis was challenged on several counts including the authors' failure to account for diverse organochlorine compounds, which exhibit antiestrogenic activity.[17,18] For example, women in Seveso, Italy, accidentally exposed in 1976 to high levels of 2,3,7,8-tetrachlorodibenzo-*p*-dioxin (TCDD) exhibited a lower incidence of breast and endometrial cancer in the early 1990s.[19] TCDD is the most toxic member of a class of compounds that includes other PCDDs, PCDFs, and PCBs, and this review will describe their inhibition of 17β-estradiol (estrogen, E2)-induced responses, the molecular mechanism of action of these chemicals, and the development of a new class of mechanism-based indirect antiestrogens for treatment of breast cancer.[20]

8.1.2 TCDD AND RELATED COMPOUNDS: BIOCHEMICAL AND TOXIC RESPONSES

TCDD has been used extensively as a prototype for investigating the biochemical and toxic responses elicited by halogenated aromatic hydrocarbons (HAHs).[20–25] TCDD induces a diverse spectrum of phase I and phase II drug-metabolizing enzymes including CYP1A1, CYP1A2, CYP1B1 and their dependent activities,[26] glutathione S-transferase,[27,28] glucuronosyl transferase,[29] and NAD(P)H quinone:oxidoreductase.[30] TCDD also increases expression of other genes/gene products, including aldehyde-3-dehydrogenase,[31] transforming growth factor α (TGFα),[32,33] δ-aminolevulinic acid synthetase,[34] plasminogen activator inhibitor 2,[35] interleukin 1β,[35] c-*fos* and c-*jun* protooncogenes,[36] and prostaglandin endoperoxide H synthase-2.[37] It has also been reported that TCDD decreases expression of several genes/gene products such as c/EBPα,[38] peroxisome proliferator receptor γ,[38] lipoprotein lipase,[38] estrogen receptor, urophorphyrinogen decarboxylase,[39,40] rat liver aldolase B,[41] phosphoenol pyruvate carboxykinase,[42] pyruvate carboxylase,[43] hydroxysteroid sulfotransferase a,[44] and adenosine deaminase.[45] The list of genes or gene products that are modulated after treatment with TCDD is continually expanding; however, these responses are highly tissue specific. For example, although TCDD induces interleukin 1β and plasminogen activator inhibitor-2 in human keratinocytes,[35] no induction was observed in Sprague-Dawley rat liver.[46]

TCDD and related compounds also elicit a diverse spectrum of toxic responses, and these include acute lethality, a wasting syndrome, tissue-/cell-specific hypo- and hyperplastic effects, immunotoxicity, thymic atrophy, developmental and reproductive toxicity, carcinogenesis, hepatotoxicity, porphyria, chloracne, and related dermal lesions.[20–26] The acute lethal toxicity of TCDD and related compounds is observed in most species; however, the LD_{50} values vary from 2.0 µg/kg for the highly responsive guinea pig to 5051 and 7200 µg/kg for the resistant hamster and Hann/Wistar rat, respectively. In contrast, many other toxic responses are highly species, sex, and age specific. For example, long-term dietary exposure to male and female Sprague-Dawley rats to TCDD (0.001, 0.01, and 0.1 µg/kg/day) resulted in development of hepatocellular carcinomas in female (but not male) rats. This type of response variability is typical for halogenated aromatics, and the mechanisms associated with tissue-/species-specific responsiveness or nonresponsiveness are poorly understood.

8.1.3 IDENTIFICATION OF THE ARYL HYDROCARBON RECEPTOR (AhR)

Poland, Nebert, and coworkers extensively investigated induction of hepatic CYP1A1-dependent aryl hydrocarbon hydroxylase (AHH) activity in genetically inbred strains of mice by TCDD and 3-methylcholanthrene (MC).[47-49] Both TCDD and MC induced hepatic microsomal AHH activity in Ah-responsive mice typified by the C57BL/6 strain, and TCDD was approximately 10^4 times more potent than MC. The differences in potency were attributed to the higher rate of metabolism of MC. In contrast, TCDD but not MC induced the same response in DBA/2 mice, a prototypical Ah-nonresponsive strain; however, the effective dose of TCDD was at least 10 times higher. It was suggested that these strain differences may be related to differential expression or structure of an intracellular receptor or acceptor protein. Support for the role of a receptor protein was derived from other studies that showed that for a number of halogenated aromatics, there was a correlation between structure-induction (AHH activity) versus other structure-activity relationships.[50] Poland and coworkers were the first to identify a hepatic cytosolic protein in C57BL/6 mice that bound [^{3}H]TCDD with high affinity.[51] Subsequent studies identified the AhR in multiple species/tissues, and photoaffinity labeling using 2-azido-3[^{125}I]iodo-7,8-dibromodibenzo-*p*-dioxin and hepatic cytosol from various species gave the following apparent molecular masses for the AhR: 95-kD (mouse), 101-kD (chicken), 103-kD (guinea pig), 104-kD (rabbit), 106-kD (rat and human), 113-kD (monkey), and 124-kD (hamster).[52]

Treatment of Ah-responsive cells/animals with TCDD results in the rapid formation of a liganded 190- to 210-kD nuclear AhR complex that contained the AhR and a second protein that was subsequently identified as the AhR nuclear translocator (Arnt) protein.[53,54] Genes for both the AhR and Arnt have been cloned, and sequence analysis has demonstrated that both proteins are members of the basic helix-loop-helix (bHLH) family of nuclear transcription factors.[55-60] The AhR and Arnt genes encode for proteins that exhibit several common structural domains (Figure 8.1), which include the DNA-binding bHLH region; two A/B repeats; a PAS domain common to the Per, Arnt, and Sim proteins; a ligand-binding domain (within the AhR); and Q-rich transactivation domains in the C-terminal region of both proteins. There is high sequence homology in the bHLH (N-terminal) and PAS domain of AhR proteins from different species and considerable variability in the C-terminal Q-rich regions. For example, Ema and coworkers compared the sequence of the AhR from Ah-responsive C57BL/6 and less-responsive DBA/2 mice and humans.[56] The major differences between the two strains of mice were associated with the length of the C-terminal regions and a critical alanine[375]-valine change in the ligand-binding domain, which is associated with the decreased binding affinity for TCDD for the AhR from DBA/2 mice. Interestingly, the ligand-binding region from the human

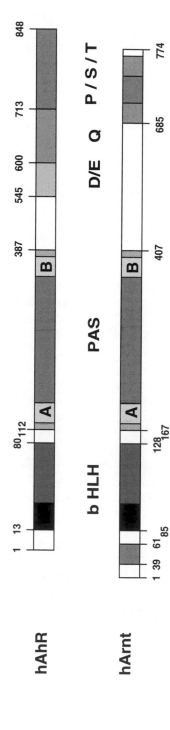

FIGURE 8.1 Structural domains of the AhR and Arnt proteins.

AhR resembles that described for the less Ah-responsive DBA/2 mouse strain.[56] Recent studies by Wilson and coworkers have identified a 39-kDa Arnt splice variant expressed in several estrogen receptor (ER)-negative human breast cancer cell lines and in some human mammary tumors.[61] This splice variant contains a large deletion in the transactivation domain and has been designated as TAD⁻Arnt.

8.1.4 MOLECULAR MECHANISMS OF AhR-MEDIATED TRANSACTIVATION

The heterodimeric nuclear AhR complex is ligand-induced transcription factor, and *cis*-genomic sequences were initially identified by several groups in the 5′-promoter regions of the rodent and human CYP1A1 genes.[62–68] The CYP1A1 gene promoter contains one or more copies of dioxin or xenobiotic responsive elements (DREs or XREs), which contain the following core binding sequence:

5′ - T - GCGTG - 3′
3″ - A - CGCAC - 5″

The core binding sequence is required for binding the nuclear AhR complex and transactivation; however, additional nucleotides are required for transactivation, and the following sequence has been proposed for a functional DRE/XRE:[69,70]

5′ - T/G N GCGTG A/C N G/C NNN - 3′
3′ - A/C N CGCAC T/G N C/G NNN - 5′

These enhancer elements have been identified in promoter regions of several Ah-responsive genes including CYP1A2,[71] CYP1B1,[72] NAD(P) quinone:oxidoreductase,[30] aldehyde-3-dehydrogenase,[31] glutathione S-transferase,[27,28] and glucuronyl transferase.[29] The generally accepted mechanism of AhR-mediated transactivation (Figure 8.2) is comparable to that described for other ligand-induced transcription factor complexes, namely, initial binding of ligand to the AhR, heterodimer formation, binding of the nuclear AhR complex with promoter elements (XRE/DRE), and interaction of the DNA-bound transcription factor complex with general transcription factors, coactivators, and other nuclear proteins required for transactivation (Figure 8.2).

Studies with Arnt- or AhR-defective mouse Hepa-1 cells have demonstrated that both proteins are required for induction of CYP1A1 gene expression by TCDD;[73–76] however, many other factors may play an important role in Ah-responsiveness. For example, proteins that bind a negative regulatory element (NRE) may modulate AhR-mediated transactivation in some cell lines.[77,78] Superinduction of CYP1A1 after treatment with cycloheximide suggests that labile inhibitory proteins may regulate induction of CYP1A1 in some cells.[79]

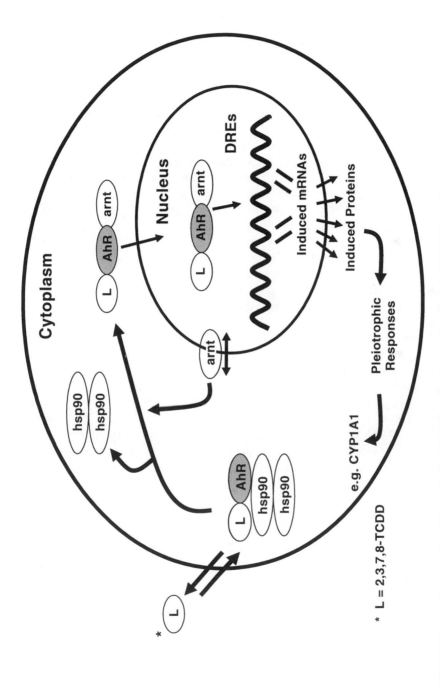

FIGURE 8.2 Proposed mechanism of ligand-induced AhR-mediated genes based on the CYP1A1 model.

8.1.5 MODULATION OF AH-RESPONSIVENESS BY THE ER IN HUMAN BREAST CANCER CELL LINES

Initial studies with both ER-negative and ER-positive breast cancer cell lines showed that while both cell lines express the AhR and Arnt and form a nuclear AhR complex after treatment with TCDD, induction of CYP1A1 was observed only in cells expressing the ER.[80,81] The requirement for ER expression on Ah-responsiveness was further investigated in transient transfection studies in both ER-negative MDA-MB-231[82] and Hs578T[83] cells transiently transfected with pRNH11c, a construct containing the -1142 to +2434 region of the CYP1A1 gene promoter linked to a bacterial chloramphenicol acetyl transferase (CAT) gene. The results (Figure 8.3) illustrate the cell-type specific restoration of Ah-responsiveness in cells cotransfected with pRNH11c and expression plasmids for the wild-type ER (hER), an N-terminal deletion variant containing the ligand-binding domain and activator function-2 (AF-2, HE19) and a C-terminal deletion variant containing AF-1 (HE15). TCDD induces CAT activity in MDA-MB-231 cells cotransfected with hER, HE15, or HE19; however, only HE19 restored inducibility in Hs578T cells. Crosstalk between the ER and AhR-mediated responses was further investigated in MDA-MBA-231 cells stably transfected with the ER. TCDD did not induce CYP1A or GST-P gene expression or their dependent activities; moreover, in transient transfection assays using pRNH11c or a construct containing a GST-P gene promoter insert, TCDD did not induce reporter gene activity.[84] These data suggest that cellular factors in addition to the ER are also required for restoring Ah-responsiveness in breast cancer cells.

The complexity of ER-AhR crosstalk was further complicated by results showing that there was not a strict correlation between ER expression and AhR-mediated gene expression. Treatment of ER-negative MDA-MB-468 breast cancer cells with TCDD resulted in formation of a nuclear AhR complex that also bound [^{32}P]DRE in a gel mobility shift assay to form an AhR-DRE retarded band.[85] TCDD also induced CYP1A1 gene expression and dependent activity, and the results showed that MDA-MB-468 cells represented the first ER-negative Ah-responsive human breast cancer cell line. Long-term culture of ER-positive MCF-7 cells in 1 μM benzo[a]pyrene resulted in isolation of resistant clones that exhibited altered genotypes.[86] BaP-resistant cells were E2 responsive and expressed the AhR and Arnt; however, TCDD did not induce CYP1A1 gene expression in this variant cell line. The nuclear AhR complex for BaP-resistant MCF-7 cells did not exhibit DNA binding in gel mobility shift assays, and the reasons for this defective binding are currently being investigated.

Wang and co-workers[87] extensively characterized the AhR from seven human cancer cell lines including both ER-positive MCF-7 and ER-negative MDA-MB-231 breast cancer cells. Photoaffinity labeling studies identified a 110-kDa protein in all cell lines; however, the sedimentation coefficient for the nuclear AhR complex from MDA-MB-231 cells was significantly lower (6.62 S) than observed for MCF-7 cells (7.23 S). Subsequent RT-PCR analysis for Arnt mRNA in MDA-MB-231 cells identified a major 1.3 kb transcript, whereas the expected 2.6 kb transcript was detected in MCF-7 cells.[61] The truncated Arnt protein was also observed by Western blot analysis using Arnt antibodies, and sequence analysis of the gene indicated that

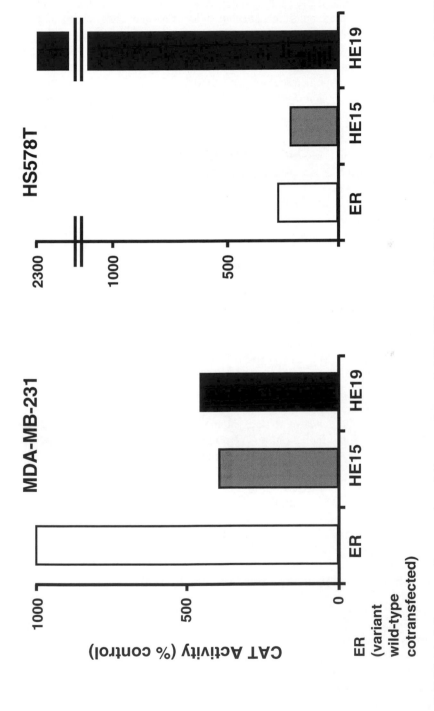

FIGURE 8.3 Cell-type-specific restoration of Ah-responsiveness in MDA-MB-231 and Hs578T human breast cancer cells treated with TCDD and transiently transfected with pRNH11c and wild-type (ER) or variant (HE15 or HE19) ER expression plasmids.

a splice variant transcript was expressed in which a major region of the C-terminal transactivation domain (TAD) had been deleted. The 36-kDa TAD⁻Arnt variant binds the AhR and forms a nuclear heterodimer that interacts with [^{32}P]DRE in gel mobility shift assay. However, the results indicate that deletion of the TAD region of Arnt results in loss of Ah-responsiveness. In contrast, the TAD⁻Arnt protein binds H1F1α and growth of MDA-MB 231 cells under conditions of hypoxia results in upregulation of hypoxia-responsive genes.[88] Thus, the TAD⁻Arnt protein interacts with H1F1α to form a functional heterodimer, and therefore the TAD is not required for hypoxia-responsiveness. Ongoing studies are probing the tissue- and cell-specific expression of TAD⁻Arnt to delineate the biological role of the Arnt variant.

8.2 INHIBITION OF ER-MEDIATED RESPONSES BY AHR AGONISTS: A NEW CLASS OF ANTIESTROGENS

8.2.1 INTRODUCTION

Several studies have reported that TCDD and related compounds inhibit diverse hormone/growth factor-mediated responses in animal and cellular models.[20] For example, TCDD inhibits epidermal growth factor (EGF) receptor binding or autophosphorylation in multiple species/tissues; however, the role of this response in AhR-mediated toxicity has not been determined.[89–94] Treatment of human keratinocytes[35] or MDA-MB-468[85] human breast cancer cells with TCDD increases TGFα mRNA and protein levels, and this is also accompanied by inhibition of MDA-MB-468 cell growth.[85] Subsequent studies showed that the growth-inhibitory response by TCDD was directly related to induction of TGFα, which exhibits antimitogenic activity in this cell line. In contrast, TCDD inhibits the mitogenic activity of TGFα, EGF, and insulin-like growth factor-1 (IGF-1) in MCF-7 or T47D cells.[95–97] TCDD modulates several steps in metabolism of cholesterol to various steroid hormones,[98,99] and induction of CYP1A1, CYP1A2, and CYP1B1 is associated with increased 2- and 4-steroid hydroxylase activities.[100–103] The antiestrogenic activity of AhR agonists has been intensively investigated in several laboratories, and this chapter primarily focuses on this response, which involves complex interactions between the AhR and ER signaling pathways.

8.2.2 ANTIESTROGENIC AND ANTIMITOGENIC ACTIVITY OF AhR AGONISTS

8.2.2.1 Inhibition of Mammary Tumor Growth by TCDD

Kociba and co-workers[104] first reported that female Sprague-Dawley rats administered TCDD (0.1, 0.01, or 0.001 μg/kg/day) developed hepatocellular carcinomas, whereas this response was not observed in male rats. A high incidence of spontaneous mammary and endometrial tumors was observed in control female rats; however, in animals treated with TCDD, there was a dose-dependent decrease in both tumors. Since formation of rodent mammary and endometrial cancer is E2-dependent, these results suggest that TCDD exhibits antiestrogenic activity, and this has been con-firmed in rodent models. TCDD inhibited 7,12-dimethylbenzanthracene (DMBA)-induced mammary tumor formation and growth in female Sprague-Dawley rats,[105] and similar results were reported in animals initiated with diethylnitrosamine.[106] Gierthy and coworkers also reported that TCDD inhibited mammary tumor growth in athymic B6D2F1 mice implanted with E2 pellets and bearing MCF-7 cell xenografts.[107] The antiestrogenic activity of TCDD observed in rodent tumor models has also been reported in individuals exposed to TCDD after an industrial accident in Seveso, Italy, in 1976. Serum levels of TCDD in some Seveso residents were among the highest ever reported (> 70,000 ppt). Severe chloracne was observed in many of the more highly exposed groups, and there was a high mortality in the exposed rodent population. Health surveys in Seveso have not shown significant long-term adverse health effects, although a recent study reported a higher female/male ratio in offspring of highly exposed individuals.[108,109] In addition, the incidence of both endometrial and breast cancer were lower than expected in women exposed to TCDD in the Seveso accident,[19] and these results were consistent with rodent studies.

8.2.2.2 Antiestrogenic Activity of TCDD and Related Compounds in Laboratory Animals

The rodent uterus is particularly sensitive to both estrogens and antiestrogens, and is extensively utilized as an *in vivo* bioassay. Gallo and co-workers first reported the antiestrogenic activity of TCDD and related compounds in the CD-1 mouse uterus, showing that TCDD blocked E2-induced uterine wet weight increase and decreased cytosolic and nuclear ER levels.[110–113] Johnson and co-workers also showed that while TCDD alone did not affect implantation in the hypophysectomized female rat, there was a 35% inhibition of estrone-induced implantation in animals cotreated with the hormone plus TCDD.[114] Brown and Lamartiniere also showed that after treatment of pubertal female Sprague-Dawley rats with TCDD, proliferation and development of the mammary gland were inhibited.[115]

Research in this laboratory has focused on the antiestrogenic activity of halo-genated aromatic hydrocarbons in the immature 25-day-old female Sprague-Dawley rat.[92,116–120] TCDD alone decreased gene expression/activities of several E2-regulated responses including uterine wet weight, peroxidase activity, cytosolic PR binding, c-*fos* mRNA, and EGF receptor mRNA levels. TCDD-induced effects were dose dependent, with the following order of sensitivity: EGF receptor mRNA > c-*fos* mRNA > peroxidase activity > uterine wet weight > cytosolic PR binding. The dose-dependent antiestrogenic activity of TCDD for these same responses was not deter-mined over a range of doses; however, the antiestrogenic potency of TCDD followed a comparable response-dependent order of sensitivity. The results were similar to those recently reported by Hyder and coworkers using the direct-acting antiestrogen ICI 182, 780.[121] Their studies showed that E2 induced both vascular endothelial growth factor (VEGF) and c-*fos* gene expression in the rodent uterus, and ICI 182,780 inhibited both responses but at different doses.

3,3',4,4',5-Pentachlorobiphenyl is the most potent AhR agonist among the PCBs, and the effects of this compound on cyclicity and ovarian follicles was determined in female Sprague-Dawley rats treated with different doses (0.025 to 7,500 ng/kg) on days 17 to 19 post-conception.[122] Vaginal opening and the start of estrous cyclicity was delayed in the offspring of the exposed animals, and several other responses including altered follicles and decreased serum hormone levels were observed. It was suggested that these responses may be related, in part, to inhibitory AhR-ER crosstalk. Buchanan and coworkers have also investigated the antiestrogenic activity of TCDD in the uterus using knockout mice and tissue recombination studies.[123,124] Their results suggest that inhibition of E2-induced uterine epithelial responses may be due to activation of stromal AhR pathways, which subsequently alter induced epithelial effects. Similar stromal-epithelial interactions have previously been reported for ERα-dependent hormone-induced uterine responses in mice. These data suggest that inhibitory AhR-ER crosstalk is functional in multiple hormone-response tissues/cells in rodent models.

8.2.2.3 Antiestrogenic Activity of TCDD and Related Compounds in Human Breast Cancer Cells

8.2.2.3.1 MCF-7 and T47D Cells

MCF-7 human breast cancer cells have been used extensively as an *in vitro* model for investigating E2-regulated responses and gene expression, effects, and mechanism of action of antiestrogens.[125,126] MCF-7 cells express relatively high levels of ERα, and E2 induces cell proliferation and expression of several genes and related activities. Both the AhR and Arnt proteins are also expressed in MCF-7 cells, and, after treatment with TCDD and related HAHs, a nuclear AhR complex is rapidly formed, resulting in induction of CYP1A1 mRNA levels and CYP1A1-dependent activities.[87,127] Based on the Ah- and E2-responsiveness of this cell line, studies on the crosstalk between the AhR- and ER-mediated signaling pathways have been investigated. Gierthy and coworkers first showed that TCDD inhibited E2-induced secretion of tissue plasminogen activator activity and postconfluent focus production in MCF-7 cells.[128,129] Subsequent studies have shown that TCDD and related compounds inhibit E2-induced cell proliferation in ER-positive MCF-7 and T47D cells, and a diverse spectrum of other responses were also inhibited by AhR agonists. TCDD inhibits E2-induced secretion of tissue plasminogen activator activity, pS2, 160-, 52-, and 34-kDa proteins; progesterone receptor (PR) binding; lactate formation; pS2, cathepsin D, prolactin receptor, and PR mRNA levels; postconfluent focus production; cell proliferation; and reporter gene activity in cells transiently transfected with plasmids containing inserts derived from the pS2, cathepsin D, and vitellogenin A2 genes.[127–140] Ongoing studies in this laboratory have shown that several other E2-induced genes or their derived E2-responsive plasmids are inhibited after cotreatment with TCDD, and these include TGFα, bcl-2, insulin-like growth factor binding protein 4 (IGFBP-4), c-fos, retinoic acid receptor α1, cyclin D1, E2F1, heat shock protein 27 (Hsp 27), and creatine kinase B (unpublished results). These data clearly demonstrate that crosstalk between the AhR and ER results in inhibition of diverse E2-regulated genes and responses, which is comparable to that observed for direct-acting "pure antiestrogens" such as ICI 164,384 and 182,780.[141] A functional iDRE has been identified near the start site of the Hsp27 gene promoter[142]; however, there is also evidence for iDRE-independent pathways.

8.2.2.3.2   Inhibition of Growth Factor-Induced Responses

Research in this laboratory has also shown that TCDD inhibits TGFα, EGF, IGF-1, and insulin-induced proliferation of MCF-7 or T47D human breast cancer cells and E2-induced IGFBP-4 expression in MCF-7 cells.[95–97,143] Figure 8.4 illustrates results of recent studies that demonstrate both the antiestrogenic and antimitogenic activities of TCDD using MCF-7 cells. Although mechanisms of growth factor-AhR crosstalk are unknown, TCDD modulates components of growth factor signaling. For example, TCDD alone did not affect IGF-1 receptor mRNA levels or K_D values; however, TCDD significantly decreased IGF-1-induced IGF receptor binding sites.[97] TCDD alone did not affect K_D and B_{max} values for binding of [^{125}I]insulin to the insulin receptor (IR) but decreased the K_D value for IR-ligand binding and increased B_{max} in cells cotreated with TCDD and insulin.[143] TCDD also inhibited insulin-induced phosphorylation of the IR. Differentiation of ovarian granulosa cells is accompanied by increased expression of luteinizing hormone receptor (LHR), and both follicle-stimulating hormone (FSH) and IGF-1 enhance LH mRNA levels in granulosa cells in culture. However, treatment with TCDD decreases basal and induced LH mRNA levels, thereby compromising ovarian granulosa cell function.[144] Current studies are focused on determining the mechanism of growth factor-AhR crosstalk and the role of the ER in mediating these interactions.

8.2.2.3.3   Inhibition of ER-Negative Breast Cancer Cell Growth by TCDD[85]

The antiestrogenic activities of AhR agonists have primarily been investigated in E2-responsive human breast cancer cell lines, and most studies have demonstrated a correlation between Ah- and E2-responsiveness. These results suggest that the potential clinical utility of AhR agonists for treatment of breast cancer would be limited to ER-positive tumors. However, after screening a number of ER-negative breast cancer cell lines, it was shown that ER-negative MDA-MB-468 cells expressed the AhR, and TCDD induced CYP1A1 gene expression, ethoxyresorufin *O*-deethylase (EROD) activity, and CAT activity in cells transiently transfected with pRNH11c. These data established MDA-MB-468 cells as the first ER-negative Ah-responsive breast cancer cell line. Previous studies showed that cytotoxic drugs and EGF inhibited growth of MDA-MB-468 cells, and the unusual antimitogenic activity of EGF was accompanied by increased expression of EGF receptor, c-*myc* and c-*fos* protooncogene levels, and increased apoptosis. TCDD also significantly decreased growth of MDA-MB-468 cells and increased EGF receptor mRNA levels; however, TCDD did not induce c-*fos* or *myc* gene expression and was significantly less active than EGF as an inducer of apoptosis. EGF protein and mRNA levels are expressed at low levels in this cell line, and TCDD did not significantly modulate this response. Subsequent studies showed that TCDD increased TGFα mRNA and immunoreactive protein levels in MDA-MB-468 cells, and antibodies directed against the EGF receptor blocked the antimitogenic activity of TCDD. Since TGFα

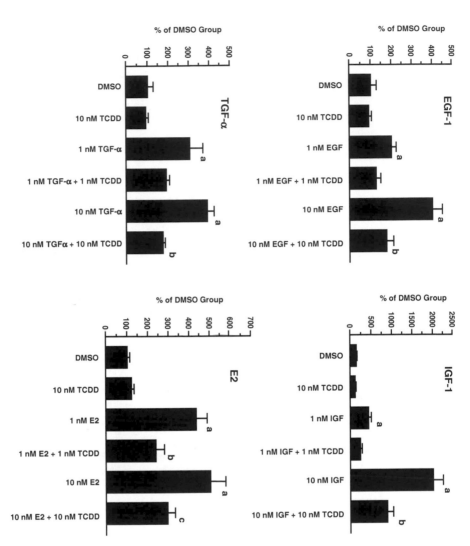

FIGURE 8.4 Effects of EGF, IGF-1, TGF-α, and E2 on proliferation of MCF-7 cells and the growth inhibitory activity of TCDD.

protein alone also inhibited proliferation of MDA-MB-468 cells, the results of this study showed that the antimitogenic activity of TCDD in this ER-negative cell line was associated with induction of TGFα protein. These data illustrate the unusual breast cancer cell-specific antimitogenic activity of TCDD, which inhibits TGFα and growth factor-induced proliferation of ER-positive breast cancer cells (Figure 8.4) but induces TGFα protein, which is antimitogenic in ER-negative MDA-MB-468 cells.

TCDD and related compounds inhibit growth of ER-independent pancreatic and prostate cancer cell lines, and in the former cells, this was associated with upregulation of p21 expression.[145,146] In parallel studies, AhR expression and function has

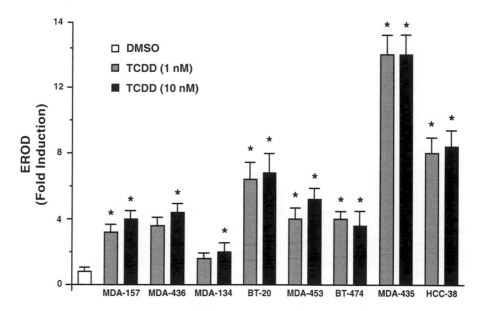

FIGURE 8.5 Ah-responsiveness of ER-negative breast cancer cells. Several ER-negative cell lines were treated with 1 or 10 nM TCDD for 24 hours and EROD activity was determined fluorimetrically. Significant ($p < 0.05$) induction compared to DMSO control is indicated by an asterisk.

been investigated in several ER-negative breast cancer cell lines. Results illustrated in Figure 8.5 show that TCDD induces AhR-dependent ethoxyresorufin *O*-deethylase activity in MDA-MB-157, MDA-MB-436, MDA-MB-134, BT-20, MDA-MB-453, BT-474, MDA-MB-435, and HCC-38 cells, and in parallel studies, TCDD and related compounds also inhibited proliferation of these ER-negative breast cancer cell lines. However, the mechanisms of TCDD-induced growth inhibition are not related to modulation of p21, other cell cycle regulated genes, or kinase activities, and current studies are investigating other potential AhR-dependent pathways that influence ER-negative breast cancer cell proliferation.

8.2.2.3.4 Inhibition of E2-Induced Cell Cycle Enzymes by TCDD

Recent studies in this laboratory have also focused on ER-AhR crosstalk associated with cell cycle enzymes. Several studies have reported that E2 decreases cells in G0/G1 and increases cells in S phase,[147–150] and the pure antiestrogen ICI 182,780 inhibits many of these estrogenic responses. The specific cell cycle enzymes in MCF-7 cells, which are modulated by E2, show some variability between studies; however, cyclin-dependent kinase 2 (cdk2) and cdk4-associated activities are increased, and retinoblastoma (RB) protein phosphorylation, E2F1 protein, cyclin D1 mRNA, and protein levels are elevated. Results of recent studies in this laboratory showed that in addition to these responses, E2 also affected the cdk-activating kinase (CAK) that contains cyclin H/cdk7 proteins and plays an important role in phosphorylation (and activation) of both cdk2 and cdk4 at threonine-160 and threonine-170, respectively.[151]

Although E2 did not affect levels of cyclin H protein, cdk7 levels were increased 2.1-fold 24 hours after treatment. Activation of cdk2/cdk4 is also dependent on cdc25 phosphatase-mediated hydrolysis of tyrosine 15, and in MCF-7 cells treated with E2 there was a significant increase (> twofold) in cdc 25 protein. Thus, treatment with cells with E2 activates multiple cell cycle proteins and related activity and thereby offers multiple targets for the indirect antiestrogenic activity of TCDD. Like ICI 182,780, TCDD inhibits cells from E2-induced progression into S phase and, in MCF-7 cells cotreated with E2 plus TCDD, there was selective inhibition of hormone-induced effects on cell cycle enzymes. For example, TCDD significantly inhibited the following E2-induced responses in MCF-7 cells: E2F1 protein, cyclin D protein and mRNA levels, phosphorylation of RB, and inhibition of cdk2-, cdk4, and cdk-7 associated kinase activities. Interestingly, TCDD alone had minimal effects on most cell cycle enzymes; however, in cells cotreated with E2 plus TCDD, there was a significant increase in p21 levels, and this response may contribute to decreased cdk2- and cdk4-associated activities. Ongoing studies in this laboratory are focused on delineating the molecular mechanisms of AhR crosstalk with hormone-regulated cell cycle enzymes in both *in vitro* and *in vivo* models.

8.2.2.4 Mechanisms of AhR-Mediated Antiestrogenicity

8.2.2.4.1 Role of the AhR

Several different approaches have been utilized to demonstrate that the antiestrogenic activities of TCDD and related compounds are mediated via binding to the AhR and formation of a functional nuclear AhR complex. Structure-antiestrogenicity relationships have been observed for several *in vivo* and *in vitro* responses, including inhibition of E2-induced uterine wet weight increase, uterine PR binding and peroxidase activity (*in vivo*), downregulation of the ER, and secretion of procathepsin D in MCF-7 breast cancer cells.[92,117,136,137,140,152] In all of these studies, there was an excellent rank order correlation between structure-antiestrogenicity and structure receptor binding affinities (or AhR-mediated activities) for several HAHs. Cell lines with known defects in AhR signaling have also been utilized in these studies. For example, TCDD inhibited E2-induced reporter gene activity in wild-type Ah-responsive mouse Hepa-1 cells transiently cotransfected with an hER expression plasmid and E2-responsive constructs derived from the vitellogenin A2, cathepsin D, or pS2 genes.[133,137,140] In contrast, antiestrogenic activities were not observed in Ah-defective Hepa-1 variant cell lines. Gillesby and coworkers also showed that TCDD did not affect reporter gene activity induced by E2 in Hepa-1 C4 (Arnt-defective) or C12 (AhR-defective) cells transiently transfected with an E2-responsive pS2-luc plasmid.[137] However, the antiestrogenic activity of TCDD in C4 and C12 cells was restored in these cells after cotransfection with Arnt or AhR expression plasmids, respectively.

BaP[r] MCF-7 cells express both the AhR and Arnt; however, this cell line is Ah-nonresponsive due to failure of the nuclear AhR to bind DNA as determined in gel mobility shift assays using [^{32}P]DRE.[86] Utilizing both wild-type and variant BaP[r] MCF-7 cells, it was shown that E2 induced cell proliferation, secretion of cathepsin D, and CAT activity (in cells transiently transfected with a plasmid containing an

E2-responsive vitellogenin A2 gene promoter insert); however, in cells treated with TCDD plus E2, antiestrogenic responses were observed only in wild-type but not BaP[r] cells. Results from both structure-activity relationships and Ah-defective cell lines strongly support a role for the nuclear AhR in mediating the antiestrogenic activity of TCDD and related HAHs.

8.2.2.4.2 Induction of E2 Hydroxylase Activities

TCDD induces CYP1A1 and CYP1B1 gene expression in MCF-7 cells, and this is accompanied by an increased rate of E2 metabolism and E2 2-, 4-, 15α-, and 16-hydroxylase activities.[100–103,153] Spink and co-workers[100–103,153] suggested that induced hormone metabolism and subsequent depletion of cellular E2 levels may be responsible for the antiestrogenic activity of TCDD. While this response may contribute to AhR-mediated antiestrogenic activity in cell culture studies, there is ample evidence showing antiestrogenic responses that are independent of induced E2 metabolism. For example, (a) several weak AhR agonists such as 6-methyl-1,3,8-triCDF (6-MCDF) and indole-3-carbinol (I3C) exhibit antiestrogenic activity at concentrations that do not induce CYP1A1;[120] (b) TCDD induces cathepsin D gene expression and glucose ÷ lactate conversion at time points (# 2 hours) that precede induction of CYP1A1 protein-dependent activities;[134] (c) induction of ERE-regulated reporter gene activities in transient transfection experiment are not inhibited by TCDD, indicating that increased oxidative metabolism of E2 is not accompanied by an antiestrogenic response;[140] (d) transient transfection studies using a construct derived from the pS2 gene promoter and various ligand (E2)-dependent or -independent chimeric ERs showed that TCDD inhibited reporter gene activity using ligand-independent chimeras (HE15 and ER$_c$VP16);[137] and (e) circulating E2 levels were not affected after *in vivo* treatment of rodents with TCDD. These results and additional data from mechanistic studies suggest that induced oxidative metabolism of E2 is not a primary mechanism of AhR-mediated antiestrogenicity.[154]

8.2.2.4.3 Inhibitory DREs (iDREs) as Genomic Targets for the AhR

Results of preliminary screening studies in this laboratory showed that some E2-inducible genes or constructs containing promoter inserts were inhibited by TCDD within 2 to 4 hours after treatment, suggesting that the inhibitory response was probably not related to induction of a new gene product. For example, in nuclear run-on assays with nuclei from cells treated with E2 for 24 hours and TCDD for 60 minutes, there was a > 70% decrease in cathepsin D mRNA levels induced by E2.[133] These results suggested that the inhibitory response may be mediated directly by the nuclear AhR complex, which is formed rapidly after treatment of MCF-7 cells with TCDD. Subsequent studies in this laboratory identified 3 E2-responsive enhancer sequences in the proximal region of the cathepsin D gene promoter, including an Sp1(N)$_{23}$ERE-half site at -199 to -165, an imperfect palindromic ERE at -119 to -107 and a GC-rich Sp1 binding site -145 to -135 (Figure 8.5A).[133,155,156]

Two unusual motifs that involve formation of a transcriptionally active ER/Sp1 protein complex mediate E2-induced transactivation. The Sp1(N)$_{23}$ERE(2) sequence binds nuclear extracts from MCF-7 cells to form a protein-DNA complex that requires intact Sp1 and ERE(2) sequences; the GC-rich site binds only the Sp1 protein; however, the ER mediates transactivation via ER-Sp1 (protein-protein) interactions, which may involve other proteins that stabilize ER/Sp1 complex formation. Studies in this laboratory have identified other E2-responsive GC-rich sites on the c-*fos* protooncogene and retinoic acid receptor α1 gene promoters. The Sp1 binding site at within the −145 to −135 region of the cathepsin D gene promoter forms an ER/Sp1-DNA complex (binding to the GC-rich site) but also requires cooperative interactions with an adjacent core DRE site that binds unliganded nuclear AhR complex. Results of transient transfection and gel mobility shift assays using wild-type and mutant oligonucleotides show that E2-responsiveness of this region of the promoter involves an ER/Sp1-AhR/Arnt complex interacting with an Sp1(N)$_4$DRE motif.[156]

At least two function iDREs have been identified within the −200 to −100 region of the cathepsin D gene promoter; and iDRE1 has been extensively characterized using the wild-type Sp1(N)$_{23}$ERE(2) oligonucleotide in gel mobility shift and transient transfection assays (see Figure 8.5B). Interaction of the liganded AhR complex with iDRE1 results in disruption of the ER/Sp1-DNA complex and loss of transactivation in transient transfection assays. Moreover, using a bromodeoxyuridine-substituted Sp1(N)$_{23}$ERE(2) oligonucleotide, the AhR complex could be crosslinked to the DNA sequence.[133] In contrast, an Sp1(N)$_{23}$ERE(2) oligonucleotide containing a mutant iDRE motif bound nuclear extracts to form an ER/Sp1-DNA complex and was E2-responsive in transient transfection assays; however, the inhibitory effects of the AhR complex were not observed in these studies. A comparable approach has also been utilized for characterizing other functional iDREs in the pS2, Hsp 27, and c-*fos* gene promoters. Current research is focused on identifying functional iDREs in other genes and investigating alternative mechanisms associated with AhR-mediated antiestrogenic activity.

8.2.2.4.4   AhR-Dependent Activation of ERα Degradation by Proteasomes

Several studies have reported that AhR agonists induce degradation of ERα in breast cancer cells and in the rodent uterus.[152,157–159] Both TCDD and E2 induce rapid degradation of ERα in ZR-75, T47D, and MCF-7 breast cancer cell lines, and TCDD (but not E2) also induces AhR degradation. Ligand-dependent degradation of both receptors was inhibited by proteasome but not protease inhibitors. AhR-ERα crosstalk was observed in cells cotreated with both E2 plus TCDD, and this resulted in extremely low levels of cellular ERα expression. Subsequent studies showed that in cells cotreated with E2 plus different concentrations of TCDD, there was a correlation between decreasing levels of ERα and decreased E2-induced transactivation using an ERE promoter construct. These results suggest that for some E2-regulated genes, the inhibitory effects of TCDD and other AhR agonists may be due, in part, to limiting levels of ERα expression.

8.2.2.4.5   Other Mechanisms of Inhibitory AhR-ERα Crosstalk

It has been reported that the AhR and ER interact with common nuclear coactivators such as the steroid receptor coactivators, and it is possible that inhibitory AhR-ERα crosstalk may be related to competition for limiting levels of common coactivators.[160-165] For example, a recent report showed activation of ERE- or DRE-dependent promoters can be inhibited or squelched by cotransfection with wild-type or deletion mutant AhR or ERα expression plasmids.[165] Rogers and Denison[166] reported that inhibitory interactions of the AhR and ERα in BG-1 ovarian cancer cells may involve induction of an inhibitory factor (protein) by TCDD, since the effects were blocked by the protein synthesis inhibitor cycloheximide. Ongoing studies in this laboratory with several E2-responsive genes including E2F1, carbamoylphosphate synthetase/aspartate transcarbamylase/dihydroorotase (cad), and retinoic acid receptor α show that inhibition by TCDD is cell context dependent and not due to limiting levels of ERα. The inhibitory mechanisms have not yet been determined but evidence suggests that competition by AhR and ERα for Sp1 binding may be important. A recent report[167] showed a new and unexpected interaction between the AhR and ERα in which AhR agonists induced estrogenic activities in breast/endometrial cancer cell lines and in the mouse uterus. Most of the studies used 3-methylcholanthrene (MC) as the AhR ligand, and in some experiments MC induced estrogenic activity but also inhibited E2-induced responses in cotreatment studies. Recent studies in this laboratory[168] showed that in the absence of the AhR, TCDD exhibited estrogenic activity, and it is possible that the estrogenic responses observed for MC may also be due to direct activation of ERα. The estrogenic mechanisms associated with MC and other AhR agonists is currently being investigated.

8.2.3 DEVELOPMENT OF AhR-BASED ANTIESTROGENS FOR TREATMENT OF BREAST CANCER

8.2.3.1 Introduction

Results reported in this review clearly demonstrate that AhR agonists exhibit antiestrogenic activities in the rodent uterus/mammary and in human breast cancer cell lines. There is also evidence from human studies that the AhR agonists exhibit antiestrogenic activities. For example, women in Seveso, Italy, exposed to TCDD following an industrial accident in 1976, exhibit lower incidence of mammary and endometrial tumors.[19] Epidemiology studies have shown that the incidence of endometrial cancer is significantly reduced among cigarette smokers,[169,170] and this corresponds to their exposure to AhR agonists such as PAHs.[171] The effects of cigarette smoking in breast cancer incidence is variable, and this may be due to protective (antiestrogenic) effects of PAHs in smoke and the genotoxicity of the same compounds. The major problems for development of clinically useful AhR-based antiestrogens are comparable to the design of other drugs, namely the compounds should exhibit maximal efficacy in target organs (breast and endometrium) but minimal toxic side effects in non-target tissues. The following two classes of AhR-based antiestrogens have been developed in this laboratory; namely, alternate-substituted alkyl PCDFs and substituted diindolylmethanes (DIMs) and their low toxicity coupled with high antitumorigenic activity indicate that these compounds are promising new drugs for treatment of breast cancer in women.

8.2.3.2   Alternate-Substituted PCDFs

A series of 6-alkyl-1,3,8-trichlorodibenzofurans (triCDFs) were originally synthesized for investigating their activities as partial AhR antagonists, and 6-methyl-1,3,8-
trichlorodibenzofuran (6-MCDF) was used as a prototype for this series of compounds. 6-MCDF competitively bound with moderate affinity to the rodent cytosolic
AhR but was a relatively weak agonist for several AhR-mediated biochemical and
toxic responses including induction of CYP1A1 and CYP1A2 in rats and cells in
culture; porphyria, immunotoxicity, and cleft palate (teratogenicity) in mice.[118,172–175]
Since 6-MCDF was a weak AhR agonist, it was hypothesized that 6-MCDF may be
a partial AhR antagonist. This was confirmed in several studies that showed that 6-
MCDF inhibited induction of CYP1A1 and CYP1A2 by TCDD in rats and fetal
cleft palate, porphyria, and immunotoxicity in C57BL/6 mice.

Results of preliminary studies showed that 6-MCDF did not antagonize TCDD-
induced antiestrogenicity in the female rat uterus but appeared to be a relatively
potent antiestrogen. Astroff and Safe[118] reported that both TCDD and 6-MCDF
caused a dose-dependent decrease in nuclear and cytosolic ER and PR binding in
21- to 25-day-old female Sprague-Dawley rats, and that 6-MCDF was only 300 to
570 times less active than TCDD as an antiestrogen. In contrast, TCDD was
> 157,000 times more potent than 6-MCDF as an inducer of hepatic CYP1A1 in
the same animals (a surrogate for toxic potency). Subsequent studies showed that
6-MCDF and related compounds inhibited E2-induced hypertrophy, peroxidase
activity, cytosolic ER and PR binding, and EGF receptor and c-fos mRNA levels in
the rat uterus.[92,118,119,176] 6-MCDF is also active in MCF-7 human breast cancer cells
and, at concentrations of 10^{-7} to 10^{-6} M, inhibits a diverse spectrum of E2-induced
responses.[177]

An extensive structure-antiestrogenicity study of 15 alternate-substituted
(2,4,6,8- and 1,3,6,8-) alkyl-PCDFs was carried out in MCF-7 cells using three
E2-induced responses, namely cell proliferation, induction of CAT activity in cells
transiently transfected with an E2-responsive Vit-CAT plasmid, and induction of
EROD activity.[178] The results showed that the antiestrogenic activities of these
congeners were response specific, and ten of the compounds were active in only
one of the assays for antiestrogenicity (i.e., inhibition of E2-induced cell growth or
CAT activity). Five compounds were active in both assays: 6-MCDF, 6-ethyl-1,3,8-
triCDF, 6-isopropyl-1,3,8-triCDF, 3-isopropyl-6-methyl-1,8-diCDF, and 6-methyl-
2,4,8-triCDF.

The *in vivo* antiestrogenic activity of a series of alkyl-substituted PCDFs has
been investigated in the immature female Sprague-Dawley rat uterus.[179] The compounds utilized in this study contain two, three, or four lateral substituents and
include 6-MCDF, 6-ethyl-1,3,8-triCDF, 6-*n*-propyl-1,3,8-triCDF, 6-*i*-propyl-1,3,8-
triCDF, 6-*t*-butyl-1,3,8-triCDF, and 8-MCDF (two lateral substituents); 6-methyl-
2,3,8-triCDF, 6-methyl-2,3,4,8-tetraCDF, 8-methyl-1,3,7-triCDF, and 8-methyl-
1,2,4,7-tetraCDF (three lateral substituents); and 8-methyl-2,3,7-triCDF and
8-methyl-2,3,4,7-tetraCDF (four lateral substituents). Two additional compounds,
8-methyl-2,3,7-trichlorodibenzo-*p*-dioxin and 8-methyl-2,3,7-tribromodibenzo-*p*-
dioxin (four lateral substituents), were also investigated. All alkyl-substituted

compounds inhibited estrogen-induced uterine wet weight increase and cytosolic and nuclear PR and ER binding. Quantitative structure-antiestrogenicity relationships were determined using 6-*i*-propyl-1,3,8-triCDF, 6-methyl-2,3,4,8-tetraCDF, and 8-methyl-2,3,4,7-tetraCDF as representative congeners containing two, three, and four lateral substituents, respectively. The ED_{50} values for antiestrogenicity were similar for the three compounds; however, the ED_{50} values for induction of hepatic CYP1A1-dependent activity were 73,600 (estimated), 8.52, and 5.31 μmol/kg for 6-*i*-propyl-1,3,8-triCDF, 6-methyl-2,3,4,8-tetraCDF, and 8-methyl-2,3,4,7-tetraCDF, respectively. Based on results of previous studies, CYP1A1 can be used as a surrogate for toxic potency in the rat; therefore, high ED_{50} (induction)/ED_{50} (antiestrogenicity) ratios would be indicative of low toxicity and high antiestrogenic potency. The ratio was 13,990 to 17,100 for 6-*i*-propyl-1,3,8-triCDF, whereas corresponding ratios for the compounds with three and four lateral substituents varied from 0.64 to 3.34. These data suggest that alternate 1,3,6,8-substituted alkyl PCDFs are useful structural models for developing new AhR-mediated antiestrogens for treatment of breast cancer.

The *in vivo* antitumorigenic activity of 6-MCDF, 8-MCDF, and 6-cyclohexyl-1,3,8-triCDF (6-CHDF) were investigated in the DMBA rat mammary tumor model.[180] At doses of 5, 10, or 25 mg/kg/week, 6- and 8-MCDF significantly inhibited mammary tumor growth, and at the 5 mg/kg/week dose, > 50% growth inhibition was observed for both isomers. In contrast, 6-CHDF was inactive at the 5 mg/kg/week dose, and the structure-antitumorigenicity relationships (6-/8-MCDF >> 6-CHDF) correlated with structure-antiestrogenicity (rat uterus) studies and the relative binding affinities of these compounds for the AhR. The antitumorigenic activity of 6- or 8-MCDF in the mammary was not accompanied by any significant changes in liver/body weight ratios, liver morphology, or induction of hepatic CYP1A1-dependent activity, which is one of the most sensitive indicators of exposure to AhR agonists. RT-PCR and Western blot analysis of mammary tumor mRNA and protein extracts, respectively, confirmed the presence of the AhR, suggesting that AhR-mediated signaling pathways are functional in rat mammary tumors.

The effects of other alternate-substituted PCDFs have also been investigated. The results (Figure 8.6) clearly demonstrate that CH_3-substituted 1,3,6,8- and 2,4,6,8-PCDFs and other 6-alkyl PCDFs were potent antitumorigenic compounds. Dose-response studies with 6-isopropyl-1,3,8-triCDF showed that inhibition of mammary tumor growth was observed at doses as low as 0.5 mg/kg/week. Ongoing studies are investigating other alternated-substituted PCDFs to delineate specific congeners that can be further developed for clinical applications.

8.2.3.3 Substituted DIMs

Indole-3-carbinol (I3C) is found as a conjugate in cruciferous vegetables such as broccoli, Brussels sprouts, and cauliflower,[181] and results of several studies indicate that I3C is both anticarcinogenic and antiestrogenic in several bioassays.[182-191] For example, I3C, related compounds, and Brussels sprouts inhibit carcinogen-induced mammary tumors in female Sprague-Dawley rats;[188,189] dietary I3C decreases spontaneous mammary tumor incidence in C3H/OuJ mice; and I3C also inhibits spon-

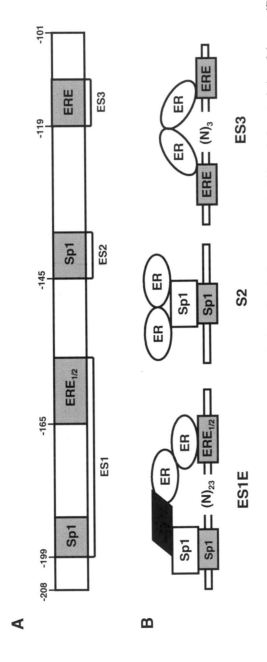

FIGURE 8.6 Identification of three E2 responsive enhancer elements in the cathepsin D gene promoter (A), and characteristics of the core iDRE (-175 to -181) in the same promoter (B).

taneous endometrial cancer formation in female Donryu rats.[191] I3C was administered either prior to or during carcinogen administration and the anticarcinogenic effects are associated, in part, with induction of both phase I and phase II drug-metabolizing enzymes, including CYP1A1, CYP1A2, CYP2B1, CYP3A1, epoxide hydrolase, glutathione S-transferase, glucuronyl transferase, and NAD(P)H:quinone oxidoreductase.[189,192–206]

I3C is unstable in an acidic environment (such as the gut) and rapidly undergoes oligomerization to give a mixture of condensation products, including diindolylmethane (DIM) (dimer), 5,6,11,12,17,18-hexahydrocyclononal[1,2-b:4,5-b′:7,8-b″]triindole, [2-(indol-3-ylmethyl)indol-3-yl]indol-3-ylmethane, 3,3′-bis(indol-3-ylmethyl)indolenine, cyclic and linear tetramers of I3C, and indolo[3,2-b]carbazole (ICZ).[193,197,202,206,207] I3C binds weakly to the AhR, and the higher molecular weight condensation products exhibit increased binding affinity for this receptor.[201,206]

Previous studies have demonstrated that incubation of I3C with breast cancer cells results in formation of DIM, and both compounds induce CYP1A1 gene expression;[202–204] however, the concentrations required for an induction response were > 30 (DIM) or > 100 µM (I3C).[208] Ongoing studies in this laboratory have focused on the AhR agonist activities of DIM in MCF-7 cells.[209] The results show that after treatment of cells with DIM, there is depletion of cytosolic AhR, which rapidly translocates into the nucleus and forms an AhR-[^{32}P]DRE complex in a gel mobility shift assay; nuclear extracts form a 200-kDa crosslinked band after photo-induced crosslinking with bromodeoxyuridine-substituted DRE. These results are consistent with a ligand-induced AhR-mediated response (e.g., Figure 8.2). However, it is clear from the results that antiestrogenic responses are observed at concentrations lower (0.1 to 60 µM) than required for induction of CYP1A1 gene expression (30 to 100 µM). Moreover, at a concentration of 10 µM, nuclear extracts from cells treated with DIM form a retarded band with [^{32}P]DRE and, like MCDF, DIM forms a nuclear AhR complex at concentrations that exhibit antiestrogenic activity but do not induce CYP1A1.

The antitumorigenic activity of DIM in the DMBA-induced rat mammary tumor model[209] was similar to that previously observed for alternate-substituted alkyl PCDFs.[180] At an oral dose of 5 mg/kg every second day, DIM significantly inhibited mammary tumor growth (Figure 8.7), but this was not accompanied by any changes in body or organ weights and histopathology (kidney, spleen, heart, uterus, or liver). Moreover, DIM did not induce hepatic microsomal EROD activity. Results of preliminary studies with other substituted-DIM and some I3C analogs show that these compounds inhibit rat mammary tumor growth at doses between 1 and 5 mg/kg (every other day), and current studies are focused on development of substituted-I3C/DIM compounds that can be used for clinical treatment of breast cancer in women.

The antiestrogenic/antitumorigenic activity of alternate-substituted PCDFs and DIM analogs is observed *in vivo* at doses that do not induce hepatic CYP1A1, which is one of the most sensitive indicators of exposure to toxic AhR agonists such as HAHs. Ligand-dependent differences in activity have been observed for other compounds that bind steroid hormone such as the ER. A possible mechanism for AhR ligand-dependent differences is illustrated in Figure 8.8 using MCDF and TCDD as

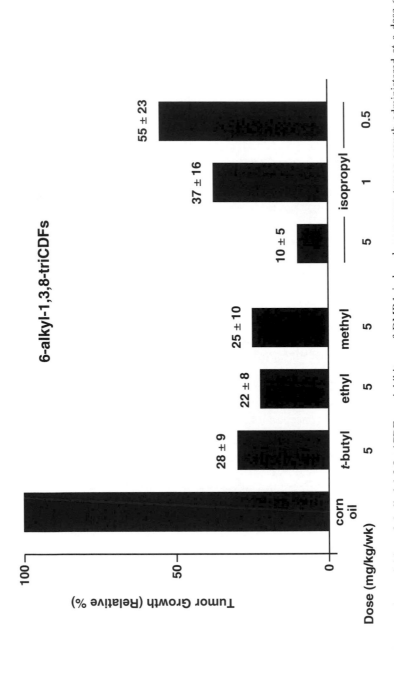

FIGURE 8.7 Comparative activities of 6-alkyl-1,3,8-triCDFs as inhibitors of DMBA-induced mammary tumor growth administered at a dose of 5 mg/kg/week.

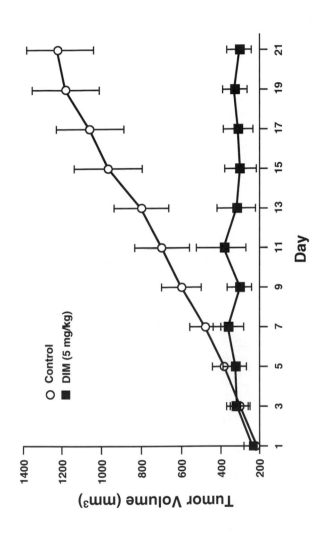

FIGURE 8.8 Inhibition of mammary tumor growth in vehicle (○) or DIM (■, 5 mg/kg every second day) treated female Sprague-Dawley rats initiated with DMBA.

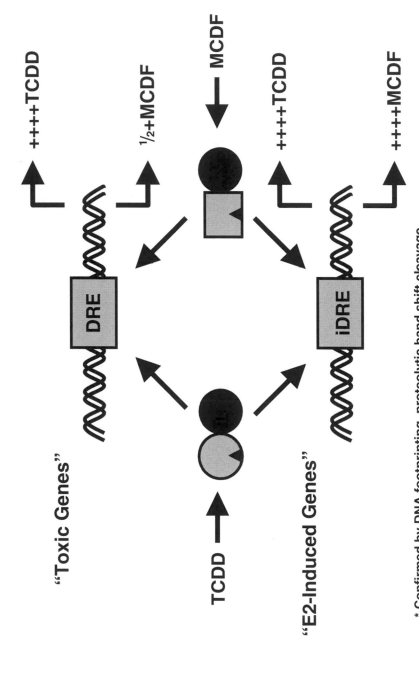

FIGURE 8.9 Proposed mechanism for ligand-dependent differences in the mechanisms of action of TCDD and MCDF.

models. Both ligands induce rapid formation of a nuclear AhR complex, and TCDD induces a complete spectrum of AhR-mediated responses including antiestrogenicity, induction of CYP1A1, and toxicity. In contrast, MCDF (or DIM) exhibits antiestrogenic activity at doses/concentrations that do not induce CYP1A1 and are not toxic. This suggests that MCDF (or DIM) induces conformational changes in the nuclear AhR complex that allow binding to iDREs associated with inhibition of E2-induced genes; in contrast, the MCDF-AhR complex exhibits ineffective binding to DREs in promoters of CYP1A1 and other genes that play a role in toxic response pathways.

Santostefano and Safe[210] studied ligand-dependent (e.g., TCDD versus MCDF) differences in properties of the transformed cytosolic or nuclear AhR complex using a proteolytic clipping band shift assay. The results showed that there were significant differences in the pattern of degraded protein-DNA products using nuclear AhR complexes derived from mouse Hepa 1c1c7 cells treated with TCDD or MCDF, confirming ligand-dependent differences in the conformation of the nuclear AhR complex. Moreover, results of *in vivo* DNA footprinting studies show that in Hepa 1c1c7 cells treated with TCDD, a footprint was observed in the CYP1A1 gene promoter DRE whereas 6-MCDF and I3C did not induce this footprint.[211] Current studies are focused on further development of relatively non-toxic AhR-based antiestrogens for clinical applications and studies that delineate mechanisms of crosstalk between AhR- and ER-mediated signaling pathways.

ACKNOWLEDGMENTS

The financial assistance of the National Institutes of Health (ES09106 and ES04176), Avax Technologies (Kansas City), and the Texas Agricultural Experiment Station is gratefully acknowledged. Stephen Safe is a Sid Kyle Professor of Toxicology at Texas A&M University.

REFERENCES

1. Kutz, F.W., Wood, P.H., and Bottimore, D.P., Organochlorine pesticides and polychlorinated biphenyls in human adipose tissue, *Rev. Environ. Contamin. Toxicol.*, 120, 1, 1991.
2. Rappe, C., Dietary exposure and human levels of PCDDs and PCDFs, *Chemosphere*, 25, 231, 1992.
3. Rappe, C., Sources of exposure, environmental concentrations and exposure assessment of PCDDs and PCDFs, *Chemosphere*, 27, 211, 1993.
4. Colborn, T., vom Saal, F.S., and Soto, A.M., Developmental effects of endocrine-disrupting chemicals in wildlife and humans, *Environ. Health Perspect.*, 101, 378, 1993.
5. Sharpe, R.M. and Skakkebaek, N.F., Are oestrogens involved in falling sperm counts and disorders of the male reproductive tract, *Lancet*, 341, 1392, 1993.
6. Sharpe, R.M., Reproductive biology. Another DDT connection, *Nature*, 375, 538, 1995.
7. Wolff, M.S. et al., Blood levels of organochlorine residues and risk of breast cancer, *J. Natl. Cancer Inst.*, 85, 648, 1993.

8. Falck, F. et al., Pesticides and polychlorinated biphenyl residues in human breast lipids and their relation to breast cancer, *Arch. Environ. Health*, 47, 143, 1992.

9. Davis, D.L. et al., Medical hypothesis: xenoestrogens as preventable causes of breast cancer, *Environ. Health Perspect.*, 101, 372, 1993.

10. Davis, D.L. and Bradlow, H.L., Can environmental estrogens cause breast cancer, *Sci. Am.*, 273, 166, 1995.

11. Wolff, M.S., Pesticides—how research has succeeded and failed in informing policy: DDT and the link with breast cancer, *Environ. Health Perspect.*, 103 Suppl 6, 87, 1995.

12. Krieger, N. et al., Breast cancer and serum organochlorines: a prospective study among white, black, and Asian women, *J. Natl. Cancer Inst.*, 86, 589, 1994.

13. López-Carrillo, L. et al., Dichlorodiphenyltrichloroethane serum levels and breast cancer risk: a case-control study from Mexico, *Cancer Res.*, 57, 3728, 1997.

14. Van't Veer, P. et al., DDT (dicophane) and postmenopausal breast cancer in Europe: case control study, *Br. J. Med.*, 315, 81, 1997.

15. Hunter, D.J. et al., Plasma organochlorine levels and the risk of breast cancer, *New Engl. J. Med.*, 337, 1253, 1997.

16. Gammon, M.D. et al., Environmental toxins and breast cancer on Long Island. II. Organochlorine compound levels in blood, *Cancer Epidemiol. Biomarkers. Prev.*, 11, 686, 2002.

17. Safe, S., Environmental and dietary estrogens and human health — is there a problem?, *Environ. Health Perspect.*, 103, 346, 1995.

18. Safe, S., Is there an association between exposure to environmental estrogen and breast cancer?, *Environ. Health Perspect.*, 105(S3), 675, 1997.

19. Bertazzi, P.A. et al., Cancer incidence in a population accidentally exposed to 2,3,7,8-tetrachlorodibenzo-*p*-dioxin, *Epidemiology*, 4, 398, 1993.

20. Safe, S., Modulation of gene expression and endocrine response pathways by 2,3,7,8-tetrachlorodibenzo-*p*-dioxin and related compounds, *Pharmacol. Therap.*, 67, 247, 1995.

21. Goldstein, J.A. and Safe, S., Mechanism of action and structure-activity relationships for the chlorinated dibenzo-*p*-dioxins and related compounds, in *Halogenated Biphenyls, Naphthalenes, Dibenzodioxins and Related Compounds*, Kimbrough, R.D. and Jensen, A.A., Eds., Elsevier-North Holland, Amsterdam, 1989, 239.

22. Poland, A., Greenlee, W.F., and Kende, A.S., Studies on the mechanism of action of the chlorinated dibenzo- *p*-dioxins and related compounds, *Annu. N. Y. Acad. Sci.*, 320, 214, 1979.

23. Poland, A. and Knutson, J.C., 2,3,7,8-Tetrachlorodibenzo-*p*-dioxin and related halogenated aromatic hydrocarbons. Examinations of the mechanism of toxicity, *Annu. Rev. Pharmacol. Toxicol.*, 22, 517, 1982.

24. Safe, S., Comparative toxicology and mechanism of action of polychlorinated dibenzo-*p*-dioxins and dibenzofurans, *Annu. Rev. Pharmacol. Toxicol.*, 26, 371, 1986.

25. Whitlock, J.P., Jr., Mechanistic aspects of dioxin action, *Chem. Res. Toxicol.*, 6, 754, 1993.

26. Whitlock, J.P. et al., Induction of cytochrome P4501A1: a model for analyzing mammalian gene transcription, *FASEB J.*, 10, 809, 1996.

27. Rushmore, T.H. and Pickett, C.B., Glutathione *S*-transferases, structure, regulation, and therapeutic implications, *J. Biol. Chem.*, 268, 11475, 1993.

28. Pimental, R.A. et al., Dioxin receptor and C/EBP regulate the function of the glutathione S-transferase Ya gene xenobiotic response element, *Mol. Cell. Biol.*, 13, 4365, 1993.

29. Emi, Y., Ikushiro, S., and Iyanagi, T., Xenobiotic responsive element-mediated transcriptional activation in the UDP glucuronosyl transferase family 1 gene complex, *J. Biol. Chem.*, 271, 3952, 1996.

30. Jaiswal, A.K., Human NAD(P)H:quinone oxidoreductase: gene structure, activity and tissue-specific expression, *J. Biol. Chem.*, 269, 14502, 1994.

31. Asman, D.C. et al., Organization and characterization of the rat class 3 aldehyde dehydrogenase gene, *J. Biol. Chem.*, 268, 12530, 1993.

32. Choi, E.J. et al., Dioxin induced transforming growth factor-α in human keratinocytes, *J. Biol. Chem.*, 266, 9591, 1991.

33. Gaido, K.W. et al., 2,3,7,8-Tetrachlorodibenzo-*p*-dioxin-dependent regulation of transforming growth factors-α and β_2 expression in a human keratinocyte cell line involves both transcriptional and post-transcriptional control, *J. Biol. Chem.*, 267, 24591, 1992.

34. Poland, A. and Glover, E., 2,3,7,8-Tetrachlorodibenzo-*p*-dioxin: a potent inducer of δ-aminolevulinic acid synthetase, *Science*, 179, 476, 1973.

35. Sutter, T.R. et al., Targets for dioxin: genes for plasminogen activator inhibitor-2 and interleukin-1β, *Science*, 254, 415, 1991.

36. Puga, A., Nebert, D.W., and Carrier, F., Dioxin induces expression of c-*fos* and c-*jun* proto-oncogenes and a large increase in transcription factor AP-1, *DNA Cell Biol.*, 11, 269, 1992.

37. Kraemer, S.A. et al., Regulation of prostaglandin endoperoxide H synthase-2 expression by 2,3,7,8,-tetrachlorodibenzo-p-dioxin, *Arch. Biochem. Biophys.*, 330, 319, 1996.

38. Liu, P.C., Phillips, M.A., and Matsumura, F., Alteration by 2,3,7,8-Tetrachlorodibenzo-p-dioxin of CCAAT/enhancer binding protein correlates with suppression of adipocyte differentiation in 3T3-L1 cells, *Mol. Pharmacol.*, 49, 989, 1996.

39. Wang, X. et al., Mechanism of 2,3,7,8-tetrachlorodibenzo-*p*-dioxin (TCDD)-mediated decrease of the nuclear estrogen receptor in MCF-7 human breast cancer cells, *Mol. Cell. Endocrinol.*, 96, 159, 1993.

40. Lu, Y.-F., Wang, X., and Safe, S., Interaction of 2,3,7,8-tetrachlorodibenzo-*p*-dioxin and retinoic acid in MCF-7 human breast cancer cells, *Toxicol. Appl. Pharmacol.*, 127, 1, 1994.

41. Ishii, Y. et al., Significant suppression of rat liver aldolase B by a toxic coplanar polychlorinated biphenyl, 3,3′,4,4′,5-pentachlorobiphenyl, *Toxicology*, 116, 193, 1997.

42. Stahl, B.U., 2,3,7,8-Tetrachlorodibenzo-p-dioxin blocks the physiological regulation of hepatic phosphoenolpyruvate carboxykinase activity in primary rat hepatocytes, *Toxicology*, 103, 45, 1995.

43. Ryu, B.W. et al., Ah receptor involvement in mediation of pyruvate carboxylase levels and activity in mice given 2,3,7,8-tetrachlorodibenzo-*p*-dioxin, *J. Biochem. Toxicol.*, 10, 103, 1995.

44. Runge-Morris, M. and Wilusz, J., Suppression of hydroxysteroid sulfotransferase-a gene expression by 3-methylcholanthrene, *Toxicol. Appl. Pharmacol.*, 125, 133, 1994.

45. Muralidhara, Matsumura, F., and Blankenship, A., 2,3,7,8-Tetrachlorodibenzo-*p*-dioxin (TCDD)-induced reduction of adenosine deaminase activity *in vivo* and *in vitro*, *J. Biochem.*, 249, 1994.

46. Fox, T.R. et al., Gene expression and cell proliferation in rat liver after 2,3,7,8-tetrachlorodibenzo-*p*-dioxin exposure, *Cancer Res.*, 53, 2265, 1993.

47. Poland, A. et al., Genetic expression of aryl hydrocarbon hydroxylase activity. Induction of monooxygenase activities and cytochrome, P-450 formation by 2,3,7,8-tetrachlorodibenzo-*p*-dioxin in mice generally 'nonresponsive' to other aromatic hydrocarbons, *J. Biol. Chem.*, 249, 5599, 1975.

48. Poland, A. and Glover, E., Genetic expression of aryl hydrocarbon hydroxylase by 2,3,7,8- tetrachlorodibenzo-*p*-dioxin: evidence for a receptor mutation in genetically nonresponsive mice, *Mol. Pharmacol.*, 11, 389, 1975.

49. Nebert, D.W. et al., Genetic expression of aryl hydrocarbon hydroxylase activity in the mouse, *J. Cell. Physiol.*, 85, 393, 1976.

50. Poland, A. and Glover, E., Chlorinated dibenzo-*p*-dioxins: potent inducer of δ-aminolevulinic acid synthetase and aryl hydrocarbon hydroxylase. II. A study of the structure-activity relationship, *Mol. Pharmacol.*, 9, 736, 1973.

51. Poland, A., Glover, E., and Kende, A.S., Stereospecific, high affinity binding of 2,3,7,8- tetrachlorodibenzo-*p*-dioxin by hepatic cytosol: evidence that the binding species is receptor for induction of aryl hydrocarbon hydroxylase, *J. Biol. Chem.*, 251, 4936, 1976.

52. Poland, A. and Glover, E., Variation in the molecular mass of the Ah receptor among vertebrate species and strains of rats, *Biochem. Biophys. Res. Commun.*, 146, 1439, 1987.

53. Elferink, C.J., Gasiewicz, T.A., and Whitlock, J.P., Jr., Protein-DNA interactions at a dioxin-responsive enhancer. Evidence that the transformed Ah receptor is heteromeric, *J. Biol. Chem.*, 265, 20708, 1990.

54. Gasiewicz, T.A., Elferink, C.J., and Henry, E.C., Characterization of multiple forms of the Ah receptor: recognition of a dioxin-responsive enhancer involves heteromer formation, *Biochemistry*, 30, 2909, 1991.

55. Ema, M. et al., cDNA cloning and structure of the putative Ah receptor, *Biochem. Biophys. Res. Commun.*, 184, 246, 1992.

56. Ema, M. et al., Dioxin binding activities of polymorphic forms of mouse and human aryl hydrocarbon receptors, *J. Biol. Chem.*, 269, 27337, 1994.

57. Dolwick, K.M. et al., Cloning and expression of a human Ah receptor cDNA, *Mol. Pharmacol.*, 44, 911, 1993.

58. Schmidt, J.V., Carver, L.A., and Bradfield, C.A., Molecular characterization of the murine *Ahr* gene: organization, promoter analysis, and chromosomal assignment, *J. Biol. Chem.*, 268, 22203, 1993.

59. Burbach, K.M., Poland, A.B., and Bradfield, C.A., Cloning of the Ah-receptor cDNA reveals a distinctive ligand- activated transcription factor, *Proc. Natl. Acad. Sci. USA*, 89, 8185, 1992.

60. Hoffman, E.C. et al., Cloning of a factor required for activity of the Ah (dioxin) receptor, *Science*, 252, 954, 1991.

61. Wilson, C.L. et al., Aryl hydrocarbon (Ah)-nonresponsiveness in estrogen receptor-negative MDA-MB-231 cells is associated with expression of a variant Arnt protein, *Arch. Biochem. Biophys.*, 346, 65, 1997.

62. Gonzalez, F.J. and Nebert, D.W., Autoregulation plus upstream positive and negative control regions associated with transcriptional activation of the mouse cytochrome P_1-450 gene, *Nucleic Acids Res.*, 13, 7269, 1985.

63. Jones, P.B. et al., Control of cytochrome P_1-450 gene expression by dioxin, *Science*, 227, 1499, 1985.

64. Jones, P.B. et al., Control of cytochrome P_1-450 gene expression: analysis of a dioxin-responsive enhancer system, *Proc. Natl. Acad. Sci. USA*, 83, 2802, 1986.

65. Jones, P.B. et al., Control of gene expression by 2,3,7,8-tetrachlorodibenzo-*p*-dioxin: multiple dioxin-responsive domains 5′-ward of the cytochrome P_1-450 gene, *J. Biol. Chem.*, 261, 6647, 1986.

66. Neuhold, L.A. et al., Regulation of mouse CYP1A1 gene expression by dioxin: requirement of two *cis*-acting elements during induction, *Mol. Cell. Biol.*, 9, 2378, 1989.

67. Sogawa, K. et al., Location of regulatory elements responsible for drug induction in the rat cytochrome P-450c gene, *Proc. Natl. Acad. Sci. USA*, 83, 8044, 1986.

68. Fujisawa-Sehara, A. et al., Regulatory DNA elements localized remotely upstream from the drug-metabolizing cytochrome P-450c gene, *Nucleic Acids Res.*, 14, 1465, 1986.

69. Yao, E.F. and Denison, M.S., DNA sequence determinants for binding of transformed Ah- receptor to a dioxin-responsive enhancer, *Biochemistry*, 31, 5060, 1992.

70. Shen, E.S. and Whitlock, J.P., Protein-DNA interactions at a dioxin-responsive enhancer - mutational analysis of the DNA-binding site for the liganded Ah receptor, *J. Biol. Chem.*, 267, 6815, 1992.

71. Quattrochi, L.C., Vu, T., and Tukey, R.H., The human *CYP1A2* gene and induction by 3-methylcholanthrene: a region of DNA that supports Ah-receptor binding and promoter-specific induction, *J. Biol. Chem.*, 269, 6949, 1994.

72. Wo, Y.-Y.P., Stewart, J., and Greenlee, W.F., Functional analysis of the promoter for the CYP1B1 gene, *J. Biol. Chem.*, 272, 26702, 1997.

73. Hankinson, O., Single-step selection of clones of a mouse hepatoma line deficient in aryl hydrocarbon hydroxylase, *Proc. Natl. Acad. Sci. USA*, 76, 373, 1979.

74. Hankinson, O., Unstable aryl hydrocarbon hydroxylase-deficient variants of a rat hepatoma line, *Somatic Cell Genet.*, 6, 751, 1980.

75. Hankinson, O., Dominant and recessive aryl hydrocarbon hydroxylase-deficient mutants of mouse hepatoma line, Hepa-1, and assignment of recessive mutants to three complementation groups, *Somatic Cell Genet.*, 9, 497, 1983.

76. Israel, D.I. and Whitlock, J.P., Jr., Induction of mRNA specific for cytochrome P_1-450 in wild type and variant mouse hepatoma cells, *J. Biol. Chem.*, 258, 10390, 1983.

77. Boucher, P.D., Ruch, R.J., and Hines, R.N., Specific nuclear protein binding to a negative regulatory element on the human *CYP*1A1 gene, *J. Biol. Chem.*, 268, 17384, 1993.

78. Sterling, K. et al., Rat *CYP1A1* negative regulatory element: biological activity and interaction with a protein from liver and hepatoma cells, *Mol. Pharmacol.*, 44, 560, 1993.

79. Israel, D.I. et al., Superinduction of cytochrome P_1-450 gene transcription by inhibition of protein synthesis in wild type and variant mouse hepatoma cells, *J. Biol. Chem.*, 260, 5648, 1985.

80. Vickers, P.J., Dufresne, M.J., and Cowan, K.H., Relation between cytochrome P4501A1 expression and estrogen receptor content of human breast cancer cells, *Mol. Endocrinol.*, 3, 157, 1989.

81. Thomsen, J.S. et al., Differences in 2,3,7,8-tetrachlorodibenzo-*p*-dioxin-inducible CYP1A1 expression in human breast carcinoma cell lines involve altered transacting factors, *Eur. J. Biochem.*, 197, 577, 1991.

82. Thomsen, J.S. et al., Restoration of Ah responsiveness in MDA-MB-231 human breast cancer cells by transient expression of the estrogen receptor, *Carcinogenesis*, 15, 933, 1994.

83. Wang, W.L. et al., Effect of transient expression of the estrogen receptor on constitutive and inducible CYP1A1 in Hs578T human breast cancer cells, *Br. J. Cancer*, 73, 316, 1996.

84. Hoivik, D. et al., Studies on the relationship between estrogen receptor content, glutathione S-transferase π expression and induction by 2,3,7,8-tetrachlorodibenzo-*p*-dioxin and drug resistance in human breast cancer cells, *Arch. Biochem. Biophys.*, 1998, (in press).

85. Wang, W. et al., Mechanism of inhibition of MDA-MB-468 breast cancer cell growth by 2,3,7,8-tetrachlorodibenzo-*p*-dioxin, *Carcinogenesis*, 18, 925, 1997.

86. Moore, M. et al., Benzo[a]pyrene-resistant MCF-7 human breast cancer cells. A unique aryl hydrocarbon-nonresponsive clone, *J. Biol. Chem.*, 269, 11751, 1994.

87. Wang, X. et al., Comparative properties of the nuclear Ah receptor complex from several human cell lines, *Eur. J. Pharmacol.*, 293, 191, 1995.

88. Wilson, C.L., *Identification and characterization of an aryl hydrocarbon receptor nuclear translocator protein variant*, Ph.D. Thesis, Texas A&M University, College Station,TX, 1997,

89. Kärenlampi, S.O. et al., Effects of cytochrome P_1-450 inducers on the cell-surface receptors for epidermal growth factor, phorbol 12,13-dibutyrate, or insulin of cultured mouse hepatoma cells, *J. Biol. Chem.*, 258, 10378, 1983.

90. Madhukar, B.V., Brewster, D.W., and Matsumura, F., Effects of *in vivo*-administered 2,3,7,8-tetrachlorodibenzo-*p*- dioxin on receptor binding of epidermal growth factor in the hepatic plasma membrane of rat, guinea pig, mouse, and hamster, *Proc. Natl. Acad. Sci. USA*, 81, 7407, 1984.

91. Madhukar, B.V. et al., 2,3,7,8-Tetrachlorodibenzo-*p*-dioxin causes an increase in protein kinases associated with epidermal growth factor receptor in the hepatic plasma membrane, *J. Biochem. Toxicol.*, 3, 261, 1988.

92. Astroff, B. and Safe, S., 2,3,7,8-Tetrachlorodibenzo-*p*-dioxin as an antiestrogen: effect on rat uterine peroxidase activity, *Biochem. Pharmacol.*, 39, 485, 1990.

93. Lin, F.H. et al., The effects of 2,3,7,8-tetrachlorodibenzo-*p*-dioxin (TCDD) on the hepatic estrogen and glucocorticoid receptors in congenic strains of Ah-responsive and Ah-nonresponsive C57BL/6 mice, *Toxicol. Appl. Pharmacol.*, 108, 129, 1991.

94. Sunahara, G.I. et al., Characterization of 2,3,7,8-tetrachlorodibenzo-*p*-dioxin-mediated decreases in dexamethasone binding to rat hepatic cytosolic glucocorticoid receptor, *Mol. Pharmacol.*, 36, 239, 1989.

95. Fernandez, P. and Safe, S., Growth inhibitory and antimitogenic activity of 2,3,7,8-tetrachlorodibenzo-*p*-dioxin (TCDD) in T47D human breast cancer cells, *Toxicol. Lett.*, 61, 185, 1992.

96. Fernandez, P. et al., High passage T47D human breast cancer cells: altered endocrine and 2,3,7,8-tetrachlorodibenzo-*p*-dioxin responsiveness, *Eur. J. Pharmacol.*, 270, 53, 1994.

97. Liu, H. et al., Inhibition of insulin-like growth factor-I responses in MCF-7 cells by 2,3,7,8-tetrachlorodibenzo-*p*-dioxin and related compounds, *Mol. Cell. Endocrinol.*, 87, 19, 1992.

98. Mebus, C.A. and Piper, W.N., Decreased rat adrenal 21-hydroxylase activity associated with decreased adrenal microsomal cytochrome P-450 after exposure to 2, 3,7,8-tetrachlorodibenzo-*p*-dioxin, *Biochem. Pharmacol.*, 35, 4359, 1986.

99. Kleeman, J.M., Moore, R.W., and Peterson, R.E., Inhibition of testicular steroidogenesis in 2,3,7,8- tetrachlorodibenzo-*p*-dioxin-treated rats: evidence that the key lesion occurs prior to or during pregnenolone formation, *Toxicol. Appl. Pharmacol.*, 106, 112, 1990.

100. Spink, D.C. et al., 2,3,7,8-Tetrachlorodibenzo-*p*-dioxin causes an extensive alteration of 17β-estradiol metabolism in human breast cancer cells, *Proc. Natl. Acad. Sci. USA*, 87, 6917, 1990.

101. Spink, D.C. et al., 17β-Estradiol hydroxylation catalyzed by human cytochrome P4501A1: a comparison of the activities induced by 2,3,7,8- tetrachlorodibenzo-*p*-dioxin in MCF-7 cells with those from heterologous expression of the cDNA, *Arch. Biochem. Biophys.*, 293, 342, 1992.

102. Spink, D.C. et al., Stimulation of 17β-estradiol metabolism in MCF-7 cells by bromochloro- and chloromethyl-substituted dibenzo-*p*-dioxins and dibenzofurans: correlations with antiestrogenic activity, *J. Toxicol. Environ. Health*, 41, 451, 1994.

103. Hayes, C.L. et al., 17β-Estradiol hydroxylation catalyzed by human cytochrome P450 1B1, *Proc. Natl. Acad. Sci. USA*, 93, 9776, 1996.

104. Kociba, R.J. et al., Results of a 2-year chronic toxicity and oncogenicity study of 2,3,7,8- tetrachlorodibenzo-*p* -dioxin (TCDD) in rats, *Toxicol. Appl. Pharmacol.*, 46, 279, 1978.

105. Holcombe, M. and Safe, S., Inhibition of 7,12-dimethylbenzanthracene-induced rat mammary tumor growth by 2,3,7,8-tetrachlorodibenzo-*p*-dioxin, *Cancer Letters*, 82, 43, 1994.

106. Tritscher, A.M. et al., Persistence of TCDD-induced hepatic cell proliferation and growth of enzyme altered foci after chronic exposure followed by cessation of treatment in DEN initiated female rats, *Carcinogenesis*, 16, 2807, 1995.

107. Gierthy, J.F. et al., Correlation of *in vitro* and *in vivo* growth suppression of MCF-7 human breast cancer by 2,3,7,8-tetrachlorodibenzo-*p*-dioxin, *Cancer Res.*, 53, 3149, 1993.

108. Reggiani, G., Acute human exposure to TCDD in Seveso, Italy, *J. Toxicol. Environ. Health*, 6, 27, 1980.

109. Mocarelli, P. et al., Change in sex ratio with exposure to dioxin, *Lancet*, 348, 409,1996.

110. Umbreit, T.H. and Gallo, M.A., Physiological implications of estrogen receptor modulation by 2,3,7,8-tetrachlorodibenzo-*p*-dioxin, *Toxicol. Lett.*, 42, 5, 1988.

111. Umbreit, T.H. et al., Effects of TCDD-estradiol interactions in three strains of mice, *Toxicol. Lett.*, 40, 1, 1988.

112. Umbreit, T.H. et al., Alteration of the acute toxicity of 2,3,7,8-tetrachlorodibenzo-*p*-dioxin (TCDD) by estradiol and tamoxifen, *Toxicology*, 59, 163, 1989.

113. Gallo, M.A. et al., Interactive effects of estradiol and 2,3,7,8-tetrachlorodibenzo- *p*-dioxin on hepatic cytochrome P-450 and mouse uterus, *Toxicol. Lett.*, 32, 123, 1986.

114. Johnson, D.C., Sen, M., and Dey, S.K., Differential effects of dichlorodiphenyltrichloroethane analogs, chlordecone, and 2,3,7,8-tetrachlorodibenzo-*p*-dioxin on establishment of pregnancy in the hypophysectomized rat, *Proc. Soc. Exp. Biol. Med.*, 199, 42, 1992.

115. Brown, N.M. and Lamartiniere, C.A., Xenoestrogens alter mammary gland differentiation and cell proliferation in the rat, *Environ. Health Perspect.*, 103, 708, 1995.

116. Romkes, M. and Safe, S., Comparative activities of 2,3,7,8-tetrachlorodibenzo-*p*-dioxin and progesterone on antiestrogens in the female rat uterus, *Toxicol. Appl. Pharmacol.*, 92, 368, 1988.

117. Romkes, M., Piskorska-Pliszczynska, J., and Safe, S., Effects of 2,3,7,8-tetrachlorodibenzo-*p*-dioxin on hepatic and uterine estrogen receptor levels in rats, *Toxicol. Appl. Pharmacol.*, 87, 306, 1987.

118. Astroff, B. and Safe, S., Comparative antiestrogenic activities of 2,3,7,8- tetrachlo-rodibenzo-*p*-dioxin and 6-methyl-1,3,8- trichlorodibenzofuran in the female rat, *Toxicol. Appl. Pharmacol.*, 95, 435, 1988.

119. Astroff, B. et al., 2,3,7,8-Tetrachlorodibenzo-*p*-dioxin inhibition of 17β-estradiol-induced increases in rat uterine EGF receptor binding activity and gene expression, *Mol. Cell. Endocrinol.*, 72, 247, 1990.

120. Astroff, B., Eldridge, B., and Safe, S., Inhibition of 17β-estradiol-induced and con-stitutive expression of the cellular protooncogene c-*fos* by 2,3,7,8- tetrachlorodibenzo-*p*-dioxin (TCDD) in the female uterus, *Toxicol. Lett.*, 56, 305, 1991.

121. Hyder, S.M. et al., Selective inhibition of estrogen-regulated gene expression *in vivo* by the pure antiestrogen ICI 182,780, *Cancer Res.*, 57, 2547, 1997.

122. Muto, T. et al., Estrous cyclicity and ovarian follicles in female rats after prenatal exposure to 3,3′,4,4′,5-pentachlorobiphenyl, *Toxicol. Lett.*, 143, 271, 2003.

123. Buchanan, D.L. et al., Antiestrogenic effects of 2,3,7,8-tetrachlorodibenzo-*p*-dioxin in mouse uterus: critical role of the aryl hydrocarbon receptor in stromal tissue, *Toxicol. Sci.*, 57, 302, 2000.

124. Buchanan, D.L. et al., Dioxin inhibition of estrogen-induced mouse uterine epithelial mitogenesis involves changes in cyclin and transforming growth factor-β expression, *Toxicol. Sci.*, 66, 62, 2002.

125. Brooks, S.C., Locke, E.R., and Soule, H.D., Estrogen receptor in a human cell line (MCF-7) from breast carcinoma, *J. Biol. Chem.*, 248, 6251, 1973.

126. Levenson, A.S. and Jordan, V.C., MCF-7: the first hormone-responsive breast cancer cell line, *Cancer Res.*, 57, 3071, 1997.

127. Harris, M. et al., Structure-dependent induction of aryl hydrocarbon hydroxylase in human breast cancer cell lines and characterization of the Ah receptor, *Cancer Res.*, 49, 4531, 1989.

128. Gierthy, J.F. et al., Suppression of estrogen-regulated extracellular plasminogen acti-vator activity of MCF-7 cells by 2,3,7,8-tetrachlorodibenzo-*p*-dioxin, *Cancer Res.*, 47, 6198, 1987.

129. Gierthy, J.F. and Lincoln, D.W., Inhibition of postconfluent focus production in cultures of MCF- 7 breast cancer cells by 2,3,7,8-tetrachlorodibenzo-*p*-dioxin, *Breast Cancer Res.*, 12, 227, 1988.

130. Biegel, L. and Safe, S., Effects of 2,3,7,8-tetrachlorodibenzo-*p*-dioxin (TCDD) on cell growth and the secretion of the estrogen-induced 34-, 52- and 160- kDa proteins in human breast cancer cells, *J. Steroid Biochem. Mol. Biol.*, 37, 725, 1990.

131. Krishnan, V. and Safe, S., Polychlorinated biphenyls (PCBs), dibenzo-*p*-dioxins (PCDDs) and dibenzofurans (PCDFs) as antiestrogens in MCF-7 human breast cancer cells: quantitative structure-activity relationships, *Toxicol. Appl. Pharmacol.*, 120, 55, 1993.

132. Krishnan, V., Narasimhan, T.R., and Safe, S., Development of gel staining techniques for detecting the secretion of procathepsin D (52-kDa protein) in MCF-7 human breast cancer cells, *Anal. Biochem.*, 204, 137, 1992.

133. Krishnan, V. et al., Molecular mechanism of inhibition of estrogen-induced cathepsin D gene expression by 2,3,7,8-tetrachlorodibenzo-*p*-dioxin (TCDD) in MCF-7 cells, *Mol. Cell. Biol.*, 15, 6710, 1995.

134. Moore, M. et al., Interaction of 2,3,7,8-tetrachlorodibenzo-*p*-dioxin, 12-*O*-tetrade-canoylphorbol-13-acetate (TPA) and 17β-estradiol in MCF-7 human breast cancer cells, *J. Steroid Biochem. Mol. Biol.*, 44, 251, 1993.

135. Narasimhan, T.R. et al., Effects of 2,3,7,8-tetrachlorodibenzo-*p*-dioxin on 17β-estra-diol-induced glucose metabolism in MCF-7 human breast cancer cells: ^{13}C-nuclear magnetic resonance studies, *Mol. Pharmacol.*, 40, 1029, 1991.

136. Harper, N. et al., Inhibition of estrogen-induced progesterone receptor in MCF-7 human breast cancer cells by aryl hydrocarbon (Ah) receptor agonists, *Mol. Cell. Endocrinol.*, 104, 47, 1994.

137. Zacharewski, T.R. et al., Antiestrogenic effects of 2,3,7,8-tetrachlorodibenzo-*p*-dioxin on 17β-estradiol-induced pS2 expression, *Cancer Res.*, 54, 2707, 1994.

138. Lu, Y.-F. et al., Inhibition of prolactin receptor gene expression by 2,3,7,8-tetrachlo-rodibenzo-*p*-dioxin in MCF-7 human breast cancer cells, *Arch. Biochem. Biophys.*, 332, 35, 1996.

139. Gillesby, B. et al., Identification of a motif within the 5'-regulatory region on pS2 which is responsible for Ap1 binding and TCDD-mediated suppression, *Biochemistry*, 36, 6080, 1997.

140. Nodland, K.I., Wormke, M., and Safe, S., Inhibition of estrogen-induced activity by 2,3,7,8-tetrachlorodibenzo-*p*-dioxin (TCDD) in the MCF-7 human breast cancer and other cell lines transfected with vitellogenin A2 gene promoter constructs, *Arch. Biochem. Biophys.*, 338, 67, 1997.

141. Parker, M.G., Action of "pure" antiestrogens in inhibiting estrogen receptor action, *Breast Cancer Res. Treat.*, 26, 131, 1993.

142. Porter, W. et al., Transcriptional activation of heat shock protein 27 gene expression by 17β-estradiol and modulation by antiestrogens and aryl hydrocarbon receptor agonists: estrogenic activity of ICI 164,384, *J. Mol. Endocrinol.*, 26, 31, 2001.

143. Liu, H. and Safe, S., Effects of 2,3,7,8-tetrachlorodibenzo-*p*-dioxin (TCDD) on insu-lin-induced responses in MCF-7 human breast cancer cells, *Toxicol. Appl. Pharma-col.*, 138, 242, 1996.

144. Minegishi, T. et al., Effect of IGF-1 and 2,3,7,8-tetrachlorodibenzo-*p*-dioxin (TCDD) on the expression of LH receptors during cell differentiation in cultured granulosa cells, *Mol. Cell. Endocrinol.*, 202, 123, 2003.

145. Koliopanus, A. et al., Increased aryl hydrocarbon receptor expression offers a potential therapeutic target in pancreatic cancer, *Oncogene*, 21, 6059, 2002.

146. Jana, N.R. et al., Cross-talk between 2,3,7,8-tetrachlorodibenzo-*p*-dioxin and test-osterone signal transduction pathways in LNCaP prostate cancer cells, *Biochem. Biophys. Res. Commun.*, 256, 462, 1999.

147. Foster, J.S. and Wimalasena, J., Estrogen regulates activity of cyclin-dependent kinases and retinoblastoma protein phosphorylation in breast cancer cells, *Mol. Endo-crinol.*, 10, 488, 1996.

148. Prall, O.W.J. et al., Estrogen-induced activation of Cdk4 and Cdk2 during G_1-S phase progression is accompanied by increased cyclin D1 expression and decreased cyclin-dependent kinase inhibitor association with cyclin E-Cdk2, *J. Biol. Chem.*, 272, 10882, 1997.

149. Planas-Silva, M.D. and Weinberg, R.A., Estrogen-dependent cyclin E-cdk2 activation through p21 redistribution, *Mol. Cell. Biol.*, 17, 4059, 1997.

150. Musgrove, E.A. et al., Growth factor, steroid, and steroid antagonist regulation of cyclin gene expression associated with changes in T-47D human breast cancer cell cycle progression, *Mol. Cell. Biol.*, 13, 3577, 1993.

151. Wang, W., Smith, R., and Safe, S., Aryl hydrocarbon receptor-mediated antiestroge-nicity in MCF-7 cells: modulation of hormone-induced cell cycle enzymes, *Arch. Biochem. Biophys.*, 356, 239, 1998.

152. Harris, M., Zacharewski, T., and Safe, S., Effects of 2,3,7,8-tetrachlorodibenzo-*p*-dioxin and related compounds on the occupied nuclear estrogen receptor in MCF-7 human breast cancer cells, *Cancer Res.*, 50, 3579, 1990.

153. Gierthy, J.F. et al., Enhancement of 2- and 16α-estradiol hydroxylation in MCF-7 human breast cancer cells by 2,3,7,8-tetrachlorodibenzo-*p*-dioxin, *Biochem. Biophys. Res. Commun.*, 157, 515, 1988.

154. Shiverick, K.T. and Muther, T.F., Effects of 2,3,7,8-tetrachlorodibenzo-*p*-dioxin on serum concentrations and the uterotrophic actions of exogenous estrone in rats, *Toxicol. Appl. Pharmacol.*, 65, 170, 1982.

155. Wang, F. et al., Identification of a functional imperfect estrogen responsive element in the 5′-promoter region of the human cathepsin D gene, *Biochemistry*, 36, 7793, 1997.

156. AnonymousPanc-28 cell reference, *xxx*, 2003.

157. Wormke, M. et al., The aryl hydrocarbon receptor mediates degradation of the estrogen receptor α through activation of proteasomes, *Mol. Cell. Biol.*, 23, 1843, 2003.

158. Safe, S. and Wormke, M., Inhibitory aryl hydrocarbon-estrogen receptor a crosstalk and mechanisms of action, *Chem. Res. Toxicol.*, 16, 807, 2003.

159. Wormke, M. et al., Crosstalk between estrogen receptor α and the aryl hydrocarbon receptor in breast cancer cells involves unidirectional activation of proteosomes, *FEBS Lett.*, 478, 109, 2000.

160. Nguyen, T.A. et al., Interactions of nuclear receptor coactivator/corepressor proteins with the aryl hydrocarbon receptor complex, *Arch. Biochem. Biophys.*, 367, 250, 1999.

161. Kumar, M.B. and Perdew, G.H., Nuclear receptor coactivator SRC-1 interacts with the Q-rich subdomain of the AhR and modulates its transactivation potential, *Gene Expr.*, 8, 273, 1999.

162. Kumar, M.B., Tarpey, R.W., and Perdew, G.H., Differential recruitment of coactivator RIP140 by *Ah* and estrogen receptors: absence of a role for LXXLL motifs, *J. Biol. Chem.*, 274, 22155, 1999.

163. Kobayashi, A. et al., CBP/p300 functions as a possible transcriptional coactivator of Ah receptor nuclear translocator (Arnt), *J. Biochem.*, 122, 703, 1997.

164. Beischlag, T.V. et al., Recruitment of the NCoA/SRC-1/p160 family of transcriptional coactivators by the aryl hydrocarbon receptor/aryl hydrocarbon receptor nuclear translocator complex, *Mol. Cell. Biol.*, 22, 4319, 2002.

165. Reen, R.K., Cadwallader, A., and Perdew, G.H., The subdomains of the transactivation domain of the aryl hydrocarbon receptor (AhR) inhibit AhR and estrogen receptor transcriptional activity, *Arch. Biochem. Biophys.*, 408, 93, 2002.

166. Rogers, J.M. and Denison, M.S., Analysis of the antiestrogenic activity of 2,3,7,8-tetrachlorodibenzo-*p*-dioxin in human ovarian carcinoma BG-1 cells, *Mol. Pharmacol.*, 61, 1393, 2002.

167. Ohtake, F. et al., Modulation of oestrogen receptor signalling by association with the activated dioxin receptor, *Nature*, 423, 545, 2003.

168. Abdelrahim, M., Smith, R. 3rd, and Safe, S., Aryl hydrocarbon receptor gene silencing with small inhibitory RNA differentially modulates Ah-responsiveness in MCF-7 and HepG2 cancer cells, *Mol. Pharmacol.*, 63, 1373, 2003.

169. Baron, J.A., La Vecchia, C., and Levi, F., The antiestrogenic effect of cigarette smoking in women, *Am. J. Obstet. Gynecol.*, 162, 502, 1990.

170. Lesko, S.M. et al., Cigarette smoking and the risk of endometrial cancer, *N. Engl. J. Med.*, 313, 593, 1985.

171. Chaloupka, K., Krishnan, V., and Safe, S., Polynuclear aromatic hydrocarbon carcinogens as antiestrogens in MCF-7 human breast cancer cells. Role of the Ah receptor, *Carcinogenesis*, 13, 2223, 1992.

172. Harris, M. et al., Partial antagonism of 2,3,7,8-tetrachlorodibenzo-*p*-dioxin- mediated induction of aryl hydrocarbon hydroxylase by 6-methyl-1,3,8-trichlorodibenzofuran: mechanistic studies, *Mol. Pharmacol.*, 35, 729, 1989.

173. Bannister, R. et al., 6-Methyl-1,3,8-trichlorodibenzofuran (MCDF) as a 2,3,7,8- tetrachlorodibenzo-*p*-dioxin antagonist in C57BL/6 mice, *Toxicology*, 54, 139, 1989.

174. Yao, C. and Safe, S., 2,3,7,8-Tetrachlorodibenzo-*p*-dioxin-induced porphyria in genetically inbred mice: partial antagonism and mechanistic studies, *Toxicol. Appl. Pharmacol.*, 100, 208, 1989.

175. Astroff, B. et al., 6-Methyl-1,3,8-trichlorodibenzofuran as a 2,3,7,8-tetrachlorodibenzo-*p*-dioxin antagonist: inhibition of the induction of rat cytochrome P-450 isozymes and related monooxygenase activities, *Mol. Pharmacol.*, 33, 231, 1988.

176. Astroff, B. and Safe, S., 6-Alkyl-1,3,8-trichlorodibenzofurans as antiestrogens in female Sprague-Dawley rats, *Toxicology*, 69, 187, 1991.

177. Zacharewski, T. et al., 6-Methyl-1,3,8-trichlorodibenzofuran (MCDF) as an antiestrogen in human and rodent cancer cell lines: evidence for the role of the Ah receptor, *Toxicol. Appl. Pharmacol.*, 13, 311, 1992.

178. Sun, G. and Safe, S., Antiestrogenic activities of alternate substituted polychlorinated dibenzofurans in MCF-7 human breast cancer cells, *Cancer Chemother. Pharmacol.*, 40, 239, 1997.

179. Dickerson, R., Howie-Keller, L., and Safe, S., Alkyl polychlorinated dibenzofurans and related compounds as antiestrogens in the female rat uterus: structure-activity studies, *Toxicol. Appl. Pharmacol.*, 135, 287, 1995.

180. McDougal, A., Wilson, C., and Safe, S., Inhibition of 7,12-dimethylbenz[*a*]anthracene-induced rat mammary tumor growth by aryl hydrocarbon receptor agonists, *Cancer Lett.*, 120, 53, 1997.

181. Preobrazhenskaya, M.N. et al., Ascorbigen and other indole-derived compounds from *Brassica* vegetables and their analogs as anticarcinogenic and immunomodulating agents, *Pharmacol. Therap.*, 60, 301, 1993.

182. Wattenberg, L.W. and Loub, W.D., Inhibition of aromatic hydrocarbon-induced neoplasia by naturally occurring indoles, *Cancer Res.*, 38, 1410, 1978.

183. Nixon, J.E. et al., Inhibition of aflatoxin B_1 carcinogenesis in rainbow trout by flavone and indole compounds, *Carcinogenesis*, 5, 615, 1984.

184. Kim, D.J. et al., Biphasic modifying effect on indole-3-carbinol on diethylnitrosamine-induced preneoplastic glutathione S-transferase placental form-positive liver cell foci in Sprague-Dawley rats, *Jpn. J. Cancer Res.*, 85, 578, 1994.

185. Morse, M.A. et al., Effects of indole-3-carbinol on lung tumorigenesis and DNA methylation induced by 4-(methylnitrosamino)-1-(3-pyridl)-1-butanone (NNK) and on the metabolism and disposition of NNK in A/J mice, *Cancer Res.*, 50, 1613, 1990.

186. Tanaka, T. et al., Inhibitory effects of the natural products indole-3-carbinol and sinigrin during initiation and promotion phases of 4-nitroquinoline 1-oxide-induced rat tongue carcinogenesis, *Jpn. J. Cancer Res.*, 83, 835, 1992.

187. Tanaka, T. et al., Inhibitory effect of sinigrin and indole-3-carbinol in diethylnitrosamine-induced hepatocarcinogenesis in male ACI/N rats, *Carcinogenesis*, 11, 1403, 1990.

188. Stoewsand, G.S., Anderson, J.L., and Munson, L., Protective effect of dietary brussels sprouts against mammary carcinogenesis in Sprague-Dawley rats, *Cancer Lett.*, 39, 199, 1988.

189. Grubbs, C.J. et al., Chemoprevention of chemically-induced mammary carcinogenesis by indole-3-carbinol, *Anticancer Res.*, 15, 709, 1995.

190. Bradlow, H.L. et al., Effects of dietary indole-3-carbinol on estradiol metabolism and spontaneous mammary tumors in mice, *Carcinogenesis*, 12, 1571, 1991.

191. Kojima, T., Tanaka, T., and Mori, H., Chemoprevention of spontaneous endometrial cancer in female Donryu rats by dietary indol-3-carbinol, *Cancer Res.*, 54, 1446, 1994.

192. Stresser, D.M. et al., Indole-3-carbinol induces a rat liver glutathione transferase subunit (Yc2) with high activity toward aflatoxin B_1 *exo*-epoxide: association with reduced levels of hepatic aflatoxin-DNA adducts *in vivo*, *Drug Metab. Dispos.*, 22, 392, 1994.

193. Wortelboer, H.M. et al., Acid reaction products of indole-3-carbinol and their effects on cytochrome P450 and phase II enzymes in rat and monkey hepatocytes, *Biochem. Pharmacol.*, 43, 1439, 1992.

194. Bradfield, C.A. and Bjeldanes, L.F., Effect of dietary indole-3-carbinol on intestinal and hepatic monooxygenase, glutathione *S*-transferase and epoxide hydrolase activities in the rat, *Food Chem. Toxicol.*, 22, 977, 1984.

195. Wortelboer, H.M. et al., Effects of indole-3-carbinol on biotransformation enzymes in the rat: *in vivo* changes in liver and small intestinal mucosa in comparison with primary hepatocyte cultures, *Food Chem. Toxicol.*, 30, 589, 1992.

196. Baldwin, W.S. and LeBlanc, G.A., The anti-carcinogenic plant compound indole-3-carbinol differentially modulates P450-mediated steroid hydroxylase activities in mice, *Chem. Biol. Interact.*, 83, 155, 1992.

197. De Kruif, C.A. et al., Structure elucidation of acid reaction products of indole-3-carbinol: detection *in vivo* and enzyme induction *in vitro*, *Chem. Biol. Interact.*, 80, 303, 1991.

198. Tiwari, R.K. et al., Selective responsiveness of breast cancer cells to indole-3-carbinol, a chemopreventative agent, *J. Natl. Cancer Inst.*, 86, 126, 1994.

199. Vang, O., Jensen, H., and Autrup, H., Induction of cytochrome P-450IA1, IA2, IIB1, IIB2 and IIE1 by broccoli in rat liver and colon, *Chem. Biol. Interact.*, 78, 85, 1991.

200. Vang, O., Jensen, M.B., and Autrup, H., Induction of cytochrome P450IA1 in rat colon and liver by indole-3-carbinol and 5,6-benzoflavone, *Carcinogenesis*, 11, 1259, 1990.

201. Jellinck, P.H. et al., Ah receptor binding properties of indole carbinols and induction of hepatic estradiol hydroxylation, *Biochem. Pharmacol.*, 43, 1129, 1993.

202. Niwa, T., Swaneck, G., and Bradlow, H.L., Alterations in estradiol metabolism in MCF-7 cells induced by treatment with indole-3-carbinol and related compounds, *Steroids*, 59, 523, 1994.

203. Michnovicz, J.J. and Bradlow, H.L., Induction of estradiol metabolism by dietary indole-3-carbinol in humans, *J. Natl. Cancer Inst.*, 82, 947, 1990.

204. Jellinck, P.H., Michnovicz, J.J., and Bradlow, H.L., Influence of indole-3-carbinol on the hepatic microsomal formation of catechol estrogens, *Steroids*, 56, 446, 1991.

205. Jellinck, P.H. et al., Distinct forms of hepatic androgen 6β-hydroxylase induced in the rat by indole-3-carbinol and pregnenolone carbonitrile, *J. Steroid Biochem. Mol. Biol.*, 51, 219, 1994.

206. Bjeldanes, L.F. et al., Aromatic hydrocarbon responsiveness-receptor agonists generated from indole-3-carbinol *in vitro* and *in vivo* - comparisons with 2,3,7,8-tetrachlorodibenzo-*p*-dioxin, *Proc. Natl. Acad. Sci. USA*, 88, 9543, 1991.

207. Grose, K.R. and Bjeldanes, L.F., Oligomerization of indole-3-carbinol in aqueous acid, *Chem. Res. Toxicol.*, 5, 188, 1992.

208. Chen, I., Safe, S., and Bjeldanes, L., Indole-3-carbinol and diindolylmethane as aryl hydrocarbon (Ah) receptor agonists and antagonists in T47D human breast cancer cells, *Biochem. Pharmacol.*, 51, 1069, 1996.
209. Chen, I. et al., Aryl hydrocarbon receptor-mediated antiestrogenic and antitumorigenic activity of diindolylmethane, *Carcinogenesis*, 19, 1631, 1998.
210. Santostefano, M. and Safe, S., Characterization of the molecular and structural properties of the transformed and nuclear aryl hydrocarbon (Ah) receptor complexes by proteolytic digestion, *Chem. Biol. Interact.*, 100, 221, 1996.
211. Arellano-Johnson, L., unpublished results, 1997.

Section II

Effect on the Male
Reproductive System

9 Endocrine Disruptors and Male Infertility

Suresh C. Sikka, Ph. D., H.C.L.D., Muammer Kendirci, M.D., and Rajesh Naz, Ph.D.

CONTENTS

0-8493-2281-2/05/$0.00+$1.50
© 2005 by CRC Press

9.1 INTRODUCTION

Endocrine disruptors are estrogen-like and antiandrogenic chemicals in the environment that have potential hazardous effects not only on a variety of aquatic flora, wildlife, and human health, but on overall ecological well-being. These chemicals have been called "endocrine disruptors" because they are thought to mimic natural hormones, inhibit the action of hormones, or alter the normal regulatory function of the endocrine systems. Reduced fertility in males is one of the major endpoints, besides testicular and prostate cancers, abnormal sexual development, alteration in pituitary and thyroid gland functions, immune suppression, and neurobehavioral effects. Interference with the action of androgen during development can cause male reproductive system abnormalities that include reduced sperm production capability.

Indeed, the evidence of the past 20 years has shown disturbing trends in male reproductive health. During a recent U.S. Congressional hearing, a startling but controversial finding reported that "each man in this room is half the man his grandfather was." Another report from Scotland revealed that men born after 1970 had a sperm count 25% lower than those born before 1959 — an average decline of 2.1% a year. Nelson and Bunge reported that semen quality might have deteriorated during the 1950s and 1960s.[1] A meta-analysis revealed a decline in sperm concentrations of healthy men from 113×10^6/ml in 1938 to 66×10^6/ml in 1990.[2] The lower sperm count was also associated with poor semen quality.[3,4] After repeated semen analysis by Olsen et al. and Swan et al., the main conclusion remained the same: In the 1950s sperm concentrations were higher than in the 1970s.[5,6] Swan et al. confirmed the declining trend in semen parameters in the United States and Europe.[7]

According to a meta-analysis of 61 papers, Carlsen et al. reported that sperm counts were decreased by 50% over the past 50 years.[2] Semen quality in healthy men was evaluated in many countries because endocrine-disrupting chemicals, in particular weak estrogenic chemicals that contaminate food, plant, and industrial materials, were suspected to be one of the causes of the impairment of male reproductive function.[8] Thus, while some environmentalists believe that the human species is approaching a fertility crisis, others think that the available data are insufficient to deduce worldwide conclusions.[9,10] Though these assertions have been disputed, the fact remains that one in six couples have trouble conceiving, with males equally responsible for their infertility. Adverse trends in male reproductive health are of concern. Prospective international studies are needed to analyze the etiology of the reproductive health problems, and environmental causes, including endocrine disruptors, should be extensively studied. Genetic susceptibility to endocrine disruption may vary, but identification of any new risk factors would give us possibilities for prevention.

When the reason for the poor quality of sperm cannot be identified, patients are treated with empirical methods. However, the development of intra-cytoplasmic sperm injection (ICSI), a technique introduced at the beginning of the 1990s, is beyond doubt the most important recent breakthrough in the treatment of male infertility. This has been made possible by many well-controlled clinical studies and basic scientific discoveries in the physiology, biochemistry, and molecular and cellular biology of the male reproductive system. This has helped in the identification of greater numbers of men with male factor problems. Newer tools for the detection of Y-chromosome deletions have further strengthened the hypothesis that the decline in male reproductive health and fertility may be related to the presence of certain toxic chemical compounds in the environment. These chemicals mimic or otherwise disrupt the estrogens or the androgen balance in the body by binding to hormone receptors during fetal and neonatal development. This may give rise to reproductive abnormalities, including low sperm counts.

Because of these effects, such endocrine disruptors are also popularly known as "gender benders." However, the evidence that such environmental chemicals cause infertility is still largely circumstantial. There are many missing links in the causal chain that would connect receptor binding to changes in reproductive health with decreased fertility. With recent discoveries of deformed frogs in Minnesota lakes, and fertility problems in alligators found in Lake Apopka in Florida[11] attributed to embryonic exposure to pollutants, a myriad of environmental agents have been classified as male reproductive toxicants. This has been the subject of a number of reviews,[12–16] suggesting that etiology, diagnosis, and treatment of male factor infertility remains a real challenge.

9.2 BACKGROUND

Several investigators have expressed serious concerns for the estrogenic effects of environmental xenobiotic chemicals, such as polychlorinated biphenyls (PCBs), dichlorodiphenyl-trichloroethane (DDT), dioxin, and some pesticides.[17–20] The potential hazards these chemicals may have on human health and ecological well-being include reproductive tract cancers, reduced male fertility, and abnormality in sexual development.[19,21–22]

In the mid-1970s, it was determined that dibromochloropropane (DBCP) exposure impaired fertility in the absence of any other clinical signs of toxicity, suggesting that the male reproductive system was the most sensitive target system. Reduced fertility, embryo/fetal loss, birth defects, childhood cancer, and other postnatal structural or functional problems were the most common outcomes from such exposures. However, the database for establishing safe exposure levels or risk assessment for such outcomes remains very limited. Declining semen quality is not the only indicator that human reproduction is at risk. A marked increase in the incidence of testicular cancer in young men has been associated with other abnormalities (including undescended testis, Sertoli-cell-only pattern, and hypospadias) that cause poor gonadal function and low fecundity rates.

The human male produces relatively fewer sperm on a daily basis compared with many of the animal species used for toxicity testing. A less dramatic decrease in sperm numbers or semen quality in humans can have serious consequences for reproductive potential. In fact, in many men over age 30, the lower daily sperm production rate already places them close to the subfertile or infertile range.[23,24] Decreased semen quality (low sperm number, motility, and structure) over the past 50 years has been attributed to environmental toxicants, many of which act as "estrogens."[25] This "estrogen hypothesis" has inspired a number of debates and serious investigations. Does that make men less fertile? After all, it takes only one sperm to fertilize an egg! Problems in the production, maturation, and fertilizing ability of sperm are the single most common cause of male infertility. Although produced in adequate numbers, sperm can have poor motility, viability, and morphology; immature lacking acrosome; and characteristics that will prevent them from fertilizing an oocyte. Normal sperm can also be produced in abnormally low numbers, thus diminishing the chances of fertilization.

A dramatic increase in knowledge of reproductive toxicity and subsequent changes in fertility has resulted from advances in the understanding of gonadal function and dysfunction. Although any discussion of gonadal function and toxicity is of special relevance to man, much of this understanding has been obtained from research using animal species and various experimental models.

9.3 ENDOCRINE DISRUPTORS AND TARGET SITES

An environmental agent could disrupt endocrine function in the male at several potential target sites. The most important are the testes, the male gonads, which usually exist in pairs and are the sites of spermatogenesis and androgen production. Spermatozoa are the haploid germ cells responsible for fertilization and species propagation. There are paracrine and autocrine regulations in various compartments of the testis that are under endocrine influences from the pituitary and hypothalamus. About 80% of the testicular mass consists of highly coiled seminiferous tubules within which spermatogenesis takes place. The remaining 20% consists of Leydig cells and Sertoli cells, whose main job is to establish normal spermatogenesis.

9.3.1 LEYDIG CELLS

These cells arise from interstitial mesenchymal tissue between the tubules during the eighth week of human embryonic development. They are located in the connective tissue between the seminiferous tubules. Leydig cells are the endocrine cells in the testis that produce testosterone from cholesterol via a series of enzymatic pathways and steroidal intermediates under the control of luteinizing hormone (LH) from the pituitary.

9.3.2 SERTOLI CELLS

Within the testes are cells that envelope the developing sperm during spermatogenesis. These cells form a continuous and complete lining within the tubular wall and establish the blood–testis barrier by virtue of tight junctions. The luminal environment is both created and controlled by these Sertoli cells, also called "nurse cells," which are under the influence of follicle-stimulating hormone (FSH) and inhibin. These Sertoli cells have several functions; they:

Provide nourishment for the developing sperm cells
Destroy defective sperm cells

Secrete fluid that helps in the transport of sperm into the epididymis
Release the hormone inhibin that helps regulate sperm production

The differentiation of Sertoli cells and the formation of a competent blood–testis barrier are essential to the establishment of normal spermatogenesis during puberty. Thus, many irregularities of spermatogenesis due to interference by endocrine disruptors may reflect changes in the function of the Sertoli cell population and not necessarily by pathology in the germ cells themselves.

9.4 ESTABLISHMENT OF SPERMATOGENESIS

Spermatogenesis is a chronological process spanning about 42 days in the rodent and 72 days in man. During this period, relatively undifferentiated spermatogonia, the immature germ cells, cyclically develop into highly specialized spermatozoa. Spermatogonia undergo several mitotic divisions to generate a large population of cells called primary spermatocytes, which produce haploid germ cells by two meiotic cell divisions. Spermiogenesis is the transformation of spermatids into elongated flagellar germ cells capable of motility. The release of mature germ cells is known as spermiation. The germ cells comprise the majority of testicular volume, which diminishes if testicular damage has occurred. A significant characteristic of mitotic arrest is that the gonocyte becomes acutely sensitive to toxic agents, e.g., irradiation.[26] Low-dose irradiation may completely eradicate germ cells while causing little damage to developing Sertoli cells, thus creating a Sertoli-cell-only testes.

9.5 ENDOCRINE DISRUPTORS THAT AFFECT MALE REPRODUCTION

Many endocrine disruptors, also termed estrogenic pollutants, from agricultural products (phytoestrogens), industrial chemicals, and heavy metals have significant environmental consequences due to their multiple routes of exposure, their widespread presence in the environment, and their ability to bioaccumulate and resist biodegradation. In addition, many pharmacological and biological agents including radiation therapy affect male reproduction via disrupting hormone influences. Table 9.1 lists the possible adverse effects caused by these agents described below.

9.5.1 ENVIRONMENTAL AGENTS

Endocrine disruptors are usually found in the environment. These chemicals make their way to humans through food, water, and air.[27] Pesticides, for example, can leave residues on foods or be washed from fields into drinking water supplies. Some plastic packaging can also deposit harmful chemicals, such as bisphenol A and phthalates, onto foods.[27] Other endocrine-disrupting chemicals could be breathed in or absorbed through the skin. However, the vast majority of chemicals have not been tested for their endocrine-disrupting capabilities.[27] Some endocrine-disrupting chemicals also have a tendency to bioaccumulate, becoming concentrated higher up the food chain. Foods high in animal fats, such as meat, fish, eggs, and dairy products,

TABLE 9.1
Effects of Hormonal Disruptors on Male Reproduction

Class	Agent	Adverse Effects
(A) Environmental:		
Organochemicals	DBCP	[↓ fertility, ↓ libido;
and Pesticides	DDT	embryo fetal loss, birth defects,
	PCBs	cancer; estrogenic effects,
	Dioxins	poor semen quality]
	Methyl chloride	
Heavy Metals	Lead	[↓ HPG-axis, ↓ spermatogenesis,
	Mercury	CNS effects, testicular damage]
	Cadmium	
	Cobalt	
	Chromium	
Ionizing Radiations	α- and β-rays	[Direct/indirect effect on gonads]
(B) Pharmacological :		
Radiation Therapy	X-rays, γ-rays	[Germ cell and Leydig cell damage]
Drugs/Phytoestrogens		
	GnRH-analogs	[↓ HPG axis,
KTZ, Leuprolide		↓ sperm; ↓ libido,
	Cyclosporine	↓ steroidogenesis]
	Lithium, narcotics	
	Anabolic steroids	
	Ethanol, nicotine	
	Flutamide	
	Gossypol, marijuana	
(C) Biological:		
	Hyperthermia	[↑ ROS, ↓ T biosynthesis,
		↓ spermatogenesis,
		testicular damage,
		poor sperm morphology]
	Superoxide, and nitric	[↑ ROS, ↓ antioxidants
	oxide radicals	↓ sperm function]
	Oxidative stress	[↑ ROS, ↑ LPO
		↑ cytokines, ↓ T,
		↓ sperm function]

Abbreviations: DBCP (dibromochloropropane); DDT (dichlorodiphenyl-trichloroethane); KTZ (ketoconazole); ROS (reactive oxygen species); LPO (lipid peroxidation);

often contain significant levels of these contaminants.[27] Processing can also introduce endocrine disruptors into food. In addition, human breastmilk, with its high fat content, is known to store large amounts of some endocrine-disrupting contaminants. A nursing infant may receive 10 to 60 times the adult daily dose of dioxins and PCBs per pound of body weight.[28]

9.5.1.1 Agricultural and Industrial Chemicals

Agricultural chemicals implicated in male reproductive toxicity include DDT (o,p-dichlorodiphenyl-trichloroethane), epichlorhydrin, ethylene dibromide, kepone, and the dioxins.[29] Dibromochloropropane, a nematocide widely used in agriculture, is a testicular toxicant and induces hypergonadotropic hypogonadism.[30,31] DDT, a commonly used pesticide, and its metabolites (p,p'-DDT, and p,p'-DDE) have estrogenic effects in males by blocking the androgen receptors.[21] The levels of serum free/bound toxicant will influence the androgen-blocking capacity. The plasma/tissue concentration of an estrogenic toxicant depends upon the detoxification and elimination mechanisms in the organism. The fate and detoxification of these organochemicals have not been described, but these agents can disrupt the hypothalamic–pituitary–testicular axis affecting the endocrine and reproductive functions. Methyl chloride, used in the production of organosilicates and gasoline antiknock additives, is a thoroughly studied industrial chemical.[32] Such organic solvents have been reported to induce changes in semen quality, testicular size, and serum gonadotropins.[33]

Polycyclic aromatic hydrocarbons (PAHs) are ubiquitous, undefined, complex mixtures encountered in the environment because of combustion as well as the use of tobacco products.[34] Since environmental exposures tend to be mixtures of various PAHs, the effect of their combined toxicity becomes more important but has not been examined in any detailed, well-designed study. A detrimental effect of endocrine disruptors on sperm concentration, motility, and morphology may be caused by impaired spermatogenesis secondary to various hormonal alterations.[35,36] A recent study has proposed that morphological sperm abnormalities due to secretory dysfunction of the Leydig and Sertoli cells may impair the sperm-fertilizing capacity.

9.5.1.2 Heavy Metals

Metals (e.g., lead, mercury, cadmium, aluminum, cobalt, chromium, arsenic, lithium, and antimony) have been noted to exert adverse reproductive effects in humans and experimental animals. More reports are available on lead-induced toxicity than any other heavy metal. Historically, the fall of the Roman Empire has been attributed to lead poisoning.[37] Adverse effects on the reproductive capacity of men working in battery plants and exposed to toxic levels of lead have been reported.[38,39] In animals, lead exposure results in a dose-dependent suppression of serum testosterone and spermatogenesis.[40,41] Although testicular biopsies reveal peritubular fibrosis, vacuolation, and oligospermia, suggesting that lead is a direct testicular toxicant,[42] some mechanistic studies have revealed that lead exposure can disrupt the hormonal feedback mechanism at the hypothalamic–pituitary level.[13] Animal studies suggest that these effects can be reversed when lead is removed from the system. Such detailed evaluations in humans are under investigation.

Mercury exposure (during the manufacture of thermometers, thermostats, mercury vapor lamps, paint, and electrical appliances, and in mining) can alter spermatogenesis and has been found to decrease fertility in experimental animals. Boron (extensively used in the manufacture of glass, cements, soaps, carpets, crockery, and leather products) has a major adverse reproductive effect on the testes and the hypothalamic–pituitary axis in a manner similar to lead. Oligospermia and decreased libido were reported in men working in boric acid-producing factories.[43] Cadmium, another heavy metal used widely in industries (electroplating, battery electrode production, galvanizing, plastics, alloys, paint pigments) and present in soil, coal, water, and cigarette smoke, is a testicular toxicant.[44] In animal studies, cadmium has been shown to cause strain-dependent severe testicular necrosis in mice.[45] Cadmium-DNA binding and inhibition of sulfhydryl-containing proteins mediate cadmium toxicity directly or through transcription mechanisms. It can also induce the expression of heat shock proteins, oxidative stress response genes, and heme oxygenase induction mechanisms.[46] Further study is needed to delineate the specific gonadotoxic mechanisms involved. Clinical studies have associated cadmium exposure with testicular toxicity, altered libido, and infertility.

9.5.2 Pharmacologic Agents

Many pharmacologic drugs, chemotherapeutic agents, and radiation therapy are known to adversely affect male reproduction.

9.5.2.1 Anabolic Steroids

Anabolic steroids, which are mostly synthetic pharmacological agents, affect normal endocrine functions. The use or abuse of these anabolic steroids mainly among athletes has grown to epidemic proportions. This has resulted in severe oligozoospermia and decreased libido. The hypogonadotropic hypogonadism due to feedback inhibition of the hypothalamus–pituitary axis is the most common cause of severe impairment of normal sperm production in this population.[47] These defects can be reversed within four months of non-use; however, sporadic azoospermia has been reported in some young men even 1 year after cessation of chronic anabolic steroid use.[48]

9.5.2.2 Estrogens

Animals and human exposed to estregens in utero have shown developmentally estregenized male phenotype-retained or cryptorchid testes, decrease in sperm number, increase in abnormal sperm, retained Müllerian ducts, epididymal cysts, hypospadias, and prostatic disease.[49] The genes involved in the process of male genital tract morphogenesis are only now being identified. The acute or persistent modulation of the expression of developmentally critical or hormone-responsive gene in the male genital tract by estregenic compounds is currently ongoing in numerous laboratories.[49]

9.5.2.3 Chemotherapeutic Agents

Many antimicrobials (e.g., tetracycline derivatives, sulfa drugs, nitrofurantoin, and macrolide agents, like erythromycin) impair spermatogenesis and spermatozoal function.[50,51] As early as 1954, antibacterial agents were reported to be toxic to spermatozoa. Cancer chemotherapy usually damages the germinal epithelium.[52]

Mechlorethamine, extensively used as nitrogen mustard during the Second World War, causes spermatogenic arrest.[53] Many common cytotoxic agents cause a dose-dependent progressive decrease in sperm count, leading to azoospermia.[54] Postmeiotic germ cells are specifically sensitive to cyclophosphamide treatment, with abnormalities observed in progeny.[55] Chronic low-dose cyclophosphamide treatment in men may affect the decondensation potential of spermatozoa due to the alkylation of nuclear proteins or DNA. This is likely to affect pre- and post-implantation loss or contribute to congenital abnormalities in offspring.[56] Combination therapy with alkylating agents has been shown to improve survival in the treatment of Hodgkin's disease, lymphoma, and leukemia. However, such combination therapy has induced sterility in most adults, as revealed by complete germinal aplasia in testicular biopsy specimens.[57]

In general, the severity of testicular damage is related to the category of chemotherapeutic agent used, the dose and duration of therapy, and the developmental stage of the testis. The recovery of spermatogenesis is variable and depends upon the total therapeutic dose and duration of treatment.[58] The effects of cytotoxic drugs on the testicular function of children are inconclusive, due to the relative insensitivity in detecting such damage with available technology; however, the prepubertal and adolescent testes are reportedly affected less by chemo- and radiation therapy than is the postpubertal testis.[59] The use of testicular biopsy, semen analysis, and assessment of the HPG axis[52] can commonly achieve the evaluation of testicular toxicity.

9.5.2.4 Radiation Therapy

Radiotherapy is alternatively used for the treatment of seminomatous germ cell tumors and lymphomas. Testicular damage due to radiation exposure (X-rays, neutrons, and radioactive materials) is generally more severe and difficult to recover than that induced by chemotherapy. Radiation effects on the testes depend on the schedule (total dose, number of fractions, duration) of the delivered irradiation, as well as the developmental stage of the germ cell in the testes at the time of exposure.[59] In general, germ cells are the most radiosensitive. A direct dose of irradiation to the testes greater than 0.35 Gy causes aspermia. The time taken for recovery increases with larger doses, and doses in excess of 2 Gy will likely lead to permanent azoospermia. At higher radiation doses (> 15 Gy), Leydig cells will also be affected.[60] Vulnerability of the testis to irradiation depends upon the age and the pubertal status of the male. In addition to direct damage to the testes, whole body irradiation can also damage the hypothalamic–pituitary axis and affect reproductive capability.[61]

9.6 MECHANISM(S) OF ACTION OF ENDOCRINE DISRUPTORS

Due to the complexity of the interactions involved in normal gonadal function and hormonal communication, any of these loci could be involved mechanistically in a toxicant's endocrine-related effect. Such impaired hormonal control could occur as a consequence of altered hormone synthesis, storage/release, transport/clearance, receptor recognition/binding, or post-receptor responses.

9.6.1 Altered Hormone Synthesis

A number of agents possess the ability to inhibit the synthesis of various hormones. Some of these agents inhibit specific enzymatic steps in the biosynthetic pathway of steroidogenesis (e.g., aminoglutethimide, cyanoketone, ketoconazole). Some fungicides block estrogen biosynthesis by inhibiting aromatase activity. Environmental estrogens and antiandrogens alter protein hormone synthesis induced by gonadal steroids. Both estrogen and testosterone have been shown to affect pituitary hormone synthesis directly or through changes in the glycosylation of LH and FSH.[62] A decrease in glycosylation of these glycoproteins reduces the biological activity of the hormones. Any environmental compound that mimics or antagonizes the action of these steroid hormones could presumably alter glycosylation.

9.6.2 Altered Hormone Storage or Release

Steroid hormones do not appear to be stored intracellularly within membranous secretory granules. For example, testosterone is synthesized by the Leydig cells of the testis and released on activation of the LH receptor. Thus, compounds that block the LH receptor or the activation of the $3',5'$-cyclic AMP-dependent cascade involved in testosterone biosynthesis can rapidly alter the secretion of this hormone. The release of many protein hormones is dependent on the activation of second messenger pathways, such as cAMP, phosphatidylinositol 4, 5-bisphosphate (PIP_2), inositol 1, 4, 5-trisphosphate (IP_3), tyrosine kinase, and Ca^{++}. Interference with these processes consequently will alter the serum levels (availability) of many hormones. Several metal cations have been shown to disrupt pituitary hormone release, presumably by interfering with Ca^{++} flux.[63]

9.6.3 Altered Hormone Transport and Clearance

Hormones are transported from blood in the free or bound state. Steroid hormones are transported in the blood by specialized transport (carrier) proteins known as sex-steroid hormone-binding globulin (SHBG) or testosterone-estrogen-binding globulin (TEBG). Regulation of the concentration of these binding globulins in the blood is of practical significance because there may be either increases or decreases that could affect steroid hormone availability. For example, DDT analogs are potent inducers of hepatic microsomal monooxygenase activities *in vivo*.[64] Induction of this monooxygenase activity by treatment with DDT analogs could possibly cause a decrease in testicular androgen as a result of enhanced degradation. Similarly, treatment with lindane (gamma-hexachlorocyclohexane) has been reported to increase the clearance of estrogen.[65]

9.6.4 Altered Hormone Receptor Recognition/Binding

Hormones elicit responses on their respective target tissues through direct interactions with either intracellular receptors or membrane-bound receptors. Specific binding of the natural ligand to its receptor is a critical step in hormone function. Intracellular (nuclear) receptors, such as those for sex steroids, adrenal steroids, thyroid hormones, vitamin D, and retinoic acid, regulate gene transcription in a ligand-dependent manner through their interaction with specific DNA sequences (response elements). A number of environmental agents may alter this process by mimicking the natural ligand and acting as an agonist or by inhibiting binding and acting as an antagonist. The best-known examples are methoxychlor, chlordecone (Kepone), DDT, some PCBs, and alkylphenols (e.g., nonylphenols and octylphenols), which can disrupt estrogen receptor function.[66,67] The anti-androgenic action of the dicarboximide fungicide vinclozolin is the result of an affinity of this compound's metabolites for the androgen receptor.[21] Interestingly, the DDT metabolite p, p′-DDE has been found to bind also to the androgen receptor and block testosterone-induced cellular responses *in vitro*.[68]

Many of the chemicals classified as environmental estrogens can actually inhibit binding to more than one type of intracellular receptor. For example, o,p-DDT and chlordecone can inhibit endogenous ligand binding to the estrogen and progesterone receptors, with each compound having IC50s that are nearly identical for the two receptors. Receptors for protein hormones are located on and in the cell membrane. When these hormones bind to their receptors, transduction of a signal across the membrane is mediated by the activation of second messenger systems. These may include (a) alterations in G-protein/cAMP-dependent protein kinase A (e.g., after LH stimulation of the Leydig cell), (b) phosphatidylinositol regulation of protein kinase C and inositol triphosphate (e.g., after GnRH stimulation of gonadotrophs; thyrotropin releasing hormone stimulation of thyrotrophs), (c) tyrosine kinase (e.g., after insulin binding to the membrane receptor), and (d) calcium ion flux. Xenobiotics thus can disrupt signal transduction of peptide hormones if they interfere with one or more of these processes.

9.6.5 Altered Hormone Post-Receptor Activation

Once the endogenous ligand or an agonist binds to its receptor, a cascade of events is initiated, indicative of the appropriate cellular response. This includes the response necessary for signal transduction across the membrane, or in the case of nuclear receptors, the initiation of transcription and protein synthesis. A variety of environmental compounds can interfere with the membrane's second messenger systems. For example, cellular responses that are dependent on the flux of calcium ions through the membrane (and the initiation of the calcium/Calmodulin-dependent cellular response) are altered by a variety of environmental toxicants. Interestingly, the well-known antiestrogen tamoxifen also inhibits protein kinase C activity.[69] Alternatively, the phorbol esters are known to mimic diacylglycerol and enhance protein kinase C activity.

Steroid hormone receptor activation can be modified by indirect mechanisms, such as a down-regulation of the receptor (temporary decreased sensitivity to ligand) as seen after TCDD exposure (including the estrogen, progesterone, and glucocorticoid receptors).[70,71] Consequently, because of the diverse known pathways of endocrine disruption, any assessment must consider the net result of all influences on hormone receptor function and feedback regulation.

9.6.6 INDUCTION OF OXIDATIVE STRESS

"Oxidative stress" is a condition associated with an increased rate of cellular damage induced by oxygen and oxygen-derived free radicals commonly known as reactive oxygen species (ROS), which belong to the class of free radicals. Chronic disease states, aging, toxin exposure, physical injury, and exposure to many types of environmental contaminants can enhance this oxidative process and cause gonadal damage.[72] Similarly, the generation of nitric oxide (NO) and reactive nitrogen species (RNS) has recently been found to have an astounding range of biological roles including vascular tone and inflammation and as a mediator of many cytotoxic and pathological effects.[73] NO generation in response to toxic exposure associated with hormonal imbalance can contribute to poor sperm motility and function, leading to infertility.[74] Nitric oxide and superoxide radicals combine to form highly reactive peroxynitrite radicals, which induce endothelial cell injury.[75] This may result in altered blood flow to the testis and impair testicular function.

The assumption that free radicals can influence male fertility has received substantial scientific support.[76] The proposed mechanism for loss of testicular and sperm function due to oxidative stress has been shown to involve excessive generation of ROS.[77] Free radicals can damage DNA and proteins, either through oxidation of DNA bases (primarily guanine via lipid peroxyl or alkoxyl radicals) or through covalent binding to MDA, resulting in strand breaks and cross-linking.[78] ROS can also induce oxidation of critical -SH groups in proteins and DNA, which will alter cellular integrity and function with an increased susceptibility to attack by toxicants (Figure 9.1). Oxidative stress is theoretically the result of an improper balance between ROS generation and intrinsic scavenging activities. Adequate levels of superoxide dismutase (SOD), catalase, and probably glutathione (GSH) peroxidase and reductase normally maintain the free radical scavenging potential in the testes. This balance can be referred to as oxidative stress status (OSS), and its assessment may play a critical role in monitoring testicular toxicity and infertility.[14]

9.7   ASSESSMENT OF TOXICITY

Several methods are being evaluated for the assessment of the effects of toxicants on the male reproductive system. Essentially, any risk assessment usually has four components: (1) hazard identification, (2) dose-response assessment, (3) human-exposure assessment, and (4) risk characterization. The hazard identification and dose-response data are developed from experimental animal studies that may be supplemented with data from *in vitro* studies. This information is then extrapolated and integrated to characterize and assess the risk to the human population.

The most common approach to evaluate the effect of cytotoxic drugs on the testis has used testicular biopsy, semen analysis, and endocrine assessment of the hypothalamic–pituitary–testicular axis (Table 9.2). Research on testicular toxicology has been advanced significantly by the introduction of *in vitro* testing systems. *In vivo* systems, however, are still essential parts of the risk assessment process, and they are unlikely to be eliminated by *in vitro* models.

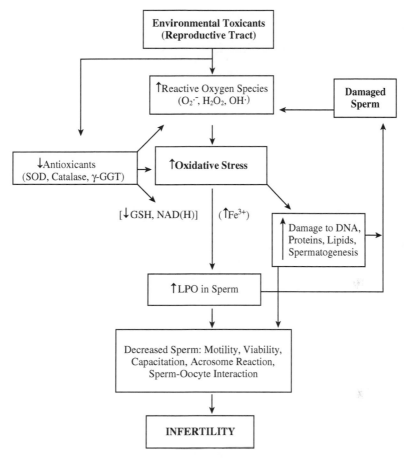

FIGURE 9.1

9.7.1 In Vitro Systems

In vitro systems are uniquely suited to investigate specific cellular and molecular mechanisms in the testis and thus improve risk assessment.[79] These *in vitro* models can be used alone or in combination with each other to test hypotheses about testicular toxicity. An original toxicant, its metabolites, the precursors, or selective inhibitors can be individually administered to isolated cell types to evaluate specific toxicity mechanisms and to note the interaction of adjacent cell types. Numerous *in vitro* model systems are described in the literature, including Sertoli-germ cell co-cultures;[80] Sertoli cell-enriched cultures;[81,82] germ cell-enriched cultures;[83] Leydig cell cultures;[40] Leydig-Sertoli cell co-cultures;[84] and peritubular and tubular cell cultures.[80,84] These *in vitro* systems are the only way to directly compare human and animal responses and to screen a class of compounds for new product development. Though these *in vitro* systems are a valuable adjunct to the *in vivo* test system, they do not replace the *in vivo* data, because they cannot provide all the facts essential

TABLE 9.2

Evaluation of Effect of Hormonal Disruptors in the Adult Male

Potential Sites	Effects	Evaluative Tests
Testis	Necrosis	Weight, Histopathology
Leydig cells	LH/PRL	Receptor analysis, RIA
	T biosynthesis/secretion	*In vitro* production and hormone assay
Sertoli cells	FSH/Inhibin/Steroids	Receptor analysis, RIA
	Sertoli/Leydig cell function	*In vitro* tests (co-culture)
	Blood-testis barrier	Morphology
Seminiferous Tubules	Spermatogonial mitosis	Germ cell count and % tubules without germ cells
	Spermatocyte meiosis	Spermatid counts and % tubules with luminal sperm
	Spermatid differentiation	Germ-cell culture, morphology
Epididymis	Sperm maturation	Histopathology, biochemical tests
Brain	Hypothalamic–pituitary axis	Pituitary cell-culture, hypothalamus perfusion, histopathology, hormone challenge, accessory sex-organ weights
Seminal Fluid	Daily sperm production	Spermatid counts and semen evaluation
Blood	HPG axis	Hormones/ABP assays

Abbreviations: LH (luteinizing hormone); PRL (prolactin); FSH (follicle-stimulating hormone); ABP (androgen binding protein); HPG (hypothalamic-pituitary-gonadal).

for hazard assessment. Moreover, certain dynamic changes associated with spermatogenesis are difficult to model *in vitro*. For example, the release of elongated spermatids by the Sertoli cells (spermiation), which is commonly inhibited by boric acid and methyl chloride, can only be studied at present by specific *in vivo* systems.

9.7.2 *IN VIVO* SYSTEMS

In vivo methods are important tools to study the integrated male reproductive system. The complete *in vivo* assessment of testicular toxicity involves multigenerational studies, now required by most regulatory agencies. These multigenerational studies have a complex design, because testicular function and spermatogenesis are very complicated processes. The spermatogenic cycle is highly organized throughout the testis. In the rat, it requires 53 days. If a toxicant affects the immature spermatogonia, the effect may not be detectable as a change in mature sperm before 7 to 8 weeks. Effects on more mature germ cells would be detected sooner. To test the sensitivity of all stages of spermatogenesis, the exposure should last the full duration of the cycle. This cannot be achieved *in vitro,* because germ cell differentiation and the physical relationship of stages within the tubules are lost in cell culture systems. The germ cells are entirely dependent upon the Sertoli cells for physical and biochemical support. Complicated endocrine and paracrine systems control Sertoli cells, Leydig cells, and germ cells.

Besides the loss of paracrine interactions, the altered metabolic activity of target or adjacent cells and difficulty in isolating and testing certain spermatogenic stages are other significant limitations of *in vitro* assessment of testicular toxicity.[79] In addition, for accurate identification of stage-specific lesions of the seminiferous epithelium, critical evaluation of morphological structures is very important. Because germ cells are continuously dividing and differentiating, the staging of spermatogenesis has proven to be an extremely sensitive tool to identify and characterize even subtle toxicological changes.

9.7.3 SPERM NUCLEAR INTEGRITY ASSESSMENT

Recent attention has been focused on assessments of sperm morphology and physiology as important endpoints in reproductive toxicology testing.[85] Structural stability of sperm nuclei varies by species, appears to be enhanced by the oxidation of protamine sulfhydryl to inter- and intra-molecular disulfide bonds, and is a function of the types of protamine present. Chemicals may disrupt the structural stability of sperm nuclei, which depend upon their unique packaging either during spermatogenesis or sperm maturation. Decondensation of an isolated sperm nucleus *in vitro* can be induced by exposure to disulfide reducing agents, and the time taken to induce extensive decondensation (assay end) is considered to be inversely proportional to the stability of the sperm nucleus. This "sperm activation assay" is also useful in the evaluation of some cases of unexplained infertility.[86] Human sperm decondenses most rapidly, followed by that of the mouse and of the hamster, while rat sperm nuclei showed a slower decondensation.[87]

Other tests, called DNA stability assay or sperm chromatin structure assay (SCSA), use direct evaluation of sperm chromatin integrity and may provide information about genetic damage to sperm. A shift in DNA pattern (from double-stranded intact DNA to denatured single-stranded) can be induced by a variety of mutagenic and chemical agents and evaluated either by DNA flow cytometric analysis or by sperm chromatin structure assay.[88,89] A single-cell gel electrophoresis (Comet) assay, which uses fluorescence intensity measurements by microscopy and image analysis, has also been recently developed.[86] A shift in the DNA pattern can also be evaluated by acridine orange staining, where double-stranded DNA is stained green and single-stranded DNA is stained red. Animals exposed to known mutagens demonstrate increased amounts of single-stranded DNA, indicating an increase in genetic damage.[90,91]

DNA flow cytometry is a very useful tool that permits rapid, objective assessment of a large number of cells, but may not be readily available. Comet assay, when combined with centrifugal elutriation, can provide a useful *in vitro* model to study differences in metabolism and the susceptibility of different testicular cell types to DNA damaging compounds. Thus, new findings through these systems should lead to greater knowledge about why a chemical or class of chemicals can cause testicular toxicity.

9.8 SCIENTIFIC DEBATE

In the wake of media coverage dealing with possible reproductive health and cancer concerns,[92] a few toxicologists have questioned whether these adverse health effects can be attributed to environmental endocrine disruption.[93,71] Arguments for a demonstrable link between hormone-disruptive environmental agents and human reproductive health effects are supported by the fact that many pesticides and other agents with estrogenic or antiandrogenic activity operate via hormone receptor mechanisms. However, in the few studies of suspected weak estrogens, like the alkylphenols, some 1000 to 10,000 times or up to 10^6 more agent is required to bind 50% of the estrogen receptor than estradiol itself.[67] Of course, crucial to risk assessment is the need to know how many receptors must be occupied before activation of a response can ensue. For some hormones such as human chorionic gonadotropin (hCG), as little as 0.5% to 5% receptor occupancy is required for full activation of response. For other hormones (those that require protein synthesis for expression of effect), higher levels of receptor occupancy are needed.

Fluctuations of hormone concentration and receptor activities, by design, absorb some environmental and physiological challenges to maintain homeostasis in adults. Only when the equilibrium control mechanisms are overwhelmed do the deleterious effects occur. An important question is whether homeostatic mechanisms are operative in the embryo and fetus.

Some investigators[94] have proposed the use of *in vitro* assays to screen for estrogenic or other hormonal activity. While steroid receptors bound to their ligand act as transcription factors for gene expression in the target tissue, simple *in vitro* screening assays based on binding to a receptor are not sufficient in themselves for measuring hormone activity. Binding of ligand to its specific receptor must be correlated with a physiologic response.

9.9 SUMMARY

The observation that humans have experienced increased incidences of developmental, reproductive, and carcinogenic effects, and the formulation of a working hypothesis that these adverse effects may be caused by environmental chemicals acting to disrupt the endocrine system that regulates these processes, is supported by observations of similar effects in aquatic and wildlife species. In other words, a common theme runs through both human and wildlife reports.

In contrast, the hypothesis that the reported increased incidence of human cancers and reproductive abnormalities and infertility can be attributed to an endocrine-disruption phenomenon is called into question for several reasons. First, secretion and elimination of hormones are highly regulated by the body, and mechanisms for controlling modest fluctuations of hormones are in place via negative feedback control of hormone concentrations. Therefore, minor increases of environmental hormones following dietary absorption and liver detoxification of these xenobiotics may be inconsequential in disrupting endocrine homeostasis.

Second, low ambient concentrations of chemicals along with low affinity binding of purported xenobiotics to target receptors probably are insufficient to activate an adverse response in adults. Whether the fetus and the young are capable of regulating minor changes to the endocrine milieu is uncertain. Finally, the data are not available for mixtures of chemicals that may be able to affect endocrine function. At the same time, in the case of environmental estrogens as endocrine disruptors, it is known that competition for binding sites by antiestrogens in the environment may moderate estrogenic effects of some chemicals. Clearly, more research to fill data gaps and to remove the uncertainty in these unknowns is needed.

With few exceptions (e.g., DES), a causal relationship between exposure to a specific environmental agent and an adverse effect on human health operating via an endocrine disruption mechanism has not been established. Short-term screening studies could be developed and validated in an effort to elucidate mechanism. Through controlled dose-response studies, it appears that these compounds (e.g., alkyl phenol ethylates and their degradation products, chlorinated dibenzodioxins and difurans, and polychlorinated biphenyls), can induce irreversible induction of male sex characteristics on females (imposex), which can lead to sterility and reduced reproductive performance.

In conclusion, a variety of extraneous and internal factors can induce testicular toxicity leading to poor sperm quality and male factor infertility. Unfortunately, several of these influences (e.g., glandular infection, environmental toxicants that are mainly estrogenic chemicals, nutritional deficiencies, aging, ischemia, and oxidative stress) disrupt the hormonal milieu and have been underestimated. Partial androgen insensitivity mainly due to altered androgen-to-estrogen balance may contribute to significant oligozoospermia. The role of chronic inflammation on the reproductive organs is not completely understood because it is asymptomatic and is difficult to demonstrate objectively.

There is an urgent need to characterize all the factors involved and to develop reliable animal models of testicular disease. No major advances have been made for the medical management of poor sperm quality. The application of assisted reproductive techniques such as ICSI to male infertility, regardless of cause, does not necessarily treat the cause and may inadvertently pass on adverse genetic consequences. Clinicians should always attempt to identify the etiology of a possible testicular toxicity, assess the degree of risk to the patients being evaluated for infertility, and initiate a plan to control and prevent exposure to others once an association between occupation/exposure and infertility has been established.

REFERENCES

1. Nelson CMK and Bunge RG: Semen analysis: Evidence for changing parameters of male fertility potential. *Fertility and Sterility*, 25: 503-507, 1974.
2. Carlsen E, Giwercman A, Keiding N, Skakkebaek NE: Evidence for decreasing quality of semen during past 50 years. *BMJ*, 305: 609-613, 1992.
3. Chapin RE, White RD, Morgan KT and Buss JS: Studies of lesions induced in the testis and epididymis of F-344 rats by inhaled methyl chloride. *Toxicol. Appl. Pharmacol.*, 76:328-343, 1984.
4. Brake A and Krause W: Decreasing quality of semen. *Br. Med. Journal*, 305:1498-1503, 1992.

5. Olsen GW, Bodner KM, Ramlow JM, Ross CE and Lipshultz LI: Have sperm counts been reduced 50 percent in 50 years? A statistical model revisited. *Fertil. Steril.*, 63:887-893, 1995.

6. Swan SH, Elkin EP, Fenster L: Have sperm densities declined? A reanalysis of global trend data. *Environ. Health Perspect.*, 105:1228-1232, 1997.

7. Swan SH, Elkin EP, Fenster L: The question of declining sperm density revisited: An analysis of 101 studies published 1934-1996. *Environ. Health Perspect.*, 108: 961-966, 2000.

8. Sharpe RM, Skakkebaek NE: Are oestrogens involved in falling sperm counts and disorders of the male reproductive tract? *Lancet*, 341: 1392–1395, 1993.

9. Fisch H, Goluboff ET, Olson JH, Feldshuh J, Broder SJ and Barad DH: Semen analyses in 1283 men from the United States over a 25-year period: No decline in quality. *Fertility and Sterility*, 65:1009-1014, 1996.

10. Parvinen M, Lahdetie J and Parvinen LM: Toxic and mutagenic influences on spermatogenesis. *Arch. Toxicol.*, 7:147-150, 1984.

11. Guillette LJ, Gross TS, Masson GR, Matter JM, Percival HF and Woodward AR: Developmental abnormalities of the gonad and abnormal sex hormone concentrations in juvenile alligators from contaminated and control lakes in Florida. *Environ. Health Prospect.*, 102(8):680-688, 1994.

12. Kavlock RJ and Perreault SD: Multiple chemical exposure and risks of adverse reproductive function and outcome. In *Toxicological of Chemical Mixtures: From Real Life Examples to Mechanisms of Toxicology Interactions.* Yang RSH (ed) Academic Press, Orlando, FL, pp. 245-297, 1994.

13. Sokol RZ: Hormonal effects of lead acetate in the male rat: Mechanism of action. *Biol. Reprod.*, 37:1135-1138, 1987.

14. Sikka SC: Gonadotoxicity. In *Male Infertility and Sexual Dysfunction,* Hellstrom WJG (ed), Springer-Verlag, NY, pp. 292-306, 1997.

15. Lamb DJ: Hormonal disruptors and male infertility: Are men at serious risk? *Reg. Toxicol. Pharmacol.*, 26:001-003, 1997.

16. Cheek AO and McLachlan JA: Environmental hormones and the male reproductive system. *J. Androl.*, 19:5-10, 1998.

17. Boris A: Endocrine studies of a nonsteroid anti-androgen and progestin. *Endocrinology,* 76:1063-1067, 1965.

18. McLachlan JA, Arnold SF: Environmental estrogens. *Am. Sci.*, 84:452-461, 1996.

19. Colborn T, vomSaal FS, Soto AM: Developmental effects of endocrine-disrupting chemicals in wildlife and humans. *Environ. Health Prospect.*, 1101(5):378-384, 1993.

20. Purdom CE, Hardiman PA, Bye VJ, Eno NC, Tyler CR and Sumpter JP: Estrogenic effects of effluents from sewage treatment works. *Chem. Ecol.*, 8:275-285, 1994.

21. Kelce WR, Monosson E, Gamcsik MP, Laws SC and Gray LE Jr.: Environmental hormone disruptors: evidence that vinclozolin developmental toxicity is mediated by antiandrogenic metabolites. *Toxicol. Appl. Pharm.*, 126:276-285, 1994.

22. Sharpe RM and Skakkebaek NE: Are estrogens involved in falling sperm counts and disorders of the male reproductive tract? *Lancet*, 351:1392-1395, 1993.

23. Sokol RZ: Toxicants and infertility: Identification and prevention. In *Management of Impotence and Infertility,* Whitehead ED and Nagler HM (eds), JB Lippincott Company, Philadelphia, 380-389, 1994.

24. Schrader SM and Kanitz MH: Occupational hazards to male reproduction. In *State of the Art Reviews in Occupational Medicine: Reproductive Hazards.* Gold E, Schenker M and Lesley B (eds), Hanley and Belfus, Inc., PA, pp. 405-414, 1994.

25. Working PK: Male reproductive toxicity: comparison of the human to animal models. *Environ. Health Prospect.*, 77:37-44, 1988.

26. Mandl AM: The radiosensitivity of germ cells. *Biol. Re.*, 39:288-294, 1964.

27. Environmental Endocrine Disruptors: What health care providers should know? http://www.psr.org.

28. World Health Organization Regional Office for Europe. Levels of PCBs, PCDDs, and PCDFs in breast milk, Copenhagen, 1989.

29. Whorton MD, Krauss RM, Marshall S: Infertility in male pesticide workers. *Lancet*, 2:1259-1261, 1977.

30. Mattison DR: The mechanisms of action of reproductive toxins. *Am. J. Indust. Med.*, 4:65-79, 1983.

31. Potashnik G and Yanai-Inbar I: Dibromochloropropane (DBCP): An 8-year reevaluation of testicular function and reproductive performance. *Fertil. Steril.*, 47:317-323, 1987.

32. Chapin RE, Gray TJB, Phelps Jl and Dutton SL: The effects of mono-(2-ethylhexyl)phthalate on rat Sertoli cell-enriched primary cultures. *Toxicol. Appl. Pharmacol.*, 96:467- 479, 1988.

33. Schrader SM: Principles of male reproductive toxicology. In *Environmental Medicine.* Brooks SM, Gochfeld M (eds), Mosby Press, St. Louis, pp. 95-100, 1995.

34. Georgellis A, Toppari J, Veromaa T, Rydstrom J and Parvinen M: Inhibition of meiotic divisions of rat spermatocytes *in vitro* by polycyclic aromatic hydrocarbons. *Mutat. Res.*, 231:125-135, 1990.

35. Vine MF, Tse CJ, Hu PC and Truong KY: Cigarette smoking and semen quality. *Fertil. Steril.*, 65:835-842, 1996.

36. Zavos PM: Cigarette smoking and human reproduction: effects on female and male fecundity. *Infertility*, 12:35-40, 1989.

37. Gilfillan SC: Lead poisoning and the fall of Rome. *J. Occup. Med.*, 7:53-60, 1965.

38. Lancranjan I, Popescu HI, Gavanescu O, Klepsch I and Serbanescu M: Reproductive ability of workmen occupationally exposed to lead. *Arch. Environ. Health*, 30:396-401, 1975.

39. Winder C: Reproductive and chromosomal effects of occupational exposure to lead in males. *Reprod. Toxicol.*, 3:221-233, 1989.

40. Ewing LL, Zirkin BR and Chubb C: Assessment of testicular testosterone production and Leydig cell structure. *Environ. Health Prospect.*, 38:19-27, 1981.

41. Foster WG, McMahon A,Young-Lai EV, Hughes EG, and Rice DC: Reproductive endocrine effects of chronic lead exposure in the male cynomolgus monkey. *Reprod. Toxicol.*, 7:203-209, 1992.

42. Braunstein GD, Dahlgren J, Loriaux DO: Hypogonadism in chronically lead poisoned men. *Infertility*, 1:33-35, 1978.

43. Weir RJ, Fisher RS: Toxicological studies on borox and boric acid. *Toxicol. Appl. Pharmacol.*, 23:251-264, 1972.

44. Friberg L, Piscator M and Nordberg GF: *Cadmium in the Environment,* 2nd ed., CRC Press, Inc., Boca Raton, FL, pp. 37-53, 1974.

45. King LM, Andrew MG, Sikka SC and George WJ: Murine strain differences in cadmium-induced testicular toxicity. *The Toxicologist*, 36, (2) pp. 186, 1997.

46. Snow ET: Metal carcinogenesis: mechanistic implications. *Pharmacol. Ther.*, 53:31-65, 1992.

47. Knuth UA, Maniera H and Nieschlag E: Anabolic steroids and semen parameters in body builders. *Fertil. Steril.*, 52:1041-1047, 1989.

48. Jarow JP and Lipshultz LI: Anabolic steroid-induced hypogonadotropic hypogonadism. *Am. J. Sports Med.*, 18:429-431, 1990.

49. McLachlan JA: Environmental signaling: What embryos and evolution teach us about endocrine disrupting chemicals. *Endocrine Rev.*, 22(3): 319-341, 2001.

50. Ericsson RJ and Baker VF: Binding of tetracycline to mammalian spermatozoa. *Nature*, 214:403-407, 1967.

51. Schlegel PN, Chang TSK, Maeshall FF: Antibiotics: Potential hazards to male fertility. *Fertil. Steril.*, 55:235-242, 1991.

52. Shalet SM: Effects of cancer chemotherapy on testicular function of patients. *Cancer Treatment Rev.*, 7:41-152, 1980.

53. Spitz S: The histological effects of nitrogen mustards on human tumors and tissues. *Cancer*, 1:383-388, 1948.

54. Meistrich ML: Quantitative correlation between testicular stem cell survival, sperm production, and fertility in mouse after treatment with different cytotoxic agents. *J. Androl.*, 3:58-68, 1982.

55. Qiu J, Hales BF and Robaire B: Adverse effects of cyclophosphamide on progeny outcome can be mediated through post-testicular mechanisms in the rat. *Biol. Reprod.*, 46:926-931, 1992.

56. Trasler JM, Hales BF and Robaire B: A time course study of chronic paternal cyclophosphamide treatment of rats: effects on pregnancy outcome and the male reproductive and hematologic systems. *Biol. Reprod.*, 37:317-326, 1987.

57. Sherins RJ and DeVita VT Jr.: Effect of drug treatment for lymphoma on male reproductive capacity. *Ann. Intern. Med.*, 79:216-220, 1973.

58. Parvinen M, Lahdetie J and Parvinen LM: Toxic and mutagenic influences on spermatogenesis. *Arch. Toxicol.*, 7:147-150, 1984.

59. Oats RD and Lipshultz LI: Fertility and testicular function in patients after chemotherapy and radiotherapy. In *Advances in Urology, vol. 2.* Lytton B (ed), Mosby Year Book, Chicago, pp. 55-83, 1989.

60. Rowley MJ, Leach DR, Warner GA and Heller CG: Effects of graded doses of ionizing radiation on the human testis. *Radiat. Res.*, 59:665-668, 1974.

61. Ogilvy-Stuart Al and Shalet SM: Effect of radiation on the human reproductive system. *Environ. Health Perspect.*, 101:109-116, 1993.

62. Wilson CA, Leigh AJ and Chapman AJ: Gonadotrophin glycosylation and function. *J. Endocrinol.*, 125:3-14, 1990.

63. Cooper RL, Goldman JM, Rehnberg GL, McElroy WK and Hein JF: Effects of metal cations on pituitary hormone secretions *in vitro. J. Biochem. Toxicol.*, 2:241-249, 1987.

64. Bulger WH, Nuccitelli RM and Kupfer D: Studies on the *in vivo* and *in vitro* estrogenic activities of methoxychlor and its metabolites role of hepatic mono-oxygenase in methoxychlor activation. *Biochem. Pharmacol.*, 27:2417-2423, 1978.

65. Welch RM, Levin W, Kuntzman R, Jocobson M and Conney AH: Effect of halogenated hydrocarbon insecticides on the metabolism and uterotropic actions of estrogens in rats and mice. *Toxicol. Appl. Pharmacol.*, 19:234-246, 1971.

66. Mueller GC and Kim UH: Displacement of estradiol from estrogen receptors by simple alkylphenols. *Endocrinology,* 102:1429-1435, 1978.

67. White TE, Rucci G, Liu Z and Gasiewicz TA: Environmentally persistent alkylphenolic compounds are estrogenic. *Endocrinology,* 135:175-182, 1994.

68. Kelce WR, Stone CR, Laws SC, Gray LE Jr., Kemppainen JA, Wilson EM: Persistent DDT metabolite p,p′-DDE is a potent androgen receptor antagonist. *Nature*, 375:581-585, 1995.

69. O'Brian CA, Liskamp RM, Solomon DH and Weinstein IB: Inhibition of protein kinase C by tamoxifen. *Cancer Res.*, 45:2462-2465, 1985.

70. Safe S, Astroff B, Harris B, Zacharewski T, Dickerson R, Romkes, M and Biegel L: 2, 3, 7, 8-Tetrachlorodibenzo-*p*-dioxin (TCDD) and related compounds as antiestrogens; characterization and mechanism of action. *Pharmacol. Toxicol.*, 69:400-409, 1991.

71. Safe SH: Environmental and dietary estrogens and human health: Is There a Problem? *Environ. Health Prospect.*, 103:346-351, 1995.

72. Sikka SC, Rajasekaran M and Hellstrom WJG: Role of oxidative stress and antioxidants in male infertility. *J. Androl.*, 16:464-468, 1995.

73. Koppenol WH, Moreno JJ, Pryor WA et al.: Peroxynitrite, a cloaked oxidant formed by nitric oxide and superoxide. *Chem. Res. Toxicol.*, 5, 834-842. 1992.

74. Rosselli M, Dubey RK, Imthurn B, Macase E and Keller PJ: Effects of nitric oxide on human spermatozoa: evidence that nitric oxide decreases sperm motility and induces sperm toxicity. *Human Reprod.*, 10:1786-1790, 1995.

75. Beckman JS, Beckman TW, Chen J, Marshall PA and Freeman BA: Apparent hydroxyl radical production by peroxynitrite: implications for endothelial injury from nitric oxide and superoxide. *Proc. Natl. Acad. Science*, 87:1620-1624, 1990.

76. Gagnon C, Iwasaki A, deLamirande E and Kavolski N: Reactive oxygen species and human spermatozoa. (Review) *Ann. NY Acad. Sci.*, 637:436-444, 1991.

77. Aitken RJ and Clarkson JS: Cellular basis of defective sperm function and its association with the genesis of reactive oxygen species by human spermatozoa. *Reprod. Fertility*, 81:459-469, 1987.

78. Alvarez JG, Touchstone JC, Blasco L and Storey BT: Spontaneous lipid peroxidation and production of hydrogen peroxide and superoxide in human spermatozoa. Superoxide dismutase as major enzyme protectant against oxygen toxicity. *J. Androl.*, 8:338-348, 1987.

79. Lamb J C IV and Chapin RE: Testicular and Germ Cell Toxicity: In-Vitro Approaches. *Reprod. Toxicol.*, 7:17-22, 1993.

80. Gray TJB: Application of *in vitro* systems in male reproductive toxicology. In *Physiology and Toxicology of Male Reproduction,* Lamb JC IV and Foster PMD (eds), Academic Press, California, pp. 250-253, 1988.

81. Chapin RE, Phelps JL, Somkuti SG and Heindel JJ: The interaction of Sertoli and Leydig cells in the testicular toxicity of tri-o-cresyl phosphate. *Toxicol. Appl. Pharmacol.*, 104:483-495, 1990.

82. Steinberger A and Clinton JP: Two-compartment cultures of Sertoli cells-Applications in testicular toxicology. In *Methods in Toxicology (part A), Male Reproductive Toxicology,* Chapin RE and Heindel JJ (eds), Academic Press, New York, pp 230-245, 1993.

83. Foster PMD, Lloyd SC and Prout MS: Toxicity and metabolism of 1,3-dinitrobenzene in rat testicular cell cultures. *Toxicol in vitro*, 1, 31-37, 1987.

84. Chapin RE, Phelps JL, Somkuti SG and Heindel JJ: The interaction of Sertoli and Leydig cells in the testicular toxicity of tri-o-cresyl phosphate. *Toxicol. Appl. Pharmacol.*, 104:483-495, 1990.

85. Darney SP: In vitro assessment of gamete integrity. In *In vitro Toxicology: Mechanisms and New Toxicology — Alternative Methods in Toxicology, Vol. 8,* Goldberg AM (ed), Ann Liebert, Inc., New York, pp 63-75, 1991.

86. Brown DB, Hayes EJ, Uchida T and Nagamani M: Some cases of human male infertility are explained by abnormal *in vitro* human sperm activation. *Fertility and Sterility*, 64:612-622, 1995.

87. Perrault SD, Barbee RR, Elstein KH, Zucker RM and Keeler CL: Interspecies differences in the stability of mammalian sperm nuclei assessed *in vivo* by sperm microinjection and *in vitro* by flow cytometry. *Biol. Reprod.*, 39:157-167, 1988.

88. Evenson DP: Flow cytometry evaluation of male germ cells. In *Flow Cytometry: Advanced Research and Clinical Applications, vol. 1*, Yen A (ed), CRC Press, Boca Raton, FL, pp. 218-246, 1989.

89. Evenson DP, Baer RK, Jost LK and Gesch RW: Toxicity of thiotepa on mouse spermatogenesis as determined by dual-parameter flow cytometry. *Toxicol. Appl. Pharmacol.*, 82:151-163, 1986.

90. Evenson DP, Jost LK, Baer RK, Turner TW and Schrader SM: Individuality of DNA denaturation patterns in human sperm as measured by the sperm chromatin structure assay. *Reprod. Toxicol.*, 5:115-125, 1991.

91. Ulbrich B and Palmer AK: Detection of effects on male reproduction - a literature survey. *J. Am. Coll. Toxicol.*, 14:293-327, 1995.

92. Raloff J: The gender benders. Are environmental "hormones" emasculating wildlife? *Sci. News*, 145:24-27, 1994.

93. Stone R: Environmental estrogens stir debate. News and Comment. *Science*, 256:308-310, 1994.

94. Soto AM, Lin TM, Justicia H, Silvia RM and Sonenschein C: An "in culture" bioassay to assess the estrogenicity of xenobiotics (E-Screen). In *Chemically Induced Alterations in Sexual and Functional Development: The Wildlife/Human Connection.* Colborn T and Clements C (eds), Princeton Scientific Publishing Co., Inc., Princeton, NJ, pp. 295-309, 1992.

10 Environmental Androgens and Antiandrogens: An Expanding Chemical Universe

L. Earl Gray Jr., Vickie Wilson, Tammy Stoker, Christy Lambright, Johnathan Furr, Nigel Noriega, Phillip Hartig, Mary Cardon, Mitch Rosen, Gerald Ankley, Andrew Hotchkiss, Edward F. Orlando, Louis J. Guillette, and William R. Kelce

CONTENTS

ABSTRACT

Within the last 10 years, awareness has grown about environmental chemicals that display antiandrogenic or androgenic activity. While studies in the early 1990s focused on pesticides that acted as androgen receptor (AR) antagonists, it soon became evident that this was not the only endocrine mode of action by which man-made chemicals could disrupt the androgen signaling pathway. Several classes of antiandrogenic toxicants have been shown to act as AR antagonists, while others inhibit Leydig cell testosterone production; other pesticides display dual endocrine-disrupting chemical (EDC) mechanisms of action, being AR antagonists and inhibitors of testosterone synthesis. Recently, we learned that toxicants can also alter sexual differentiation by inhibiting insl3 mRNA production during sexual differentiation.

The classes of chemicals known to interfere with the androgen signaling pathway include dicarboximide fungicides (e.g., vinclozolin), organochlorine-based insecticides (p,p′ DDT and DDE), conazole fungicides (prochloraz), plasticizers (phthalates), and urea-based herbicides (linuron). *In utero* exposure to these "antiandrogenic" chemicals results in profiles of effects in the offspring that are pathognomonic for each mode of action. Mixture studies reveal that these chemicals generally induce cumulative dose-additive responses when co-administered with one another.

Although we have known about estrogen-mimics for decades, androgens of anthropogenic origin were only found in the environment in 2001. Recent studies from several laboratories around the world reported that effluents from pulp and paper mills display androgenic activity, often of sufficient potency to masculinize or sex-reverse female fish. Within the last year or two we also have learned that effluent from beef cattle feedlots was androgenic and may contain 17 beta trenbolone, a steroid used to promote growth in cattle. In summary, we are only beginning to understand what classes of chemicals have the potential to act as EDCs by altering the androgen signaling pathway. Although we have little data from field studies on the effects of these chemicals or their levels in the environment, animal studies demonstrate that antiandrogens have the potential to alter male sexual differentiation and reproductive development, whereas the androgenic substances can masculinize and defeminize females.

10.1 INTRODUCTION

Wildlife populations from contaminated ecosystems display a variety of reproductive and endocrine alterations including sex reversal, vitellogenin production in male oviparous vertebrates, reduced phallus size in alligators, masculinized females with imposex in snails, male-like gonopodia in mosquitofish, and altered social behavior in birds.[1, 2] In some cases, clear cause-and-effect relationships exist between exposure to endocrine-disrupting chemicals (EDCs) and adverse effects in fish, wildlife, and domestic animals. Within the last ten years, scientists recognized that some environmental chemicals display antiandrogenic or androgenic activity.[3-6] To this end, we have investigated the *in vivo* and *in vitro* effects of suspect androgenic and antiandrogenic substances. While studies in the early 1990s focused on pesticides that acted as androgen receptor antagonists,[7-9] it soon became evident that this was not the only endocrine mode by which toxicants disrupted the androgen signaling pathway.[10-13] Several classes of toxicants disrupt sex differentiation and onset of puberty in males by inhibiting androgen synthesis in the fetal or pubertal rat testis. Some of these, like the conazole fungicide prochloraz,[14] directly inhibit Leydig cell testosterone production, whereas phthalate plasticizers alter fetal development by inhibiting Leydig cell differentiation and testosterone[11,12] and insl3[13] hormone production during sex differentiation. Linuron and prochloraz act both as AR antagonists[14,15] and inhibitors of testosterone synthesis, while only prochloraz inhibits aromatase activity.[16] Many of these hormonally active environmental substances, then, are somewhat promiscuous in their ability to interact with the endocrine system at different levels of function.

The classes of chemicals known to interfere with the androgen signaling pathway include dicarboximide fungicides (vinclozolin), organochlorine-based insecticides (p,p' DDT and DDE), conazole fungicides (prochloraz), plasticizers (phthalates), and urea-based herbicides (linuron). *In utero* exposure to these "antiandrogenic" chemicals results in profiles of effects in the offspring that are pathognomonic for each mode of action. Mixture studies with AR antagonists and phthalate esters reveal cumulative dose-additive responses with co-administration.[5,17]

Although we have known about estrogen-mimics for decades, androgens of anthropogenic origin were found in the environment only within the last few years. Since 2001, several studies from laboratories around the world reported that effluents from pulp and paper mills displayed androgenic activity,[18-22] often with sufficient potency to masculinize or sex-reverse female fish. Within the last year or two, we learned that effluent from beef cattle feedlots was androgenic, in part due to the presence of 17 beta trenbolone, a growth promoter.[23,24] In summary, we are only beginning to understand what classes of chemicals have the potential to act as EDCs by altering the androgen signaling pathway. As such, a systematic approach to EDC identification is required if we are to understand the complete spectrum of chemicals that disrupt reproductive development and function via endocrine mechanisms. Identification of such EDCs is important because animal studies demonstrate that anti-androgens have the potential to alter male sexual differentiation and reproductive development,[3,15,25-29] whereas the androgenic substances have the potential to masculinize and defeminize females[24,30] if exposure is sufficiently high during a critical period of development.

10.1.1 *In Vitro* and *In Vivo* Androgenic Effects of Pulp and Paper Mill Effluents in the Laboratory and the Field: Environmental Androgens Revealed

Environmental chemicals with androgenic activity have only been detected recently. Several independent research groups have detected androgenic activity in pulp and paper mill effluent (PME) from Florida, the Baltic Sea, the Great Lakes, and New Zealand. Two groups, including our own[18] and the laboratory of Dr. E. Wilson at the University of North Carolina, Chapel Hill (UNC),[31] found that kraft pulp and paper mill effluent from sites on the Fenholloway River in Florida include a chemical mixture that binds AR and induces androgen-dependent gene expression *in vitro*. This mode of action is consistent with the masculinized female fish (*Gambusia holbrooki*) found in this river downstream from the plant and with the physical evidence suggesting that water samples collected from sites downstream from the mill all displayed androgenic activity, whereas water samples taken upstream of the plant or from a nearby river did not display androgenicity (Figure 10.1). Although this endocrine activity was originally thought to arise from high concentrations of androstenedione in the effluent,[31, 32] it was subsequently determined that this steroid was not among the chemicals in the active fraction,[21] as evaluated in a Toxicity Identification Evaluation conducted following USEPA guidelines.

The idea that substances in the environment with androgenic activity has long been suspected because female mosquitofish from contaminated sites on this river display an anal fin that is enlarged into a male-like gonopodium,[33] an effect that was first observed in the 1970s and persists in many of the fish today (Figure 10.2). The anal fin in the male mosquitofish is modified by androgens into an elongated gonopodium, which is used by the male during mating to deposit sperm, this species having internal fertilization and bearing live young. Masculinized female mosquitofish (Figure 10.2) have an elongated, male-like anal fin that contains more segments than a normal female. In a sample of several hundred fish from contaminated sites on the Fenholloway River, the frequency distribution of anal fin ray segments ranges from normal to completely male-like, with the majority of females having anal fins that are intersex with regard to the numbers of segments in the fin (Figure 10.2). This is in stark contrast to the fewer number of fin segments in female mosquitofish taken from the cleaner Ecofina River, which does not receive effluent from the pulp mill. Masculinization of the anal fin and mating behavior has been achieved in female

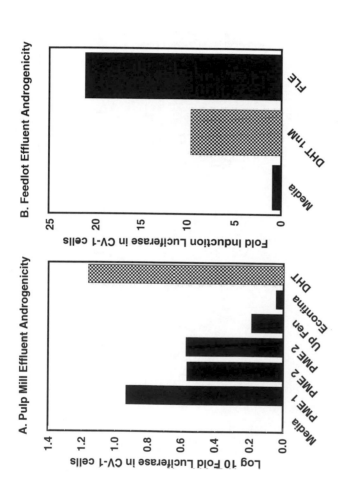

FIGURE 10.1 *In vitro* androgenic effects of pulp mill (a) and beef cattle feedlot (b) effluents. CV-1 cells, transiently cotransfected with hAR and MMTV-luc genes, are stimulated by pulp mill and feedlot effluents in an androgenic manner to about the same degree as the stimulation induced by the positive control dihydrotestosterone (DHT). In Figure A the highest level of androgenicity is displayed at site PME1 at the discharge point of the effluent into the Fenholloway River[18] (see Parks et al.[18] for details on the assays and a site map of the collection points). PME2 and PME3 are sites on the river downstream from the discharge point, with site 2 being closer to the mill than site 3. Media refers to the media control, while Up Fen is a site on the Fenholloway River upstream from the pulp mill. For analyses, all data were normalized to the media control and are described as fold induction over media. Econfina refers to a water sample collected from the Econfina River, which is near the Fenholloway River and arises from the same headwaters but is not contaminated by pulp mill effluent. Figure B displays the data from the eastern Nebraska feedlot effluent sample, termed FLE, which flows into the Elkhorn River.[35] The androgenic activity of the FLE sample is from this site is far greater than the media control but does not differ significantly from 1 nM DHT, the positive control. Data are from Orlando et al.[35]

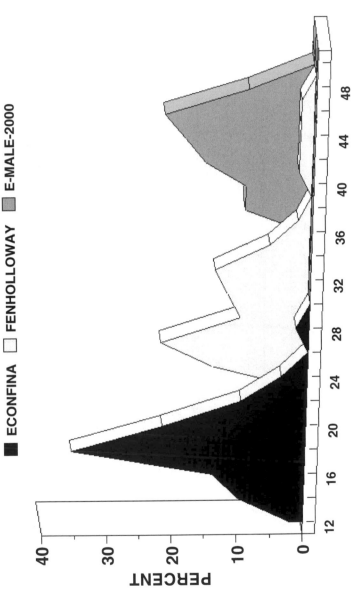

FIGURE 10.2 Population frequency histograms of anal fin ray segmentation. Female mosquitofish from the Fenholloway River display masculinized anal fins (in white) having a greater number of segments in the longest ray of the anal fin as compared to females (in black) from the Econfina River, a nearby river from the same watershed that does not receive pulp mill effluent. For comparison, the data from males (in gray) from the Econfina River also are shown to confirm the sex dimorphism of this reproductive trait. Data are from Parks et al.[18]

mosquitofish in the laboratory with exposures to pulp mill effluent from the Fenholloway River[34] and from New Zealand.[22]

The androgenic potential of a New Zealand pulp and paper mill effluent was measured by applying assays with mosquitofish (*Gambusia affinis*) and goldfish (*Carassius auratus*).[22] Female mosquitofish exposed for 21 days to untreated or secondary-treated pulp mill effluent displayed significant masculinization of the gonopodium, with the degree of gonopodial masculinization being reduced with secondary-treatment of the effluent, a process that removes some of the androgenic substances in the water. Male mating behavior also was observed in the masculinized females. *In vitro*, kraft effluent extract bound to androgen receptors from goldfish testis cytosol. The androgenic compounds androstenedione and testosterone were not detected in the extracts used for the *in vitro* component of this study.

Male-biased sex ratios of fish embryos have been reported near a pulp mill on the Swedish Baltic coast. Broods from the eelpout (*Zoarces viviparus*) were significantly male biased in the vicinity of a large kraft pulp mill on the Swedish Baltic coast, suggesting that masculinizing compounds in the effluent were affecting gonadal differentiation and promoting skewed sex ratios.[19] Investigations at 13 sites for up to 4 years showed a relatively stable sex ratio around 50/50, except at locations in close proximity to the mill. The eelpout produced male-biased broods close to the mill. Interestingly, when the mill shut down for a period of time, which coincided with the stage of development when the eelpout gonads were differentiating, the sex ratios were no longer male biased. However, the following year after the mill reopened, the male bias reappeared.

10.2 *IN VITRO* AND *IN VIVO* STUDIES WITH FEEDLOT EFFLUENTS AND TRENBOLONE, AN ANABOLIC STEROID PRESENT IN SOME CATTLE FEEDLOT EFFLUENTS

The androgenic anabolic steroid trenbolone acetate is licensed as a growth promoter for farm animals in the U.S. and several other countries. Even though it is used in several million beef cattle in the U.S., a risk assessment of its potential effects on fish and wildlife has yet to be conducted. It was recently demonstrated that this androgen was found in an active form in the environment and persists for long periods[23] in some samples. In an 8-week study, cattle were treated with trenbolone acetate and liquid manure was collected and spread on fields after several months of storage. During storage, the level of trenbolone decreased from 1700 to 1100 pg/g of the active 17 alpha-isomer, corresponding to a half-life of 267 days. In a study conducted using cattle feedlot effluent from Nebraska, we found a high level of androgenicity in the effluent (Figure 10.1), and our colleagues at the Universities of Nebraska and Florida found that wild fathead minnows (*Pimephales promelas*) displayed morphological (50% reduction in testis weight) and endocrine (abnormal testosterone/estradiol ratios)[35] alterations compared to fish from a non-contaminated reference site. At this time, we have not determined whether the androgenic activity in this sample arises from natural steroids or from trenbolone.

Wilson et al.[24] found that 17 beta trenbolone was as potent *in vitro* and *in vivo* as are the most potent natural and synthetic androgens. It displays high affinity for human and fish androgen receptors and induces androgen-dependent gene expression *in vitro* in MDA-KB2 cells at the same concentrations as dihydrotestosterone (DHT). In a short-term *in vivo* assay of androgenicity using the immature-castrate male rat, trenbolone was as potent as testosterone propionate (sc) in inducing growth of androgen-dependent muscles (the levator ani-bulbocavernosus complex). However, trenbolone was less effective than testosterone in stimulating growth of the ventral prostate. This pharmacological behavior is typical of a C19 norandrogen like trenbolone, as they are not activated to more potent androgens by 5 alpha reductase, an enzyme present in high concentrations in the prostate but not muscle. When administered (sc) *in utero*, 17 beta trenbolone masculinized female rat offspring[24] at the same concentrations as did (sc) testosterone propioniate.[30] Although the ability of trenbolone to induce reproductive tract malformations in androgen-sensitive tissues is not surprising, the developmental toxicity and multigenerational reproduction studies used in a risk assessment of the potential effects of this steroid on human health did not detect these malformations in developmentally exposed animals.

Some of the greatest concerns about the effects of trenbolone relate to its potential effects on terrestrial and aquatic ecosystems around these feedlots because they are likely to be contaminated with the highest levels of this chemical and its metabolites. In this regard, Ankley et al.[36] studied the effects of the androgenic growth promoter 17-beta-trenbolone on fecundity and reproductive endocrinology of the fathead minnow (*Pimephales promelas*). A competitive binding study with the fathead minnow androgen receptor demonstrated that 17-beta-trenbolone had a higher affinity for the receptor than did testosterone. When male and female fish were exposed for 21 days to nominal concentrations of 17-beta-trenbolone ranging from 0.005 to 50 microg/L, treated pairs displayed reduced fecundity (lowest observed effect level = 0.05 microg/L versus the measured concentrations of 0.027 microg/L). Treated females developed nuptial tubercles, structures normally present only on the heads of mature males, and had reduced plasma steroid (testosterone and 17 beta-estradiol) and vitellogenin levels. The 17-beta-trenbolone also altered reproductive hormone levels in male fathead minnows at concentrations higher than those producing effects in females. Males exposed to 17-beta-trenbolone at 41 microg/L exhibited decreased plasma concentrations of 11-ketotestosterone and increased concentrations of 17 beta-estradiol and vitellogenin. It is worthy to note that the *in vivo* effects of 17 beta trenbolone on fecundity and female fathead minnow reproductive morphology and function occurred at concentrations equivalent to those that induced luciferase in MDA-KB2 cells *in vitro,*[24] indicating that this *in vivo* fish assay is very sensitive to androgens. Ongoing studies in Dr. Ankley's laboratory are measuring trenbolone and its metabolites from water in aquatic ecosystems that receive effluent from Concentrated Animal Feedlot Operations (CAFOs). Recently, the USDA and USEPA released guidelines for CAFO effluent but these guidelines did not include monitoring of hormonally active substances like trenbolone. Further research is needed to determine if EDCs in CAFO effluents disrupt endocrine function, fecundity, population levels, or ecosystem diversity.

10.3 DICARBOXIMIDE FUNGICIDES: VINCLOZOLIN AND PROCYMIDONE

10.3.1 THE FUNGICIDE VINCLOZOLIN — *IN VITRO* AND SHORT-TERM *IN VIVO* EFFECTS OF AN AR ANTAGONIST

Vinclozolin, procymidone, iprodione, and chlozolinate are dicarboximide fungicides. Vinclozolin and procymidone are AR antagonists with equivalent potency, while iprodione and chlozolinate do not appear to be antiandrogenic *in vivo*.[37] Of the antiandrogenic EDCs, the mechanism of action of vinclozolin is the most thoroughly characterized. Vinclozolin metabolites, M1 and M2 competitively inhibit the binding of androgens to AR of several species from different vertebrate classes.[7,38] M1 and M2 also inhibit DHT-induced transcriptional activity in cells transfected with the human AR. Kelce et al.[39] subsequently demonstrated that vinclozolin treatment altered the expression of androgen-dependent genes *in vivo* in an antiandrogenic manner, similar to the antiandrogenic drug flutamide. In contrast, neither vinclozolin nor its metabolites display affinity for the estrogen receptor, although they do have weak affinity for the progesterone receptor.[40] Furthermore, vinclozolin, M1, and M2 do not inhibit 5α-reductase activity, the enzyme required for the conversion of testosterone (T) to the more active androgen DHT.[7]

In a short-term screening assay, vinclozolin inhibited the growth of androgen-dependent tissues in castrate-immature testosterone-treated[41] and pubertal male rat.[5,42] In the intact pubertal[42] and adult male rat,[43] vinclozolin treatment also alters hypothalamic–pituitary–gonadal function, causing elevations in serum LH and testosterone, although the effects seen in the adult animal are less dramatic and occur only at much higher dosage levels. In contrast to vinclozolin, treatment with other antiandrogens like p,p' DDE[9,39] and methoxychlor[44,45] fail to induce changes in serum LH or testosterone levels.

The extent to which vinclozolin interrupts the hypothalamic–pituitary–gonadal axis also is dependent on developmental stage. When fetal testis testosterone and progesterone production and insl3 mRNA levels were examined at gestational day 18, following vinclozolin treatment from day 14 to 18 of pregnancy, no effects were observed (Figure 10.3). Although vinclozolin treatment elevates testosterone production in the pubertal and adult male rat by inducing high levels of LH, this effect was not seen in the fetal rat, or was expected, because testis function is not under control of the pituitary hormones during *in utero* sex differentiation.

In mixture studies using castrate-immature testosterone-treated male rats (Hershberger assay), combinations of vinclozolin and procymidone (0, 25, 50, and 100 mg/kg/day for 7 days inhibited testosterone-induced growth of androgen-dependent tissues (ventral prostate, seminal vesicles, and levator ani-bulbocavernosus muscles) in a dose-additive fashion at 25 and 50 mg/kg/day.[5] A few years later, the results of this mixture study were replicated in another laboratory.[17] At higher dose levels, we found that vinclozolin and procymidone also increased liver and adrenal weights in a dose-additive manner.[5]

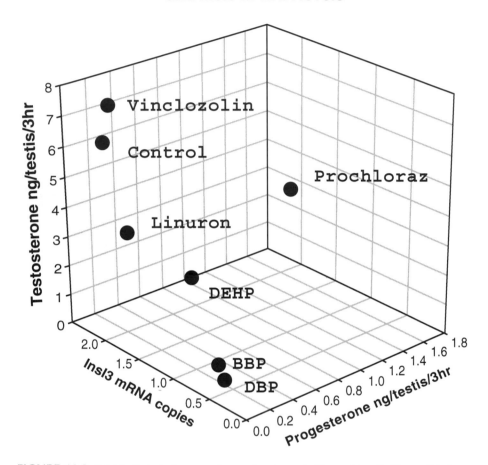

FIGURE 10.3 Fetal testis testosterone and progesterone production and insulin-like peptide hormone (insl3) mRNA (number of message copies × 10⁶ per 100 ng RNA) levels following gestational exposure to several chemicals known to alter androgen signaling in the male rat fetus. Data are from Wilson et al.[13] Testosterone and progesterone production values were measured on day 18 of pregnancy *ex vivo* after maternal treatment with the toxicant from gestational day 14 to 18 after a 3-hour incubation period. Three (insl3) mRNA levels were measured by QPCR from testes harvested after the incubation period. The androgen receptor antagonist vinclozolin has no effect on fetal testis testosterone, progesterone, or insl3 levels. This toxicant alters development by acting directly on the androgen-dependent tissues at the level of the AR, not via the testis. Linuron and prochloraz both inhibit fetal testis testosterone production, while prochloraz induces a tenfold increase in progesterone production. This indicates that these two pesticides, which also are AR antagonists, inhibit steroidogenesis, albeit at different points in the pathway. The three phthalate esters DEHP, DBP, and BBP act similarly to one another, but differ from all the above toxicants. They inhibit testosterone production and insl3 mRNA levels as well. The fact that they inhibit both steroid and peptide hormones in the fetal testis suggests that the phthalates are delaying maturation of the fetal Leydig cells rather than acting at a specific site in the steroid pathway.

10.3.2 Dose-Response Developmental Effects of Vinclozolin

Administration of vinclozolin by oral gavage at 100 or 200 mg/kg/day during sexual differentiation demasculinizes and feminizes the male offspring. Vinclozolin-treated male offspring display female-like anogenital distance at birth, retained nipples, hypospadias, suprainguinal ectopic testes, a blind vaginal pouch, epididymal granulomas, and small to absent sex accessory glands. Weights of descended testes were reduced at 200 mg/kg/day, but epididymal agenesis was rare and there were no cases of gubernacular agenesis. In contrast to their male siblings, the female offspring do not display any malformations or permanent functional alterations.

High-dose vinclozolin-treated males were capable of displaying mounting behavior as adults, but were unable to achieve intromissions due to hypospadias. When examined during pubertal life, treated male offspring did not show evidence of demasculinized brains, as they displayed normal levels of male-like rough-and-tumble play behavior.[46] Although we failed to observe alterations in androgen-dependent play behavior in vinclozolin-treated male offspring, Hotchkiss et al.[47,48] subsequently demonstrated that sc neonatal administration of vinclozolin at 200 mg/kg/day or flutamide did demasculinize aggressive play behavior when measured at 35 days of age. Female newborn rat pups injected with testosterone displayed more male-like aggressive play behavior. These studies suggest that play behavior, which is organized by androgens in the neonatal stage of life in rodents, can be disrupted in a predictable manner by the administration of antiandrogens to the male rat or androgens to the female rat when administered directly to the pup during the critical period of CNS sex differentiation. In the earlier vinclozolin studies, pups may not have been exposed to sufficient levels of M1 and M2 via the milk to demasculinize this androgen-dependent process.

When administered at lower dosage levels (0, 3.125, 6.25, 12.5, 25, 50, or 100 mg/kg/day from gestational day 14 to postnatal day 3),[28,49] vinclozolin at doses of 3.125 mg/kg/day and above reduced neonatal anogenital distance and increased the incidence of retained nipples/areolas in infant male rats. When examined at maturity, ventral prostate weight was reduced in all treatment groups (significant at 6.25, 25, 50, and 100 mg/kg/day) and permanent nipples were detected in males at 3.125 (1.4%), 6.25 (3.6%), 12.5 (3.9%), 25 (8.5%), 50 (91%), and 100 (100%) mg/kg/day. Most of the developmental effects seen in our study have since been replicated in a second laboratory.[49] In a recent risk assessment of vinclozolin, the USEPA used the permanent reduction in ventral prostate weight as the critical effect to set a No Observed Adverse Effect Level. Vinclozolin treatment at 50 and 100 mg/kg/day induced hypospadias and other reproductive tract malformations. Even though all of the effects of vinclozolin likely result from the same initial mechanism (i.e., AR binding), the affected endpoints display a wide variety of dose-response curves and ED50s and some of these dose response curves failed to display an obvious threshold. These differences in sensitivity likely reflect competing levels of ambient androgens or the strict androgen dependence of these developmental processes.

Another study was conducted to identify the most sensitive period of fetal development to the disruptive effects of vinclozolin.[50] When pregnant rats were dosed by oral gavage with 400 mg vinclozolin/kg/day on either gestational days (GD) 12 to 13, 14 to 15, 16 to 17, 18 to 19, or 20 to 21, the most pronounced effects resulted from exposure on GD 16 to 17 with less-severe effects seen in males exposed to vinclozolin on GD 14 to 15 and GD 18 to 19.

If the effects of vinclozolin are mediated via AR then one would expect co-administration of testosterone to antagonize the developmental effects of this pesticide on male offspring (i.e., increase ambient levels of testosterone to compete with the pesticide for AR androgen binding). On the other hand, vinclozolin should protect the female fetus from the masculinizing action of testosterone in the same litters. To test these hypotheses, we administered vinclozolin (gavage at 200 mg/kg/day) or testosterone propionate (TP sc at 1 mg/rat/day) alone and in combination to SD rats on to days 14 to 19.[51] As expected, in female offspring, TP-induced alterations including increased anogenital distance, fewer nipples, vaginal agenesis, and hydrometrocolpos and induced development of prostate and bulbourethral glands and levator ani muscle tissues. All of these effects were reversed by co-administration of vinclozolin with TP. In the male offspring, vinclozolin-induced alterations were only modestly antagonized by TP. Compared with the vinclozolin-treated group, vinclozolin plus TP-treated male offspring had less-well-developed nipples and a lower incidence of ectopic testis. Many of the other reproductive alterations were not attenuated by TP co-administration. We observed that the combination of vinclozolin and TP, two chemicals with opposing endocrine action, antagonized one another during sexual differentiation, especially in the female offspring.

10.3.3 PUBERTAL EFFECTS OF VINCLOZOLIN

Peripubertal administration of EDCs can alter the onset of pubertal landmarks in male and female rats. The sensitivity of this life stage to hormonally active chemicals is the basis for the consideration of using standardized pubertal assays[52,53] in the endocrine screening and testing program that is being developed by the USEPA as mandated by 1996 U.S. legislation (the Food Quality Protection Act and Safe Drinking Water Act). Androgens play a key role in pubertal maturation in young males, and antiandrogens like vinclozolin or androgens like methyltestosterone produce predictable alterations of this process. The ease with which a delay or acceleration in preputial separation (PPS), a landmark of puberty in the male rat, can be measured enables us to use this endpoint to evaluate chemicals for antiandrogenic and androgenic activity, respectively.

Monosson et al.[42] conducted a pubertal study with vinclozolin using doses of 0, 10, 30, or 100 mg/kg/day. She examined the morphological landmarks of puberty, hormone levels, and sex accessory gland development in male rats. Vinclozolin treatment delayed pubertal maturation, reduced sex accessory gland, and epididymal growth (at 30 and 100 mg/kg/day), and serum LH (significant at all dosage levels), testosterone, and 5α-androstane,3α,17-diol (at 100 mg/kg/day) levels were increased. Testis size was slightly but not significantly increased. The metabolites M1 and M2 were found in the serum of animals from the two highest dosage groups at levels well below the *in vitro* Ki values determined previously by Kelce et al.[7] These results suggest that when the vinclozolin metabolites occupy even a small percentage of available ARs; this prevents maximal AR-DNA binding and alters *in vivo* androgen-dependent gene expression and protein synthesis, resulting in obvious alterations to pubertal development in the male rat. In the recent risk assessment, a vinclozolin-induced delay in puberty of less than 2 days (as measured by age at preputial separation) was deemed as an adverse effect by the USEPA, and the data were used to limit specific exposures of children to vinclozolin.

The effects of vinclozolin also have been studied in several species of lower vertebrates including fish,[54-60] amphibians,[61] birds,[62] and reptiles[63] as well as invertebrates.[64] While many of the studies obtained positive responses, some did not flag vinclozolin as an antiandrogen. It remains to be determined whether these negative results arise from a lack of metabolic activation of vinclozolin to the antiandrogenic metabolites M1 and M2 or if the AR of the species did not bind M1 or M2 with the same affinity as does mammalian AR. It also is important to recognize that the role of androgens and AR function varies greatly from species to species; a trait or physiologial process that is androgen dependent in one species may not rely upon androgens or be sexually dimorphic in another.

Results to date by Cardon et al.[65] with recombinant AR from the rainbow trout and fathead minnow indicate that the AR from these fishes bind M1 and M2 with the same affinity as does the mammalian AR. Similarly, we compared the competitive binding of several chemicals to fish and human AR using rainbow trout androgen receptor alpha (rtAR) and human androgen receptor (hAR) expressed in transfected COS cells. Saturation ligand binding and Scatchard analysis using [^{3}H]R1881, a synthetic androgen, revealed a Kd of 0.24 nM for the rtAR and a Kd of 2.27 nM for the hAR. Binding studies in competition with [^{3}H]R1881 were conducted using steroids and a selection of environmental chemicals shown to bind mammalian AR. All the chemicals and steroids studied competed for binding in both rtAR and hAR. The relative order of binding affinities of natural and synthetic androgens for the rtAR and hAR were similar: methyltrienolone > trenbolone > 11-ketotestosterone > dihydrotestosterone (DHT) > testosterone > androstenedione, except that DHT and testosterone had higher affinity than 11-ketotestosterone in hAR than in rtAR. Other steroids and antiandrogens also were studied and the relative binding affinities were similar for the two species. Similar comparisons are now being made between hAR and the fathead minnow AR and plans to expand this project to include receptors from all vertebrate classes are under way. For invertebrates, it remains to be determined if they have functional AR or any other steroid-like nuclear transcription factor.[66, 67]

10.3.4 PROCYMIDONE — *IN VITRO* AND SHORT-TERM *IN VIVO* EFFECTS

Procymidone is a dicarboximide fungicide similar in structure to vinclozolin. Hosokawa et al.[8] demonstrated in a competitive binding assay that procymidone effectively inhibited the binding of [3H]-DHT to the androgen receptor in both rats and mice. Ostby et al.[26] demonstrated that procymidone inhibited DHT-induced transcriptional activation at 0.2 µM in CV-1 cells cotransfected with the human AR and a MMTV-luciferase reporter gene, while at 10 µM, DHT-induced transcriptional activity was completely inhibited. In addition, 1 µM procymidone blocked DHT-induced AR-DNA binding in a CHO cell promoter interference assay. Although it is likely that metabolites of procymidone, rather than procymidone itself, are the true AR antagonists, the metabolites studied to date have not displayed affinity for AR.[8]

In vivo, procymidone acts as an AR antagonist in the Hershberger assay. Administration of 25 mg/kg/day and above for 7 days to castrate-immature male rats inhibits testosterone-induced growth of the sex accessory tissues and androgen-dependent muscles.[5,17] When combined with vinclozolin in this assay, the two AR antagonists inhibit testosterone's stimulatory effects in a dose-additive manner.

As discussed above, vinclozolin alters AR-dependent gene expression *in vivo* increasing testosterone-repressed prostatic message (TRPM-2) and repressing prostatein subunit C3 (C3) mRNA levels.[39] We conducted a similar study to determine if adult male rats exposed to procymidone display effects similar to vinclozolin on TRPM-2, C3, and AR message levels using real-time reverse transcription polymerase chain reaction (QPCR).[68] An extension of this study using microarray analysis is discussed below.[69] Castrated SD rats were dosed with the vehicle + testosterone implant (T), oral vinclozolin (200 mg/kg/day) + T implant (VT), oral procymidone (200 mg/kg/day) + T implant (PT), or vehicle with an empty implant (Oil). Rats were necropsied after 20 hours, and 4 and 7 days. As expected, castration without T replacement (Oil), VT, and PT decreased androgen-dependent tissue weights and increased serum LH as compared to the T group. Serum T levels did not differ among the T, VT, and PT groups. TRPM-2 was increased at all time points in Oil, VT, and PT groups versus the T controls. At 7 days, C3 mRNA levels were reduced in the Oil, VT, and PT groups. These results demonstrate that vinclozolin and procymidone produce a nearly identical profile of morphological, endocrine, and molecular alterations of androgen-dependent processes that are similar to but less robust than those produced by elimination of T by castration.

For microarray analysis of gene expression profiles in the above study, tissue from the ventral prostate was collected at the 20-hour and 4-day time points for isolation of total RNA followed by analysis using Clontech Atlas 1.2 Toxicology arrays. As hypothesized, similar changes in gene expression were observed in the PT and VT groups at both the 20-hour and 4-day time points. While only 36 genes were affected at 20 hours, 156 genes were altered 4 days after the start of treatment. The increase in the number of genes altered over time likely reflects regression of the ventral prostate seen at 4 days, but not at 20 hours. The results of the microarray analysis compared well with the results obtained by QPCR, and several other known androgen-dependent genes also were affected. In addition, several genes that are not known to be androgen-dependent changed consistently among the groups.

10.3.5 Dose-Response Developmental Effects of Procymidone in the Male Rat

When administered by gavage at 100 mg/kg/day on gestational day 14 to day 3 after birth, procymidone reduces anogenital distance in male pups and induces retained nipples, hypospadias, cleft phallus, a vaginal pouch, and reduced sex accessory gland size in male rat offspring.[26] At 25, 50, 100, and 200 mg/kg/day, effects were detected at all dosage levels and included reduced anogenital distance (at 25 mg/kg/day and above); induced nipples (25 and above); permanently reduced size of several androgen-dependent tissues (levator ani and bulbocavernosus muscles (25 and above), prostate (50 and above), seminal vesicles (100 and above), Cowper's gland (100 and above), and glans penis (100 and above); and induced malformations including hypospadias (50 and above), cleft phallus (50 and above), exposed os penis, vaginal pouch (50 and above) and ectopic, undescended testes (200). Procymidone had a marked effect on the histology of the dorsolateral and ventral prostatic and seminal vesicular tissues (at 50 mg/kg/day and above). The effects consisted of fibrosis, cellular infiltration, and epithelial hyperplasia. In contrast to the developmental effects, procymidone had little effect, if any, on the reproductive tract of the adult male rat (2 weeks at dosage levels as high as 2000 ppm in the diet).[70]

10.4 PROCYMIDONE — *IN VITRO* AND SHORT-TERM EFFECTS

10.4.1 LINURON — *IN VITRO* AND SHORT-TERM *IN VIVO* EFFECTS

Linuron is a urea-based herbicide with an acute oral LD50 in rats of 4000 mg/kg. Existing *in vitro* data demonstrate that linuron is a weak AR ligand[15,27,71] with an EC50 between 64 and 100 µM. Lambright et al.[15] reported that linuron competed *in vitro* with androgen for rat prostatic AR (EC50 = 100-300 µM) and human AR (hAR) in a COS cell whole cell binding assay (EC50 = 20 µM). Linuron also inhibited DHT-hAR induced gene expression in CV-1 and MDA-KB2 cells (EC$_{50}$ = 10 µM).

In vivo, linuron treatment (100 mg/kg/day oral for 7 days) reduced testosterone- and DHT-dependent tissue weights in the Hershberger assay using castrate-immature testosterone propionate-treated male rats, and linuron treatment (100 mg/kg/day oral for 4 days) altered the expression of androgen-regulated genes in ventral prostate *in situ*.[15]

10.4.2 DEVELOPMENTAL EFFECTS OF LINURON IN THE MALE RAT

The effects of linuron treatment *in vivo* are difficult, if not impossible, to detect in adult animals, but are quite apparent in the offspring when administered during gestation.[27,37,72,73] In a modified multigenerational study, the only effects seen in P0 generation male rats when linuron was administered from weaning through puberty, breeding, and lactation at 0, 20, or 40 mg/kg/day by gavage in oil was a 2.5-day delay in PPS and a small reduction in seminal vesicle and cauda epididymal weights.[37] Fertility and serum testosterone, LH, FSH, and prolactin levels were unaffected in the P0 generation at dosage levels up to 40 mg/kg/day. In contrast, dramatic effects were seen in the F1 generation in the 40 mg/kg/day dose group, including malformations and subfertility. The F1 pairs sired fewer pups under continuous breeding conditions (63 pups versus 104, mated continuously over 12 breeding cycles), and the F1 males had reduced testes and epididymal weights, and lower testes spermatid numbers, effects missed in earlier studies[71] cited in the USEPA risk assessment documents.

When administered at 100 mg/kg/day from days 14 to 18 of gestation (115), anogenital distance in male offspring is reduced by about 30%, and the incidence of areolas/nipples in the male offspring as infants was increased from 0% in controls to more than 44% in the linuron-treated males. Unlike the profile seen with vinclozolin and procymidone, linuron treatment induces a low incidence of hypospadias, but relatively high levels of epididymal and testicular malformations. For example, epispadias was only found in 1 of 13 males (partial hypospadias with the urethral opening halfway down the phallus), but more than half of the males had epididymal and testicular abnormalities. Several androgen-dependent tissues were permanently reduced in size in linuron-treated male offspring as a result of this brief exposure during sex differentiation, including the seminal vesicles, ventral prostate, levator ani/bulbocavernosus muscles, and epididymides. The high incidences of epididymal and testicular malformations (> 50% of the linuron-treated males displaying agenesis or atrophy of one or both organs) combined with a low incidence of hypospadias are atypical for an AR antagonist and more closely resemble the effects seen in animals exposed *in utero* to phthalates, which inhibit fetal Leydig cell hormone production. When the ability of the fetal testis is examined on gestational day 18, after treatment with linuron at 100 mg/kg/day from gestational day 14 to 18, testosterone production is significantly reduced, while progesterone production is not markedly altered and insl3 mRNA is unaffected (Figure 10.3).

The epididymal malformations seen in treated male offspring included agenesis of the caput or corpus epididymides, while some testes were atrophic, fluid filled, and flaccid. These malformations also are produced at lower dosage levels. McIntyre et al.[27,72,73] detected malformations in male rat offspring at dosage levels of linuron as low as 12.5 mg/kg/day (days 10 to 22 of gestation), the lowest dose examined, and found that the testis abnormalities were not a direct effect of prenatal linuron and did not develop until after puberty, being caused by pressure atrophy arising from the epididymal abnormalities.

Taken together, these mechanistic data demonstrate that linuron is "antiandrogenic" via dual mechanisms of action. It is an AR antagonist and it inhibits fetal testis testosterone synthesis. The fact that linuron produces a profile of malformations that differs from the standard AR antagonist, but resembles the effects seen with DBP or DEHP treatment, suggests that the effect of linuron on fetal testosterone synthesis may be the most important of the two mechanisms of action in the fetal male.

10.5.1 IN VITRO EFFECTS AND SHORT-TERM IN VIVO EFFECTS OF p,p' DDE

Although use of DDT has been banned in some countries, it is still in use in many parts of the world, and all wildlife and humans are exposed, with some exposures in the high ppm range. A world-wide ban of this pesticide is currently being considered, but this has become very controversial because DDT is used to control vectors of malaria, a disease that accounts for many deaths. Although agricultural use of DDT is declining and will eventually end, human exposure from DDT use in the home continues. Hence, it is now more important than ever to determine the potential effects of continued usage of this pesticide on humans. In addition, high concentrations of DDT and its metabolites, especially p,p' DDE, persist in North American fields, farms, orchards, and Superfund sites. Adverse effects of p,p'

DDT/DDE exposures have been reported in humans,[74-78] but there is no clear linkage of these potential effects to the interaction of p,p′ DDE and DDT with the AR.

In 1995 Kelce et al.[79] found that p,p′-DDE displayed antiandrogenic activity both *in vivo* and *in vitro*, acting as an AR antagonist. *In vitro*, p,p′ DDE binds to the AR and prevents DHT-induced transcriptional activation in cells transfected with the human AR and inhibits androgen-dependent gene expression *in vivo*.[39]

This antiandrogen alters pubertal development in the male rat.[79] When p,p′ DDE is administered at 0, 30, or 100 mg/kg/day from weaning until about 50 days of age, the age at puberty, measured by a delay in preputial separation, was delayed about 5 days in male rats treated with the high dose. Subsequently, the antiandrogenic effects of p,p′ DDE induced were confirmed by several laboratories as part of an interlaboratory evaluation of the Hershberger assay, which uses castrate-immature androgen-treated male rats.[41,80] As expected for an AR antagonist, p,p′ DDE-treatment consistently reduced androgen-dependent tissue weights in the Hershberger assay.

10.5.2 Developmental Effects of p,p′ DDE in the Male Rat and Rabbit

When p,p′ DDE is administered to Long Evans Hooded (LE) and Sprague-Dawley (SD) male rat offspring by gavage in oil during gestation treatment at 100 mg/kg/day (days 14 to 18 of gestation), it reduces anogenital distance in newborn male rat offspring and induces hypospadias, retained nipples, and permanently smaller androgen-dependent tissues.[37,81,82] While the alterations were evident in both rat strains, the SD strain appeared to be more affected in our studies.[37] Only the SD strain displayed hypospadias, and other effects were of a greater magnitude in the treated SD than in the LE rats. It is uncertain if this reflects a true strain difference in sensitivity or if it merely results from experiment-to-experiment variation. You et al.[81,82] studied the effects of p,p′-DDE on the male offspring using the same protocol and they also found that p,p′-DDE induced antiandrogenic effects on anogenital distance and areola development in both LE and SD rat strains. They found that in oral treatment with p,p′ DDE at 100 mg/kg/day as above, fetal rat tissue p,p′ DDE levels ranged from 1 to 2 µg/g during sexual differentiation.

In the rabbit (Dutch Belted)[83] when the AR antagonist p,p′ DDT[9,84] was administered during gestation (does treated) and lactation (pups treated), reproductive abnormalities were displayed by male offspring. Infantile exposure alone resulted in delays in testicular descent in the rabbit, while combined lactational plus gestational exposure induced uni/bilateral cryptorchidism. Serum levels of p,p′ DDT and DDE in offspring were 208 ppb p,p′ DDT and 38 ppb p,p′ DDE.

10.6.1 In Vitro Effects of the Prochloraz, a Conazole Fungicide

Prochloraz is a conazole fungicide that displays several mechanisms of action capable of disrupting reproductive function and development. Prochloraz inhibits the enzyme aromatase[16] *in vitro*, and it acts as an AR antagonist, inhibiting androgen-induced gene expression *in vitro*, and retards sex accessory tissue growth in castrate-immature testosterone-treated male rats.[14] In MDA-KB2 cells stably transfected with MMTV-luc reporter genes, prochloraz concentrations above 1 µM caused a dose-dependent inhibition of DHT-induced luciferase expression with no indication of cytotoxicity except at 100 micromolar. Prochloraz also inhibited R1881 binding to the rat AR (EC_{50} approximately 60 µM using ventral prostate cytosol).

In a study in which dams were dosed with one of several "antiandrogens" from day 14 to 18 of pregnancy, Wilson et al.[13] found that prenatal prochloraz exposure reduced fetal testis testosterone and increased progesterone production on gestational day 18 over the 3-hour incubation period by about tenfold. In contrast, prochloraz did not affect testis insl3 mRNA levels (Figure 10.3). Thus prochloraz appears to alter endocrine function via several diverse mechanisms of action, one of which delays parturition and the others demasculinize the male fetus during sex differentiation.

10.6.2 IN VIVO DEVELOPMENTAL EFFECTS OF PROCHLORAZ IN THE MALE RAT

When prochloraz was administered to pregnant rat dams from gestational day 14 to 18 at doses of 62.5, 125, 250, and 500 mg/kg bodyweight/day, maternal weight gain was inhibited at 500 mg/kg/day, and parturition was delayed in a dose-related manner.[85] The delay in delivery may be related to an inhibition of aromatase activity (estrogen synthesis) as estrogen levels rise near term in this species. In male rat offspring, prenatal prochloraz treatment reduced anogenital distance and induced female-like areolas in male offspring at frequencies of 33%, 71%, and 100% in 62.5, 125, and 250 mg/kg groups, respectively. A high percentage of males in the 250 mg/kg treatment group also displayed hypospadias. In contrast, the epididymides and gubernacular ligaments were generally not affected. No reproductive effects were noted in the female offspring.

The results of prenatal administration of prochloraz differs considerably from those obtained with prenatal linuron treatment even though both pesticides are AR antagonists and both inhibit fetal testosterone synthesis.[13] The profile of effects in the male rat offspring induced by prenatal prochloraz more closely resembles that of an AR antagonist like vinclozolin, whereas the profile of effects obtained with linuron is more phthalate-like, suggesting that linuron is primarily affecting fetal male tract development by inhibiting testosterone synthesis, whereas prochloraz is acting as an AR antagonist. Further studies are needed to confirm these hypotheses.

10.7.1 "ANTIANDROGENIC" EFFECTS OF PHTHALATE ESTERS DURING DEVELOPMENT

Recent concerns about exposures of children to phthalates from toys and other products have resulted in a ban of phthalates in certain toys by the European Union. Although industry has repeatedly assured the safety of these chemicals, most of them have never been rigorously examined by the manufacturers for multigenerational reproductive effects. Currently, the population considered to potentially be at greatest risk are children on dialysis, because they receive some of the highest exposures from dialysis tubing. Children and women of childbearing age[86,87] have higher levels than other groups in general, and on occasion incredibly high levels are found in humans.[88]

The phthalates represent a class of toxicants that alter reproductive development via a mechanism of action that does not involve AR or ER binding.[10-12] Although many of the same effects are seen in animals exposed in utero to AR antagonists, in vitro studies found that neither the diesters nor their active monoester metabolites compete with androgens for binding to AR. While some have suggested that some of the effects are estrogenic, based upon in vitro work,[89,90] these observations are inconsistent[89] and it is evident that diagnostic estrogen effects are not seen in in vivo studies.[37] For example, we have found that di-n-butyl phthalate (DBP) did not produce any signs of estrogenicity in the ovariectomized female rat. DBP (sc at 200 or 400 mg/kg/day or by gavage at 1000 mg/kg/day, administered for 2 days, followed on the third day by 0.5 mg progesterone sc) did not induce a uterotropic response or increase estrogen-dependent sex behavior (lordosis). In addition, phthalate-treatment did not increase uterine weight in juvenile female rats, and oral DBP-treatment (250, 500, or 1000 mg/kg/day from weaning through adulthood) failed to accelerate vaginal opening or to induce in constant estrus in intact female rats.

Within the last 5 years several laboratories have demonstrated that perinatal exposure to different phthalate esters alters development of the male rat reproductive tract in an antiandrogenic manner. In particular, prenatal DBP, BBP, or DEHP treatment causes underdevelopment and agenesis of the epididymis and testicular abnormalities. At higher dosage levels, in utero DINP also induces malformations in male rats. Among the "antiandrogenic" EDCs, the phthalates are unique in their ability to induce agenesis of the gubernacular cords.[29] Differentiation of the gubernaculum is dependent upon the Leydig cell peptide hormone insulin-like peptide 3 (insl3) during sexual differentiation.[91-93] Knockout mice lacking insl3 display undescended, freely moving testis due to gubernacular agenesis. In contrast, this lesion is not displayed in AR knockout mice. Taken together, these results suggested that the phthalates DBP, BBP, and DEHP were inhibiting insl3 levels in addition to inhibiting fetal testis androgen production. Wilson et al.[13] confirmed this hypothesis. When the effects of these three phthalate esters on fetal testis endocrine function were compared to vinclozolin, linuron, and prochloraz, only the phthalates reduced both insl3 mRNA and testosterone levels (Figure 10.3). It is also evident from these data that insl3 is not dependent upon testosterone, as both linuron and prochloraz reduced testosterone production without affecting insl3 mRNA. Coupled with in vitro assays to identify AR antagonism, the endocrine profiles from the fetal testes are consistent with the profiles of malformations seen in the male offspring after in utero treatment. Only the phthalates cause gubernacular agenesis, while all of these toxicants alter differentiation of the androgen-dependent tissues.

To date, there are no published multigenerational studies that have included 1) relatively low dosage levels of DEHP; 2) developmental exposure; 3) an examination of sensitive endpoints; and 4) an adequate number of adult offspring. We recently completed a study that was designed to begin to address this data gap. Pregnant SD rats were dosed by gavage with DEHP from gestational day 8 to day 17 of lactation with 0, 11, 33, 100, or 300 mg/kg/day. In half of the males (PUB cohort), dosing was continued from 18 to 63–65 days of age while the rest (IUL cohort) were not dosed directly. The PUB cohort was necropsied at 63 to 65 days of age, while the IUL cohort was necropsied at full maturity. The 300 mg/kg/day IUL group displayed permanent reductions in reproductive organ weights and permanent nipples. In the high-dose group, more than a quarter of the males displayed testicular or epididymal abnormalities. These abnormalities also were displayed at a low incidence in the 11, 33, and 100 mg/kg/day dose groups, along with subtle reductions in reproductive organ weights. In the PUB group, puberty was delayed (100 and 300) and reproductive organ weights (300 mg) were reduced in size. Liver and adrenal weights were affected in all dose groups including 11 mg/kg/day (by one-tailed t-test), the lowest dose tested. The most serious effects (malformations and irreversible effects on organ weights and function) are induced by *in utero* exposure to the phthalate esters at dosage levels that do not induce severe or permanent testicular lesions in pubertal male rats.

Mylchreest et al.[25] observed similar malformations in male rat progeny after prenatal oral exposure (day 10 to 22 of gestation) to DBP with effects occurring at dosage levels as low as 100 mg/kg/day. In our multigenerational assessment of the reproductive effects of DBP on the male and female parents and their progeny, daily oral administration of 500 mg/kg/day by gavage delayed puberty in P0 male rats and reduced fertility in both male and female P0 rats,[37] while 250 mg/kg/day induced reproductive tract malformations and reduced fecundity in the F1 offspring. In addition, when P0 dams were dosed by gavage with 500 mg DBP/kg or DEHP (750 mg/kg/day) only during sexual differentiation (GD14 –to PND 4) the male offspring were profoundly malformed. More limited dosing in "pulses" during 4-day periods of gestation demonstrated that DBP at 500 mg/kg/day was most effective on days 16 to 19,[37] coincident with the known development of androgendependent tissues. Within the last few years, several laboratories have examined male rats late in fetal life,[94-96] or after birth[3, 97-99] following *in utero* phthalate treatment, and the results of these studies are remarkably consistent when exposure was late in pregnancy, when androgen-dependent tissues are being formed.

DBP also disrupts reproductive function in the rabbit.[100] Rabbits were exposed to 0 or 400 mg DBP/kg/day *in utero* (gestation days 15 to 29) or during adolescence (postnatal weeks [PNW] 4 to 12), and male offspring were examined at 6, 12, and 25 weeks of age. Another group was exposed only after puberty (for 12 weeks). The most pronounced reproductive effects were observed in male rabbits exposed *in utero*. Male offspring in this group exhibited reduced numbers of ejaculated sperm (down 43%), testis weights (at 12 weeks, down 23%), and reduced accessory sex gland weights (at 12 and 25 weeks, down 36% and 27%, respectively). Serum testosterone levels were reduced at 6 weeks by 32%; there was a slight increase in histological alterations of the testis and a doubling (from 16 to 30%, $p < 0.01$) of abnormal sperm; and 1 of 17 males manifested hypospadias, hypoplastic prostate, and cryptorchid testes with carcinoma *in situ*-like cells. In the DBP group exposed during adolescence, basal serum testosterone levels were reduced at 6 weeks ($p < 0.01$), while at 12 weeks testosterone production *in vivo* failed to respond normally to a GnRH challenge ($p < 0.01$). In addition, the weight of accessory sex glands was reduced at 12 weeks but not at 25 weeks after a recovery period; there was a slight increase in the percentage of abnormal sperm in the ejaculate; and 1 of 11 males was unilaterally cryptorchid. In both of these DBP-treated groups, daily sperm production, epididymal sperm counts, mating ability, and body and non-reproductive organs weights were unaffected. Thus, DBP induces lesions in the reproductive system of the rabbit, with the intrauterine period being the most sensitive stage of life.

The delay in the age at puberty in the male rat has been a consistent finding with phthalate esters like DBP,[37] BBP,[101] and DEHP and is not unexpected for a class of chemicals generally viewed as being "antiandrogenic" *in utero* and during pubertal development. The effects of these phthalate esters on androgen-dependent tissues is limited to the developing animal, as the testicular and reproductive effects of phthalate administration beginning in adulthood are minimal.[43,102] However, inexplicably a recent publication[103] claimed that DEHP elevated androgen levels in the male rat and, based on these results, the authors proposed a model indicating that phthalate administration during puberty would accelerate puberty rather than delay puberty. They also proposed that DEHP might accelerate puberty in females because serum estradiol levels were elevated in males in their study. As they did not actually determine the age at puberty or measure any androgen-dependent tissues in their study, it is difficult to evaluate the biological significance of the changes in the levels of testosterone and estradiol that they report. Clearly, however, their "androgen model" is not consistent with any of the published literature on either the effects of phthalates on the age at puberty or with the consistent reductions seen in androgen-dependent tissues in phthalate-treated male rats.

10.8.1 Antiandrogenic Effects of PBDE-71[104]

While there has been a decline in environmental and tissue levels of many contaminants like the organochlorine-based pesticides, the polychlorinated biphenyls, and dioxins in fish, wildlife, and human populations, tissue levels of polybrominated diphenyl ethers (PBDEs) are increasing in all species,[105-109] including humans.[109-111] PBDEs are synthesized in large quantities as flame retardants for commercial products. The detection of PBDEs in tissues from wildlife species and in human milk and plasma has raised concerns about possible adverse effects. Recently, Stoker et al. showed that one PBDE mixture (DE-71) delayed the age at puberty in male rats when administered at 30, 60, and 120 mg/kg/day by 3, 4, and 5 days, respectively, and suppressed ventral prostate and seminal vesicle growth. Although these effects occurred concurrently with reduced serum thyroxin levels, serum testosterone was not reduced, suggesting DE-71 might be acting as an androgen receptor antagonist. To elucidate the potential antiandrogenic effects of this mixture, DE-71 and DE-100 (2,2', 4,4',6-pentaBDE), one of the congeners in this DE-71 mixture, were examined *in vivo* and *in vitro*.[104] Stoker et al.[104] found that DE-100 acted as a competitive inhibitor in an AR binding assay (rat ventral prostate cytosol) with an IC50 of

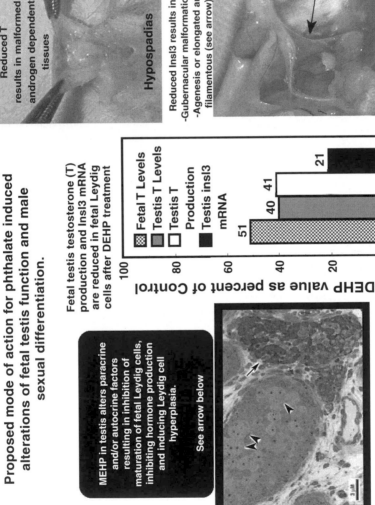

FIGURE 10.4 Proposed mode of action for phthalate induced alterations of fetal testis function and male rat sexual differentiation.

approximately 5 microM. In addition, both DE-71 and DE-100 inhibited DHT-induced transcriptional activation in MDA-KB2 cells. *In vivo*, DE-71 was antiandrogenic in castrate-immature testosterone propionate-treated rats (Hershberger assay), reducing sex accessory tissue growth without affecting body weight. In conclusion, DE-71 and DE-100 appear to be AR antagonists. Additional studies are in progress to determine if DE-71 can alter sexual differentiation of the male rat when administered during pregnancy.

10.9.1 Mixtures of "Antiandrogens": AR Antagonists versus Inhibitors of Steroidogenesis

Although risk assessments are typically conducted on a chemical-by-chemical basis, the 1996 Food Quality Protection Act mandated that the USEPA consider cumulative risk from chemicals that act via a common mechanism. Our studies begin to provide a framework for assessing the cumulative effects of "antiandrogenic" EDCs.[5,112] SD rats were dosed orally on days 14 to 18 of gestation with EDCs singly or in pairs at dosage levels equivalent to about 50% the ED50 for hypospadias or epididymal agenesis including (1) two AR antagonists (vinclozolin plus procymidone, each at 50 mg/kg/day), (2) two phthalate esters with a common metabolite (DBP and BBP, each at 500 mg/kg/day), (3) two phthalate esters with different active metabolites (DEHP and DBP (500)), (4) a phthalate ester plus an AR antagonist (DBP [500] plus procymidone [50]), and (5) linuron (75 mg/kg/day) plus BBP (500). We expected that individually each chemical would not induce hypospadias or high levels of other malformations using this dosing regimen, but mixing any two together would induce reproductive tract malformations in about 50% of the males and induce cumulative effects on other androgen-dependent organs. In the current study, all combinations produced cumulative effects on every androgen-dependent tissue. However, only the phthalate ester combinations caused agenesis of the insl3-dependent gubernacular ligaments. The effects of DBP and DEHP in one study and vinclozolin plus procymidone were cumulative, indicating that toxicants need not have a common active metabolite to produce cumulative adverse effects. Rather, these mixtures represent combinations of chemicals with a common "toxicophore" or "pharmacophore." We also found that EDCs that alter differentiation of the same reproductive tissues during sexual differentiation produce cumulative and apparently dose-additive effects when combined, even if they do not share a common toxicophore, as was the case with the mixture of procymidone plus BBP. It is important to note that the relative potency factors among the chemicals varied from tissue to tissue based upon the mechanism and mode of toxicity. These results indicate that a single toxicity equivalent factor for each chemical will not accurately predict the results of certain mixtures.

REFERENCES

1. Colborn, T., The wildlife/human connection: modernizing risk decisions. *Environ Health Perspect* **1994,** 102 Suppl 12, 55-9.
2. Colborn, T.; vom Saal, F. S.; Soto, A. M., Developmental effects of endocrine-disrupting chemicals in wildlife and humans. *Environ Health Perspect* **1993,** 101, (5), 378-84.
3. Foster, P. M.; Mylchreest, E.; Gaido, K. W.; Sar, M., Effects of phthalate esters on the developing reproductive tract of male rats. *Hum Reprod Update* **2001,** 7, (3), 231–5.
4. Gray, L. E., Jr., Xenoendocrine disrupters: laboratory studies on male reproductive effects. *Toxicol Lett* **1998,** 102–103, 331–5.
5. Gray, L. E.; Ostby, J.; Furr, J.; Wolf, C. J.; Lambright, C.; Parks, L.; Veeramachaneni, D. N.; Wilson, V.; Price, M.; Hotchkiss, A.; Orlando, E.; Guillette, L., Effects of environmental antiandrogens on reproductive development in experimental animals. *Hum Reprod Update* **2001,** 7, (3), 248–64.
6. Kelce, W. R.; Gray, L. E.; Wilson, E. M., Antiandrogens as environmental endocrine disruptors. *Reprod Fertil Dev* **1998,** 10, (1), 105–11.
7. Kelce, W. R.; Monosson, E.; Gamcsik, M. P.; Laws, S. C.; Gray, L. E., Jr., Environmental hormone disruptors: evidence that vinclozolin developmental toxicity is mediated by antiandrogenic metabolites. *Toxicol Appl Pharmacol* **1994,** 126, (2), 276–85.
8. Hosokawa, S.; Murakami, M.; Ineyama, M.; Yamada, T.; Yoshitake, A.; Yamada, H.; Miyamoto, J., The affinity of procymidone to androgen receptor in rats and mice. *J Toxicol Sci* **1993,** 18, (2), 83–93.
9. Kelce, W. R.; Stone, C. R.; Laws, S. C.; Gray, L. E.; Kemppainen, J. A.; Wilson, E. M., Persistent DDT metabolite p,p′-DDE is a potent androgen receptor antagonist. *Nature* **1995,** 375, (6532), 581–5.
10. Mylchreest, E.; Foster, P. M., DBP exerts its antiandrogenic activity by indirectly interfering with androgen signaling pathways. *Toxicol Appl Pharmacol* **2000,** 168, (2), 174–5.
11. Mylchreest, E.; Sar, M.; Wallace, D. G.; Foster, P. M., Fetal testosterone insufficiency and abnormal proliferation of Leydig cells and gonocytes in rats exposed to di(n-butyl) phthalate. *Reprod Toxicol* **2002,** 16, (1), 19–28.
12. Parks, L. G.; Ostby, J. S.; Lambright, C. R.; Abbott, B. D.; Klinefelter, G. R.; Barlow, N. J.; Gray, L. E., Jr., The plasticizer diethylhexyl phthalate induces malformations by decreasing fetal testosterone synthesis during sexual differentiation in the male rat. *Toxicol Sci* **2000,** 58, (2), 339–49.
13. Wilson, V. S.; Lambright, C.; Furr, J.; Ostby, J.; Wood, C.; Held, G.; Gray, L. E., Jr., Phthalate ester-induced gubernacular lesions are associated with reduced insl3 gene expression in the fetal rat testis. *Toxicol Lett* **2004,** 146, (3), 207–15.
14. Vinggaard, A. M.; Nellemann, C.; Dalgaard, M.; Jorgensen, E. B.; Andersen, H. R., Antiandrogenic effects *in vitro* and *in vivo* of the fungicide prochloraz. *Toxicol Sci* **2002,** 69, (2), 344–53.
15. Lambright, C.; Ostby, J.; Bobseine, K.; Wilson, V.; Hotchkiss, A. K.; Mann, P. C.; Gray, L. E., Jr., Cellular and molecular mechanisms of action of linuron: an antiandrogenic herbicide that produces reproductive malformations in male rats. *Toxicol Sci* **2000,** 56, (2), 389–99.
16. Vinggaard, A. M.; Hnida, C.; Breinholt, V.; Larsen, J. C., Screening of selected pesticides for inhibition of CYP19 aromatase activity *in vitro*. *Toxicol in vitro* **2000,** 14, (3), 227–34.

17. Nellemann, C.; Dalgaard, M.; Lam, H. R.; Vinggaard, A. M., The combined effects of vinclozolin and procymidone do not deviate from expected additivity *in vitro* and *in vivo*. *Toxicol Sci* **2003,** 71, (2), 251–62.

18. Parks, L. G.; Lambright, C. S.; Orlando, E. F.; Guillette, L. J., Jr.; Ankley, G. T.; Gray, L. E., Jr., Masculinization of female mosquitofish in Kraft mill effluent-contaminated Fenholloway River water is associated with androgen receptor agonist activity. *Toxicol Sci* **2001,** 62, (2), 257–67.

19. Larsson, D. G.; Forlin, L., Male-biased sex ratios of fish embryos near a pulp mill: temporary recovery after a short-term shutdown. *Environ Health Perspect* **2002,** 110, (8), 739–42.

20. Larsson, D. G.; Kinnberg, K.; Sturve, J.; Stephensen, E.; Skon, M.; Forlin, L., Studies of masculinization, detoxification, and oxidative stress responses in guppies (Poecilia reticulata) exposed to effluent from a pulp mill. *Ecotoxicol Environ Saf* **2002,** 52, (1), 13–20.

21. Durhan, E. J.; Lambright, C.; Wilson, V.; Butterworth, B. C.; Kuehl, O. W.; Orlando, E. F.; Guillette, L. J., Jr.; Gray, L. E.; Ankley, G. T., Evaluation of androstenedione as an androgenic component of river water downstream of a pulp and paper mill effluent. *Environ Toxicol Chem* **2002,** 21, (9), 1973–6.

22. Ellis, R. J.; van den Heuvel, M. R.; Bandelj, E.; Smith, M. A.; McCarthy, L. H.; Stuthridge, T. R.; Dietrich, D. R., *In vivo* and *in vitro* assessment of the androgenic potential of a pulp and paper mill effluent. *Environ Toxicol Chem* **2003,** 22, (7), 1448–56.

23. Schiffer, B.; Daxenberger, A.; Meyer, K.; Meyer, H. H., The fate of trenbolone acetate and melengestrol acetate after application as growth promoters in cattle: environmental studies. *Environ Health Perspect* **2001,** 109, (11), 1145–51.

24. Wilson, V. S.; Lambright, C.; Ostby, J.; Gray, L. E., Jr., *In vitro* and *in vivo* effects of 17beta-trenbolone: a feedlot effluent contaminant. *Toxicol Sci* **2002,** 70, (2), 202–11.

25. Mylchreest, E.; Cattley, R. C.; Foster, P. M., Male reproductive tract malformations in rats following gestational and lactational exposure to Di(n-butyl) phthalate: an antiandrogenic mechanism? *Toxicol Sci* **1998,** 43, (1), 47–60.

26. Ostby, J.; Kelce, W. R.; Lambright, C.; Wolf, C. J.; Mann, P.; Gray, L. E., Jr., The fungicide procymidone alters sexual differentiation in the male rat by acting as an androgen-receptor antagonist *in vivo* and *in vitro*. *Toxicol Ind Health* **1999,** 15, (1–2), 80–93.

27. McIntyre, B. S.; Barlow, N. J.; Wallace, D. G.; Maness, S. C.; Gaido, K. W.; Foster, P. M., Effects of *in utero* exposure to linuron on androgen-dependent reproductive development in the male Crl:CD(SD)BR rat. *Toxicol Appl Pharmacol* **2000,** 167, (2), 87–99.

28. Gray, L. E., Jr.; Ostby, J.; Monosson, E.; Kelce, W. R., Environmental antiandrogens: low doses of the fungicide vinclozolin alter sexual differentiation of the male rat. *Toxicol Ind Health* **1999,** 15, (1–2), 48–64.

29. Gray, L. E., Jr.; Ostby, J.; Furr, J.; Price, M.; Veeramachaneni, D. N.; Parks, L., Perinatal exposure to the phthalates DEHP, BBP, and DINP, but not DEP, DMP, or DOTP, alters sexual differentiation of the male rat. *Toxicol Sci* **2000,** 58, (2), 350–65.

30. Wolf, C. J.; Hotchkiss, A.; Ostby, J. S.; LeBlanc, G. A.; Gray, L. E., Jr., Effects of prenatal testosterone propionate on the sexual development of male and female rats: a dose-response study. *Toxicol Sci* **2002,** 65, (1), 71–86.

31. Jenkins, R.; Angus, R. A.; McNatt, H.; Howell, W. M.; Kemppainen, J. A.; Kirk, M.; Wilson, E. M., Identification of androstenedione in a river containing paper mill effluent. *Environ Toxicol Chem* **2001,** 20, (6), 1325–31.

32. Jenkins, R. L.; Wilson, E. M.; Angus, R. A.; Howell, W. M.; Kirk, M., Androstenedione and progesterone in the sediment of a river receiving paper mill effluent. *Toxicol Sci* **2003,** 73, (1), 53–9.

33. Howell, W.; Black, D.; Bortone, S., Abnormal expression of secondary sex characters in a population of mosquitofish, *Gambusia affinis holbrooki*: evidence for environmentally induced masculinization. *Copeia* **1980,** 4, 676–681.

34. Davis, W.; Bortone, S., *Effects of kraft mill effluent on sexuality in fishes. An environmental early warning?* Chemically-Induced Alterations in Sexual and Functional Development: The Human/Wildlife Connection, Colborn, T. and Clements, C. (eds), Princeton Scientific Publishing Co, Inc: Princeton, NJ, 1992; Vol. XXI, p 113–128.

35. Orlando, E.; Kolok, A.; Binzcik, G.; Gates, J.; Horton, M.; Lambright, C.; Gray, L.; Soto, A. M.; Guillette, L., Endocrine disrupting effects of cattle feedlot effluent on an aquatic sentinel species the fathead minnow. *Environ Health Perspect* **2003,** doi:10.1289.ehp.6591, 1–31.

36. Ankley, G. T.; Jensen, K. M.; Makynen, E. A.; Kahl, M. D.; Korte, J. J.; Hornung, M. W.; Henry, T. R.; Denny, J. S.; Leino, R. L.; Wilson, V. S.; Cardon, M. C.; Hartig, P. C.; Gray, L. E., Effects of the androgenic growth promoter 17-beta-trenbolone on fecundity and reproductive endocrinology of the fathead minnow. *Environ Toxicol Chem* **2003,** 22, (6), 1350–60.

37. Gray, L. E., Jr.; Wolf, C.; Lambright, C.; Mann, P.; Price, M.; Cooper, R. L.; Ostby, J., Administration of potentially antiandrogenic pesticides (procymidone, linuron, iprodione, chlozolinate, p,p′-DDE, and ketoconazole) and toxic substances (dibutyl- and diethylhexyl phthalate, PCB 169, and ethane dimethane sulphonate) during sexual differentiation produces diverse profiles of reproductive malformations in the male rat. *Toxicol Ind Health* **1999,** 15, (1–2), 94–118.

38. Wong, C.; Kelce, W. R.; Sar, M.; Wilson, E. M., Androgen receptor antagonist versus agonist activities of the fungicide vinclozolin relative to hydroxyflutamide. *J Biol Chem* **1995,** 270, (34), 19998–20003.

39. Kelce, W. R.; Lambright, C. R.; Gray, L. E., Jr.; Roberts, K. P., Vinclozolin and p,p′-DDE alter androgen-dependent gene expression: *in vivo* confirmation of an androgen receptor-mediated mechanism. *Toxicol Appl Pharmacol* **1997,** 142, (1), 192–200.

40. Laws, S. C.; Carey, S. A.; Kelce, W. R.; Cooper, R. L.; Gray, L. E., Jr., Vinclozolin does not alter progesterone receptor (PR) function *in vivo* despite inhibition of PR binding by its metabolites *in vitro*. *Toxicology* **1996,** 112, (3), 173–82.

41. Yamasaki, K.; Sawaki, M.; Ohta, R.; Okuda, H.; Katayama, S.; Yamada, T.; Ohta, T.; Kosaka, T.; Owens, W., OECD validation of the Hershberger assay in Japan: phase 2 dose response of methyltestosterone, vinclozolin, and p,p′-DDE. *Environ Health Perspect* **2003,** 111, (16), 1912–9.

42. Monosson, E.; Kelce, W. R.; Lambright, C.; Ostby, J.; Gray, L. E., Jr., Peripubertal exposure to the antiandrogenic fungicide, vinclozolin, delays puberty, inhibits the development of androgen-dependent tissues, and alters androgen receptor function in the male rat. *Toxicol Ind Health* **1999,** 15, (1–2), 65–79.

43. O'Connor, J. C.; Frame, S. R.; Ladics, G. S., Evaluation of a 15-day screening assay using intact male rats for identifying antiandrogens. *Toxicol Sci* **2002,** 69, (1), 92–108.

44. Gray, L. E., Jr.; Ostby, J.; Ferrell, J.; Rehnberg, G.; Linder, R.; Cooper, R.; Goldman, J.; Slott, V.; Laskey, J., A dose-response analysis of methoxychlor-induced alterations of reproductive development and function in the rat. *Fundam Appl Toxicol* **1989,** 12, (1), 92–108.

45. Gray, L. E., Jr.; Ostby, J.; Cooper, R. L.; Kelce, W. R., The estrogenic and antiandrogenic pesticide methoxychlor alters the reproductive tract and behavior without affecting pituitary size or LH and prolactin secretion in male rats. *Toxicol Ind Health* **1999,** 15, (1–2), 37–47.

46. Gray, L. E., Jr.; Ostby, J. S.; Kelce, W. R., Developmental effects of an environmental antiandrogen: the fungicide vinclozolin alters sex differentiation of the male rat. *Toxicol Appl Pharmacol* **1994,** 129, (1), 46–52.

47. Hotchkiss, A. K.; Ostby, J. S.; Vandenbergh, J. G.; Gray, L. E., Jr., An environmental antiandrogen, vinclozolin, alters the organization of play behavior. *Physiol Behav* **2003,** 79, (2), 151–6.

48. Hotchkiss, A. K.; Ostby, J. S.; Vandenburgh, J. G.; Gray, L. E., Jr., Androgens and environmental antiandrogens affect reproductive development and play behavior in the Sprague-Dawley rat. *Environ Health Perspect* **2002,** 110 Suppl 3, 435–9.

49. Hellwig, J.; van Ravenzwaay, B.; Mayer, M.; Gembardt, C., Pre- and postnatal oral toxicity of vinclozolin in Wistar and Long-Evans rats. *Regul Toxicol Pharmacol* **2000,** 32, (1), 42–50.

50. Wolf, C. J.; LeBlanc, G. A.; Ostby, J. S.; Gray, L. E., Jr., Characterization of the period of sensitivity of fetal male sexual development to vinclozolin. *Toxicol Sci* **2000,** 55, (1), 152–61.

51. Wolf, C. J.; LeBlanc, G. A.; Gray, L. E., Jr., Interactive Effects of Vinclozolin and Testosterone Propionate on Pregnancy and Sexual Differentiation of the Male and Female SD Rat. *Toxicol Sci* **2004.**

52. Goldman, J. M.; Laws, S. C.; Balchak, S. K.; Cooper, R. L.; Kavlock, R. J., Endocrine-disrupting chemicals: prepubertal exposures and effects on sexual maturation and thyroid activity in the female rat. A focus on the EDSTAC recommendations. *Crit Rev Toxicol* **2000,** 30, (2), 135–96.

53. Stoker, T. E.; Parks, L. G.; Gray, L. E.; Cooper, R. L., Endocrine-disrupting chemicals: prepubertal exposures and effects on sexual maturation and thyroid function in the male rat. A focus on the EDSTAC recommendations. Endocrine Disrupter Screening and Testing Advisory Committee. *Crit Rev Toxicol* **2000,** 30, (2), 197–252.

54. Baatrup, E.; Junge, M., Antiandrogenic pesticides disrupt sexual characteristics in the adult male guppy *Poecilia reticulata. Environ Health Perspect* **2001,** 109, (10), 1063–70.

55. Bayley, M.; Junge, M.; Baatrup, E., Exposure of juvenile guppies to three antiandrogens causes demasculinization and a reduced sperm count in adult males. *Aquat Toxicol* **2002,** 56, (4), 227–39.

56. Bayley, M.; Larsen, P. F.; Baekgaard, H.; Baatrup, E., The effects of vinclozolin, an anti-androgenic fungicide, on male guppy secondary sex characters and reproductive success. *Biol Reprod* **2003,** 69, (6), 1951–6.

57. Kinnberg, K.; Toft, G., Effects of estrogenic and antiandrogenic compounds on the testis structure of the adult guppy (*Poecilia reticulata*). *Ecotoxicol Environ Saf* **2003,** 54, (1), 16–24.

58. Kiparissis, Y.; Metcalfe, T. L.; Balch, G. C.; Metcalfe, C. D., Effects of the antiandrogens, vinclozolin and cyproterone acetate on gonadal development in the Japanese medaka (Oryzias latipes). *Aquat Toxicol* **2003,** 63, (4), 391–403.

59. Makynen, E. A.; Kahl, M. D.; Jensen, K. M.; Tietge, J. E.; Wells, K. L.; van der Kraak, G.; Ankley, G. T., Effects of the mammalian antiandrogen vinclozolin on development and reproduction of the fathead minnow (*Pimephales promelas*). *Aquatic Toxicol* **2000**, 48, (4), 461–475.

60. Stanton, M. E.; Crofton, K. M.; Gray, L. E.; Gordon, C. J.; Boyes, W. K.; Mole, M. L.; Peele, D. B.; Bushnell, P. J., Assessment of offspring development and behavior following gestational exposure to inhaled methanol in the rat. *Fundam Appl Toxicol* **1995**, 28, (1), 100–10.

61. van Wyk, J. H.; Pool, E. J.; Leslie, A. J., The effects of anti-androgenic and estrogenic disrupting contaminants on breeding gland (nuptial pad) morphology, plasma testosterone levels, and plasma vitellogenin levels in male *Xenopus laevis* (African clawed frog). *Arch Environ Contam Toxicol* **2003**, 44, (2), 247–56.

62. McGary, S.; Henry, P. F.; Ottinger, M. A., Impact of vinclozolin on reproductive behavior and endocrinology in Japanese quail (*Coturnix coturnix japonica*). *Environ Toxicol Chem* **2001**, 20, (11), 2487–93.

63. Crain, D. A.; Guillette, L. J., Jr.; Rooney, A. A.; Pickford, D. B., Alterations in steroidogenesis in alligators (*Alligator mississippiensis*) exposed naturally and experimentally to environmental contaminants. *Environ Health Perspect* **1997**, 105, (5), 528–33.

64. Tillmann, M.; Schulte-Oehlmann, U.; Duft, M.; Markert, B.; Oehlmann, J., Effects of endocrine disruptors on prosobranch snails (*Mollusca: Gastropoda*) in the laboratory. Part III: Cyproterone acetate and vinclozolin as antiandrogens. *Ecotoxicology* **2001**, 10, (6), 373–88.

65. Cardon, M.; Hartig, P.; Gray, L.; Wilson, V., Rainbow trout androgen receptor alpha and human androgen receptor: Comparisons in the COS whole cell binding assay. *The Toxicologist* **2003**, 71, 132.

66. Thornton, J. W.; Need, E.; Crews, D., Resurrecting the ancestral steroid receptor: ancient origin of estrogen signaling. *Science* **2003**, 301, (5640), 1714–7.

67. Thornton, J. W.; DeSalle, R., A new method to localize and test the significance of incongruence: detecting domain shuffling in the nuclear receptor superfamily. *Syst Biol* **2000**, 49, (2), 183–201.

68. Wilson, V.; Wood, C.; Held, G.; Lambright, C.; Ostby, J.; Furr, J.; Gray, L., Comparison of the effects of two AR antagonists on tissue weights and hormone levels in male rats and on expression of three androgen dependent genes in the ventral prostate. *The Toxicologist* **2003**, 71, 131.

69. Rosen, M.; Wilson, V.; Schmid, J.; Gray, L., Gene array analysis of the ventral prostate in rats exposed to either vinclozolin or procymidone. *The Toxicologist* **2003**, 71, 94.

70. Hosokawa, S.; Murakami, M.; Ineyama, M.; Yamada, T.; Koyama, Y.; Okuno, Y.; Yoshitake, A.; Yamada, H.; Miyamoto, J., Effects of procymidone on reproductive organs and serum gonadotropins in male rats. *J Toxicol Sci* **1993**, 18, (2), 111–24.

71. Cook, J. C.; Mullin, L. S.; Frame, S. R.; Biegel, L. B., Investigation of a mechanism for Leydig cell tumorigenesis by linuron in rats. *Toxicol Appl Pharmacol* **1993**, 119, (2), 195–204.

72. McIntyre, B. S.; Barlow, N. J.; Foster, P. M., Male rats exposed to linuron *in utero* exhibit permanent changes in anogenital distance, nipple retention, and epididymal malformations that result in subsequent testicular atrophy. *Toxicol Sci* **2002**, 65, (1), 62–70.

73. McIntyre, B. S.; Barlow, N. J.; Sar, M.; Wallace, D. G.; Foster, P. M., Effects of *in utero* linuron exposure on rat Wolffian duct development. *Reprod Toxicol* **2002**, 16, (2), 131–9.

74. Longnecker, M. P.; Klebanoff, M. A.; Brock, J. W.; Zhou, H.; Gray, K. A.; Needham, L. L.; Wilcox, A. J., Maternal serum level of 1,1-dichloro-2,2-bis(p-chlorophenyl)ethylene and risk of cryptorchidism, hypospadias, and polythelia among male offspring. *Am J Epidemiol* **2002**, 155, (4), 313–22.

75. Longnecker, M. P.; Klebanoff, M. A.; Zhou, H.; Brock, J. W., Association between maternal serum concentration of the DDT metabolite DDE and preterm and small-for-gestational-age babies at birth. *Lancet* **2001,** 358, (9276), 110–4.

76. Longnecker, M. P.; Rogan, W. J.; Lucier, G., The human health effects of DDT (dichlorodiphenyltrichloroethane) and PCBs (polychlorinated biphenyls) and an overview of organochlorines in public health. *Annu Rev Public Health* **1997,** 18, 211–44.

77. Chen, A.; Rogan, W. J., Nonmalarial infant deaths and DDT use for malaria control. *Emerg Infect Dis* **2003,** 9, (8), 960–4.

78. Rogan, W. J., The DDT question. *Lancet* **2000,** 356, (9236), 1189.

79. Kelce, W. R.; Monosson, E.; Gray, L. E., Jr., An environmental antiandrogen. *Recent Prog Horm Res* **1995,** 50, 449–53.

80. O'Connor, J. C.; Frame, S. R.; Davis, L. G.; Cook, J. C., Detection of the environmental antiandrogen p,p-DDE in CD and Long-Evans rats using a tier I screening battery and a Hershberger assay. *Toxicol Sci* **1999,** 51, (1), 44–53.

81. You, L.; Brenneman, K. A.; Heck, H., *In utero* exposure to antiandrogens alters the responsiveness of the prostate to p,p'-DDE in adult rats and may induce prostatic inflammation. *Toxicol Appl Pharmacol* **1999,** 161, (3), 258–66.

82. You, L.; Casanova, M.; Archibeque-Engle, S.; Sar, M.; Fan, L. Q.; Heck, H. A., Impaired male sexual development in perinatal Sprague-Dawley and Long-Evans hooded rats exposed *in utero* and lactationally to p,p'-DDE. *Toxicol Sci* **1998,** 45, (2), 162–73.

83. Veeramachaneni, D. N., Deteriorating trends in male reproduction: idiopathic or environmental? *Anim Reprod Sci* **2000,** 60–61, 121–30.

84. Waller, C. L.; Juma, B. W.; Gray, L. E., Jr.; Kelce, W. R., Three-dimensional quantitative structure—activity relationships for androgen receptor ligands. *Toxicol Appl Pharmacol* **1996,** 137, (2), 219–27.

85. Noriega, N.; Ostby, J.; Lambright, C.; Wilson, V.; Gray, L., Prenatal exposure to the fungicide prochloraz alters the onset of parturition in the dam and sexual differentiation in male rat offspring. *The Toxicologist* **2004,** 73.

86. Blount, B. C.; Silva, M. J.; Caudill, S. P.; Needham, L. L.; Pirkle, J. L.; Sampson, E. J.; Lucier, G. W.; Jackson, R. J.; Brock, J. W., Levels of seven urinary phthalate metabolites in a human reference population. *Environ Health Perspect* **2000,** 108, (10), 979–82.

87. Brock, J. W.; Caudill, S. P.; Silva, M. J.; Needham, L. L.; Hilborn, E. D., Phthalate monoesters levels in the urine of young children. *Bull Environ Contam Toxicol* **2002,** 68, (3), 309–14.

88. Hauser, R.; Duty, S.; Godfrey-Bailey, L.; Calafat, A., Medications as a source of human exposure to phthalates: A case report. *Environ Health Perspect* **2004,** doi:10.1289/ehp.6804.

89. Zacharewski, T. R.; Meek, M. D.; Clemons, J. H.; Wu, Z. F.; Fielden, M. R.; Matthews, J. B., Examination of the *in vitro* and *in vivo* estrogenic activities of eight commercial phthalate esters. *Toxicol Sci* **1998,** 46, (2), 282–93.

90. Harris, C. A.; Henttu, P.; Parker, M. G.; Sumpter, J. P., The estrogenic activity of phthalate esters *in vitro*. *Environ Health Perspect* **1997,** 105, (8), 802–11.

91. Ivell, R.; Bathgate, R. A., Reproductive biology of the relaxin-like factor (RLF/INSL3). *Biol Reprod* **2002,** 67, (3), 699–705.

92. Nef, S.; Parada, L. F., Cryptorchidism in mice mutant for Insl3. *Nat Genet* **1999**, 22, (3), 295–9.

93. Zimmermann, S.; Steding, G.; Emmen, J. M.; Brinkmann, A. O.; Nayernia, K.; Holstein, A. F.; Engel, W.; Adham, I. M., Targeted disruption of the Insl3 gene causes bilateral cryptorchidism. *Mol Endocrinol* **1999**, 13, (5), 681–91.

94. Ema, M., Antiandrogenic effects of dibutyl phthalate and its metabolite, monobutyl phthalate, in rats. *Congenit Anom Kyoto* **2002**, 42, (4), 297–308.

95. Ema, M.; Miyawaki, E., Effects on development of the reproductive system in male offspring of rats given butyl benzyl phthalate during late pregnancy. *Reprod Toxicol* **2002**, 16, (1), 71–6.

96. Ema, M.; Miyawaki, E.; Hirose, A.; Kamata, E., Decreased anogenital distance and increased incidence of undescended testes in fetuses of rats given monobenzyl phthalate, a major metabolite of butyl benzyl phthalate. *Reprod Toxicol* **2003**, 17, (4), 407–12.

97. Arcadi, F. A.; Costa, C.; Imperatore, C.; Marchese, A.; Rapisarda, A.; Salemi, M.; Trimarchi, G. R.; Costa, G., Oral toxicity of bis(2-ethylhexyl) phthalate during pregnancy and suckling in the Long-Evans rat. *Food Chem Toxicol* **1998**, 36, (11), 963–70.

98. Foster, P. M.; Cattley, R. C.; Mylchreest, E., Effects of di-n-butyl phthalate (DBP) on male reproductive development in the rat: implications for human risk assessment. *Food Chem Toxicol* **2000**, 38, (1 Suppl), S97–9.

99. Moore, R. W.; Rudy, T. A.; Lin, T. M.; Ko, K.; Peterson, R. E., Abnormalities of sexual development in male rats with *in utero* and lactational exposure to the anti-androgenic plasticizer Di(2-ethylhexyl) phthalate. *Environ Health Perspect* **2001**, 109, (3), 229–37.

100. Higuchi, T. T.; Palmer, J. S.; Gray, L. E., Jr.; Veeramachaneni, D. N., Effects of dibutyl phthalate in male rabbits following *in utero*, adolescent, or postpubertal exposure. *Toxicol Sci* **2003**, 72, (2), 301–13.

101. Nagao, T.; Ohta, R.; Marumo, H.; Shindo, T.; Yoshimura, S.; Ono, H., Effect of butyl benzyl phthalate in Sprague-Dawley rats after gavage administration: a two-generation reproductive study. *Reprod Toxicol* **2000**, 14, (6), 513–32.

102. Sjoberg, P.; Lindqvist, N. G.; Ploen, L., Age-dependent response of the rat testes to di(2-ethylhexyl) phthalate. *Environ Health Perspect* **1986**, 65, 237–42.

103. Akingbemi, B. T.; Ge, R.; Klinefelter, G. R.; Zirkin, B. R.; Hardy, M. P., Phthalate-induced Leydig cell hyperplasia is associated with multiple endocrine disturbances. *Proc Natl Acad Sci U S A* **2004**, 101, (3), 775–80.

104. Stoker, T.; Cooper, R.; Lambright, C.; Gray, L., *in vivo* and *in vitro* anti-androgenic effects of DE-71, a commercial polybrominated diphenyl ether (PBDE) mixture. *The Toxicologist* **2004**, 73.

105. Marsh, G.; Athanasiadou, M.; Bergman, A.; Asplund, L., Identification of hydroxylated and methoxylated polybrominated diphenyl ethers in Baltic Sea salmon (Salmo salar) blood. *Environ Sci Technol* **2004**, 38, (1), 10–8.

106. Lind, Y.; Darnerud, P. O.; Atuma, S.; Aune, M.; Becker, W.; Bjerselius, R.; Cnattingius, S.; Glynn, A., Polybrominated diphenyl ethers in breast milk from Uppsala County, Sweden. *Environ Res* **2003**, 93, (2), 186–94.

107. Akutsu, K.; Kitagawa, M.; Nakazawa, H.; Makino, T.; Iwazaki, K.; Oda, H.; Hori, S., Time-trend (1973–2000) of polybrominated diphenyl ethers in Japanese mother's milk. *Chemosphere* **2003**, 53, (6), 645–54.

108. Rayne, S.; Ikonomou, M. G.; Antcliffe, B., Rapidly increasing polybrominated diphenyl ether concentrations in the Columbia River system from 1992 to 2000. *Environ Sci Technol* **2003**, 37, (13), 2847–54.

109. Sjodin, A.; Patterson, D. G., Jr.; Bergman, A., A review on human exposure to brominated flame retardants—particularly polybrominated diphenyl ethers. *Environ Int* **2003,** 29, (6), 829–39.
110. Schecter, A.; Pavuk, M.; Papke, O.; Ryan, J. J.; Birnbaum, L.; Rosen, R., Polybrominated diphenyl ethers (PBDEs) in U.S. mothers' milk. *Environ Health Perspect* **2003,** 111, (14), 1723–9.
111. Sjödin, A.; Jones, R.; Focant, J.-F.; Lapeza C.; Wang, R. Y.; McGahee, E. I.; Zhang Y.; Turner, W.; Slazyk, B.; Needham, L.; Patterson, D. J., Retrospective time trend study of polybrominated diphenyl ether and polybrominated and polychlorinated biphenyl levels in human serum from the United States. *Environ Health Perspect* **2004,** doi:10.1289/ehp.6826., Online 14 January 2004.
112. Gray, L.; Ostby, J.; Furr, J.; Lambright, C.; Hotchkiss, A.; Wilson, V., Cumulative effects of endocrine disrupters (EDCs): synergy or additivity? *The Toxicologist* **2004,** 74.

11 Endocrine Disruptors and Male Sexual Dysfunction

Suresh C. Sikka, Ph. D., H.C.L.D.,
Muammer Kendirci, M.D., and
Rajesh Naz, Ph.D.

CONTENTS

11.1   INTRODUCTION

Erectile dysfunction (ED) can be defined as the inability to achieve or maintain an erection sufficient for satisfactory sexual intercourse. It is estimated that 20 to 30 million Americans suffer from ED [1]. The onset of ED is mostly very gradual, interrupted by seemingly partial recoveries. The Massachusetts Male Aging Study (MMAS) reported that 52% of men aged 40 to 70 experienced some degree of ED and that with advancing age there is a progressive decline in libido, frequency of nocturnal or morning erections, and sexual intercourse [1]. However, sexual satisfaction did not decline, suggesting that men accommodate for age-related changes in sexual capacity by altering expectations. The decline in libido with age has been associated with a similar decrease in the male hormone testosterone. This association between low libido, declining androgen, and the onset of ED is not clear at present. In order to understand the complexity of this process and the role of hormonal disruptors, it is important to first focus on what is currently known about male sexual function, with penis being the most important target organ. The association between hypogonadism and ED has not been clarified. There appears to be a direct relationship between serum androgen levels and libido but the association with sexual function is less clear. It is well known that libido can have a significant impact as a "conditioner" for sexual function, and thus androgens may play an important role in both libido and the pathophysiology of ED.

11.2 PHYSIOLOGY OF ERECTION

Penile erection is a result of passive dilation of the lacunar spaces and relaxation of the smooth musculature of the cavernosal arteriovenous bed and trabecular network. Three neuroeffector pathways coordinate the smooth muscle tone in the corpora cavernosa. These are the adrenergic, cholinergic, and non-adrenergic/non-cholinergic (NANC) pathways [2]. Penile flaccidity is maintained by the adrenergic-mediated sympathetic tone of the cavernosal smooth muscle. Erection is triggered by stimulation of a dual-innervated neuronal pathway involving both cholinergic and NANC mediators. The primary mediator of penile erections is nitric oxide (NO), originating from NANC neurons, cavernosal smooth muscle cells, and cholinergic-stimulated endothelial cells [2]. Nitric oxide synthase (NOS) generates NO from its precursor, L-arginine. NO acts on the enzyme guanylate cyclase to increase cGMP levels. Cyclic GMP is the active second messenger responsible for smooth muscle relaxation that initiates this first phase of erection [3]. This is followed by the emissary veins and subtunical venules compression against the fibroelastic tunica albuginea, leading to the "steady-state," where arterial inflow and venous outflow both decrease. The contraction of the bulbocavernosus and ischiocavernosus muscles results in the rigidity of the erection [4]. Finally, a sympathetic stimulation leads to seminal emission, ejaculation, and contraction of the lacunar space followed by detumescence and return of the basal adrenergic-mediated cavernosal smooth muscle tone. Other neurotransmitters have also been postulated to play some role in penile tumescence/detumescence [5]. Any agent including hormonal disruptors causing imbalances between vasoconstrictive mediator (e.g., endothelin-1) and cavernosal smooth muscle relaxation, especially in an aging male, may, therefore, play a significant role in ED.

11.3 ENDOCRINOLOGY OF SEXUAL FUNCTION

In order to understand role of endocrine disruptors in ED, it is important to consider how endocrine system interacts with sexual function.

11.3.1 Testosterone and Development of Male Reproductive System

Before birth, testosterone secretion by the fetal testes is responsible for masculinizing the reproductive tract and external genitalia and for promoting descent of the testes into the scrotum. After birth, testosterone secretion ceases, and the testes and other parts of reproductive system remain small and nonfunctional until puberty (see Figure 11.1). Environmental chemicals acting as antiandrogen can disrupt this normal sexual development during fetal life [6]. At the onset of puberty, the Leydig cells once again start secreting testosterone, and spermatogenesis is initiated in the seminiferous tubules for the first time. Testosterone is responsible for the growth and maturation of the entire male reproductive system. Ongoing testosterone secretion is essential for spermatogenesis and for maintaining a mature male reproductive tract throughout adulthood. Potent hormonal disruptors in the environment can

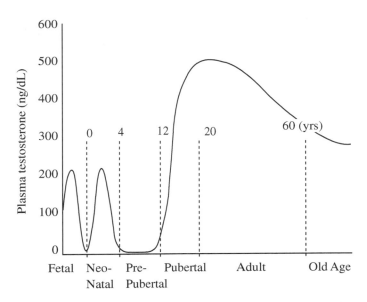

FIGURE 11.1 Plasma testosterone profile in a male from fetal stage until old age. Unlike the female sex hormone estrogen, testosterone does not peak and fall in a monthly cycle.

impair normal development of these organs of the male reproductive system and can affect sperm production [7]. Other effects of testosterone include development of libido at puberty; maintenance of adult male sex drive; control secretion of LH by the anterior pituitary via feedback mechanisms, development and maintenance of male secondary sexual characteristics, and general protein anabolic effects including bone growth and induction of aggressive behavior. How environmental toxicants alter these effects in the male is not clear.

Testosterone seems to act centrally and at local level, at least in animals. In rodents, the neurons of anterior hypothalamus, specifically median preoptic area (MPOA), have the capacity of accumulating isotopically labeled sex steroids as evidenced by autohistoradiographic studies. These neurons play an essential role in male sexual behavior [8]. The appetitive elements of sexual behavior (sexual motivation) would be under control of other neuronal systems, also able to accumulate sex steroids (amygdala, lateral septum, ventral striatum), and MPOA is also involved in these appetitive aspects [8, 9]. Androgen receptors have been detected in the human temporal cortex [10].

In spinal animals, postural reactions to sexual stimulation are facilitated by testosterone [11, 12]. Certain spinal motor neurons accumulate androgens [13]. The major pelvic ganglion, which is an important intermediary of the autonomic innervation to the penis, is also a target for androgens [14]. Testosterone stimulates the tyroxine hydroxylase and choline acetyl-transferase activities in its neurons [15]. Recent animal model data suggests that androgens may have a direct effect upon the penis [16, 17]. Reilly and colleagues demonstrated that castration obliterated the penile erectile response to pelvic ganglionic stimulation via both NO- and non-NO-dependent pathways in a rat model [18, 19]. They reported that androgen mediated the erectile response by stimulating the expression of the neuronal isoform of NO and by alternative pathway, including one that is independent of NO but involves the synthesis of cyclic GMP.

11.3.2 Testosterone as the Sex Hormone – Role in Erectile Function

Testosterone is the main sex hormone in men. Low testosterone levels have a strong correlation with decreased libido, which suggests a major role for androgens in sexual function. With advancing age, bioavailable testosterone shows a typical pattern (Figure 11.1). Testosterone levels have been shown to correlate significantly with nocturnal penile tumescence [20]. Studies have demonstrated a significant decline in penile NO synthase activity in castrated animals that can be reversed by androgen supplementation, especially with dihydrotestosterone (DHT). Increases in NOS mRNA have been demonstrated with androgen supplementation [21]. These studies suggest active biochemical pathways for the influence of androgens on erectile function and dysfunction. However, the clinical use of androgens for the treatment of erectile response not resulting from hypogonadism is controversial.

Androgens are clearly required for sexual interest in men. In hypogonadal men supplemented with androgens, cessation of supplementation results in a progressive decline of sexual interest, sexual fantasies, and arousal, starting after 2 or 3 weeks after withdrawal. Surgical or drug-induced castration following the administration of LHRH agonists [22] or antagonists [23] result in the same effects. Sexual interest and arousal return to the previous level about 2 weeks after reintroduction of androgens or cessation of anti-LHRH or anti-androgen therapy. These observations suggest that the effect of testosterone on sexual function in man is centrally mediated through libido.

The relationship between androgens and penile erection are more complicated. Spontaneous erections, either nocturnal or morning, are clearly androgen dependent. Nocturnal Penile Tumescence and Rigidity (NPTR) monitoring using a Rigiscan device shows a significant reduction in frequency, amplitude, and rigidity of the erections in men with marked hypogonadism while they are not reduced in moderate decrease of serum testosterone [24, 25].

Nocturnal erections are highly correlated with the serum testosterone level, and constitute the most sensitive clinical criterion of well-balanced androgen production. However, nocturnal erections may require up to 6 to 12 months of androgen supplementation to regain complete normality [26]. Nocturnal erections are also highly correlated with sexual interest. Studies in paraphilic men [25] or sexual aggressors [27] treated with antiandrogens report a significant decrease of erections parallel with that of sexual interest. Psychogenic erections, that is, induced by visual stimuli or fantasies, are only partly androgen dependent. In young hypogonadal men, several studies reported complete erectile response to a strong audio-visual sexual stimulation (AVSS) as induced with erotic movies despite cessation of androgen supplementation, without increase of the response after restarting androgens. Several other studies conclude to some partial dependence on androgens. The penile rigidity induced by visual sexual stimulation did not differ between hypogonadal men and controls. However, regarding both duration and maximum level of rigidity, there was a significant increase following androgen replacement in the hypogonadal men, suggesting that erectile response to AVSS may also be influenced by androgen-sensitive mechanisms [24]. Lange et al. also found a borderline significant relationship between the erectile response to AVSS and the serum testosterone level [28]. All together, these studies support the fact that the psychogenic erections are only partly androgen dependent, although the level of evidence is lower than that of the studies having established the androgen dependence of the nocturnal erections, due to a less rigorous methodology. There have been some evidences in terms of the relationship between androgens and ejaculation. Castration or removal of androgen supplementation results in delayed ejaculation and a reduction of the ejaculated volume. Subsequently, ejaculation and orgasm disappear in many cases and return to normal with androgen replacement [11, 29].

The investigations related to serum testosterone levels and erectile function have indicated that the minimum levels of testosterone (i.e., 350 ng/dl) for erectile functions were the levels below which sexual behavior is impaired but there were normal nocturnal penile tumescence (NPT), and there were still lower threshold values (i.e., 150 ng/dl) below which NPT are also impaired [30]. Other authors have suggested a level of 200 ng/dl as threshold for sleep-related erection [31]. It appears that the plasma testosterone levels required for normal libido and sexual activity are rather low. In controlled studies, the effects of testosterone injections upon sexual function definitely correlate with the serum testosterone level only up to a certain level. Salminies et al. suggested that between 200 and 450 ng/dl effect is maximal [32]. No marked increase in sexual interest or activity occurred over this limit. Buena et al. did not observe changes in sexual function when the serum testosterone levels of normal men were pharmacologically changed by means of testosterone injections following pituitary desensitization with an LHRH-agonist [33]. Indeed, after suppressing testosterone levels with GnRH analogues, which resulted in a marked decrease in frequency of sexual desire and activity, androgen replacement at a dose maintaining testosterone levels approximately half the basal levels was found to be appropriate for sustaining normal libido and sexual activity [23].

Different methodological flaws could explain the discordant results of these studies, including: small number of patients in certain series, and limited information resulting from only single testosterone determinations. Several studies also reported a significant increase in sexual interest and arousal following injection of large doses of androgens to eugonadal males [34, 35], including males referred for lack of sexual interest [36], though in all these studies this effect was too modest to lead to an increase in sexual activity. In eugonadal men, amplitude and duration of NPTR proved to be modestly but significantly increased following injection of large doses of testosterone esters [24]. Furthermore, Buvat et al. observed a borderline significant improvement in satisfying sexual intercourse by increasing the circulating level of testosterone with injections of chorionic gonadotropins in eugonadal males referred for erectile dysfunction or low sexual interest [37].

This body of data thus supports a highly significant relationship between the serum testosterone level and sexual interest and activity up to a certain limit, probably individually different, but with values not exceeding 200 to 450 ng/dl. Beyond this level a weaker relationship may exist, but the most extensive studies suggest no therapeutic effect of androgen administration in eugonadal men [35, 36].

11.4 MECHANISM OF ACTION OF HORMONAL DISRUPTORS

Natural sex hormones (estrogens or androgens) travel in the bloodstream searching out compatible receptor sites located in the nucleus of specific cells. The hormones enter the cell, lock onto a specific receptor, and turn on specific genes. The genes tell the cell to make new proteins or other substances that can change cell functions (grow, divide, or make more enzyme). Unlike some hormones that act in seconds or minutes, this process may take hours to complete.

Although natural steroid hormones generally function by binding to specific receptor sites, synthetic environmental estrogens can affect the hormonal system in a number of different ways:

1. They bind to specific receptor sites inside the nucleus of a cell that mimic or evoke a proper hormone response.
2. They block or inhibit a normal hormone response.
3. They mimic and block hormones (PCBs do both).
4. They elicit a weaker or a stronger hormone response or make a totally new response.
5. They bind to other receptors and create a novel reaction or interfere indirectly with normal hormonal action.
6. They alter production and breakdown of hormone receptors and natural hormones, which changes hormonal blood concentrations and endocrine responses.

Thus, several normal and abnormal responses can occur when any imposter binds with specific hormone receptors.

11.4.1 Effect on Specific Receptors

The action of androgen, mediated via androgen receptors (ARs), is essential for normal development of the mammalian male reproductive system. Under normal physiological conditions, testosterone and DHT are the primary androgens that activate the AR. Three classes of chemicals, when administered during the developmental period, that influence androgen levels are (a) those that have antagonistic properties with the AR (antiandrogens); (b) those that interact with the estrogen receptor; and (c) those that interact with the aromatic hydrocarbon (Ah) receptor.

11.4.1.1 Antiandrogens

Chemicals that can bind to the AR without activating it and simultaneously prevent binding of true androgens are called antiandrogens. Examples of antiandrogens include hydroxyflutamide, the pesticides procymidone [36] and vinclozolin [38], and the DDT metabolite p,p′-DDE [39]. O,p′-DDT has weak estrogenic activity.

Estradiol and DES have some affinity for the AR [39, 40]. Therefore, the mechanism by which estrogenic chemicals impair development of the male reproductive system may be via antiandrogenic properties rather than or in addition to activity related to estrogen receptor activation.

Failure to activate the AR due to low androgen levels or antiandrogen activity (e.g., due to fungicide vinclozolin) would produce results similar to the less severe alterations seen in individuals with defective ARs. The range of those effects is seen clearly in human 45XY genetic males who have defects in the AR (androgen-insensitivity syndrome) [41]. Similar effects have been observed in genotypic males exposed prenatally to DES. Gray et al. (1994) administered DES to pregnant rats from gestation day 14 to postnatal day 3. Male offspring had a variety of reproductive effects that are characteristic of interference with AR action, including reduction of ano-genital distance to that characteristic of females, impaired penis development, existence of vaginal pouches, prostate gland agenesis, delayed preputial separation, and reduced or absent sperm production as judged by seminiferous tubule atrophy [38].

11.4.1.2   Estrogen Receptor Interactions

Exposure *in utero* to exogenous chemicals (octyphenol, octyphenol phenoxylate, and butyl benzyl phthalate as well as DES) with estrogenic activity can reduce sperm production, and can cause improper development of the penis, cryptorchidism, and testicular tumors [42, 43]. Male offspring exposed to DES *in utero* had increased incidence of genital malformations, including epididymal cysts (nonmalignant; 21% versus 5% for controls) and testicular abnormalities (11% versus 3%) including small (hypoplastic) testes, and microphallus [44, 45]. In considering these results, it is important to note that DES is a potent synthetic estrogen that also has antiandrogen properties. With exposure *in utero* to relatively high levels of a potent exogenous estrogen, about one third of the men who were recontacted have clinically detectable reproductive system effects. The types of effects that were observed are consistent with those that would be predicted from studies with rodents, but men appear to be less sensitive.

11.4.1.3   Aryl Hydrocarbon (Ah) Receptor Agonists

Dioxin (2, 3, 7, 8-TCDD) and other halogenated aromatic hydrocarbons that cause male reproductive system abnormalities can activate the Ah receptor [46, 47]. The effects seen during development appear to result from the ability of dioxin to impair testosterone biosynthesis and normal sexual differentiation. The low androgen level is not accompanied by increased LH levels, indicating impairment of the feedback mechanism for control of LH synthesis and release. Observed effects include decreased anogenital distance, delayed testis descent, impaired spermatogenic function, decreased accessory sex gland weights, and feminization of male sexual behavior.

11.4.2 Effect on Receptor Gene Expression

Abnormality in the expression of the genome or interference with the action of gene products, as well as acceleration of the rate of cell division, can be induced in male reproductive organs by chemicals having endocrine activity. Because the male reproductive endocrine system involves components from the hypothalamus and pituitary (affecting gonadotropin production), as well as the testes (affecting testosterone production), opportunities for disruption exist at multiple levels and with a variety of types of endocrine action [47]. Thus, chemicals with estrogenic, antiandrogenic, or aryl hydrocarbon receptor binding activity are primary disruptor suspects, as are chemicals that influence the synthesis or release of FSH, LH, or prolactin [48].

Although disruption of the endocrine balance will adversely affect the adult male reproductive system, the developing male reproductive system pre- and postnatally appears to be particularly susceptible and uniquely sensitive. In mammals, including humans, development of the male phenotype requires activation of the SRY gene on the Y chromosome. In the absence of expression of that gene, the female phenotype develops. The mechanisms of action of the SRY gene and the cascade of events that follow have not been elucidated fully. However, any interference with Mullerian ducts to regress will result in the presence of rudimentary components of the female reproductive tract in general. Depending on the extent and the timing of that interference, the consequences would be complete or partial failure of the development of the male reproductive system, which could limit androgen production, delay or prevent onset of the puberty, and affect sexual behavior in adults [48].

11.4.3 Effect on Ion Channels

The research currently being conducted using cavernosal smooth muscle cells in primary culture has shown the importance of ion channels on the surface of penile smooth muscle cells (Sikka et al., presented at AUA Annual Meeting, 2004). Two ion channels of particular significance are calcium and potassium. Simply speaking, calcium ion is responsible for smooth muscle contraction (i.e., penile flaccidity) and potassium ion is responsible for smooth muscle relaxation (i.e., erection). Alteration of those two ion channels by hormonal disruptors and other toxic agents represents important venues of future research.

11.5 HOW ENVIRONMENTAL ESTROGENS DIFFER FROM NATURAL HORMONES

Environmental estrogens are a diverse group of synthetic chemicals and natural plant compounds that may act like estrogen hormones in animals and humans. Although most are weaker than natural estrogens, some have been associated with reproductive and developmental problems in wildlife and laboratory animals. Natural hormones and phytoestrogens are short-lived, do not accumulate in tissue, and are easily broken down by our bodies. Most natural estrogens stay in the bloodstream only minutes or at most a few hours [49]. Although opinions vary about their benefits, the health effects associated with phytoestrogens are influenced by the age of the individual during exposure (for instance, fetus, child, or adult) and the length and concentration of exposure. The estrogenic drugs, such as ethynylestradiol, are more stable and remain in the body longer than natural estrogens, like estradiol. However, pesticides and other environmental estrogens are not easily or readily broken down, are more persistent, and are long-lived, remaining intact in the environment and in living organisms for many years [49].

In most cases, the chemical structures of natural hormones and the synthetic environmental estrogens are strikingly different. Chains of carbon rings form the backbone of the sex steroid hormones (estrogens, androgens, progestins). Each hormone differs only in the location and number of attachments to the main stem. Environmental estrogens (e.g., PCBs), on the other hand, come in all shapes and sizes. Many of the compounds have carbon rings stacked in various ways (polycyclic, or many rings). Some have chlorine atoms or other side chains extending off the main structure. Still others contain no rings or chlorine. These structural differences between natural hormones and environmental estrogens may lead to functional difference [49].

11.6 AGING AND ED

While it is undeniable that aging brings changes to every man's sexual life, it is equally undeniable that plenty of men enjoy healthy, active sex lives through their 50s, 60s, 70s, and even into their 80s! In spite of continuing good health, all men have to accept some loss in their sensitivity to touch and in the tone of their penile smooth muscle. As early as 1948, Kinsey [50] reported that by age 75, about 25% of men become impotent, and that the incidence of impotence increases with age, but later studies (e.g., Baltimore Longitudinal Study of Aging, and the Charleston Heart Study Cohort) increased this number to 55%. As men get older, it usually takes longer for them to achieve an erection. Older men also have longer refractory periods. Some early warning signs of sexual dysfunction include fewer morning erections, fewer spontaneous erections, increasing inability to induce an erection, increasing inability to maintain an erection, and increasing inability to assume sexual positions.

11.6.1 ROLE OF HYPOGONADISM

Male hypogonadism is defined by decreased androgen effect, which is most commonly due to impaired testicular secretion of testosterone and decreased bioavailability of circulating androgens through an increase in serum binding proteins. Normal serum androgen levels are critical for the maintenance of sexual functions in the aging male. Cellular senescence results in increased deposition of a less-compliant collagen subtype in the corpora cavernosa and tunica albuginea. This can lead to veno-occlusive dysfunction and decreased neuronal transmission to the cavernosal smooth muscle [51]. Aging also is believed to result in altered endothelial function, which manifests in decreased basal nitric oxide release and increased basal endothelin-1 [52, 53]. There is evidence for up-regulation of endothelin-1 mRNA with aging [53]. Correlations have been demonstrated between androgen levels and mRNA levels for nitric oxide synthase [54]. Thus, any hormonal control of this balance between NO and endothelin may play a significant role in the onset of impotence in the aging male. How endocrine disruptors directly alter this balance is not known.

Recent studies have shown an increased prevalence of ED, reduced libido, delays in achieving erection, orgasm, and prolonged latency time in the aged men, where hypogonadism is more frequent than in young men [55–58]. Investigations document an age-related decrease in serum androgen levels, which is associated with an age-related decrease in sexual function. Pfeiffer et al. demonstrated an inverse relationship between age and sexual intercourse frequency and sexual interest [59]. These evidences correspond with a well-described decrease in serum androgen levels with age [55, 60–62]. However, it remains unclear whether there is a causal relationship between age and decreased androgens.

11.6.2 CONTROVERSIES RELATED TO HYPOGONADISM AND ED

There is lot of debate going on related to decline of human male sexual response with age and its relationship with hypogonadism. Korenman et al. observed an increased prevalence of hypogonadism among older men when compared with young controls in a cohort-controlled study of 267 men with ED and 107 controls [63]. However, when corrected for age, there was no association between hypogonadism and ED in the older population. They concluded that both hypogonadism and ED were common conditions in the aging male but that they might not be causally related. Current evidence further suggests that hormonal factors do not play a substantial role in the age-associated increased prevalence of ED observed in man. Other causes of ED increase with age. Although the predominant etiological factor of ED in older men appears to be vasculogenic disease, the diminution of libido associated with age most likely has an endocrinological basis. Table 11.1 lists such clinical manifestations that may be associated with hypogonadism in aging males. Androgen replacement therapy may not be sufficient to restore normal sexual function in aging men due to the presence of other etiological factors.

In men there is no sharp decline or break-off point in serum sex steroid levels. Studies have documented a gradual age-related decline in serum testosterone concentrations in healthy adult men [60]. Furthermore, the existence of an age-related gradual decline in bioactive testosterone levels is now generally accepted, which was confirmed by longitudinal data [61, 64]. Highest plasma levels are observed in the age group 20 to 30 years, but levels start to decrease around age 35 years and are very low at age 75 (the mean free testosterone levels are only 50% [0.22 nMol/l] of levels at age 25 years [0.45 nMol/l]) [65].

The exact prevalence of hypogonadism among aged men is not known and is dependent upon the definition of hypogonadism that is utilized. One definition that has been utilized is to select the population with the lowest quintile of serum testosterone and the highest quintile of gonadotropins. Using this definition, the prevalence of hypogonadism in the Massachusetts Male Aging Study is 4% among men 40 to 70 years old [60]. The prevalence of hypogonadism among men over 55 years increases to 20% when hypogonadism is defined as having a serum testosterone

TABLE 11.1
Clinical Manifestations Associated with
Hypogonadism in the Aging Male

Affected System	Clinical Manifestations
Psychological	Lack of mental energy
	Decreased of cognitive functions
	Decrease of the feeling of general well-being
	Irritability
	Inability of concentration
	Depressive symptoms
	Nervousness
Physical	Generalized weakness
	Lack of physical energy
	Decrease in muscle mass and strength
	Ostopenia
	Gynecomastia
	Decreased body hair
	Abdominal obesity
Vasomotor	Excessive sweating
	Occasional hot flushes
	Insomnia
	Palpitation
Sexual	Decrease in sexual activity
	Loss of libido
	Erectile dysfunction
	Lengthening of refractory period
	Less-well-defined quality of orgasm
	Poor intensity of ejaculation
	Decrease in volume of ejaculate

concentration below the normal range of serum testosterone for healthy young adult men. The prevalence of testosterone deficiency among older men increases dramatically if hypogonadism is defined by the amount of bioavailable testosterone in the serum, and it has been estimated by some authors to be as high as 50% [60]. In an investigation of 300 healthy men applying a definition of hypogonadism as a morning level of testosterone below the lower limit of normal (12 nmol/L), Vermeulen and Kaufman [66] reported that none of the men aged 20 to 40 years had testosterone levels within the hypogonadal range, but 7% of those aged 40 to 60 years, 21% of those aged 60 to 80 years, and 35% of those over the age of 80 had hypogonadism. Thus, the definition of hypogonadism in aging men remains unclear. For instance, a decrease of serum testosterone from 800 ng/dl to 400 ng/dl (although both values are within the normal range) may represent a physiologically significant decline in androgen levels for that individual, establishing a state of hypogonadism, who may then respond positively to androgen replacement therapy. This may not be true for

TABLE 11.2
Commercially Available Testosterone Preparations

Preparation	Generic Name	Trade Name	Dose
Injectable	Testosterone cypionate	Depo-testosterone	200–400 mg every 3–4 weeks
	Testosterone enanthate	Delatesrtryl	200–400 mg every 3–4 weeks
Oral	Fluoxymesterone	Halotestin	5–20 mg daily
	Methyltestosterone	Metandren	10–30 mg daily
	Testosterone undecanoate	Andriol	120–160 mg daily
Transdermal	Testosterone patch	Androderm	6 mg daily
	Testosterone patch	Testoderm	10–20 mg daily
	Testosterone gel	Androgel	2.5–5 mg daily

most of the population. Table 11.2 lists such commercially available testosterone preparations that have shown some promise in improving ED in hypogonadal men. However, in the absence of longitudinal data it is impossible to state with certainty whether or not this is the case.

The large interindividual variability of androgen levels in healthy men is attributable to genetic, socioeconomic, and environmental factors. Meikle et al. attributes about 30% of the variability to genetic factors [67]. Circadian and ultradian pulsatile variations in androgen levels also play a role in the variability of the measured values. Among the more personal factors, obesity, probably via the induced hyperpinsulinemia and low SHBG levels, is accompanied by decreased testosterone levels and in morbid obesity, even decreased free testosterone level, whereas several studies suggest that a vegetarian diet is accompanied by lower free testosterone levels [68]. Smokers have a higher free testosterone level than non-smokers. Physical or psychological stress is generally accompanied by decreased testosterone levels. This androgen deficiency in elderly men is generally moderate and some authors suggest using the term: Partial Androgen Deficiency of the Aging Male (PADAM).

The hypothalamus–pituitary system of the elderly is more sensitive to sex hormone feedback [69-71], whereas the decrease of the androgen receptor concentration in the corpora cavernosa or pubic skin suggests a decreased sensitivity at this level [72, 73]. Unfortunately, a more reliable parameter of androgen action is not available. Histological studies in man demonstrated that decreased number and volume of Leydig cells might be responsible for hypogonadism [66]. Zirkin and colleagues observed similar findings in aging rat model, where both spermatogenesis and steroidogenesis decrease in an age-dependent manner similar to that observed in the human condition [74]. The primary defect in these aged rats is Leydig cell dysfunction. However, several human studies have demonstrated abnormalities in the hypothalamus–pituitary axis, which showed an increased SHBG level was a primary event leading to low levels of bioavailable testosterone in older men [63, 66]. Thus, the hypogonadism present in elderly men is multifactorial and may be collectively termed as "andropause."

11.7 HORMONAL CAUSES OF MALE SEXUAL DYSFUNCTION

11.7.1 PRIMARY HYPOGONADISM

Total testosterone is usually found to be normal in ED patients. The average value of total testosterone does not differ or is slightly decreased than in that of men with normal erectile function [75-82]. In series of 2722 patients referred for ED, 2.1 to 21% of patients (average 8.3%) were found to have a serum total testosterone level lower than 300 ng/dl [11, 83-88]. The prevalence of the low testosterone levels increases with age. In a series of 1022 unselected ED patients, 9% of patients older than 50 years had a serum testosterone less than 300 ng/dl and 2.6% had 200 ng/dl, compared to 4% and 0.8% of those less than 50 years, respectively [88]. Free testosterone or non-sex hormone binding globulin (nSHBG)-bound testosterone (bioavailable testosterone) is considered as the only fractions of serum testosterone available to the target cells. Buvat et al. assessed the prevalence of the decreases of both fractions in over 400 ED patients according to their age [89]. Free testosterone was decreased in 22.6% before the age of 50 and in 37.1% after age 50. nSHBG-bound testosterone was reduced in 3.9% before and in 24.4% after age 50. Korenman et al. reported on a substantial prevalence of low levels of nSHBG-bound testosterone in the older men with ED [63]. However, Pirke et al. found no difference between their groups of ED patients and controls regarding the mean value of serum free testosterone [78]. Additionally, the decrease in the levels of nSHBG-bound testosterone was not different whether the older men were with ED or not [63]. In contrast, Buvat-Herbaut et al. found a significant decline in the mean value of free testosterone and nonSHBG-bound testosterone in ED patients compared to age-matched controls [80]. These results suggest the occurrence of an inconsistency with the levels of bioavailable testosterone between normal and ED patients.

For thousands of years, it was known that castration decreased sexual interest and activity, revealing the essential role of the testicles. A fascinating fact is that men with nonfunctioning testicles and low testosterone may sometimes continue to have normal desire and erections. In most cases, however, reduced libido and sexual performance accompany a decrease in testosterone [90]. The extent to which less-than-optimal testosterone, especially in the aging male, impairs sexual function is influenced by the state of penile blood flow and nerve conduction (refer to Table 11.1). A younger man in good health except for diminished testosterone may often continue to have good erections, but an older man whose penile blood flow is beginning to be reduced by arteriosclerosis, or whose nerve conduction is diminished by diabetes or other neuropathy, even a moderate decrease in testosterone may interfere with erections, with improvement following supplementation [91]. Different studies estimate that up to 30% of men with sexual dysfunction have hormonal causes, with the majority having hypogonadism [92]. The most frequent cause of hypogonadism is age-related primary testicular failure.

While many studies have documented the restoration of serum testosterone levels with androgen supplementation (using injection, patch, implant, or oral routes as shown in Table 11.2), few have evaluated its efficacy in the management of erectile dysfunction [93]. One study reported significant improvements in frequency, duration, and rigidity of nocturnal penile tumescence with testosterone supplementation [21]. Sexual desire and arousal was also significantly improved. However, only 35 to 60% of men can expect a measurable improvement in sexual performance with restoration of normal serum testosterone levels [94, 95].

11.7.2 SECONDARY HYPOGONADISM

Low testosterone not accompanied by elevated gonadotropins suggests defective pituitary or hypothalamic function, also known as secondary hypogonadism. The most frequent cause of secondary hypogonadism in the population of impotent men is idiopathic LH deficiency, probably resulting from hypothalamic dysfunction [96]. A hypothalamic cause is suggested and a pituitary cause made less likely by observing LH rise after stimulation testing with GnRH [90, 92].

11.7.3 ROLE OF EXCESSIVE ESTROGEN IN THE MALE

Estrogens belong to a family of steroid hormones that regulate and sustain female sexual development and reproductive function and stimulate tissue growth by (a) promoting cell proliferation (DNA synthesis and cell division) in female sex organs (breasts, uterus); (b) promoting hypertrophy in female breast and male muscle during puberty; and (c) initiating the synthesis of specific proteins [97]. Under these guidelines, any natural steroid, plant compound, or synthetic chemical that elicits these responses in laboratory tests is considered estrogenic. Estrogen excess causes LH suppression with resulting diminished testosterone production, which is most often seen in obese men [98]. This is probably a result of adipose tissue conversion of testosterone to estrogen. Chronic liver disease can also produce estrogen excess, both because of hepatic aromatization of testosterone to estrogen and because of increased sex hormone binding globulin, which can result in a reduced amount of active testosterone in the circulation [99].

A rarer cause of estrogen excess during occupational exposure is production of an adrenal androgen, DHEA, which is also converted to estrogen in the liver and adipose tissue. These men may have gynecomastia and feminine fat distribution, and blood tests reveal low testosterone and LH accompanied by elevated total estrogen (estrone + estradiol) [99]. Measurement of estradiol alone is not sufficient, since much of the estrogen in men is in the form of estrone. Hormonal ablation therapy using LHRH agonists or estrogens to reduce circulating testosterone to castrate levels is the mainstay of therapy for metastatic prostate cancer. However, this leads to a decrease in libido and erectile dysfunction.

11.8 METABOLIC DISORDERS AND ED

11.8.1 NEUROLOGICAL CAUSES OF MALE SEXUAL DYSFUNCTION

Agents that affect the central or peripheral nervous system or alter the pituitary–hypothalamic–gonadal axis may directly impair sexual function by altering endocrine function [96, 97]. GnRH release from the hypothalamus is suppressed by stress-induced increases in catecholamines, prolactin, corticotropin-releasing factor, and opiates. Cranial irradiation may lead to irradiation-induced hypothalamic dysfunction with hyperprolactinemia, resulting in impotence [100]. Hyperprolactinemia decreases the secretion of GnRH, resulting in low testosterone levels [90]. Erectile dysfunction (88%) and decreased libido (80%) are the most common presenting symptoms of hyperprolactinemia [100]. Oral bromocriptine can normalize prolactin levels and restore normal erections.

11.8.2 DIABETES MELLITUS

Diabetes mellitus has been one of the most common cause of ED. Fifty percent of diabetic men are impotent after 10 years of diabetes [101]. Age, duration of diabetes, and diabetic complications can predict ED in most diabetic patients. While glycosylated hemoglobin has been suggested as a predictor of the association of ED and diabetes, other factors, such as alcohol intake, age, and antihypertensive medications are more accurate predictors [102–104]. The pathophysiology of ED in diabetics is dependent upon neuropathy, microangiopathy, and generalized vascular disease [105]. Since diabetes is associated with a risk of hypogonadism, a serum testosterone should also be evaluated routinely.

11.8.3 OBESITY

Obese men who are otherwise healthy have been found to have low serum testosterone levels with a progressive fall in serum testosterone [106]. Despite this low serum testosterone, obese men might not display clinical evidences of hypogonadism [107]. They have normal libido, potency, testicular size, and spermatogenesis. This paradox is partially explained by the finding that most obese men have normal free testosterone levels. This is due to a decrease in the SHBG, which reduces the protein-bound testosterone. There are some men with marked obesity (> 250% of ideal body weight) that have subnormal free testosterone levels. Obese men have elevated estradiol and estrone levels [108]. The high estrogen levels may reflect the ability of the adipose tissue to convert androgens to estrogens. When these obese men lose weight and their adipose tissue, the abnormal androgen and estrogen levels revert to normal [109]. Serum gonadotropins are normal in obese men.

11.8.4 RENAL DISEASE

Chronic renal failure impairs sexual function in about 50% of men [110], and hemodialysis does not seem to improve it. Patients with renal failure have elevations of LH and FSH and some decrease in serum testosterone, hormone levels that are characteristic of a primary testicular dysfunction [111, 112]. This evidence has been supported by the observation that hCG stimulation testing in these patients fails to elevate serum testosterone levels [113]. Elevated prolactin levels may also be seen in men with chronic renal failure [114, 115]

In some patients, renal transplantation may reverse the low serum testosterone levels seen pretransplant and improve sexual function in about 80% of patients [116]. Dialysis rarely improves the sexual dysfunction [117]. If potency does not improve post-transplantation, the etiology of the dysfunction is most likely non-endocrine such as an abnormal vascular supply to the penis. Therefore, in patients with chronic renal failure, a lowered serum testosterone level may be the cause of the sexual dysfunction, and these patients may be candidates for exogenous androgen therapy. If exogenous testosterone fails to improve the dysfunction, that is usually what occurs in this setting, then a vasculopathy or neuropathy as the etiology of the dysfunction should be addressed [118].

11.8.5 THYROID DISEASE

Increased thyroid hormone secretion has been associated with an increase in total testosterone but with normal free testosterone. This is due to the elevation in the SHBG or, as it is occasionally referred to, testosterone-estrogen binding globulin (TEBG) associated with hyperthyroidism. The elevation in SHBG causes a relative decline in the free testosterone levels, which cause an elevation of serum LH and further increase in serum testosterone and, by peripheral conversion, an increase in serum estradiol. Due to increased estrogens, the patients with hyperthyroidism may complain or present with gynecomastia and a decrease in libido [119]. The libido does not respond to exogenous testosterone therapy that may also make the gynecomastia worse.

Treatment of the thyrotoxicosis reverses the symptoms and signs of the disorder. In hypothyroidism, LH and FSH are usually increased due to testicular resistance to gonadotropins. Serum testosterone and SHBG are usually decreased. Free testosterone may be increased, decreased, or normal. Potency is usually normal in hypothyroidism but ED and decrease in libido were reported in some men. If hypothyroid men complain of ED, replacement with thyroxin rarely improves the potency [120].

11.8.6 HYPERPROLACTINEMIA

Hyperprolactinemia is a common endocrine cause of erectile dysfunction. Men with hyperprolactinemia tend to have decreased libido and have ED. Serum gonadotropins and testosterone are usually decreased in men with hyperprolactinemia. Hyperprolactinemia can decrease gonadotropins by inhibition of GnRH secretion, and larger nonfunctioning tumors cause hypogonadism by direct damage to the gonadotrophs [121]. The abnormalities of testosterone metabolism have been demonstrated in hyperprolactinemia [122]. Other mechanisms might be responsible for diminishing erectile activity in hyperprolactinemia, including direct suppression of the libido center or decreased relaxation of the corpus cavernosum through mechanisms that are independent of testosterone action [123]. Men with acquired hypogonadotropic hypogonadism, such as pituitary tumor, commonly complain of decreased erectile function. These tumors commonly secrete prolactin, and high serum prolactin levels can interfere with the hypothalamic–pituitary–gonadal axis at many levels. In macroadenomas, the LH and FSH deficiencies are not always restored to normal with dopamine agonist therapy even if the prolactin levels return to normal. Prolactin interferes with brain neurotransmission and may impair libido.

In addition, it may also have adverse effects on sexual function in men separate from that of testosterone suppression, since treatment of these patients with exogenous testosterone does not always reverse ED until the prolactin levels have been returned to normal levels [124]. If medical therapy fails to control the effects of the tumor, surgical adenectomy may be indicated. Depression and anxiety are common in men with pituitary hyperprolactinemia independent of the lowered testosterone levels and may play a role in the decreased libido seen in these men [125]. Besides an ademona, hyperprolactinemia may also be caused by certain drugs and in some patients with chronic renal failure [100].

11.8.7 OTHER MISCELLANEOUS FACTORS

Nutritional disorders such as protein malnutrition and severe obesity may be associated with hypogonadotropic hypogonadism. Androgen production can be restored after weight correction. However, it may be difficult to differentiate the role of these conditions in loss of libido and causing ED. Sickle cell anemia has been found to cause hypoandrogenism, due to testicular damage [126] that may lead to ED. Testosterone supplementation can be useful for anemia and sexual problems. Chronic liver diseases are associated with increased SHBG and hormonal abnormalities such as low androgens, elevated estrogens, and hyperprolactinemia. ED and gynecomastia are commonly encountered in chronic liver diseases. Although total serum testosterone is low or normal, due to concomitant elevation of SHBG, the free testosterone is usually low. High circulating estrogens may play a role in the inhibition of LH secretion. Prolactin can be elevated. Gynecomastia can be explained by the increased estrogen/testosterone ratio that could affect sexual function. Acute illnesses such as sepsis, respiratory failure, or myocardial infarction are accompanied by decreased testosterone levels due to temporary inhibition of androgen production [127]. Hypogonadism can be both primary and secondary. The factors that cause hypogonadism and associated sexual disorders in acute illnesses can be hypoandrogenism, hyperprolactinemia, or hyperestrogenemia. Hemochromatosis, the disease characterized with excessive iron deposition in a variety of tissues including liver and pituitary gland, is also associated with selective gonadotrophic failure without affecting the rest of pituitary function, thus affecting normal hormone balance.

11.9 ENDOCRINE DISRUPTORS AND ED

An environmental hormone disruptor, in general, may be defined as an exogenous agent that interferes with the synthesis, secretion, transport, binding, action, or elimination of natural hormones that are responsible for the maintenance of homeostasis, reproduction, development, or behavior in the body. Endocrine disruptors are usually either natural products or synthetic chemicals that mimic, enhance (an agonist), or inhibit (an antagonist) the action of biological hormones. Dose, duration, and timing of exposure at critical periods of life are important considerations for assessing the adverse effects of endocrine disruptor. Effects may be reversible or irreversible, immediate (acute) or latent and not expressed for a period of time. Table 11.3 lists many such disruptors directly or indirectly affecting sexual function as described below [128].

TABLE 11.3
Hormonal Disruption and Male Sexual Dysfunction

Class	Agent/Condition	Effects
(A) Pharmacological		
Antiandrogen	Cimetidine, cyproterone, spironolacton ketoconazole, finasteride, flutamide, progestins, anabolic steroids	↓DHT, altered HPG-axis, ↓libido Impotence
Estrogen	Estradiol, estriol, DES	↓T; gynecomastia
Phytoestrogens	Flavonoids, lignans, alkaloids	↓libido, delayed orgasm, gynecomastia
Antihypertensives	Calcium channel blockers, thiazides, β-blockers, methyldopa, digoxin	Impotence, libido
Antidepressants	Trazodone, Prozac, lithium, Sertraline	Delayed ejaculation, priapism, ↓orgasm
(B) Environmental		
Chemicals	DBCP, DDT, PCBs, dioxins, methyl chloride, vinclozolin,	↓HPG-axis, ↓T, ↓Libido, Deformities of sex-organs.
Heavy Metals	Lead, mercury, cadmium, cobalt lithium	Central, gonadal, ↓HPG-axis
Radiations	∝-and β-rays; X-and ∝-rays	Nerve damage, impotence, low ejaculatory volume
(C) Recreational	Alcohol, nicotine, marijuana valium, cocaine, morphine	Depression, impotence
(D) Physiological	Cardiac/hepatic/pulmonary/renal failure; genitourinary conditions	↓libido, impotence
(E) Disease States		
Hypertension/Diabetes	Nerve/vascular/muscular damage	Organic impotence_____
Depression, Sickness, Death,	Emotional stress	Psychogenic impotence, ↓libido
Other Endocrine Disorders	Testicular feminization, hyperthyroidism, hyperprolactinemia, hypogonadism, pituitary tumor	↓T, ↓libido, impotence altered HPG-axis

Abbreviations: DBCP (dibromochloropropane); DDT (dichlorodiphenyl-trichloroethane); DHT (dihydrotestosterone); DES (diethyl stilbestrol); PCBs (polychlorinated biphenyls); T (testosterone)

11.9.1 Environmental Chemicals

Recent reports suggest that many chemicals released into the environment can affect normal endocrine function. Some deleterious effects observed in animals have been attributed to persistent organic chemicals, such as polychlorinated biphenyls (PCBs), dichlorodiphenyl-trichloroethane (DDT), dioxin, and some pesticides [6]. These chemicals existing in the environment may mimic natural hormones and disrupt bodily functions if ingested, even in minute quantities. Convincing evidences exist that chemical exposures in rodents have led to increased estrogenic activity or reduced androgen levels or otherwise have interfered with the action of androgen during development, causing male reproductive system abnormalities [129]. Results obtained from the observation of men exposed to DES *in utero* demonstrate that environmental agents may alter neuroendocrine function both during development and in the sexually mature organism [130]. Testing for the endocrine-disrupting potential of environmental chemicals should include the ability to detect antiandrogenic activity as well as estrogenic activity. Testing also should be able to detect alteration in androgen receptor and all receptor function as reflected in genome expression [131].

11.9.1.1 Organochlorines

PCBs are a group of commercially produced organic chemicals used since the 1940s in industrial applications and throughout the nuclear weapons complex. PCBs are found in many gaskets and large electrical transformers and capacitors in the gaseous diffusion plants. Many studies and reviews have found PCBs to be toxic to both humans and laboratory animals [6, 128, 130, 132].

11.9.1.2 Pesticides

Vinclozolin, a fungicide used on grapes, and p,p′-DDE, the major persistent metabolite of DDT, have been shown to feminize the reproductive systems of male (rat) pups born in a multigenerational study [39, 133]. These pups had a very small analgenital distance, which is an androgen-dependent measure, and the external genitalia of older animals had female characteristics, suggesting that these agents inhibited the action of androgens. For the male reproductive tract to develop, a number of proteins have to be synthesized, and that synthesis depends on androgens secreted by the testes during development. These chemicals interfere with androgens by binding to the androgen receptor and prevent the transcription of DNA. On the other hand, testicular cancer, undescended testis, and urethral abnormalities can arise during fetal development in the female. These medical conditions may be due to altered exposure to estrogens during pregnancy and not due to androgen interference. Whereas androgens normally act like keys that open doors to reproductive development, certain androgenic toxicants may act like keys that jam the locks. In spite of the recent wave of publicity about endocrine disruptors, most men are still unaware that their reproductive health is under scrutiny.

In addition to chemical exposure, many drugs and medications, disease states, and environmental factors are likely to disturb the endocrine profile resulting in decreased sexual performance (Table 11.1).

11.9.2 Pharmacological Agents

Many prescription and non-prescription drugs directly or indirectly act as hormonal disruptors and can affect sexual functioning in both men and women. In men, loss of libido (sexual desire), impotence, delayed (or absent) orgasm, failure of ejaculation, and priapism (prolonged painful erection) are common consequences of many drugs [134, 135]. Women are often less affected but can experience loss of libido, inhibition of orgasm, or lack of orgasm from medicines. Unfortunately, many patients blame old age and low hormonal activity for diminishing sexual abilities, when, in truth, the problem may be the direct consequence of a drug.

11.9.2.1 Antihypertensives

About one third of men who take thiazide diuretics (hydrochlorothiazide, chlorthalidone, beneroflumethiaide) as therapy for high blood pressure have problems with libido, erection, and ejaculation, but the mechanism is not known [136]. Spironolactone (Aldactone) at high doses blocks androgen receptors and lowers the sex drive, leading to impotence and gynecomastia [137]. Digoxin, a cardiac drug similar in structure to sex steroids, decreases testosterone and increases estrogen and is associated with erectile failure and gynecomastia [138]. Methyldopa (Aldomet), a synthetic relative of the neurotransmitter dopamine, is a well-documented cause of erectile problems [136]. Guanethidine and clonidine, which oppose the action of the sympathetic nervous system, also cause impotence. Clonidine (Catapress), an α_2-agonist, impairs erectile function and decreases libido in up to 40% of patients. β-blockers are used for many cardiovascular problems as well as for high blood pressure. Men taking propranolol (Inderal), the most common β-blocker, complained of loss of libido and erection. When a β-blocker causes problems, a drug of a different class should immediately replace it. Although loss of libido can be attributed to hypogonadism, reduced perfusion pressure of the lacunar spaces after antihypertensive therapy is probably the main cause of reduced penile rigidity.

11.9.2.2 Depression and Related Drugs

Depression itself is associated with impaired sexual function in terms of lost desire and performance. However, most antidepressant drugs such as serotonin reuptake inhibitors, clomipramine, lithium carbonate, and monoamine oxidase inhibitors are associated with higher rates of impotence than other antidepressant classes [139]. Ejaculation and orgasmic difficulties, as well as alterations in libido, arousal, and erectile function, are prominent adverse effects of taking these medications [139, 140]. The new antidepressants selective serotonin reuptake inhibitor (Prozac) has negative effects on men's potency, but found to be useful in delaying premature ejaculation.

11.9.2.3 Other Brand-Name Drugs

Over extended periods of usage these drugs can cause impotence, possibly due to altered hormone synthesis or action. Some of these listed drugs are included in the Table 11.3.

Alcoholism drugs: Antabuse; *Antifungal drugs:* – Ketoconazole; *Arthritis drugs:* Indocin; *Bleeding drugs:* Amicar; *Epilepsy drugs:* Dilantin; *Gastrointestinal drugs:* Antrocol, Arco-Lase, Butabell, Pro-Banthene, Probocon, Regian, Tagamet, Uretron, Zantac; *Glaucoma drugs:* Diamox; *Headache drugs:* Sansert; *Infection drugs,* Flagyl, Satiric; *Muscle spasm drugs:* Flexural, Norflex, Norgesic, X-Otag; *Parkinson's disease drugs:* Akineton, Artane, Cogentin, Kemadrin, Pagitane; *Prostrate drugs:* Estrace, Eulexin, Lupron, Proscar, Zoladex; *Tuberculosis drugs:* Trecator-SC [136].

11.9.3 RECREATIONAL AGENTS

Many recreational agents in our daily environment directly or indirectly affect hormonal profile and can cause partial or complete impotence.

11.9.3.1 Marijuana

Cannabinoids are psychoactive chemicals found in marijuana. In a frequent marijuana user, THC (tetrahydrocannabinol) and other cannabinoids are stored in body fat and released slowly over time. This slow release could disturb hormonal profile, leading to decreased fertility and sexual function. Marijuana use also decreases blood testosterone levels [136]. The National Institute on Drug Abuse reports that new cultivation and breeding techniques produce plants many times more potent than the pot smoked 3 decades ago. The extent of the actual damage caused by these drugs is still unclear, but there is the belief that the damage is irreversible.

11.9.3.2 Smoking

Smoking in itself does not appear to be a direct cause of impotence, but chemical substances (nicotine) in tobacco smoke and its metabolite cotinine cause arterial constriction that may lead to impotence [141]. Men with treated heart disease who smoke are almost three times more likely to be completely impotent than those who do not. Similarly, men with treated high blood pressure and untreated arthritis who smoke are more than twice as likely to be completely impotent as those who do not. However, such interactions and the role of altered hormonal profile leading to decreased libido or sexual performance in smokers is not clearly understood.

11.9.3.3 Alcohol

Nominal alcohol consumption often leads to changes in sexual behavior for a majority of people. Alcohol use is likely to increase subjective sexual desire, arousal, and pleasure, while lowering physiological arousal. Alcohol provokes the desire, but it takes away the performance. After drinking even moderate amounts of alcohol, many men find it difficult to achieve or maintain an erection. Alcohol abuse can cause hypogonadism and increased risk of sexual dysfunction [132, 135]. Experimental rats given a large dose of ethyl alcohol are almost incapable of having an erection. High estrogen and low testosterone levels are often found in alcoholic men.

11.9.3.4 Street Drugs

Heroin, morphine, methadone, cocaine, LSD, marijuana, amphetamines, and barbiturates are widely known to affect a man's sexual performance [136, 141]. To what extent these may have any direct or indirect interactions with hormone secretion causing sexual impairment needs to be investigated. Street drugs in relatively small quantities are considered to act as aphrodisiacs for some men within a few hours of ingestion, either through their own action or through a placebo effect.

11.9.4 Sexual Stimulants

Many men and women have chosen to go back to nature in search of sexual well-being. Recently, some more new herbal products have emerged, claiming to help control hormonal imbalance and increase sexual potency. Herbal products are commonly used to improve health and prevent disease. Garlic, ginseng, and Ginkgo biloba are some of the most commonly ingested herbs. Though some studies suggest their effectiveness for improving libido and sexual performance in humans, actual scientific data established in a controlled environment is lacking.

11.9.4.1 Herbal

"Ginseng" in traditional Chinese medicine and "Shilajeet" in the Indian Ayurvedic system have been used for centuries to enhance stamina, capacity, and androgenicity to cope with fatigue and physical stress. These are thought to improve libido and sexual function. However, their mechanism of action is unclear. Recent studies have suggested that the antioxidant potential of vitamin E, especially in diabetes [142], and organ-protective actions of ginseng [143] may help prevent onset of impotence. Enhanced NO synthesis thus could contribute to ginseng-associated vasodilatation and perhaps also to an aphrodisiac action of this root. Further controlled scientific studies are needed to confirm or refute these claims.

11.9.4.2 Other Phytoproducts

Dietary phytoestrogens and their interactions in the body at the endocrine level may significantly affect various functions [143, 144]. A unique combination of rainforest botanicals has recently become available as a natural sexual stimulant for men. It is referred to as "Rainforce Touchfire." It has a long documented history of use by the rainforest Indians. It is formulated to nutritionally support male sexual function and desire. It includes several herbal male tonics combined with Nettle Root, which has recently been documented to increase bioavailable testosterone levels in the bloodstream by as much as ten times. Another powerful natural product designed to enhance sexual desire in men is extract of Muira puma, also known as Potency

Wood. Muira puma has recently been the subject of clinical research (unpublished data). In two recent clinical trials performed at the Institute of Sexology in Paris, an herbal extract of Muira puma was shown very effective. It is likely that more clinical trials will be needed to test the effects of herbal substances on human sexuality.

Proanthocyanidins occur naturally in many fruits and vegetables and in high concentrations in both pine bark and grape seeds. *Pycnogenols*, another phytoproduct, constitute the most potent antioxidants known to man, up to 50 times more potent than vitamin E and 20 times more than vitamin C. These are considered to strengthen the immune system, help protect against the damage of free radicals, and support collagen, and are natural protectors against aging. Because of their association in the maintenance of a healthy body, they may play an important role in human sexuality, possibly via increased hormonal output.

Jatoba tea is a unique treasure of the Amazon rainforest. Different tribes in the Amazon have been drinking this herbal tea for hundreds of years as an energizer to help them feel strong and vigorous. It has been used for the treatment of fatigue and as a tonic for the respiratory and urinary systems to fight fungus and yeast-like candida albicans. Its wonderful health-producing benefits have been associated with increased sexual desire and potency.

11.9.4.3 Pheromones

The richness of olfactosexual behavior has been recognized throughout human experience, even in cultures that found the idea embarrassing [145]. All releaser effects of odors in man tend to be more variable than in lower mammals because of the large variety of human signal systems and the size of the override from learned or conditioned behavior. This is almost certainly in part genetic, but psychoanalytic writers have documented the possibility of a special role for odor in psychosexual development. The known candidates for pheromones are those self-selected by man and used in perfumery (muskone, civet one, castoreum, and synthetics such as exaltolide); those derived from steroids and observed incidentally, such as boar paint; and a few special cases (*cis*-4-hydroxydodeca-6-enoic acid lactone) in deer tarsal gland odor. The substances of initial choice as probable releasers and possible sexual primers in man are all musk odors (steroids, large-ring cycloketones, and lactones). The part played by 6, 8, and 10-carbon acids and lactones is unknown. Odors fixed from a partner might also have a playback function as hormonal releasers.

11.9.5 Environment and ED

Our daily environment plays a significant role in supporting or undermining normal sexual performance. Physical and mental illness due to many disease states, divorce, death in the family, depression, anxiety, stress, etc., all can disturb the hormonal status and contribute to impaired sexual performance.

11.9.5.1 Physical Condition

Physically ill men, especially if they are cigarette smokers, are six times more likely to be impotent than healthy men. The medical conditions most often associated with impotence, according to the Massachusetts Male Aging Study, are cardiovascular disease, diabetes, hypertension, an untreated ulcer, arthritis, and allergy [1]. It is usually hard to tell whether the medical condition itself is the most important risk factor or the medication being taken for it or a combination of the two. Men who have had coronary bypass surgery or who suffer from myocardial infarction, stroke, or peripheral blood disease most likely have problems with the supply of arterial blood to the penis. Radiation therapy of the pelvic area frequently causes scarring that results in the penile arteries losing their ability to dilate. With age and the ingestion of toxic agents, neurotransmitter levels may be lower, and the sense of touch decreases. The most frequent neurological disorders associated with impotence are prostate surgery, spinal cord injury, multiple sclerosis, and peripheral neuropathy [1]. Also in an obese man, the body elastin is progressively replaced by less elastic collagen. This may affect the framework of the smooth muscle in the penis, although the MMAS found no correlation between overweight (obesity) and impotence. Thus, most of these conditions do alter the endocrine system.

11.9.5.2 Psychological or Emotional Risk Factors

More than 80% of all cases of persistent impotence can be traced to one or more *physical* causes. The remaining 20% are caused by unknown physical or psychological factors [146]. However, even when the cause is wholly psychological or emotional, it is expressed in *physical* terms. That is, some message does not travel along a nerve or a specific hormone is not secreted into the bloodstream. Psychiatrists divide sexual dysfunction into sexual desire disorders, sexual arousal disorders, orgasm disorders, sexual pain disorders, and a miscellaneous category [50, 147]. Many men occasionally pass through a phase of low interest in sex. It is natural that a man should wonder if his impotence problem has a physical or psychological cause.

11.10 CONCLUSION

The endocrine disruptor story gets more and more complicated as new research findings are revealed. One of the biggest and probably most complex mysteries is how substances with different shapes and structures produce similar physiological results. Certain substances can mimic hormones by binding to specific hormone receptors inside cells; e.g., DDT, some PCBs, and many phytoestrogens bind to estrogen receptors. Not all endocrine disruptors alter hormonal action by binding to hormone receptors, however. Some relay molecular messages through a complex array of cellular proteins, hormone and nonhormone response elements that indirectly turn genes on/off and alter cell growth and division. DDT, at or below levels found in human breast fat tissue, can bypass the estrogen receptor and stimulate a complex mixture of cell signaling proteins (growth factor receptors) and processes that eventually will lead to cell division. DDT can also bind to the androgen receptor and inhibit androgen binding. Thus, the same chemical can influence the endocrine system in more than one way. If understood, these complex modes of action of endocrine disruptors may be able to answer the questions of how different molecules impact the endocrine system and other functions especially the least understood sexual dysfunction.

REFERENCES

1. Feldman, H.A., et al. Impotence and its medical and psychosocial correlates: results of the Massachusetts Male Aging Study. *J Urol*, 1994. **151**(1): p. 54–61.
2. Rajfer, J., et al. Nitric oxide as a mediator of relaxation of the corpus cavernosum in response to nonadrenergic, noncholinergic neurotransmission. *N Engl J Med*, 1992. **326**(2): p. 90–4.
3. Gonzalez-Cadavid, N.F., R.J., Nitric oxide and other neurotransmitters of the corpus cavernosum, in Infertility and Sexual Dysfunction, W.J.G. Hellstrom (ed.). Springer-Verlag, New York, 1997: p. 425–439.
4. Wagner, G., Vascular mechanisms involved in erection and erectile disorders. *Clin Endocrinol Metab,* 1982. **11**(3): p. 717–23.
5. Saenz de Tejada, I., Molecular mechanisms for the regulation of penile smooth muscle contractility. *Int J Impot Res*, 2000. **12 Suppl 4**: p. S34–8.
6. Cheek, A.O. and J.A. McLachlan, Environmental hormones and the male reproductive system. *J Androl*, 1998. **19**(1): p. 5–10.
7. Thomas, K.B. and C.T, Organochlorine endocrine disruptors in human tissue, in Chemically-Induced Alterations in Sexual and Functional Development: The Wildlife/Human Connection, T. Colborn and C. Clements (eds.). 1992, New Jersey: Princeton Science Publishing Co., Inc. 365–394.
8. Everitt, B.J., Neuroendocrine mechanisms underlying appetitive and consummatory elements of masculine sexual behavior, in "The Pharmacology of Sexual Function and Dysfunction," I.B. J (ed.), 1995, Esteve Foundation Symposia, Elsevier Science: Amsterdam. p. 15–31.
9. Baum, M. Reassessing the role of medial preoptic area/anterior hypothalamic neurons in appetitive aspects of masculine sexual behavior, in "Esteve Foundation Symposia." 1995. Amsterdam: Excepta Medica., Elsevier Science.
10. Puy, L., et al. Immunocytochemical detection of androgen receptor in human temporal cortex characterization and application of polyclonal androgen receptor antibodies in frozen and paraffin-embedded tissues. *J Steroid Biochem Mol Biol*, 1995. **55**(2): p. 197–209.
11. Buvat, J., Neurotransmetteurs cérébraux et contrôle ducomportement sexuel masculin. Andrologie, 1996. **6**(184–199).
12. Hart, B.L., Effects of testosterone propionate and dihydrotestosterone on penile morphology and sexual reflexes of spinal male rats. *Horm Behav*, 1973. **4**(3): p. 239–46.
13. Breedlove, S. and A. Arnold, Hormone accumulation in a sexually dimorphic motor nucleus of the rat spinal cord. *Science*, 1980. **210**: p. 564–566.
14. Dail, W.G., A.P. Evan, and H.R. Eason, The major ganglion in the pelvic plexus of the male rat: a histochemical and ultrastructural study. *Cell Tissue Res*, 1975. **159**(1): p. 49–62.

15. Melvin, J.E. and R.W. Hamill, The major pelvic ganglion: androgen control of postnatal development. *J Neurosci*, 1987. **7**(6): p. 1607–12.

16. Giuliano, F., et al. Autonomic control of penile erection: modulation by testosterone in the rat. *J Neuroendocrinol*, 1993. **5**(6): p. 677–83.

17. Mills, T.M., V.S. Stopper, and V.T. Wiedmeier, Effects of castration and androgen replacement on the hemodynamics of penile erection in the rat. *Biol Reprod*, 1994. **51**(2): p. 234–8.

18. Reilly, C.M., et al. Androgenic maintenance of the rat erectile response via a non-nitric-oxide-dependent pathway. *J Androl*, 1997. **18**(6): p. 588–94.

19. Reilly, C.M., et al. Androgenic regulation of NO availability in rat penile erection. *J Androl*, 1997. **18**(2): p. 110–5.

20. Schiavi, R.C., et al. Hormones and nocturnal tumescence in healthy aging men. *Arch Sex Behav*, 1993. **22**: p. 207.

21. Morales, A., et al. Testosterone supplementation for hypogonadal impotence: assessment of biochemical measures and therapeutic outcomes. *J Urol*, 1997. **157**(3): p. 849–54.

22. Rousseau, L., et al. Sexuality changes in prostate cancer patients receiving antihormonal therapy combining the antiandrogen flutamide with medical (LHRH agonist) or surgical castration. *Arch Sex Behav*, 1988. **17**: p. 87–98.

23. Bagatelle, C., et al. Effects of endogenous testosterone and estradiol on sexual behaviour in normal young men. *J Clin Endocrinol Metab*, 1994. **78**: p. 711–716.

24. Carani, C., et al. Testosterone and prolactin: behavioural and psychophysiological approaches in men, in "Esteve Foundation Symposia." 1995. Amsterdam: Elsevier Science.

25. Rosen, R. Pharmacological effects on Nocturnal Penile Tumescence (NPT), in "Esteve Foundation Symposia." 1995. Amsterdam: Elsevier Science.

26. Burris, A.S., et al. A long-term, prospective study of the physiologic and behavioral effects of hormone replacement in untreated hypogonadal men. *J Androl*, 1992. **13**(4): p. 297–304.

27. Cooper, A.J., et al. Medroxyprogesterone acetate, nocturnal penile tumescence, laboratory arousal, and sexual acting out in a male with schizophrenia. *Arch Sex Behav*, 1990. **19**(4): p. 361–72.

28. Lange, J.D., et al. Serum testosterone concentration and penile tumescence changes in men. *Horm Behav*, 1980. **14**(3): p. 267–70.

29. Bancroft, J., Sexual desire and the brain. J Sex Marit Ther, 1988. **3**: p. 11–27.

30. Carani, C., et al. Prolactin and testosterone: their role in male sexual function. *Int J Androl*, 1996. **19**(1): p. 48–54.

31. Granata, A.R., et al. Relationship between sleep-related erections and testosterone levels in men. *J Androl*, 1997. **18**: p. 522–527.

32. Salminies, S., et al. Effects of testosterone replacement on sexual behavior in hypogonadal men. *Arch Sex Behav*, 1982. **11**: p. 345–353.

33. Buena, F., et al. Sexual function does not change when serum testosterone levels are pharmacologically varied within the normal male range. *Fertil Steril*, 1993. **59**(5): p. 1118–23.

34. WHO, Task Force on Psychosocial Research in Family Planning. Hormonal contraception for men: acceptability and effects onsexuality. Studies in Family Planning, 1982. **13**: p. 328–342.

35. Anderson, R.A., et al. The effects of exogenous testosterone on sexuality and mood of normal men. *J Clin Endocrinol Metab*, 1992. **75**: p. 1503–1507.

36. O'Carroll, R. and J. Bancroft, Testosterone therapy for low sexual interest and erectile dysfunction in men: a controlled study. *Br J Psych*, 1984(145): p. 146–151.

37. Buvat, J., A. Lemaire, and M. Buvat-Herbaut, Human chorionic gonadotropin treatment of nonorganic erectile failure and lack of sexual desire: a double-blind study. *Urology*, 1987. **30**(3): p. 216–9.

38. Gray, L.E., Jr., J.S. Ostby, and W.R. Kelce, Developmental effects of an environmental antiandrogen: the fungicide vinclozolin alters sex differentiation of the male rat. *Toxicol Appl Pharmacol*, 1994. **129**(1): p. 46–52.

39. Kelce, W.R., et al. Persistent DDT metabolite p,p'-DDE is a potent androgen receptor antagonist. *Nature*, 1995. **375**(6532): p. 581–5.

40. Newbold, R.R. and J.A. McLachlan, Diethylstilbestrol associated defects in murine genital tract development, in "Estrogens in the Environment," E.B.J.A. McLachlan (ed.). 1985, Elsevier Science: Holland: p. 288–318.

41. Quigley, R., et al. Stimulation of proximal convoluted tubule phosphate transport by epidermal growth factor: signal transduction. *Am J Physiol*, 1995. **269**(3 Pt 2): p. F339–44.

42. Sharpe, R.M. and N.E. Skakkebaek, Are oestrogens involved in falling sperm counts and disorders of the male reproductive tract? Lancet, 1993. **341**(8857): p. 1392–5.

43. Sharpe, R.M., Declining sperm counts in men—is there an endocrine cause? *J Endocrinol*, 1993. **136**(3): p. 357–60.

44. Gill, W.B., G.F.B. Schumacher, and M. Bibbo, Structural and functional abnormalities in the sex organs of male offspring of mothers treated with diethylstilbestrol (DES). *J Reprod Med*, 1976. **16**: p. 147–153.

45. Gill, W.B., et al. Association of diethylstilbestrol exposure in utero with cryptorchidism, testicular hypoplasia and semen abnormalities. *J Urol*, 1979. **122**: p. 36–39.

46. Whitlock, J.P., The aromatic hydrocarbon receptor, dioxin action, and endocrine homeostasis. *Trends Endocrinol Metab*, 1994. **5**: p. 183–188.

47. Safe, S., et al. 2,3,7,8-Tetrachlorodibenzo-*p*-dioxin (TCDD) and related compounds as antioestrogens: characterization and mechanism of action. *Pharmacol Toxicol*, 1991. **69**(6): p. 400–9.

48. Klyde, B.J., Hormonal causes of male sexual dysfunction, in "Management of Impotence and Infertility," H.M. Whitehead (ed). 1994, J.B. Lippincott Co.: Philadelphia. p. 115.

49. Lieberman, S., Are the differences between estradiol and other estrogens, naturally occurring or synthetic, merely semantical? *J Clin Endocrinol Metab*, 1996. **81**(2): p. 850–1.

50. Kinsey, A.C., Sexual Behavior in the Human Male, W.B. Pomeroy, C.E. Martin (eds). 1948, W.B. Saunders: Philadelphia. p. 236.

51. Gonzalez-Cadavid, N.F. and J. Rajfer, Nitric oxide and other neurotransmitters of the corpus cavernosum, in "Infertility and Sexual Dysfunction," W.J.G. Hellstrom (ed.) 1997, Springer-Verlag: New York. p. 425–439.

52. Garban, H., et al. Effect of aging on nitric oxide-mediated penile erection in rats. *Am J Physiol*, 1995. **268**(1 Pt 2): p. H467–75.

53. Saenz de Tejada, I., et al. Endothelin: localization, synthesis, activity, and receptor types in human penile corpus cavernosum. *Am J Physiol*, 1991. **261**(4 Pt 2): p. H1078–85.

54. Lugg, J.A., J. Rajfer, and N.F. Gonzalez-Cadavid, Dihydrotestosterone is the active androgen in the maintenance of nitric oxide-mediated penile erection in the rat. *Endocrinology*, 1995. **136**(4): p. 1495–501.

55. Davidson, J.M., et al. Hormonal changes and sexual function in aging men. *J Clin Endocrinol Metab*, 1983. **57**(1): p. 71–7.
56. Finkle, A.L., et al. Sexual potency and aging males. *JAMA*, 1959. **170**: p. 1391–1393.
57. Kinsey A.C., W.B. Pomeroy, and C.F. Martin, "Sexual Behavior in the Human Male." 1948, Philadelphia: Saunders.
58. Martin, C.E., Factor affecting sexual functioning in 60-79-year-old married males. *Arch Sex Behav*, 1981. **10**(5): p. 399–420.
59. Pfeiffer, E., A. Verwoerdt, and H.S. Wang, Sexual behavior in aged men and women. *Arch Gen Psychiatry*, 1968. **19**: p. 753–758.
60. Tenover, J.L., Testosterone and the aging male. *J Androl*, 1997. **18**(2): p. 103–6.
61. Morley, J.E., et al. Longitudinal changes in testosterone, luteinizing hormone, and follicle-stimulating hormone in healthy older men. *Metabolism*, 1997. **46**(4): p. 410–3.
62. Vermeulen, A., R. Rubens, and L. Verdonck, Testosterone secretion and metabolism in male senescence. *J Clin Endocrinol Metab*, 1972. **34**(4): p. 730–5.
63. Korenman, S.G., et al. Secondary hypogonadism in older men: its relation to impotence. *J Clin Endocrinol Metab*, 1990. **71**(4): p. 963–9.
64. Pearson, U.J.D., et al. Effect of age and cigarette smoking on longitudinal changes in androgens and SHBG in healthy males, in "77th Ann Meet Endocrin Soc." Bethesda, MD.
65. Veldhoen, N. and C.C. Helbing, Detection of environmental endocrine-disruptor effects on gene expression in live Rana catesbeiana tadpoles using a tail fin biopsy technique. *Environ Toxicol Chem*, 2001. **20**(12): p. 2704–8.
66. Kaufman, J.M. and A. Vermeulen, Androgens in Male Senescence, in "Testosterone,Testosterone, Action, Deficiency, Substitution," Nieschlag, E. (ed.). 1998, Springer: Berlin. p. 437–471.
67. Meikle, A.W., et al. Quantitating genetic and nongenetic factors that determine plasma sex steroid variation in normal male twins. *Metabolism*, 1986. **35**(12): p. 1090–5.
68. Vermeulen, A. and J.M. Kaufman, Role of the hypothalamo-pituitary function in hypoandrogenism of healthy aging. *J Clin Endocrinol Metab*, 1992. **74**: p. 1226.
69. Desylpere, J.P., et al. Influence of age on pulsatile luteinizing hormone release and responsiveness of the gonadotrophs to sex hormone feedback. *J Clin Endocrinol Metab*, 1987. **64**: p. 68–73.
70. Winters, S.J., R.J. Sherins, and P. Troen, The gonadotropin-suppressive activity of androgen is increased in elderly men. *Metabolism*, 1984. **33**(11): p. 1052–9.
71. Winters, S.J. and L. Atkinson, Testoderm Study Group. Serum LH concentrations in hypogonadal men during transdermal testosteone replacement through scrotal skin: further evidence that aging enhances testosterone negative feed back. *Clin Endocrinol*, 1997. **47**: p. 317–322.
72. Rajfer, J., P.C. Namkun, and H. Petrap, Identification, partial characterization of age associated changes in a cytoplasmatic androgen receptor in the rat penis. *J Ster Biochem*, 1980. **13**: p. 1489–1492.
73. Gonzales-Kadavid, N.F., et al. Expression of androgen receptor gene in rat penile tissue and cells during sexual maturation. *Endocrinology*, 1991. **129**: p. 1671–1678.
74. Zirkin, B.R., H. Chen, and L. Luo, Leydig cell steroidogenesis in aging rats. *Exp Gerontol*, 1997. **32**(4–5): p. 529–37.
75. Ansari, J.M., A study of 65 impotent males. *Br J Psychiatry*, 1975. **127**: p. 337–41.
76. Davies, T.F., et al. Reduced 'gonadotrophin response to releasing hormone' after chronic administration to impotent men. *Clin Endocrinol (Oxf)*, 1977. **6**(3): p. 213–8.

77. Lawrence, D.M. and G.I. Swyer, Plasma testosterone and testosterone binding affinities in men with impotence, oligospermia, azoospermia, and hypogonadism. *Br Med J*, 1974. **1**(904): p. 349–51.

78. Pirke, K.M., et al. Pituitary gonadal system function in patients with erectile impotence and premature ejaculation. *Arch Sex Behav*, 1979. **8**: p. 41–48.

79. Racey, P.A., et al. Proceedings: Testosterone in impotent men. *J Endocrinol*, 1973. **59**(2): p. 23.

80. Buvat-Herbaut, M., et al. Serum bioavailable testosterone is decreased in 39% and serum free testosterone in 28% of the impotent patients who have normal serum total testosterone, in "Proceedings of the 3rd Biennal World Meeting on Impotence." Boston. I988.

81. Forti, G., et al. Radioimmunoassay of plasma testosterone. *Clin Endocrinol (Oxf)*, 1974. **3**(1): p. 5–17.

82. Raboch, J., J. Mellan, and L. Starka, Plasma testosterone in male patients with sexual dysfunction. *Arch Sex Behav*, 1975. **4**(5): p. 541–5.

83. Spark, R.F., R.A. White, and P.B. Connolly, Impotence is not always psychogenic. Newer insights into hypothalamic-pituitary-gonadal dysfunction. *Jama*, 1980. **243**(8): p. 750–5.

84. Nickel, J.C., et al. Endocrine dysfunction in impotence: incidence, significance and cost-effective screening. *J Urol*, 1984. **132**(1): p. 40–3.

85. Maatman, T.J. and D.K. Montague, Routine endocrine screening in impotence. *Urology*, 1986. **27**(6): p. 499–502.

86. Kropman, R.F., et al. Routine endocrine screening in impotence: significance and cost effectiveness. *Int J Impot Res*, 1991. **3**(87–94).

87. Johnson, A.R., 3rd and J.P. Jarow, Is routine endocrine testing of impotent men necessary? *J Urol*, 1992. **147**(6): p. 1542–3; discussion 1543–4.

88. Buvat, J. and A. Lemaire, Endocrine screening in 1,022 men with erectile dysfunction: clinical significance and cost-effective strategy. *J Urol*, 1997. **158**(5): p. 1764–7.

89. Buvat, J., A. Lemaire, and J. Ratajczyk, Role des hormones dans les dysfonctions sexuelles, l'homosexualité, le transsexualisme et les comportements sexuels deviants: Consequences diagnostiques et therapeutiques. *Contracept Fertil Sex*, 1996. **24**: p. 834–846.

90. Pogach, L.M. and V. JL., Endocrine disorders associated with erectile dysfunction, in "Male Sexual Dysfunction," R. J. Krane (ed.). 1983, Little Brown: Boston. p. 63–76.

91. Tenover, J.S., Effects of testosterone supplementation in the aging male. *J Clin Endocrinol Metab*, 1992. **75**(4): p. 1092–8.

92. Schdrmeyer, T.H. and H. RD., Endocrinology of impotence, in "Erectile Dysfunction," U. Jonas (e). 1991, Springer-Verlag: Berlin, p. 78–90.

93. Eardley, I., New oral therapies for the treatment of erectile dysfunction. *Br J Urol*, 1998. **81**(1): p. 122–7.

94. Ben-Galim, E., R.E. Hillman, and V.V. Weldon, Topically applied testosterone and phallic growth. Its effects in male children with hypopituitarism and microphallus. *Am J Dis Child*, 1980. **134**(3): p. 296–8.

95. Findlay J.C., V. Place, and S. PJ., Treatment of primary hypogonadism in men by the transdermal administration of testosterone. *J Clin Endocrinol Metabol*, 1989. **68**: p. 369.

96. Guay, A.T., S. Bansal, and M.B. Hodge, Possible hypothalamic impotence. Male counterpart to hypothalamic amenorrhea? *Urology*, 1991. **38**(4): p. 317–22.

97. Marcus, R. and S.G. Korenman, Estrogens and the human male. *Annu Rev Med*, 1976. **27**: p. 357–70.
98. Wortsman, J., A. Hamidinia, and W. SJ., Hypogonadism following long-term treatment with diethylstilbestrol. *Am J Med Sci*, 1989. **297**: p. 364.
99. Adlercreutz, H., Hepatic metabolism of estrogens in health and disease. *NEJM*, 1974. **290**: p. 1081.
100. Leonard, M.P., C.J. Nickel, and A. Morales, Hyperprolactinemia and impotence: why, when and how to investigate. *J Urol*, 1989. **142**(4): p. 992–4.
101. Minhas, S. and I. Eardley, Diabetic Impotence, in "Textbook of Erectile Dysfunction," K.R. Carson, C.C. Goldstein (ed.), 1998, Isis Medical Publishers: Oxford. p. 531–540.
102. McCulloch, D.K., et al. The natural history of impotence in diabetic men. *Diabetologia*, 1984. **26**(6): p. 437–40.
103. Naliboff, B.D. and M. Rosenthal, Effects of age on complications in adult onset diabetes. *J Geriatr Soc*, 1989. **37**: p. 838–842.
104. Klein, R., B.E. Klein, and K.E. Lee, Prevalence of self-reported erectile dysfunction in people with long term IDBM. *Diabetes Care*, 1996. **19**: p. 135–141.
105. Hakim, L.S. and I. Goldstein, Diabetic sexual dysfunction. *Endocrinol Metab Clin North Am*, 1996. **25**(2): p. 379–400.
106. Glass, A.R., et al. Low serum testosterone and sex hormone-binding globulin in massively obese men. *J Clin Endocrinol Metabol*, 1977. **45**: p. 1211–1219.
107. Strain, G.W., et al. Mild hypogonadotropic hypogonadism in obese men. *Metabolism*, 1982. **31**: p. 871–875.
108. Schneider, G., et al. Increased estrogen production in obese men. *J Clin Endocrinol Metab*, 1979. **48**: p. 633–638.
109. Stanik, S., et al. The effect of weight loss on reproductive hormones in obese men. *J Clin Endocrinol Metab*, 1981. **53**: p. 828–832.
110. Rodger, R.S., et al. Prevalence and pathogenesis of impotence in one hundred uremic men. *Uremia Invest*, 1984. **8**(2): p. 89–96.
111. Lim, V.S. and V.S. Fang, Gonadal dysfunction in uremic men. A study of the hypothalamo-pituitary-testicular axis before and after renal transplantation. *Am J Med*, 1975. **58**: p. 655–662.
112. Handelsman, D.J. and Q. Dong, Hypothalamo-pituitary gonadal axis in chronic renal failure. *Endocrinol Metab Clin North Am*, 1993. **22**(1): p. 145–61.
113. Coppola, A. and G. Cuomo, [Pituitary-testicular evaluation in patients with chronic renal insufficiency in hemodialysis treatment]. *Minerva Med*, 1990. **81**(6): p. 461–4.
114. Weizman, R., A. Weizman, and J. Levi, Sexual dysfunction associated with hyperprolactinemia in males and females undergoing hemodialysis. *Psychosom Med Clin (Barc)*, 1983. **45**: p. 259–269.
115. Gura, V., et al. Hyperprolactinemia: a possible cause of sexual impotence in male patients undergoing chronic hemodialysis. *Nephron*, 1980. **26**(1): p. 53–4.
116. Nghiem, D.D., et al. Factors influencing male sexual impotence after renal transplantation. *Urology*, 1983. **21**(1): p. 49–52.
117. Procci, W.R. and D.J. Martin, Effect of maintenance hemodialysis on male sexual performance. *J Nerv Ment Dis*, 1985. **173**(6): p. 366–72.
118. Lawrence, I.G., et al. Correcting impotence in the male dialysis patient: experience with testosterone replacement and vacuum tumescence therapy. *Am J Kidney Dis*, 1998. **31**(2): p. 313–9.
119. Kidd, G.S., A.R. Glass, and R.A. Vigersky, The hypothalamic-pituitary-testicular axis in thyrotoxicosis. *J Clin Endocrinol Metab*, 1979. **48**(5): p. 798–802.

120. Wortsman, J., W. Rosner, and M.L. Dufau, Abnormal testicular function in men with primary hypothyroidism. *Am J Med*, 1987. **82**(2): p. 207–12.

121. Molitch, M.E., Prolactin, in "The Pituitary," S. Melmed (ed.). 1995, Blackwell: Cambridge, MA. p. 133–186.

122. Bouloux, P.M.G. and J.A.H. Wass, Endocrinology, in "Impotence: Diagnosis and Management of Male Erectile Dysfunction," R.S. Kirby, C.C. Carson, and G.D. Webster (Eds.). 1991, Butterworth-Heinemann Ltd.: Oxford. p. 44–54.

123. Sato, F., et al. Suppressive effects of chronic hyperprolactinemia on penile erection and yawning following administration of apomorphine to pituitary-transplanted rats. *J Androl*, 1997. **18**(1): p. 21–5.

124. Carter, J.N., et al. Prolactin-screening tumors and hypogonadism in 22 men. *N Engl J Med*, 1978. **299**(16): p. 847–52.

125. Swerdloff, R.S. and C. Wang, Influence of pituitary disease on sexual development and functioning. *Psychother Psychosom*, 1998. **67**(3): p. 173–80.

126. Zonszein, J., Diagnosis and management of endocrine disorders of erectile dysfunction. *Urol Clin North Am*, 1995. **22**(4): p. 789–802.

127. Spratt, D.I., et al. Both hyper- and hypogonadotropic hypogonadism occur transiently in acute illness: bio- and immunoactive gonadotropins. *J Clin Endocrinol Metab*, 1992. **75**(6): p. 1562–70.

128. Sikka, S.C., Drug, environment, and chemical exposures in the realm of sexuality, in "The Handbook of Sexual Dysfunction," W.J.G. Hellstrom (ed.). 1999, The American Society of Andrology, San Francisco. p. 27–34.

129. Kavlock, R. and S. Perreault, Multiple chemical exposure and risks of adverse reproductive function and outcome, in "Toxicological of Chemical Mixtures: From Real Life Examples to Mechanisms of Toxicology Interactions," R.S.H. Yang (ed.). 1994, Academic Press: Orlando, FL. p. 245–297.

130. Zaebst, D., S. Tanaka, and M. Haring, Occupational exposure to estrogens-problems and approaches, in "Estrogens in the Environment," M.A. McLachlan (ed.). 1980, Elsevier/North-Holland: New York. p. 377–389.

131. Soto, A., et al. An "in culture" bioassay to assess the estrogenicity of xenobiotics (E-Screen), in "Chemically Induced Alterations in Sexual and Functional Development: The Wildlife/Human Connection," T. Colborn and C. Clements (eds.). 1992, Princeton Scientific Publishing Co., Inc.: Princeton, NJ. p. 295–309.

132. Sikka, S.C., Gonadotoxicity, in "Male Infertility and Sexual Dysfunction," W.J.G. Hellstrom (ed.). 1997, Springer-Verlag: New York. p. 292–306.

133. Kelce, W., et al. Environmental hormone disruptors: Evidence that vinclozolin developmental toxicity is mediated by antiandrogenic metabolites. *Jr Toxicol Appl Pharm*, 1993. **126**: p. 1392–1395.

134. Mills, L.C., Drug-induced impotence. Am Fam Physician, 1975. **12**(2): p. 104–6.

135. Horowitz, J.D. and A.J. Goble, Drugs and impaired male sexual function. *Drugs*, 1979. **18**(3): p. 206–17.

136. Abramowicz, M., ed. Drugs that cause sexual dysfunction: An update. "The Medical Letter on Drugs and Therapeutics," Vol. 34. 1992, The Medical Letter, Inc.: New Rochelle, NY. 73–78.

137. Greenblatt, D.J. and J. Koch-Weser, Gynecomastia and impotence: complications of spironolactone therapy. *Jama*, 1973. **223**(1): p. 82.

138. Neri, A., et al. The effect of long-term administration of digoxin on plasma androgens and sexual dysfunction. *J Sex Marital Ther*, 1987. **13**(1): p. 58–63.

139. Mitchell, J.E. and M.K. Popkin, Antipsychotic drug therapy and sexual dysfunction in men. *Am J Psychiatry*, 1982. **139**(5): p. 633–7.

140. Blay, S.L., M.P. Ferraz, and H.M. Calil, Lithium-induced male sexual impairment: two case reports. *J Clin Psychiatry*, 1982. **43**(12): p. 497–8.
141. Xie, Y., et al. Effect of long-term passive smoking on erectile function and penile nitric oxide synthase in the rat. *J Urol*, 1997. **157**(3): p. 1121–6.
142. Sikka, S.C., et al. Role of vitamin E and oxidative stress in the pathophysiology of diabetic impotence. *J Urol*, 1996. **155**(5): p. 623.
143. Chen, X. and T.J. Lee, Ginsenosides-induced nitric oxide-mediated relaxation of the rabbit corpus cavernosum. *Br J Pharmacol*, 1995. **115**(1): p. 15–8.
144. Chapin, R.E., et al. Endocrine modulation of reproduction. *Fundam Appl Toxicol*, 1996. **29**(1): p. 1–17.
145. Morris, N.M. and J.R. Udry, Pheromonal influences on human sexual behavior: an experimental search. *J Biosoc Sci*, 1978. **10**(2): p. 147–57.
146. Carroll, J.L., D.J. Ellis, and D.H. Bagley, Age-related changes in hormones in impotent men. Jefferson Sexual Function Center. *Urology*, 1990. **36**(1): p. 42–6.
147. Ryan, G., Reclaiming male sexuality, in "A Guide to Potency, Vitality and Prowess," A. Melman (ed.). 1997, M. Evans and Co., Inc.: New York.

12 Prostate Development: Mechanisms for Opposite Effects of Low and High Doses of Estrogenic Chemicals

Catherine A. Richter, Barry G. Timms, and Frederick S. vom Saal

CONTENTS

12.1 INTRODUCTION

The prostate is one of the male accessory glands that contributes to seminal fluid. In male mice, removal of this organ reduces fertility.[1] There has been speculation for some time that estrogen plays a role in normal development as well as subsequent disease of the prostate.[2,3] One basis for this speculation is that embryologists recognized that the region of the developing urogenital sinus (UGS) just caudal to the bladder, from which the prostatic ducts emerge during fetal life, develops into a portion of the vagina in females. It thus seemed reasonable to speculate that, since the vagina is an estrogen-responsive organ, portions of the prostate might also be responsive to estrogen. This led to speculation that estrogen might play a role in regulating prostate development and subsequent function, as well as diseases associated with aging.

In contrast to the above prediction that estrogen might play a role in normal prostate development, there are numerous reports that prenatal or neonatal exposure to high, pharmacological doses of estradiol or the estrogenic drug diethylstilbestrol (DES) dramatically interfere with prostate development in mice and rats.[4] More recently there have been studies concerning the effects of endogenous estradiol as well as very low doses of estrogenic chemicals on prostate development. Many questions have been raised regarding the potential for environmental chemicals with estrogenic activity to alter prostate development at concentrations encountered in the environment (referred to as environmentally relevant doses of chemicals). It is likely that very high doses of DES do not serve as a model for potential effects of low doses of these chemicals. This conclusion is based on the generally greater potency of DES relative to most "environmental estrogens" and, most importantly, high doses of a hormone can lead to "down-regulation" of the capacity for tissues to respond to the hormone, while low doses of the same hormone can stimulate or "up-regulate" response capacity.[5,6] The idea that dose is important is not a new concept in endocrinology, toxicology, or pharmacology. However, prior to recent findings based on manipulating estrogen levels within a physiological range in fetal mice, physiologically relevant low doses of estrogen had simply not been examined.[7,8] One reason for this was the difficulty associated with measuring estradiol in very small volumes of serum from fetal and neonatal rats and mice, in which levels of other lipids are very high and the free, biologically active fraction (0.2 to 0.3% of total serum estradiol) is extremely low; total estradiol measured by radioimmunoassay consists of free estradiol as well as estradiol bound to plasma proteins.[8,9]

In humans, the prostate is notable for its vulnerability to disease. Prostate cancer is one of the most common cancers in men in the United States.[10] Benign prostatic hyperplasia (BPH) is a common condition beginning in middle age in men. Nearly half of middle-aged men can expect to develop urinary problems associated with BPH during their lifetime.[11] We review *in vivo* and *in vitro* studies showing that exposure to a very small increase in circulating estradiol or to very low doses of estrogenic chemicals present in the environment during fetal life in male mice can lead to differences in prostate differentiation that persist into adulthood. The potential for environmentally relevant concentrations of environmental estrogens to impact human prostate pathogenesis is of immense importance as a public health issue.

However, there are no human data at this time to assess whether any aspect of prostate disease in men is related to developmental exposure to manmade estrogenic chemicals present in the environment. The marked similarity in effects in mice and humans of exposure during sexual differentiation to high doses of DES, and the conclusion from this literature that the mouse is the best animal model for predicting the effects of developmental exposure to estrogen in humans is cause for concern, based on the effects on the mouse prostate that we describe below.

12.2 HISTORICAL OVERVIEW OF THE PROSTATE

Pathology of the prostate was attributed in 1685 by Samuel Collins to "indulgence in venery" (the pursuit of sexual pleasure). Collins recognized that prostate enlargement was important with regard to urethral obstruction; this was also discussed in 1769 by Giambattista Morgagni.[2,3] Franks[3] noted that Morgagni identified the site of origin of hyperplasia within the prostate and also examined the prevalence of this disease in old men.

John Hunter observed in 1786 that the prostate (and other accessory reproductive organs) underwent involution following castration. Zuckerman[2] comments on the remarkable fact that even though the implication of this observation would suggest that castration might serve as a treatment to relieve the effects of prostatic enlargement on urethral obstruction, which results in death due to uremic poisoning if untreated, the implication of this observation was not grasped until almost a hundred years later. Castration as a treatment for enlargement of the prostate was finally proposed in 1893, after which it became the method of treating this disease. However, this approach was soon abandoned, because at that time, mortality associated with surgery was unacceptably high. In addition, although it might seem surprising today, at the end of the nineteenth century there was still considerable controversy concerning the role of the testes in accessory reproductive organ function. This controversy is interesting in that it had been reported in the middle of the nineteenth century that testicular grafts reversed the effects of castration in cockerels, which led to attempts to reverse impotence in aging men by means of grafting animal testicular tissue. At this time it was believed that any effects of the testes on organs such as the prostate were probably mediated by nerves, not secreted substances. However, in 1927 methods for extracting gonadal steroids were described, and testosterone was finally identified as the most potent of the testicular hormones in 1935. Prostate growth in castrated rats was being routinely used as a bioassay for potency of testicular hormones by this time.[12,13]

Our current understanding of prostate development and anatomy appears to have progressed steadily during the past 60 years, but has been partially hindered by reliance on old anatomical descriptions.[14-16] Lowsley's[17] description of prostatic lobes has been replaced by the now widely accepted concept that the human prostate is better described as consisting of zones.[18] The recent advancement in computer technology now allows organ structure to be visualized by three-dimensional (3-D) reconstruction, from digitized serial sections. Three-dimensional reconstruction requires tracing, digitizing and axial alignment of identified objects (anatomical structures) within each section. This provides a powerful tool for examining anatomy, including that of the prostate. This technique has been particularly useful in understanding the complex pattern of ductal morphogenesis, a feature that is extremely difficult to grasp when viewing two-dimensional histological sections in a microscope.[16,19] Also, the digitized information used to reconstruct the prostate provides the basis for making quantitative comparisons of experimental manipulations on the developing prostate.[8,19]

12.3 PROSTATE ANATOMY AND HOMOLOGY AMONG SPECIES

12.3.1 PROSTATE DEVELOPMENT

The prostate ducts begin forming as epithelial buds at about 10 weeks of gestation in humans and gestation day 17 in mice.[20] These outgrowths begin as solid epithelial buds that branch during late fetal life in humans, forming a compound tubulo-alveolar gland structure.[21] In mice, birth occurs within 2 days of the beginning of prostate differentiation, and extensive ductal branching occurs throughout infancy and adolescence. The adult structure is not achieved until approximately postnatal day 50.[22] In humans, the pubertal reawakening of androgen secretion by the testes results in the prostatic glandular ducts forming a patent lumen within the terminal acini. The epithelial lining becomes highly differentiated, after which androgen-dependent secretory activity begins.

As shown in Figure 12.1, the anatomy of the human prostate is now described in terms of zones.[18] The transition zone is composed of short glandular ducts and surrounds the urethra above the intersection of the ejaculatory ducts; the central zone surrounds the transition zone just under the bladder and is traversed by the ejaculatory ducts; and the peripheral zone lies outside the posterior of the central zone and extends along the urethra below the intersection of the ejaculatory ducts.[23] The morphology of the mouse prostate, which is divided into dorsolateral and ventral lobes, has been described in a series of papers by Sugimura.[22,24,25] Individual prostatic glandular ducts extend from the urethra and branch into terminal ducts that are lined with pseudostratified columnar epithelium. In humans, a continuous layer of basal cells underlies the epithelium, while in rodents basal cells are dispersed along the epithelial basement membrane.[26] The epithelial glandular ducts of the prostate are surrounded by a layer of smooth muscle cells. In humans, this layer of smooth muscle is much thicker than in rodents.[26]

The ejaculatory ducts form from the embryonic Wolffian ducts. The ejaculatory ducts enter the prostatic urethra caudal and lateral to the site of the utricle, which is the remnant of the Müllerian ducts as they merge and enter the posterior UGS (Figure 12.2). The utricle becomes enclosed in the central zone of the human prostate. Each ejaculatory duct (vas deferens) merges with the ipsilateral seminal vesicle duct, which differentiates during the 13th week of embryonic life in humans from the Wolffian duct proximal to the UGS. The ejaculatory ducts lead into the prostatic urethra next to an enlarged portion of the urethral crest, the verumontanum (also referred to as the colliculus seminalis) in the posterior wall of the urethra (Figure 12.1).

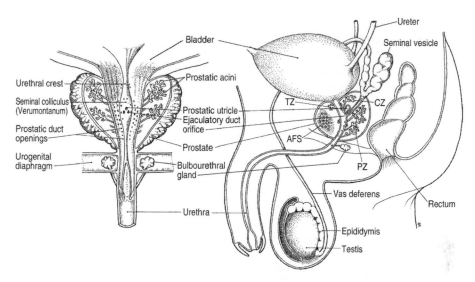

FIGURE 12.1 Diagrams of frontal and sagittal sections of the male urogenital complex showing the anatomical position of the adult prostate and associated structures. The prostatic zones are: central zone (CZ), peripheral zone (PZ), and transition zone (TZ). The anterior fibromuscular stroma (AFS) is also shown. From Reference 16.

The prostatic urethra is divided into a proximal segment (from bladder neck to verumontanum) and distal segment (from verumontanum to external sphincter), forming a 35 to 40° angle from the horizontal at the verumontanum. The proximal urethra is surrounded by circular smooth muscle, which is referred to as the preprostatic sphincter and functions to stop retrograde ejaculation into the bladder. In the proximal portion of the urethra in humans closest to the bladder neck, short prostatic ducts that mingle with sphincteric stroma have been proposed as the potential site for pathogenesis of BPH.[27] Hyperplasia of the short ducts in the transition zone during development of BPH impinges on the urethra and can lead to obstruction.

McNeal introduced the hypothesis of a reawakening of embryonic inductive interactions to describe the inappropriate new ductal budding that occurs during the onset of BPH in old age. This was thought to result from non-prostatic stroma (the proximal urethral sphincter) inducing adjacent transition zone ducts to begin new ductal formation in areas of stromal proliferation. Tissue recombination studies have confirmed that adult human prostatic epithelium is capable of undergoing proliferation and differentiation in response to stromal signals.[26] A very interesting aspect of prostate carcinoma is that it is predominantly found in glands originating from the caudal and posterior region of the prostatic urethra. In contrast to the short glands in the transition zone that are predominantly the site of BPH, these are long ducts that branch and extend in the peripheral zone of the prostate in men. The portion of the embryonic UGS from which these different prostate ducts originate is thus highly predictive of the type of pathology observed in the ducts during aging.

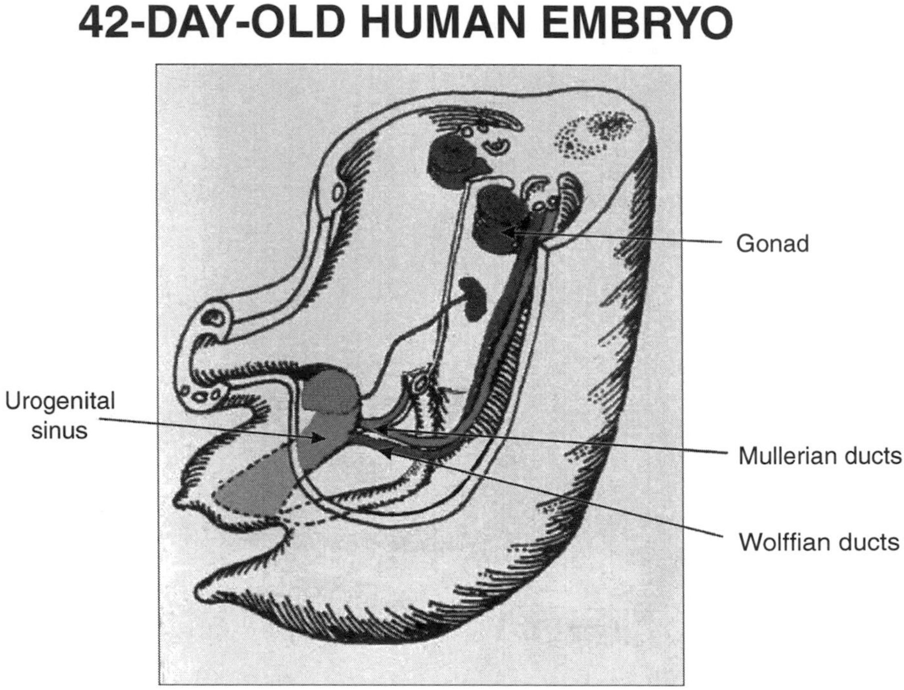

42-DAY-OLD HUMAN EMBRYO

FIGURE 12.2 Genital ducts prior to differentiation. Drawing of a human embryo at about 42 days of age with the upper half and left body wall cut away to demonstrate the gonads, associated Wolffian (mesonephric) and Müllerian (paramesonephric) ducts, and urogenital sinus (UGS). The prostate differentiates from the cranial UGS. The gut and its mesentery have been removed. Modified from Reference 140.

12.3.2 EVIDENCE FOR HOMOLOGY OF THE RODENT DORSOLATERAL AND HUMAN PROSTATE

It has been proposed that the variety of interspecies differences observed in the structure of the adult prostate gland reflects a diversity that makes it difficult to find a suitable animal model for the study of human prostatic disease.[27] Using a computer-assisted three-dimensional approach to visualize the microanatomy of prostate development, Timms[19] has compared the ductal budding patterns during prostate morphogenesis in rat, mouse, and human (Figure 12.3 and Figure 12.4). The three-dimensional reconstruction procedure revealed marked similarities among rodents and human prostate gland genesis.

When different species share similar regulatory systems and a common pattern of development of a structure, this is taken as evidence that the structure in the different species is homologous, even though the final form in the adult might appear markedly different (the classic example is the wing of a bat, hand of a human, and fin of a dolphin). Timms proposed that the prostatic ducts that originate from similar regions of the UGS in rats, mice, and humans are homologous structures.[19] First, the ducts that develop into the dorsolateral lobe in rodents show a pattern of budding

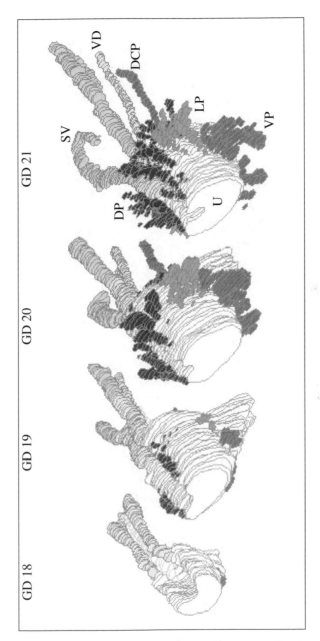

FIGURE 12.3 Serial section reconstructions of the rat urogenital complex on gestation day (GD) 18, 19, 20, and 21, illustrating the stages of early prostate development. Prostate morphogenesis begins at GD 18 and by GD 19 the dorsal, ventral, lateral, and dorsocranial (coagulating gland) buds are visible. On GD 21 (the day before birth), prostate budding from the UGS is essentially complete. U: urethra; DP: dorsal prostate; LP: lateral prostate; VP: ventral prostate; CG: coagulating [dorsocranial] gland; SV: seminal vesicle; VD: vas deferens. From Reference 141.

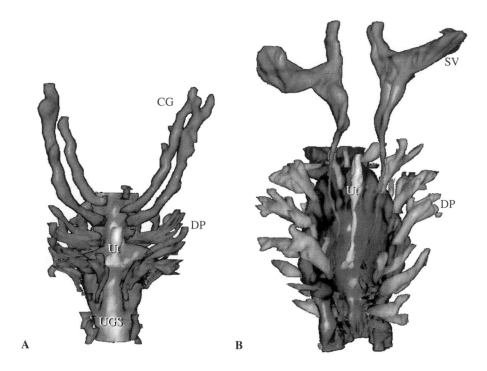

FIGURE 12.4 Panel A: Dorsal view of a newborn mouse urogenital sinus (UGS) reconstruction showing the dorsal prostate outgrowths (DP) aligned with the paired prostatic sulci. The seminal vesicles and ejaculatory ducts have been removed from this reconstruction to clearly illustrate that the most cranial ducts form the long paired coagulating glands (CG). These glands extend and attach to the anterior surface of the mouse seminal vesicles during subsequent development. Panel B: Dorsal view of a 13-week male human fetus showing a similar paired pattern of prostatic duct outgrowths along the UGS. The most cranial dorsal prostate outgrowths correspond to the equivalent anatomical location of the mouse coagulating glands At these stages of fetal growth, the mouse and human prostate budding patterns demonstrate striking similarities. Ut: utricle; SV: seminal vesicles.

similar to that in the human (Figure 12.3). This finding is significant in that Price[28] observed that the relationship of prostate ductal openings into the urethra persists in the adult in the same relative position as in the fetus. A difference between rodents and humans is that, unlike rodents, the human prostate does not exhibit significant postnatal duct development in the ventral region of the UGS. The ventral region of the mouse prostate is thus likely to be less relevant for investigating factors that might impact the pathology of the human prostate relative to the rodent dorsolateral prostate. The coagulating glands are the most cranial ducts that develop from the urethra, and these appear homologous to the most dorsocranial prostate ducts in humans.

Dogs and cats have homogenous prostate tissue similar to the peripheral zone in humans, while the seminal vesicles and the central zone of the prostate are absent.[29] The glandular ducts that form the zones of the prostate prone to BPH in men, the transition and central zones,[27,30,31] are thus absent in dogs. Homology also involves functional similarities, and a focus of research is on regulatory factors that mediate development in humans and animal models.[32,33] However, mesenchyme from the mouse prostate has been shown to produce the appropriate regulatory factors that induced differentiation of human bladder epithelium into epithelium characteristic of the human prostate,[34] providing evidence for the similarity of regulatory factors required to identify homologous structures. As lobe-specific or zone-specific molecular determinants of development emerge, further insight into homology between species will be realized.

12.4 REGULATION OF PROSTATE DEVELOPMENT

12.4.1 TESTOSTERONE AND 5α-DIHYDROTESTOSTERONE (DHT)

Between the seventh and eighth week of gestation in humans, and around gestation day 12 in mice, Leydig cells in the developing testes begin production of androgens, with testosterone being the major androgen secreted throughout sexual differentiation.[35-37] Testosterone secreted by each testis mediates differentiation of the ipsilateral Wolffian (mesonephric) duct system. Testosterone in the circulation mediates development of the UGS and external genitalia (Figure 12.2). Secretion of Müllerian-inhibiting hormone (MIH) by the Sertoli cells, which line the seminiferous tubules, suppresses the development of the Müllerian (paramesonephric) duct ipsilateral to each testis. Estrogen antagonizes the action of MIH, while testosterone facilitates the action of MIH.[38]

Testosterone produced by the testes is delivered to target tissues through the blood. Within some androgen-target organs, testosterone is converted to 5α-dihydrotestosterone (DHT) by the enzyme 5α-reductase. Testosterone and DHT are both ligands for the androgen receptor. DHT has a higher affinity than testosterone for the androgen receptor, thus enabling it to induce the same response as testosterone at a lower concentration. Expression of 5α-reductase in the Wolffian ducts occurs after sexual differentiation in most species, thus providing one basis for high levels of testosterone achieved by diffusion from the ipsilateral testis being required for development of each Wolffian duct into the epididymis, vas deferens, and seminal vesicle. Production of DHT by 5α-reductase in mesenchymal tissue is required for normal masculinization of the cranial UGS into the prostate as well as development of the penis and scrotum.[39] This is revealed by studies in which testosterone levels in the fetal blood are in a normal range and androgen receptor numbers in fetal tissues are normal, but 5α-reductase activity is inhibited by administration of drugs such as finasteride. Genetic defects may also produce a deficiency in the capacity to produce DHT, and in this condition normal masculinization of the prostate and external genitalia does not occur.[40] There is some evidence that testosterone and DHT have distinct roles in regulation of gene expression in the adult prostate.[41]

12.4.2 GROWTH FACTOR SIGNALING BETWEEN MESENCHYME AND EPITHELIUM

Development of the prostate begins with outgrowths (glandular buds) of the urothelium lining the lumen of the UGS. The first detectable molecular event in prostate development is the expression of the homeobox gene Nkx3.1 in UGS epithelium, which precedes formation of epithelial buds. Nkx3.1 expression is dependent on activity of the sonic hedgehog (Shh) gene. The homeobox transcription factors HoxA10, HoxA13, and HoxD13 are also required for prostate development.[21]

Tissue recombination studies have shown that the developing prostatic epithelium is dependent on androgen-induced paracrine secretions from the mesenchyme.[42] In turn, the epithelium influences the architecture of the mesenchyme.[26] DHT binds to androgen receptor expressed in UGS mesenchyme, which induces the initial formation and development of epithelial buds from the urethra. The epithelial buds show little capacity to bind androgen, and functional androgen receptor in the epithelium is not required for initial prostate development.[42-44] Since the interactions of the mesenchyme and epithelium are hormone dependent and are central to the development of the prostate, we discuss below evidence that they represent a point of vulnerability to perturbation by chemicals in the environment referred to as "endocrine disruptors."

An important and as-yet-unanswered question in prostate development is the identity of the paracrine factor(s), or andromedins, that induce epithelial development. The simplest model of andromedin action is that transcription of a single growth factor expressed only in prostate mesenchyme is directly up-regulated by liganded androgen receptors, and the andromedin acts directly on receptors in epithelial cells to induce proliferation and budding. The expected properties of an andromedin is thus that it is produced by mesenchyme cells in an androgen-dependent manner, that it induces proliferation of epithelial cells, and that it is able to induce prostate epithelial development in epithelium lacking androgen receptors. No single factor with all these properties has yet been found. In fact, a more complex picture, involving an array of permissive and restrictive signals, is emerging.[21] The controls on epithelial duct development in the prostate appear to be closely related to developmental signals in other organs derived from branched epithelial structures, including the pancreas, salivary gland, lung, kidney, and mammary gland.[45] A potential mechanism of feedback of growth factor signaling on androgen receptor activity is phosphorylation of androgen receptors. Specifically, epidermal growth factor (EGF) induces phosphorylation of androgen receptors at ser-650.[46] EGF can enhance the transcriptional activity of androgen receptors in response to androgen.[47]

The family of fibroblast growth factors (FGFs) offers several members with andromedin-like properties. FGF-7, also known as keratinocyte growth factor (KGF), is expressed in mesenchyme and its receptor, FGFR2(iiib) is expressed in epithelium. FGF-7 stimulates epithelial development. However, FGF-7 mRNA is not induced by testosterone *in vivo*, and stimulation of epithelial development by FGF-7 can be blocked by an antiandrogen.[48] Another andromedin candidate, FGF-10, is expressed by prostate mesenchyme and is necessary for prostate development, as revealed by the lack of a prostate in FGF-10 knockout mice.[49] However, FGF-10 is not directly regulated by androgen receptors, and addition of FGF-10 is not sufficient to stimulate formation of epithelial buds in the absence of testosterone.[49,50] These results suggest that an additional, androgen-dependent factor is required to support stimulation of epithelial growth by FGF-10. The available data support the hypothesis that FGF-10 has distinct roles in the initial process of formation of epithelial buds, which requires both FGF-10 and androgen, and in further growth and branching of the epithelial ducts, which can be stimulated by FGF-10 alone.[49,50] FGF-10 is highly expressed in the ventral mesenchymal pad (VMP) of the developing UGS in both males and females.[50] As epithelial buds grow into the VMP, they undergo extensive growth and branching to form the ventral prostate.

Insulin-like growth factor-1 (IGF-1)-deficient mice develop prostates with reduced size, reduced number of duct tips, and reduced branch points.[51] The observation that initial formation of prostatic buds occurs in IGF-1 knockout animals suggests that IGF-1 stimulates prostate development at a later point in development than FGF-10. A discontinuous smooth muscle layer that differentiates within the UGS mesenchyme separates the outer layer of mesenchyme, including the VMP, from the epithelium early in development. In females, this smooth muscle layer thickens and becomes continuous, potentially blocking the epithelium from receiving proliferative signals from the mesenchyme. Testosterone induces thinning of the smooth muscle layer, and thus may function to maintain communication between the mesenchyme and epithelium; this would allow the action of mesenchymal growth factors such as FGF-7 and FGF-10 on the epithelium.[32]

Epidermal growth factor and transforming growth factor α (TGF-α) both bind the EGF receptor, and are both expressed in developing prostate in humans and rodents.[52] Androgens do not directly regulate TGF-α, but EGF treatment up-regulated TGF-α in mesenchyme cells.[53] Disruption of the EGF gene in mice did not alter formations of prostatic buds. However, disruption of both EGF and TGF-α resulted in significantly fewer buds in the dorsolateral region, and disruption of TGF-α alone resulted in significantly more buds in the dorsolateral region.[52] These results suggest a partially redundant and partially antagonistic relationship between EGF and TGF-α in regulation of formation of prostatic buds.

Epithelial buds extending from different regions of the urethra, organized as lobes in mice and zones in humans, form distinct regional architectures. These changes in organization of the epithelium are produced by different balances of branching, proliferation, and differentiation, which are controlled by different regions of mesenchyme surrounding the UGS. One molecule that may contribute to some of these differences is fucosyltransferase1, an enzyme that synthesizes the H antigenic determinant carbohydrate structure on certain proteins and lipids. Fucosyltransferase1 supports epithelial proliferation and is found in a restricted distribution within the developing prostatic epithelium.[54]

Proliferation signals in the developing prostate epithelium must be balanced by signals that limit inappropriate proliferation. Members of the transforming growth factor β (TGF-β) family, including TGF-β's, activins, and bone morphogenic proteins (bmp's) are negative regulators of epithelial growth.[55,56] Bmp-4 is expressed in prostate mesenchyme immediately adjacent to the epithelial ducts.[57] Bmp-4 expression is attenuated at the tips of epithelial ducts.[57] During growth and branching of epithelial ducts, bmp-4 is localized to branching points, while FGF-10 is localized to the growing tips of the epithelial ducts.[49] Defects in bmp-4 expression in mice lead to increased branching in the ventral prostate and coagulating glands (dorsocranial prostate).[57]

12.5 ESTROGEN MODULATES PROSTATE DEVELOPMENT

12.5.1 INHIBITORY EFFECTS OF HIGH, PHARMACOLOGICAL DOSES OF ESTROGEN

An extensive literature relating to the effects of exposure to synthetic estrogens during differentiation of the prostate and other accessory reproductive organs in rodents consistently has shown inhibitory effects of very high, pharmacological levels of estrogen on prostate function. For example, exposure to a high dose of DES or estradiol caused abnormal development and lesions throughout the reproductive system in males.[58-66] Administration of high, supra-physiological levels of androgen during sexual differentiation has similar effects.[67] High doses of estrogens act directly on the developing prostate to inhibit epithelial proliferation and branching, and disrupt differentiation of the stroma and epithelium,[68] and androgen receptor expression is permanently suppressed.[5,64] Squamous metaplasia of prostatic and coagulating gland (dorsocranial prostate) ductal epithelium in male mice and rats has been reported after exposure to exogenous estrogen during early life.[69-71] Similar effects of high doses of estrogen on rat[72] and mouse[5] prostate in primary culture have been reported.

Administration of the high (200 µg/kg/day) dose of DES to pregnant mice completely inhibited the formation of ducts in the dorsal and lateral prostate in male fetuses. Relative to the negative controls, the high dose of DES caused a very different pattern of budding in the ventral UGS, with numerous abnormal short buds being apparent throughout the entire length of the urethra that we examined.

The literature using high doses of DES was stimulated by the finding that similar high doses of DES resulted in a rare vaginal cancer in the female offspring of women treated with DES during pregnancy.[73] This led to extensive research on the DES daughters, as well as on both male and female rats and mice exposed to DES during sexual differentiation. Unfortunately, studies of DES sons have been much smaller and not of sufficient power to adequately assess the possibility of abnormalities of the prostate.[74] Epidemiological studies of DES daughters and experimental evidence concerning DES-exposed female mice has revealed that there is over 90% concordance for effects.[73] Prostate abnormalities would thus be expected in DES sons given the findings that tumors (albeit at a low frequency) occur in mid-life following developmental exposure to DES in male rats and mice.[69,70]

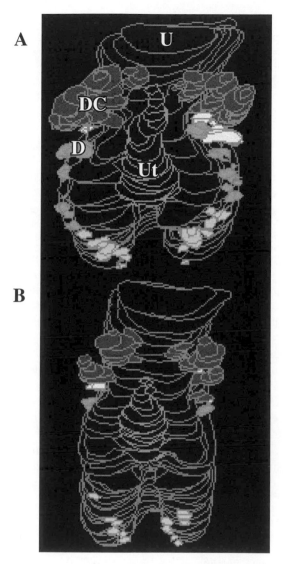

FIGURE 12.5 These computer-assisted, serial-section reconstructions show the dorsal portion of the prostate from two mouse fetuses. The top prostate (Panel A) is reconstructed from a male fetus exposed to 0.32 pg/ml free serum estradiol. The prostate from an untreated male with 0.21 pg/ml free serum estradiol is shown below in Panel B. Glandular buds that form into the dorsocranial (DC) and dorsal (D) glands in the adult prostate can be seen as outgrowths of the fetal urogenital sinus (ventral buds are not visible). The utriculus (Ut) is the remnant of the regressing embryonic female reproductive tract (Müllerian ducts). Compared to controls, estradiol significantly increased the number and size of prostatic glandular buds and caused a reduction in the size of the lumen of the urethra, which passes through the prostate. From Reference 8.

12.5.2 STIMULATORY EFFECTS OF LOW, PHYSIOLOGICAL DOSES OF ESTROGEN

In contrast to the early studies of responses to high doses of estrogens that led to the initial view that estrogen inhibited prostate development, we found that male mouse and rat fetuses exposed *in utero* to the highest levels of endogenous estradiol (i.e., within a physiological range) showed an increase in prostate size, associated with an increase in prostatic androgen receptors.[75,76] We subsequently administered increasing doses of both estradiol (via Silastic capsule) and DES (via feeding) to pregnant female mice and examined the prostate in male offspring in adulthood. Following fetal exposure to both estradiol and DES, we found an inverted-U dose-response relationship for adult prostate weight.[8] Specifically, as serum estradiol concentrations were increased in male mouse fetuses via maternal Silastic implants from 50 to 800% relative to controls, first an increase and then a decrease in adult prostate weight was observed in male offspring.

The lowest dose of estradiol that we administered to pregnant mice via Silastic capsule resulted in a 50% increase in free serum estradiol in male mouse fetuses from 0.2 pg/ml (in controls) to 0.3 pg/ml (measured on gestation day 18). This 0.1 pg/ml increase in free serum estradiol was associated with an increase in total serum estradiol of 52 pg/ml (from 94 pg/ml in controls to 146 pg/ml); the percentage free estradiol in fetal mouse serum is 0.2%. The 0.1 pg/ml increase in free serum estradiol increased the number of developing prostate glands (by 40%) based on three-dimensional reconstruction of the prostate collected from male fetuses on gestation day 18, 1 day after initiation of fetal prostate development (Figure 12.5). The developing prostatic glandular ducts in the dorsal region of the UGS were also enlarged in estrogen-treated males relative to control males. This effect on the prostate was permanent. In adulthood, males exposed to the 50% increase in estradiol during fetal life had enlarged prostates (by 40%) that showed a sixfold increase in prostatic androgen receptors relative to prenatally untreated males.[8]

There is also a significant enlargement of the utricule in male mouse fetuses caused by the 0.1 pg/ml increase in free serum estradiol.[8] It is well known that elevated levels of estrogen inhibit regression of the Müllerian ducts. For example, treatment of pregnant females with DES interferes with the action of Müllerian-inhibiting hormone on Müllerian duct regression in mice[70] and humans.[71] The utriculus is the Müllerian duct remnant that persists within the central zone of the human prostate,[77] and the size of this area of the prostate in men may thus correlate with fetal estradiol exposure; this portion of the Müllerian duct differentiates into the dorsocranial portion of the vagina in females.[38]

Similar to low doses of estradiol, feeding pregnant mice DES at doses of 0.02, 0.2 and 2 μg/kg/day body weight/day permanently increased prostate weight in male offspring (Figure 12.6). A DES dose of 20 μg/kg/day led to prostate weight that did not differ significantly from control males, while 200 μg/kg/day significantly decreased adult prostate weight [8]. Taken together, the above findings provide evidence that with regard to prostate development, effects seen in response to high, pharmacological/toxicological doses of natural or manmade estrogens are opposite to effects seen with low doses within the normal physiological range of estrogenic activity.[6,78]

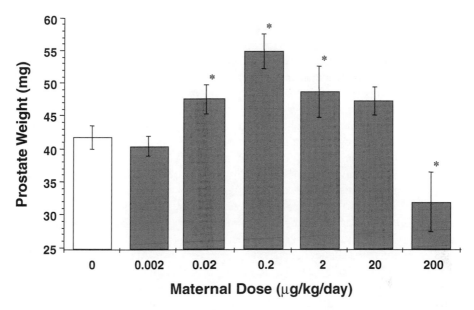

FIGURE 12.6 Mean (+SEM) prostate weight (mg) in 8-month-old CF-1 male mice produced by females fed different doses of DES from day 11 - 17 of pregnancy. Group means that differed significantly from controls are indicated by an asterisk. From Reference 8.

Using computer assisted 3-D reconstruction, we have also found that feeding pregnant mice a low, 0.1 µg/kg/day dose of DES stimulated additional prostate duct formation as well as an increase in the size of the ducts when male mouse fetuses were examined on gestation day 19 just prior to parturition. In contrast, a high 200 µg/kg/day dose of DES completely inhibited the development of ducts in the dorsolateral prostate.[79] Gupta reported virtually identical findings based on feeding pregnant mice the same low and high doses of DES. Gupta also conducted an *in vitro* experiment with fetal UGS in primary culture. She held the level of testosterone constant, and addition of 0.1 pg/ml DES stimulated an increase in prostate ducts, confirming the very high sensitivity of the developing mouse prostate to estrogen.[5]

12.5.3 MECHANISMS OF EFFECTS OF LOW DOSES OF ESTROGEN

There is considerable evidence for estrogen responsiveness (the presence of estrogen receptors) of the prostate in rodents and other mammals.[80-83] The discovery of two types of estrogen receptor (ERα and ERβ), and their differential localization in prostatic epithelium and stroma, has led to speculation about different biological effects.[84] This is particularly relevant when comparing effects of natural and environmental estrogens. For example, bisphenol A leads to different responses with ERβ present or ERα present.[85] In addition, the ligand-activation properties of ERα and ERβ differ in response to estrogenic chemicals present in plants such as soy, flax, clover, etc., such that ERβ is fully induced by some phytoestrogens that are only partial agonists for ERα.[86] The high-dose effects of estrogens on the mouse prostate, including histological changes and down-regulation of AR, appears to be mediated by ERα, which is expressed in mesenchyme, and not ERβ, which is expressed in epithelium in the mouse.[87] Our findings also show that during prostate development in fetal rats (on gestation day 20), UGS mesenchyme strongly expresses mRNA for ERα, while ERα mRNA in UGS epithelium is at background levels.[76]

In the developing human, ERα protein is not detectable in mesenchyme or epithelium during prenatal development. ERβ protein is not present in the human UGS during the initial formation of epithelial buds. However, ERβ protein is strongly expressed in epithelial basal cells beginning in mid-gestation, when prostate proliferation is most active, leading these authors to suggest that ERβ might mediate the effects of estrogen on epithelial cell proliferation in the prostate of human fetuses.[33] Since ERβ is the only estrogen receptor present in the human UGS during development, and since ERβ is more strongly activated by phytoestrogens and xenoestrogens than ERα, studies of xenoestrogen effects in the mouse, which expresses ERα in the UGS mesenchyme during development, may actually underestimate effects on the prostate in human fetuses.

In addition to the studies conducted by Gupta reviewed above, there are a number of other studies that have shown a stimulating effect of estrogen on the prostate. For example, estradiol (10 pM) stimulated androgen receptor-mediated transcriptional activity induced by dihydrotestosterone (DHT). This was demonstrated *in vitro* using UGS cells co-transfected with estrogen receptor and androgen receptor expression vectors.[88] In addition, estrogen and androgen have been shown to have a synergistic interaction in stimulating stromal cells obtained from hyperplastic human prostates,[89] and estradiol can stimulate androgen receptor transcriptional activity in the presence of the co-activator ARA70.[90] We have investigated the effects of estradiol on fetal mouse UGS mesenchyme cells in primary culture. Our results partially recapitulate the effects of estradiol observed *in vivo*. We have shown that at low, physiological doses, estradiol acts directly on cells of the UGS mesenchyme to up-regulate expression of androgen receptor mRNA.[91,92] This up-regulation of AR mRNA was observed over a wide dose range, from 1 pM to 10 µM estradiol. A dose of 100 nM estradiol induced the maximum AR expression.[91] Although the dose-response curve for AR mRNA induced by estradiol was inverted-U shaped, as expected from *in vivo* results, the dose range resulting in up-regulation of AR mRNA was much greater than expected. AR mRNA was up-regulated at both physiological and pharmacological doses. In addition, down-regulation of AR mRNA relative to the control was not observed, in contrast to *in vivo* studies, which consistently show down-regulation of AR at pharmacological doses.

Thus, the down-regulation of AR mRNA at high doses of estradiol must come about through a separate mechanism of action, distinct from the low-dose up-regulation of AR mRNA in response to estradiol. Indeed, a recent study has shown that neonatal exposure to high doses of estrogens permanently increases the rate of proteosomal degradation of androgen receptor protein in the prostate.[93] Based on these results, enhanced transcription of AR mRNA may contribute to the increase in androgen receptor activity observed at low doses of estrogen, and degradation of AR protein by the proteosome may contribute to the decrease in androgen receptor activity observed at high doses of estrogen. The report that estrogen only stimulates TGF-α at supra-physiological doses in MCF-7 breast cancer cells, and that a markedly different array of other genes is turned off and on as the doses of estrogen increase from the physiological range to the supra-physiological range, makes it likely that multiple mechanisms will be found to mediate inverted-U dose-response curves for estrogen in different tissues *in vivo*. [94]

The changes in AR mRNA levels that we observed in cells exposed to physiological levels of estradiol were relatively modest, between 20% and 50%.[91] However, androgen binding measurements both *in vivo* and *in vitro* have revealed consistently greater changes, from twofold to sevenfold, in response to physiological doses of estrogens.[5,8] Gene array analyses of gene expression patterns often use a cut-off of twofold or threefold changes when determining which genes are regulated by a treatment. However, the magnitude of change in mRNA levels is not always indicative of the magnitude of change in the physiology of the tissue or organism under study. A further complication is that different genes have different sensitivities, different-shaped dose-response curves, and different time courses.[94,95] Therefore, investigations of gene expression patterns at high doses of estrogens may not be relevant to the physiological responses observed at low doses of estrogens. The inverted-U-shaped dose-response curve observed for prostate size in mice exposed to estrogens is likely to reflect interplay between systemic and local responses. At the tissue level, each of hundreds of changes in expression of genes could contribute to dose-related differences in phenotype.

Estradiol can directly bind and activate androgen receptor (AR) in the presence of the co-activator ARA_{70}.[90] In the LNCaP prostate cancer cell line, either estrogen or androgen can activate formation of a complex of AR, estrogen receptor (ER), and Src, and thus induce cell proliferation through the Src-Ras-Erks pathway.[96] AR activates PAK6 kinase activity, and PAK6 inhibits transcriptional activation by AR and ER.[97] Estrogen receptor alpha (ERα) can directly bind AR and alter transcriptional activation by AR.[88,98] Finally, estrogen alters AR expression levels in a tissue-specific manner.[99-101] Analysis of gene expression patterns in adult human prostate stroma cells in response to a high dose of estradiol revealed hundreds of estrogen-regulated genes.[95] Estrogen treatment thus has pleiotropic effects, both *in vivo* and *in vitro*. Many "housekeeping" genes are up-regulated by estradiol, including the ribosomal protein RBP and the cytoskeleton protein vimentin.[92]

There is evidence that EGF and IGF-1 may be required to mediate the effects of estrogens on prostate epithelial proliferation.[102] EGF can mimic effects of estrogens by activating the estrogen receptor in female mice.[103] EGF is required for DES-induced growth and branching of mouse prostate organ cultures, while IGF-1 is required only for DES-induced branching.[102]

In dogs, estradiol synergizes with dihydrotestosterone to increase androgen binding in prostatic cells and thus increases prostate growth.[104] Studies have also shown that estradiol influences hypothalamic androgen receptors in adult male rats.[105] In addition, estradiol regulates the expression of receptors for a number of hormones, such as uterine oxytocin receptors and both uterine and brain progesterone receptors.[106,107] Taken together, these findings show that the physiological effects of exposure to estrogen can include changes in the functioning of a variety of tissues due to changes in the receptors for other hormones that regulate these tissues.

Importantly, when exposure to estrogen occurs during critical periods in development, effects on tissue function are permanent.

Interestingly, elevation of testosterone levels during development appears to have similar effects compared to elevation of estrogen levels. Aromatase knockout mice are unable to produce estrogen, and males exhibit increased testosterone and DHT levels in serum and tissues. These males also have enlarged prostates.[108] Thus, both an increase in serum androgen levels caused by deficient aromatase activity, and an increase in prostatic androgen receptor levels induced by elevated estrogen exposure, can lead to stimulation of prostate growth.

12.6   ENVIRONMENTAL ENDOCRINE-DISRUPTING ESTROGENIC CHEMICALS ALTER PROSTATE DEVELOPMENT

Studies now identify that many chemicals have the capacity to disrupt the functioning of the endocrine system, either by binding to endogenous hormone receptors, by interfering with enzyme activity, or via other mechanisms, such as interfering with plasma transport of hormones.[109,110] Thus, there are chemicals being used in common household products that, prior to being used to manufacture these products, were not tested for the possibility that they might be able to bind to receptors for natural steroids, such as estrogen and androgen. Because development of all organs is coordinated by endocrine signals, the disruption of endocrine signals during critical periods in organ development can lead to permanent effects on organ function. Functional effects might not be noticed based only on examination for gross malformations, which, along with cancer, has been the focus of toxicological testing.

Chemicals used as pesticides, such as methoxychlor,[78] stimulate enlargement of the prostate as a result of exposure to very low, environmentally relevant doses during development. Interestingly, the organochlorine hexachlorobenzene (HCB) enhances androgen signaling in the prostate at low doses and represses androgen signaling at high doses.[111]

We recently examined the effects of fetal exposure to bisphenol A, an estrogen-mimicking chemical. Bisphenol A is used to make polycarbonate plastic (for example, baby-feeding bottles are made from polycarbonate). Bisphenol A is also a component of the resin lining of food and beverage cans, in dental sealants, and many other plastic products. Approximately 2 billion pounds of bisphenol A are used per year, and another 100 million pounds of brominated bisphenol A are used as flame retardants in a wide variety of products.

We used a screening assay involving human breast cancer cells (MCF-7) to assess the estrogenic potency of bisphenol A. This assay revealed that the plasma binding proteins that result in a very low free, bioavailable fraction of estradiol in fetal blood show only limited binding to bisphenol A. The proportion of the unconjugated bisphenol A in blood that is bioactive is thus high relative to estradiol.[7] Our findings suggested that developing mouse fetuses would respond to doses of bisphenol A within the range that humans are exposed to this chemical, such as through the use of polycarbonate to store food, eating canned products, and having dental sealant applied to protect teeth.

Based on predictions from our *in vitro* assay, we fed pregnant mice 2 or 20 µg/kg/day bisphenol A per gram body weight per day for 7 days from gestation day 11 to 17, prior to and during the initial period of prostate development. We observed numerous effects in male offspring, including permanent enlargement of the prostate and preputial glands, a decrease in testicular sperm production, and a decrease in seminal vesicle and epididymidal size.[7,112] In female offspring, we observed abnormal body growth and an early onset of puberty.[113] Many other effects of very low doses of bisphenol A have been reported in over 60 peer-reviewed publications in mollusks, insects, fish, frogs, rats, and mice.

The Wolffian ducts and UGS express estrogen receptors during prenatal development in the mouse.[83,114] Therefore, these organs can potentially be directly affected by compounds that bind to estrogen receptors, such as bisphenol A. The decrease in the size of the epididymis and seminal vesicles suggests that bisphenol A interfered with the normal development of the Wolffian ducts as well as the testes. In contrast, bisphenol A significantly increased the size of the preputial glands and prostate relative to untreated males. The finding that an elevation in an estrogenic chemical during fetal life decreased seminal vesicle size in adulthood is consistent with our prior findings. Specifically, male mice that developed *in utero* between two female fetuses (2F males), and were thus exposed to elevated estradiol via diffusion from the adjacent females, had smaller seminal vesicles in adulthood than their siblings who developed *in utero* between two male fetuses (2M males); in contrast, 2F males had larger prostates.[75]

Subsequent studies have suggested that this effect was mediated by a permanent "imprinted" decrease in seminal vesicle 5α-reductase activity in 2F males relative to 2M males (unpublished observation). However, the larger seminal vesicles found in 2M male mice were initially thought to be due solely to the supplement in testosterone that 2M males received due to being positioned *in utero* between male fetuses. The finding that a low dose of an estrogenic chemical during fetal life can permanently decrease seminal vesicle and epididymis size provides additional evidence that suggests the elevated estradiol in 2F males may have contributed to the development of small seminal vesicles in these males. It had previously been reported that estrogen exerts an inhibitory effect on 5α-reductase activity in accessory reproductive organs.[115,116]

In contrast to findings regarding organs that differentiate from Wolffian ducts, adult 2F male mice, as well as male mice exposed experimentally as fetuses to a 50% increase in serum estradiol, exhibited enlargement of the prostate that was associated with a permanent increase in prostatic androgen receptors.[8,75] As mentioned above, the prostate develops from the UGS, while seminal vesicles develop from a different embryonic tissue, the Wolffian ducts, under different hormonal control. Taken together, these findings provide evidence that during fetal life, the specific genes influenced by estrogen are different in the Wolffian ducts and UGS. Thus, what appeared initially as contradictory findings, with some organs increasing in size and others decreasing in size, associated with a small increase in serum estradiol during fetal life, now has proven to be a consistent outcome following administration of estrogenic chemicals during fetal life.

An interesting finding is that bisphenol A stimulated proliferation of human prostate cancer (LNCaP) cells. There was an inverted-U dose-response curve, with maximum stimulation at 1 nM (~230 parts per trillion, or ppt) and lower stimulation at doses tenfold lower (23 ppt) or tenfold higher (2.3 ppb), and no stimulation at either 2.3 ppt (NOAEL) or 23 ppb. Of considerable importance is that the 23 ppb dose of bisphenol A would have been erroneously thought to be the no adverse effect level (NOAEL), if this had been the lowest dose tested in a study that had only examined higher but not lower doses.[117]

There is a mutant form of the androgen receptor in LNCaP cells that appears to show a higher binding to bisphenol A than the wild-type androgen receptor. This raises the question as to the potential for bisphenol A to exhibit significant binding to other members of the nuclear receptor superfamily, such as androgen receptors. In fact, there is a report that bisphenol A can bind to androgen receptors. Specifically, bisphenol A had an efficacy similar to the antiandrogenic drug Flutamide in inhibiting binding of DHT to androgen receptors in a yeast reporter assay. But, at the concentrations detected in human blood,[118] there should not be significant binding of bisphenol A to wild type androgen receptors. In sharp contrast, the concentration of bisphenol A that stimulated LNCaP prostate cells with the mutant form of the androgen receptor was directly within the range of bisphenol A found in human blood.

Gupta[5] reported that in CD-1 mice, oral administration of bisphenol A to pregnant mice at a dose of 50 µg/kg/day from gestation day 14 to 18 resulted in a permanent increase in prostate size and prostate androgen receptors. Bisphenol A also caused a decrease in the size of the epididymis. In this study by Gupta, male mice were examined at 3, 21, and 60 days of age. The finding that fetal exposure increased prostate androgen receptors is virtually identical to the significant increase in prostate androgen receptors produced by a small increase in fetal estradiol [8] or a maternal dose of 0.1 µg/kg/day diethylstilbestrol (DES), and also exactly replicated our findings [112] of an increase in prostate size and a decrease in epididymis size in male mice using 2 and 20 µg/kg/day bisphenol administered to pregnant cf.-1 mice.

A novel finding in the study by Gupta is that the 50 µg/kg/day dose of bisphenol A resulted in an increase in the length of the space between the anus and genital papilla (that becomes the scrotum) on postnatal days 3 and 21, similar to the increase in the size of the prostate. It is well known that the UGS (from which the prostate differentiates) and the external genitals are similar in the hormonal and enzyme activity (specifically 5α-reductase) requirements for normal differentiation during fetal life. In contrast, as described above, the development of the seminal vesicles and epididymis from the Wolffian ducts shows marked differences from the UGS in the hormonal requirements and intracellular enzymes that mediate the early period of differentiation. It is thus consistent with other findings[75] that exposure during fetal life to low doses of bisphenol A increases the size of the prostate and the anogenital distance measure, yet decreases the size of the seminal vesicles and epididymis. It is important that in these same studies Gupta found that a high dose of DES (200 µg/kg/day) administered to pregnant mice had opposite effects than a low dose

(0.1 µg/kg/day); the high dose both inhibited prostate development and decreased the anogenital distance measure, consistent with many prior findings in rats and mice.[4,8]

To determine whether effects of bisphenol A were directly on the prostate, Gupta[5,102] placed the fetal mouse prostate in primary culture. A 50 pg/ml (50 ppt) dose of bisphenol A stimulated prostate growth and gland formation, as well as androgen receptors, while a dose of 5 ppt bisphenol A did not produce a significant stimulatory effect.[5] The effect of 50 ppt bisphenol A was similar to the effect of 0.5 ppt DES examined in the same experiment, demonstrating that bisphenol A is about 100-fold less potent relative to DES. We will review other studies below also showing effects of bisphenol A at doses of 50 ppt in invertebrates.

Based on initial findings from experiments in which we observed permanent enlargement of the prostate in male offspring as a result of administering pregnant mice doses of bisphenol A,[7] DES,[8] and ethinyl estradiol,[119] as well as the findings reported by Gupta,[5] we directly compared the effects of these three estrogenic chemicals on the fetal prostate in mice using 3-D reconstruction. Figure 12.6 shows that relative to controls, DES and ethinyl estradiol at a dose of 0.1 µg/kg/day and bisphenol A at a dose of 10 µg/kg/day stimulated the formation of additional prostate ducts and epithelial hyperplasia. Epithelial hyperplasia was revealed by more than a 50% increase in staining for proliferating cell nuclear antigen (PCNA) by each of the three estrogenic chemicals based on staining of sections containing prostate buds from the 3-D reconstruction. The pattern of PCNA staining overlapped with staining for mouse keratin 5 (MK 5), a basal cell marker.

Based on the above findings, in Figure 12.7 we propose a model of potential stages and tissues in early ductal development in the UGS that are influenced by exposure to estrogenic chemicals.[79] Our findings show that proliferation of UGS epithelial cells in the dorsolateral prostate by estrogenic chemicals promotes ductal growth from the base to the distal tip through increased stimulation of cell proliferation at the proximal end of the duct. Basal cells are a subset of epithelial cells found in the undifferentiated UGS and then in the developing prostate ducts,[120] and our findings suggest that basal cells provide the proliferative pool during the initial formation of ducts. The cords of ductal cells appear to be pushed out from the UGS into the surrounding mesenchyme as a result of proliferation of the basal cells. Estrogenic chemical stimulated the formation of additional ducts and also increased the rate of epithelial proliferation in the dorsal and lateral region of the UGS, while little effect of estrogen was observed in the ventral UGS. Estrogen may act to stimulate a larger proportion of basal cells into the proliferating pool in the dorsal and lateral UGS, revealing a regional effect of estrogen within the developing UGS, which is known to express estrogen receptors at this time in development.[76,114] An interesting aspect of these findings is that once branching of the ducts begins, proliferation occurs at the ductal tip.[21]

An interesting additional observation is that these estrogenic chemicals also resulted in a significant decrease in the size of the urethra at the bladder neck, as well as a gross malformation in the region of the colliculus (Figure 12.4). These findings show that bisphenol A is approximately 100-fold less potent relative to DES, which is consistent with findings by Gupta based on both *in vivo* and *in vitro*

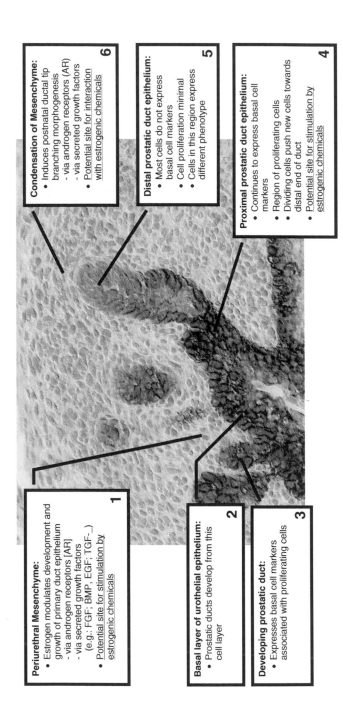

Condensation of Mesenchyme:
- Induces postnatal ductal tip branching morphogenesis
  - via androgen receptors (AR)
  - via secreted growth factors
- Potential site for interaction with estrogenic chemicals

6

Distal prostatic duct epithelium:
- Most cells do not express basal cell markers
- Cell proliferation minimal
- Cells in this region express different phenotype

5

Proximal prostatic duct epithelium:
- Continues to express basal cell markers
- Region of proliferating cells
- Dividing cells push new cells towards distal end of duct
- Potential site for stimulation by estrogenic chemicals

4

Periurethral Mesenchyme:
- Estrogen modulates development and growth of primary duct epithelium
  - via androgen receptors [AR]
  - via secreted growth factors (e.g.: FGF; BMP, EGF; TGF–)
- Potential site for stimulation by estrogenic chemicals

1

Basal layer of urothelial epithelium:
- Prostatic ducts develop from this cell layer

2

Developing prostatic duct:
- Expresses basal cell markers associated with proliferating cells

3

FIGURE 12.7 Sequence of events associated with initial development and growth of prostatic duct epithelium (1 to 6). Potential areas of action for estrogenic chemicals in the mesenchyme (blue boxes; 1 and 6) and the epithelium (red box; 4) are indicated. Each of these regions provides a unique opportunity for estrogenic effects on the relationship between mesenchyme and growth controlling factors, particularly in mesenchyme adjacent to the urethra and base of developing ducts and the epithelial-mesenchymal interface at the ductal tip. Because the proximal duct is associated with the proliferative population of cells, this is the most sensitive area for estrogenic effects on epithelium during development. FGF: fibroblast growth factor; BMP: bone morphogenic proteins; EGF: epidermal growth factor; TGF-β: transforming growth factor-beta. From Reference 79.

experiments.[5] An important aspect of these findings is that the blood levels of bisphenol A in fetal mice throughout the 24 hours after maternal administration of bisphenol A are significantly lower than mean blood levels of unconjugated bisphenol A in human fetuses.[118,121]

Finally, in primary cultures of UGS mesenchyme cells, bisphenol A also significantly increased AR mRNA levels at the lowest dose (1 nM) so far examined.[122] These findings confirm two different studies by Gupta[5,102] that bisphenol A increases androgen receptor protein in the fetal prostate in primary organ culture.

Taken together, the findings reported by Gupta, Nagel, Richter, Timms, and vom Saal are consistent in showing virtually identical effects of both bisphenol A and DES on the prostate *in vitro* and *in vivo* in outbred mice (cf.-1 and CD-1). In contrast, in inbred mice (C57BL/6N), bisphenol A was reported to not alter testis, epididymis, or seminal vesicle weight at doses of 2, 20, or 200 µg/kg/day administered at different life stages.[123] This finding is interesting in that we have found that C57BL/6J males are 1000-fold less responsive to the stimulatory effects of fetal DES exposure on prostate size relative to either cf.-1 or CD-1 male fetuses, while the effects of DES on the uterus of the female siblings of these males showed an identical response to DES (unpublished observation). Our findings, and that of Nagao et al., thus are in contrast to the findings of Spearow,[124] who reported that peripubertal administration of estradiol to C57 mice had a greater suppressing effect on testis relative to CD-1 mice. Studies to compare the response to different estrogenic chemicals at different life stages in different rat and mouse strains are needed to clarify these diverse findings.

In a study by Ramos et al.,[125] on gestation day 8 pregnant Wistar rats were implanted with Alza osmotic pumps that released bisphenol A at doses of 25 and 250 µg/kg/day. Prenatal exposure to both doses of bisphenol A increased the size of the area occupied by fibroblasts but decreased the size of the area occupied by smooth muscle in the periductal stroma of the ventral prostate of males examined when 30 days old. These changes in the cytoarchitecture of the ventral prostate were associated with a decrease in the proportion of periductal stroma cells that were positive for androgen receptors in males exposed to both doses of bisphenol A. These findings are thus different from those observed in the mouse prostate as a result of exposure during fetal life to low doses of bisphenol A. However, our findings have suggested that the ventral region of the rat and mouse prostate has a different sensitivity to estrogenic effects relative to the dorsolateral prostate.[76,79]

12.7 ESTROGEN AND ADULT PROSTATE PATHOLOGY

Exposure to supplemental estrogen (in combination with androgen) in adulthood has been related to hyperplasia of the prostate in dogs[126] and dysplasia and neoplasia in Noble rats.[127] In mice, elevation of either androgens or estrogens alone fails to produce dysplasia, but treatment with androgens and estrogens in combination resulted in prostatic dysplasia.[128] In Noble rats, neoplastic tumors can be induced to form in the dorsolateral prostatic lobes, while Sprague-Dawley rats typically do not develop tumors.[127,129-131] Although fewer than 1% of Noble rats spontaneously develop adenocarcinoma of the prostate, treatment with a combination of low doses of testosterone and estradiol-17b (via Silastic capsules) for 4 months leads to multifocal epithelial dysplasia,[131,132] and longer treatment (about 10 months) results in the transition from dysplasia to neoplastic tumors in about 20% of treated males. Histological examination of prostate tumors in Noble rats treated with androgen and estrogen showed that they primarily involved glandular epithelium, and metastases after transplantation into hosts revealed differentiated epithelial components.[129] Neoplastic development occurs in specific regions of the peripheral zone of the human prostate gland.[133] Dysplasia in the dorsolateral lobe of testosterone and estradiol treated Noble rats is almost identical to the premalignant lesions described in the human gland.

12.8 SUMMARY

There is little or no information concerning the issue of whether prostate enlargement in men might be related to exposure during fetal life to estrogenic chemicals. However, there has been a doubling of the incidence of abnormal development of the penile urethra (hypospadias) in male babies over the past 20 years in the U.S.,[134] suggesting that an environmental factor is involved.[135] There is historical evidence that male sperm counts have declined by 50% over the past 50 years, while the incidence of testicular and prostate cancer has increased; there are regional differences in sperm counts as well as prostate and testicular cancer rates. These findings suggest that environmental factors are mediating these effects,[136-138] which is supported by recent evidence correlating herbicide levels in men with sperm density.[139] Prospective studies in humans (the Children's Health Initiative) that will include examination of the relationship of exposure to chemicals during fetal life via the mother (as well as many other factors), and consequences to health, are being planned based on findings from animal studies.

At this time there have been no published human studies to raise awareness within the medical community or the Food and Drug Administration (FDA) concerning fetal exposure to bisphenol A from polycarbonate plastic food and beverage containers, tin cans, and dental sealants or in drinking water. The focus of the relatively few studies of exposure of human fetuses to ethinylestradiol during the critical period of reproductive organ development has only been on externally visible malformations at birth. Based upon generally negative findings of grossly observable external malformations at birth, DES was considered safe for administration to millions of women during pregnancy for over 2 decades, but later DES was found to result in serious long-term harm to offspring. This tragic lesson appears to have been forgotten with regard to conclusions being drawn from similar studies of ethinylestradiol. The current assumption is that the amounts of ethinylestradiol or bisphenol A to which human fetuses are exposed are safe. We propose that the data from this and other animal studies regarding the potential for ethinylestradiol and bisphenol A to be considered as risk factors during fetal development at current exposure levels is sufficient, and together with the similarity to effects of low doses of DES, warrant a thorough reevaluation of this assumption.

ACKNOWLEDGMENTS

We thank Dr. Ellen Shapiro for providing the human tissue. Funding was provided by grants to CAR from NIEHS (ES-11549), BGT from EPA R-827403, and FVS from NIEHS (ES11283).

REFERENCES

1. Pang, S., Chow, P., and Wong, T., The role of the seminal vesicles, coagulating glands and prostate on the fertility and fecundity of mice, *J. Reprod. Fertil.*, 56, 129, 1979.
2. Zuckerman, S., The endocrine control of the prostate, *Proc. R. Soc. Med.*, 29, 1557, 1936.
3. Franks, L.M., Benign nodular hyperplasia of the prostate: a review, *Annals of the Royal College Surgeons of England*, 14, 92, 1954.
4. Prins, G.S., Developmental estrogenization of the prostate gland, in *Prostate: Basic and Clinical Aspects*, Naz, R.K., CRC Press, Boca Raton, FL, 1997, pp. 247.
5. Gupta, C., Reproductive malformation of the male offspring following maternal exposure to estrogenic chemicals, *Proc. Soc. Exp. Biol. Med.*, 224, 61, 2000.
6. Welshons, W.V. et al. Large effects from small exposures. I. Mechanisms for endocrine-disrupting chemicals with estrogenic activity, *Environ. Health Perspect.*, 111, 994, 2003.
7. Nagel, S.C. et al. Relative binding affinity-serum modified access (RBA-SMA) assay predicts the relative *in vivo* bioactivity of the xenoestrogens bisphenol A and octylphenol, *Environ. Health Perspect.*, 105, 70, 1997.
8. vom Saal, F.S. et al. Prostate enlargement in mice due to fetal exposure to low doses of estradiol or diethylstilbestrol and opposite effects at high doses, *Proc. Natl. Acad. Sci. USA*, 94, 2056, 1997.
9. Montano, M.M., Welshons, W.V., and vom Saal, F.S., Free estradiol in serum and brain uptake of estradiol during fetal and neonatal sexual differentiation in female rats, *Biol. Reprod.*, 53, 1198, 1995.
10. Weir, H.K. et al. Annual report to the nation on the status of cancer, 1975-2000, featuring the uses of surveillance data for cancer prevention and control, *J. Natl. Cancer Inst.*, 95, 1276, 2003.
11. Verhamme, K.M. et al. Incidence and prevalence of lower urinary tract symptoms suggestive of benign prostatic hyperplasia in primary care—the Triumph project, *Eur. Urol.*, 42, 323, 2002.
12. Burstein, S.R., The historical background of gerontology. III. The quest for rejuvenation, *Geriatrics*, 10, 536, 1955.
13. Medvei, V.C., *A History of Endocrinology*, MTP Press, Lancaster, PA, 1982.
14. Tisell, L.-E. and Salander, H., The lobes of the human prostate, *Scand. J. Urol. Nephrol.*, 9, 185, 1975.
15. McNeal, J.E., Anatomy of the prostate: An historical survey of divergent views, *The Prostate*, 1, 3, 1980.
16. Timms, B.G., Anatomical perspectives of prostate development, in *Prostate: Basic and Clinical Aspects*, Naz, R.K., CRC Press, New York, 1997.
17. Lowsley, O.S., The development of the human prostate gland with reference to the development of other structures at the neck of the urinary bladder, *Am. J. Anat.*, 13, 299, 1912.

18. McNeal, J.E., The prostate gland: Morphology and pathobiology, *Monographs in Urology,* 4, 1, 1983.
19. Timms, B.G., Mohs, T.J., and Didio, L.J.A., Ductal budding and branching patterns in the developing prostate, *J. Urol.,* 151, 1427, 1994.
20. Takeda, H., Lasnitzki, I., and Mizuno, T., Analysis of prostatic bud induction by brief androgen treatment in the fetal rat urogenital sinus, *J. Endocrinol.,* 110, 467, 1986.
21. Marker, P.C. et al. Hormonal, cellular, and molecular control of prostatic development, *Dev. Biol.,* 253, 165, 2003.
22. Sugimura, Y., Cunha, G.R., and Donjacour, A.A., Morphogenesis of ductal networks in the mouse prostate, *Biol. Reprod.,* 34, 961, 1986.
23. Lavoipierre, A.M., Ultrasound of the prostate and testicles, *World J. Surg.,* 24, 198, 2000.
24. Sugimura, Y. et al. Whole-mount autoradiography study of DNA synthetic activity during postnatal development and androgen-induced regeneration in the mouse prostate, *Biol. Reprod.,* 34, 985, 1986.
25. Sugimura, Y., Cunha, G.R., and Donjacour, A.A., Morphological and histological study of castration-induced degeneration and androgen-induced regeneration in the mouse prostate, *Biol. Reprod.,* 34, 973, 1986.
26. Hayward, S.W. et al. Interactions between adult human prostatic epithelium and rat urogenital sinus mesenchyme in a tissue recombination model, *Differentiation,* 63, 131, 1998.
27. McNeal, J., Pathology of benign prostatic hyperplasia. Insight into etiology, *Urol. Clin. North Am.,* 17, 477, 1990.
28. Price, D., Comparative aspects of development and structure in the prostate, *Natl. Cancer Inst. Monogr.,* 12, 1, 1963.
29. McNeal, J.E., The anatomic heterogeneity of the prostate, in *Models of Prostate Cancer,* Coffey, D., Merchant, D., and Murphy, G., Liss, New York, 1980, pp. 149.
30. Hiraoka, Y. and Akimoto, M., Anatomy of the Prostate from Fetus to Adult-Origin of Benign Prostatic Hyperplasia, *Urol. Res.,* 177, 1987.
31. Aumüller, G., Morphologic and regulatory aspects of prostatic function, *Anat. Embryol.,* 179, 519, 1989.
32. Thomson, A.A. et al. The role of smooth muscle in regulating prostatic induction, *Development,* 129, 1905, 2002.
33. Adams, J.Y. et al. Expression of estrogen receptor beta in the fetal, neonatal, and prepubertal human prostate, *Prostate,* 52, 69, 2002.
34. Aboseif, S. et al. Mesenchymal reprogramming of adult human epithelial differentiation, *Differentiation,* 65, 113, 1999.
35. Block, E., Lew, M., and Klein, M., Studies on the inhibition of fetal androgen formation: Testosterone synthesis by fetal and newborn mouse testes *in vitro, Endocrinol.,* 88, 41, 1971.
36. Wilson, J.D., George, F.W., and Griffin, J.E., The hormonal control of sexual development, *Science,* 211, 1278, 1981.
37. vom Saal, F.S., Sexual differentiation in litter bearing mammals: influence of sex of adjacent fetuses *in utero, J. Anim. Sci.,* 67, 1824, 1989.
38. vom Saal, F.S., Montano, M.M., and Wang, M.H., Sexual differentiation in mammals, in *Chemically Induced Alterations in Sexual and Functional Development: The Wildlife/Human Connection,* Colborn, T. and Clement, C., Princeton Scientific Publishing Co., Princeton, NJ, 1992, pp. 17.
39. Roy, A.K. et al. Regulation of androgen action, *Vitam. Horm.,* 55, 309, 1999.

40. Bardin, C.W. and Catterall, J.F., Testosterone: a major determinant of extragenital sexual dimorphism, *Science,* 211, 1285, 1981.

41. Dadras, S.S. et al. Inhibition of 5 α-reductase in rat prostate reveals differential regulation of androgen-response gene expression by testosterone and dihydrotestosterone, *Gene Expr.,* 9, 183, 2001.

42. Cunha, G.R. and Chung, L.W., Stromal-epithelial interactions—I. Induction of prostatic phenotype in urothelium of testicular feminized (Tfm/y) mice, *J. Steroid Biochem.,* 14, 1317, 1981.

43. Shannon, J.M. and Cunha, G.R., Autoradiographic localization of androgen binding in the developing mouse prostate, *The Prostate,* 4, 367, 1983.

44. Takeda, H. et al. Autoregulation of androgen receptor expression in rodent prostate: Immunohistochemical and *in situ* hybridization analysis, *Biochem. Biophys. Res. Commun.,* 177, 488, 1991.

45. Davies, J.A., Do different branching epithelia use a conserved developmental mechanism?, *Bioessays,* 24, 937, 2002.

46. Gioeli, D. et al. Androgen receptor phosphorylation: Regulation and identification of the phosphorylation sites, *J. Biol. Chem.,* 277, 29304, 2002.

47. Gupta, C., Modulation of androgen receptor (AR)-mediated transcriptional activity by EGF in the developing mouse reproductive tract primary cells, *Mol. Cell. Endocrinol.,* 152, 169, 1999.

48. Thomson, A.A., Foster, B.A., and Cunha, G.R., Analysis of growth factor and receptor mRNA levels during development of the rat seminal vesicle and prostate, *Development,* 124, 2431, 1997.

49. Donjacour, A.A., Thomson, A.A., and Cunha, G.R., FGF-10 plays an essential role in the growth of the fetal prostate, *Dev. Biol.,* 261, 39, 2003.

50. Thomson, A.A. and Cunha, G.R., Prostatic growth and development are regulated by FGF10, *Development,* 126, 3693, 1999.

51. Ruan, W.F. et al. Evidence that insulin-like growth factor I and growth hormone are required for prostate gland development, *Endocrinol.,* 140, 1984, 1999.

52. Abbott, B.D. et al. Lack of expression of EGF and TGF-α in the fetal mouse alters formation of prostatic epithellial buds and influences the response to TCDD, *Toxicol. Sci.,* 76, 427, 2003.

53. Itoh, N., Patel, U., and Skinner, M.K., Developmental and hormonal regulation of transforming growth factor-α and epidermal growth factor receptor gene expression in isolated prostatic epithelial and stromal cells, *Endocrinol.,* 139, 1369, 1998.

54. Marker, P.C. et al. *fucosyltransferase1* and H-type complex carbohydrates modulate epithelial cell proliferation during prostatic branching morphogenesis, *Dev. Biol.,* 233, 95, 2001.

55. Ball, E.M.A. and Risbridger, G.P., New perspectives on growth factor-sex steroid interaction in the prostate, *Cytokine Growth Factor Rev.,* 14, 5, 2003.

56. Itoh, N. et al. Developmental and hormonal regulation of transforming growth factor-β1 (TGFβ1), -2, and -3 gene expression in isolated prostatic epithelial and stromal cells: epidermal growth factor and TGFβ interactions, *Endocrinol.,* 139, 1378, 1998.

57. Lamm, M.L.G. et al. Mesenchymal factor bone morphogenetic protein 4 restricts ductal budding and branching morphogenesis in the developing prostate, *Dev. Biol.,* 232, 301, 2001.

58. Kincl, F., Pi., A., and Lasso, L., Effects of estradiol benzoate treatment in the newborn male rat, *Endocrinol.,* 72, 966, 1963.

59. Arai, Y., Nature of metaplasia in rat coagulating glands induced by neonatal treatment with estrogen, *Endocrinology,* 86, 918, 1970.

60. Rajfer, J. and Coffey, D.S., Sex steroid imprinting of the immature prostate, *Invest. Urol.,* 16, 186 1978.

61. Rajfer, J. and Coffey, D.S., Effects of neonatal steroids on male sex tissues, *Invest. Urol.,* 17, 3, 1979.

62. Vannier, B. and Raynaud, J.P., Long-term effects of prenatal oestrogen treatment on genital morphology and reproductive function in the rat, *J. Reprod. Fertil.,* 59, 43, 1980.

63. Lung, B. and Cunha, G.R., Development of seminal vesicles and coagulating glands in neonatal mice. I. the morphogenetic effects of various hormonal conditions, *The Anatomical Record,* 199, 73, 1981.

64. Prins, G.S., Neonatal estrogen exposure induces lobe-specific alterations in adult rat prostate androgen receptor expression, *Endocrinology,* 130, 2401, 1992.

65. Prins, G.S. et al. Effects of neonatal estrogen exposure on prostatic secretory genes and their correlation with androgen receptor expression in the separate prostate lobes of the adult rat, *Endocrinology,* 132, 2387, 1993.

66. Santti, R. et al. Developmental estrogenization and prostatic neoplasia, *The Prostate,* 24, 67, 1994.

67. Baranao, J. et al. Effects of androgen treatment of the neonate on rat testis and sex accessory organs, *Biol. Reprod.,* 25, 851, 1981.

68. Jarred, R.A. et al. Evidence that estrogens directly alter androgen-regulated prostate development, *Endocrinology,* 141, 3471, 2000.

69. Arai, Y., Chen, C.-Y., and Nishizuka, Y., Cancer development in male reproductive tract in rats given diethylstilbestrol at neonatal age, *Jpn. J. Cancer Res.,* 69, 861, 1978.

70. McLachlan, J.A., Newbold, R.R., and Bullock, B., Reproductive tract lesions in male mice exposed prenatally to diethylstilbestrol, *Science,* 190, 991, 1975.

71. Driscoll, S.G. and Taylor, S.H., Effects of prenatal maternal estrogen on the male urogenital system, *Obstet. Gynecol.,* 56, 537, 1980.

72. Martikainen, P. et al. Interaction of male and female sex hormones in cultured rat prostate, *Prostate,* 11, 291, 1987.

73. Newbold, R., Cellular and molecular effects of developmental exposure to diethyl-stilbestrol: Implications for other environmental estrogens, *Environ. Health Perspect.,* 103, 83, 1995.

74. Swan, S.H. and vom Saal, F.S., Alterations in male reproductive development: The role of endocrine disrupting chemicals, in *Endocrine Disruptors in the Environment,* Metzler, M., Springer-Verlag, Heidelberg, 2001, pp. 131.

75. Nonneman, D.J. et al. Intrauterine position effects on steroid metabolism and steroid receptors of reproductive organs in male mice, *Biol. Reprod.,* 47, 723, 1992.

76. Timms, B.G., Petersen, S.L., and vom Saal, F.S., Prostate gland growth during development is stimulated in both male and female rat fetuses by intrauterine proximity to female fetuses, *J. Urol.,* 161, 1694, 1999.

77. Blacklock, N.J., The development and morphology of the prostate, in *The Endocrinology of Prostate Tumours,* Ghanadian, R., MTP Press, Lancaster, England, 1983, pp. 1.

78. Welshons, W.V. et al. Development of *in vitro* assays to predict activity of xenoestrogens in animals: fetal exposure to methoxychlor and other xenoestrogens increases adult prostate size in mice, *Toxicol. Ind. Health,* 15, 12, 1999.

79. Timms, B.G. et al. Estrogenic chemicals in plastic and oral contraceptives disrupt the fetal mouse prostate and urethra, *Submitted,* 2004.

80. Mawhinney, M. and Neubauer, B., Actions of estrogen in the male, *Invest. Urol.,* 16, 409, 1979.

81. Jung-Testas, I. et al. Androgen and estrogen receptors in rat ventral prostate epithelium and stroma, *Endocrinol.,* 109, 1287, 1981.
82. Cunha, G.R. et al. The endocrinology and developmental biology of the prostate, *Endocr. Rev.,* 8, 338, 1987.
83. Cooke, P.S. et al. Estrogen Receptor Expression in Developing Epididymis, Efferent Ductules, and Other Male Reproductive Organs, *Endocrinol.,* 128, 2874, 1992.
84. Kuiper, G.G.J.M. et al. Cloning of a novel estrogen receptor expressed in rat prostate and ovary, *Proc. Natl. Acad. Sci. USA,* 93, 5925, 1996.
85. Routhledge, E.J. et al. Differential effects of xenoestrogens on coactivator recruitment by estrogen receptor (ER) α and ERβ, *J. Biol. Chem.,* 46, 35986, 2000.
86. Salvatori, L. et al. Oestrogens and selective oestrogen receptor (ER) modulators regulate EGF receptor gene expression through human ER α and β subtypes via an Sp1 site, *Oncogene,* 22, 4875, 2003.
87. Prins, G.S. et al. Estrogen imprinting of the developing prostate gland is mediated through stromal estrogen receptor α: studies with αERKO and βERKO mice, *Cancer Res.,* 61, 6089, 2001.
88. Kumar, V.M., Leo, M.E., and Tindall, D.J., Modulation of androgen receptor transcriptional activity by the estrogen receptor, *J. Androl.,* 15, 534, 1994.
89. Collins, A.T. et al. Androgen and oestrogen responsiveness of stromal cells derived from the human hyperplastic prostate: oestrogen regulation of the androgen receptor, *J. Endocrinol.,* 143, 269, 1994.
90. Yeh, S. et al. From estrogen to androgen receptor: A new pathway for sex hormones in prostate, *Proc. Natl. Acad. Sci. USA,* 95, 5527, 1998.
91. Richter, C.A. and vom Saal, F.S., Dioxin interacts with estrogen and androgen response systems to disrupt prostate development, *Organohalogen Compounds,* 65, 63, 2003.
92. Richter, C.A. et al. Estradiol upregulates androgen receptor mRNA in fetal mouse urogenital sinus mesenchyme cells, *Submitted,* 2004.
93. Woodham, C., Birch, L., and Prins, G.S., Neonatal estrogen down-regulates prostatic androgen receptor through a proteosome-mediated protein degradation pathway, *Endocrinol.,* 144, 4841, 2003.
94. Coser, K.R. et al. Global analysis of ligand sensitivity of estrogen inducible and suppressible genes in MCF7/BUS breast cancer cells by DNA microarray, *Proc. Natl. Acad. Sci. USA,* 100, 13994, 2003.
95. Bektic, J. et al. Identification of genes involved in estrogenic action in the human prostate using microarray analysis, *Genomics,* 83, 34, 2004.
96. Migliaccio, A. et al. Steroid-induced androgen receptor-oestradiol receptor β-Src complex triggers prostate cancer cell proliferation, *EMBO J.,* 19, 5406, 2000.
97. Lee, S.R. et al. AR and ER interaction with a p21-activated kinase (PAK6), *Mol. Endocrinol.,* 16, 85, 2002.
98. Panet-Raymond, V. et al. Interactions between androgen and estrogen receptors and the effects on their transactivational properties, *Mol. Cell. Endocrinol.,* 167, 139, 2000.
99. Adesanya-Famuyiwa, O.O. et al. Localization and sex steroid regulation of androgen receptor gene expression in rhesus monkey uterus, *Obstet. Gynecol.,* 93, 265, 1999.
100. Esposito, T. et al. Regulation of androgen receptor mRNA expression in primary culture of Harderian gland cells: cross-talk between steroid hormones, *Comp. Biochem. Physiol. B: Biochem. Mol. Biol.,* 132, 97, 2002.

101. Suzuki, K. et al. Synergistic effects of estrogen and androgen on the prostate: Effects of estrogen on androgen- and estrogen-receptors, BrdU uptake, immunohistochemical study of AR, and responses to antiandrogens, *Prostate,* 26, 151, 1995.

102. Gupta, C., The role of estrogen receptor, androgen receptor and growth factors in diethylstilbestrol-induced programming of prostate differentiation, *Urol. Res.,* 28, 223, 2000.

103. Ignar-Trowbridge, D.M. et al. Coupling of dual signaling pathways: epidermal growth factor action involves the estrogen receptor, *Proc. Natl. Acad. Sci. USA,* 89, 4658, 1992.

104. Trachtenberg, J., Hicks, L.L., and Walsh, P.C., Androgen- and estrogen-receptor content in spontaneous and experimentally induced canine prostatic hyperplasia, *J. Clin. Invest.,* 65, 1051, 1980.

105. Roselli, C.E. and Fasasi, T.A., Estradiol increases the duration of nuclear receptor occupation in the preoptic area of the male rat treated with testosterone, *J. Steroid Bochem. Mol. Biol.,* 42, 161, 1992.

106. Challis, J.R.G. and Lye, S.J., Parturition, in *Physiology of Reproduction,* Knobil, E., Neill, J., and Pfaff, D., Raven Press, New York, 1994, pp. 985.

107. Clark, J.H. and Mani, S.K., Actions of ovarian steroid hormones, in *Physiology of Reproduction,* Knobil, E., Neill, J., and Pfaff, D., Raven Press, New York, 1994, pp. 1011.

108. McPherson, S.J. et al. Elevated androgens and prolactin in aromatase-deficient mice cause enlargement, but not malignancy, of the prostate gland, *Endocrinology,* 142, 2458, 2001.

109. Colborn, T., vom Saal, F.S., and Soto, A.M., Developmental effects of endocrine disrupting chemicals in wildlife and humans, *Environ. Health Perspect.,* 101, 378, 1993.

110. Kavlock, R.J. et al. Research needs for the risk assessment of health and environmental effects of endocrine disruptors: A report of the US EPA sponsored workshop, *Environ. Health Perspect. Suppl.,* 104, 715, 1996.

111. Ralph, J.L. et al. Disruption of androgen regulation in the prostate by the environmental contaminant hexachlorobenzene, *Environ. Health Perspect.,* 111, 461, 2003.

112. vom Saal, F.S. et al. A physiologically based approach to the study of bisphenol A and other estrogenic chemicals on the size of reproductive organs, daily sperm production, and behavior, *Toxicol. Ind. Health,* 14, 239, 1998.

113. Howdeshell, K.L. et al. Exposure to bisphenol A advances puberty, *Nature,* 401, 763, 1999.

114. Stumpf, W.E., Narbaitz, R., and Sar, M., Estrogen receptors in the fetal mouse, *J. Steroid Biochem.,* 12, 55, 1980.

115. Djoesland, O., Androgen metabolism by rat epididymis: effects of castration and antiandrogens, *Steroids,* 27, 47, 1976.

116. Tindall, V.J., French, F.S., and Nayfeh, S.N., Estradiol-17β inhibition of androgen uptake and binding in epididymis of adult male rats *in vivo*: A comparison with cyproterone acetate, *Steroids,* 37, 257, 1981.

117. Wetherill, Y.B. et al. The xenoestrogen bisphenol A induces inappropriate androgen receptor activation and mitogenesis in prostate adenocarcinoma cells, *Mol. Cancer Therap.,* 7, 515, 2002.

118. Schönfelder, G. et al. Parent bisphenol A accumulation in human maternal-fetal-placental unit, *Environ. Health Perspect.,* 110, A703, 2002.

119. Thayer, K.A. et al. Altered reproductive organs in male mice exposed prenatally to sub-clinical doses of 17α-ethinyl estradiol, *Hum. Reprod.,* 16, 988, 2001.

120. Soeffing, W.J. and Timms, B.G., Localization of androgen receptor and cell specific cytokeratins in basal cells of rat ventral prostate, *J. Androl.,* 16, 197, 1995.

121. Zalko, D. et al. Biotransformations of bisphenol A in a mammalian model: answers and new questions raised by low-dose metabolic fate studies in pregnant CD-1 mice, *Environ. Health Perspect.,* 111, 309, 2003.

122. Richter, C.A. et al. Androgen receptor mRNA is upregulated by estrogen in mouse prostate primary cell culture, *Toxicol. Sci.,* 72(S-1), 238, 2003.

123. Nagao, T. et al. Low-dose bisphenol A does not affect reproductive organs in estrogen-sensitive C57BL/6N mice exposed at the sexually mature, juvenile, or embryonic stage, *Reprod. Toxicol.,* 16, 123, 2002.

124. Spearow, J.L. et al. Genetic variation in susceptibility to endocrine disruption by estrogen in mice, *Science,* 285, 1259, 1999.

125. Ramos, J.G. et al. Prenatal exposure to low doses of bisphenol A alters the periductal stroma and glandular cell function in the rat ventral prostate, *Biol. Reprod.,* 65, 1271, 2001.

126. DeKlerk, D.P. et al. Comparison of spontaneous and experimentally induced canine prostatic hyperplasia, *J. Clin. Invest.,* 64, 842, 1979.

127. Leav, I. et al. Biochemical alterations in sex hormone-induced hyperplasia and dysplasia of the dorsolateral prostates of Noble rats, *J. Natl. Cancer Inst.,* 80, 1045, 1988.

128. Risbridger, G.P. et al. Oestrogens and prostate cancer, *Endocrine-Related Cancer,* 10, 187, 2003.

129. Noble, R.L., Prostate carcinoma of the Nb rat in relation to hormones, *Int. Rev. Exp. Pathol.,* 23, 113, 1982.

130. Leav, I. et al. Androgen supported-estrogen enhancement of epithelial proliferation in the prostate of intact Noble rats, *Prostate,* 15, 23, 1989.

131. Ofner, P., Bosland, M., and Vena, R.L., Differential effects of diethystilbestrol and estradiol-17β in combination with testosterone on rat prostate lobes, *Toxicol. Appl. Pharmacol.,* 112, 300, 1992.

132. Ho, S.-M. et al. The conjoint actions of androgens and estrogens in the induction of proliferative lesions in the rat prostate, in *Hormonal Carcinogenesis*, Li, J.J., Li, S.A., and Nandi, S., Springer-Verlag, New York, 1992.

133. McNeal, J.E. and Bostwich, D.G., Intraductal dysplasia: A premalignant lesion of the prostate, *Hum. Pathol.,* 17, 64, 1986.

134. Paulozzi, L.J., Erickson, J.D., and Jackson, R.J., Hypospadias trends in two US surveillance systems, *Pediatrics,* 100, 831, 1997.

135. Baskin, L.S., Himes, K., and Colborn, T., Hypospadias and endocrine disruption: Is there a connection?, *Environ. Health Perspect.,* 109, 1175, 2001.

136. Carlsen, E. et al. Declining semen quality and increasing incidence of testicular cancer: Is there a common cause?, *Environ. Health Perspect.,* 103 (Suppl 7), 137, 1995.

137. Hass, G.P. and Sakr, W.A., Epidemiology of prostate cancer, *CA. Cancer J. Clin.,* 47, 273, 1997.

138. Swan, S.H., Elkin, E.P., and Fenster, L., Have sperm densities declined: A reanalysis of global trend data, *Environ. Health Perspect.,* 105, 1228, 1997.

139. Swan, S.H. et al. Semen quality in relation to biomarkers of pesticide exposure, *Environ. Health Perspect.,* 111, 1478, 2003.

140. Allan, F.D., *Essentials of Human Embryology*, Oxford University Press, New York, 1960.
141. Timms, B.G., Peterson, R.E., and F.S., V.S., 2,3,7,8-Tetrachlorodibenzo-*p*-dioxin interacts with endogenous estradiol to disrupt prostate gland morphogenesis in male rat fetuses, *Tox. Sci.,* 67, 264, 2002.

13 Metal Ions as Endocrine Disruptors: Implications for Prostate Cancer

Shuk-Mei Ho

CONTENTS

13.1 ABSTRACT

Metal ions are significant contaminants of the environment. Yet, their impacts on normal and malignant prostatic functions are poorly understood. Studies implicating metal ions as environmental risk factors for the prostate are limited and have been focused mainly in the area of prostate cancer. Information on heavy-metal–ion influences on the other major prostatic diseases, such as benign prostatic hyperplasia

0-8493-2281-2/05/$0.00+$1.50
© 2005 by CRC Press

and prostatitis, is virtually non-existent. Zinc is a crucial intracellular trace element of the prostate and plays important roles in regulating androgenic action, intermediate metabolism, mitochondrial functions, and normal transcriptional activities of prostatic cells. Prostatic secretion of the metal ion into seminal plasma may affect sperm viability and male fertility. High zinc contents are found in normal and hyperplastic prostates, while a marked reduction in tissue zinc contents is noted during aging and neoplastic transformation of the gland. In parallel, serum and urinary zinc concentrations in prostate cancer patients are consistently reduced when compared with those found in healthy controls. Recent studies revealed that zinc transporters play essential roles in regulating influx and efflux of the ion in prostatic cells that may influence prostate cancer susceptibility among African American men.

Clear correlations between dietary zinc intake and prostate cancer risk have yet to be established, while the benefits of zinc supplement for prostate cancer prevention remain uncertain. Human exposure to cadmium is normally via food, air, and water contamination. In the 21st century a major source of environmental burden will come from disposal of millions of computers and electronic devices. Occupational exposure and cigarette smoking remain as major contributors of the overall bodily burden. In rodents and cell culture studies, cadmium is a proven carcinogen of the prostate. The citation exerts its carcinogenic influences via multiple mechanisms, including induction of oxidative stress and possibly DNA damage, activation of oncogenes and disruption of tumor suppressor activities, and acting as an estrogenic or androgenic mimic. The inter-relationship between cadmium and expression of various metallothioneins in prostate cells may affect tissue susceptibility to cadmium-induced carcinogenesis in the organ and the sensitivity of prostate cancer cells to drug therapies. In human studies, only weak associations have been found to exist between cadmium exposure and prostate cancer risk. However, the metal ion may have a stronger correlation with evolution of an aggressive form of prostate cancer. Of significance is the long half-life of cadmium in the human prostate and its continued accumulation in the organ with advancement of age. Finally, results from a handful of investigations suggest that both copper and arsenic may have potential carcinogenic action in the prostate. Future mechanistic and population-based studies on the roles played by heavy metals as endocrine disruptors and disease-causing agents are definitely warranted.

13.2   INTRODUCTION

The prostate is perhaps the most disease-prone organ of the aging human male. Prostatic adenocarcinoma, benign prostatic hyperplasia (BPH), and prostatitis are common disorders found in the aged human gland.[1–3] Additionally, adenosis or atypical adenomatous hyperplasia (AAH) and prostatic intraepithelial neoplasia (PIN) are often identified incidentally in autopsy, biopsy, and transurethral resection samples of the prostate.[4,5] The etiologies of these prostatic diseases or pathological conditions are poorly understood. Epidemiologic and basic research studies have, however, identified separate endogenous and exogenous risk factors for each of these conditions.[14–12] Aging appears to be the single common endogenous determinant, whereas changes in endogenous hormonal milieu also play an important role in the pathogenesis of these diseases. Studies implicating environmental factors as causative factors of prostatic diseases are scarce, and they are almost exclusively limited to prostate cancer. Among environmental factors, dietary fat, Western life style, metal ions, and environmental estrogens are likely of importance.[1] In this chapter, discussions focus only on heavy metal ions as endocrine disruptors and disease-causing agents of the prostate, with special emphasis on prostate cancer.

13.3 ZINC

13.3.1 MECHANISMS OF ZINC ACTION IN THE PROSTATE

It has long been known that the prostate has the highest concentration of zinc.[13,14] The zinc content is high in the epithelial cells and low in the stromal components.[15,16] Subcellular distribution favors the nuclear fraction, but substantial levels are also found in the cytosol[17] and mitochondria.[18] In the rat prostate, the lateral lobe contains several-fold higher zinc contents than the dorsal and ventral lobes.[18] Both testosterone and prolactin have been shown to increase zinc contents in the lateral lobe of the rat prostate gland. The precise physiological roles of zinc in the gland are unknown. *In vitro* studies have demonstrated that zinc enhances binding of androgen-androgen receptor complexes to cell nuclei[19] and increases total androgen uptake by prostatic tissues.[17] It has also been suggested that zinc inhibits mitochondrial m-aconitase activity and citrate oxidation.[18] Neutralized zinc, injected directly into the rat prostate, reduces prostatic weight and 5α-reductase activity.[20] Large quantity of zinc is apparently secreted into prostatic fluid and reaches the seminal plasma, where it plays a role in extending the functional life span of the ejaculated sperm.[14]

13.3.2 PROSTATIC ZINC CONTENT AND PROSTATE CARCINOGENESIS

When zinc contents in expressed prostatic fluids from healthy men and patients suffering from chronic prostatitis, adenoma, or adenocarcinoma were analyzed, a marked reduction (> 90%) in zinc level was observed only in fluid samples from cancer patients.[21] These findings were in accord with those reported in an earlier study on zinc contents in post-prostatic-massage urine[22] and in serum samples. Marked reductions in plasma zinc levels were noted in patients with prostate cancer when compared with healthy subjects or BPH patients.[23–28] Further declines in serum zinc levels were observed after cancer patients had undergone androgen ablation therapies.[25,28] In one study, aging was shown to associate with significant declines in tissue zinc contents. Collectively, these data clearly indicate that zinc is present in high concentrations in normal and hyperplastic human prostates, but its levels are considerably reduced with advancement of age or neoplastic transformation. Recent studies have provided several mechanistic links as to how zinc might contribute to prostate cancer primary and secondary prevention. In one report, exposure of PC-3 cells to physiological concentrations of zinc increased sensitivity of tumor cells to tumor necrosis factor-alpha- or paclitaxel-mediated cell death.[29] A second study demonstrated an inverse relationship between zinc content and prostate-specific antigen (PSA) in 28 patients.[30] This finding raises the possibility that zinc can directly regulate PSA production. It has also been proposed that a "low zinc, low citrate" phenotype represents a hypoxia-defense adaptation, which is believed to have importance implication on prostate cancer cell growth.[31]

Intracellular zinc content is now believed to be regulated by zinc transporters,[32,33] providing the first evidence that prolactin and testosterone regulated zinc intake into normal and cancerous prostatic epithelial cells. This process was subsequently shown to be mediated by a class of membrane proteins known as zinc transporters. High levels of zinc-transporter-2 were expressed in the rat lateral and dorsal prostate, where pre-cancerous and cancer lesions likely developed.[34] In human prostate cells, the zinc transporter ZIP1 is the major zinc uptake regulator.[35] The activities of these zinc transporters, via control of influx and efflux of the cation, is now believed to regulate intracellular metallothionein levels that in turn influence cellular sensitivity to various heavy metals.[36,37] Recently, expression of the zinc transporter ZnT4 in prostate specimens[38] and serum levels of a zinc binding protein zinc alpha-2-glycoprotein[39] were found to have prognostic values for prostate cancer progression. Furthermore, a recent epidemiology study demonstrated down-regulation of two zinc transporters, hZIP1 and hZIP2, in African American men when compared to white males[40] and may explain the high incidence of prostate cancer in the former group. Collectively, these findings have provided new insights to the relationship between zinc and prostate carcinogenesis, as it has become apparent that 1) the carcinogenic process, *per se*, may perturb zinc metabolism/homeostasis in the prostate, and 2) zinc content, either in circulating or at the tissue level, directly or indirectly, may predispose the gland to neoplastic transformation. Importantly, environmental influences, such as dietary habits or cadmium exposure (see next section), that affect prostatic zinc content may have major consequences in disease development of the gland.

13.3.3 DIETARY ZINC AND PROSTATE CANCER RISK

The American diet is often deficient in zinc,[13] hence a question arises as to whether dietary intake of zinc influences disease development in the prostate. Observational studies data revealed conflicting data. In a Utah study, in which 358 cases were compared to 679 controls, weekly intake of zinc was found to have little association with prostate cancer.[41] In contrast, when a Hawaii population with 452 cases of prostate cancer and 899 age-matched controls was studied, weekly zinc intake, adjusted for age and ethnicity, was found to be greater for prostate cancer cases than for healthy controls.[42] Results from this study thus implicate dietary zinc as a risk factor for prostate cancer. In contrast, when 115 prostate cancer cases were compared with 227 age-matched controls nested in the prospective CLUEII study baseline in 1989, higher zinc intake was found to slightly lower prostate cancer risk.[43] In a recent large-scale study in which supplemental zinc intake was correlated to prostate cancer risk among 46,974 American men participating in the Health Professionals Follow-Up Study (14 years), zinc intake up to 100 mg/day was found to have no effects on prostate cancer risk except when higher doses of zinc supplement was used. The higher doses slightly increased the risk of advanced prostate cancer.[44] Collectively, these observational studies provide no strong evidence in support of the notion that dietary zinc supplement offers protection against prostate cancer but a dietary deficient in this cation may have adverse effects in the long term.

13.4 CADMIUM

13.4.1 CADMIUM IS A SIGNIFICANT AND GROWING ENVIRONMENTAL CONTAMINANT

Cadmium contamination results from zinc mining and smelting, sewage-sludge disposal, various industrial usages, and combustion of municipal waste and fossil fuels.[45,46] Worldwide production in the 1970s was around 18,000 tons/year,[47] of which about 4000 tons were used in the United States. The heavy metal ion is commonly found in plated metals, pigments, batteries, stabilizers in plastics, metallurgy, and nuclear reactor rods, and as catalysts.[48] In the 21st century, the major source of cadmium contamination will come from semiconductor, electrical, and electronic equipment manufacturing.[49] One recent estimate indicates that between 1997 and 2004 over 315 million computers will become obsolete, and this will generate almost 2 million pounds of cadmium burden to the environment. Cadmium is in many computer and electronic components such as SMD chip resistors, infrared detectors, and semiconductors. Older types of cathode ray tubes also contain the metal ion. Amazingly, cadmium contamination of our food chain is quite common. A recent study showed that the Greenland marine food chains contain high levels of cadmium in addition to mercury and selenium.[50]

Cadmium compounds are classified as toxic with a possible risk of irreversible effects on human health.[51] The metal ion can be absorbed through respiration and via ingestion. It accumulates in the human body with a long biological half-life of >20 years.[52,53] An acute exposure to high dose can cause symptoms of poisoning but chronic low-dose exposure is hard to detect. Cadmium contamination in food, soil, air, and water may be high in industrial areas.[52,54, 55] Non-occupational exposure probably takes place through consumption of contaminated fish, drinking water, contaminated air, and cigarette smoking.[53,54,55] This cation is frequently found in the National Priorities List sites. The National Toxicology Program (NTP, 1991) has classified it as a substance that may reasonably be anticipated as a human carcinogen.[55,56]

13.4.2 CD IS A SUSPECTED CARCINOGEN FOR THE HUMAN PROSTATE

Cadmium exposures have been linked to prostate cancer (PCa) in some, but not all, epidemiological studies.[53,57,58,59] Occupational exposure to cadmium may be a causative factor for PCa. A recent analysis of the Swedish National Cancer Registry during 1961 to 1979 revealed that workers in occupations and industries with cadmium exposure had elevated risk for PCa.[59] Among 522 Swedish workers exposed to cadmium for at least 1 year in a nickel-cadmium battery plant, the mortality rate for PCa was increased in a dose- and latency- dependent manner.[60] A case-referent study of 345 PCa cases and 1346 referents in Netherlands found a statistically significant excess risk for subjects who reported frequent occupational exposure to cadmium.[61] In a Utah population-based case-control study, occupational exposure to cadmium was correlated with a small but significant increase in PCa risk.[62] Non-occupational exposure may also contribute to higher PCa incidence in the general population. Positive associations have been observed between cadmium in drinking water or food and PCa.[62,41,63,57] In Spain, high incidences of PCa were observed in certain areas where cadmium is naturally present in abnormally high concentrations in stream sediment.[63] In general, studies that revealed a positive correlation between cadmium exposure and PCa only indicated a weak association[62,60,64,41,63,59] but cadmium exposure might have a stronger association with aggressive PCa.[62]

Data from laboratory investigations also support a link between cadmium and PCa. Higher levels of cadmium were found in PCa specimens when compared to levels noted in normal or hyperplastic tissues,[65,26,66,67] with the highest concentration in high-grade cancers.[65] At the cellular level, cadmium was found to be rather evenly distributed between the epithelial cells and stroma of the human prostate.[65,15] Exposure of an immortalized human non-tumorigenic prostatic epithelial cell line (pRNS-1-1) to cadmium induced malignant transformation that resulted in transformants capable of forming tumors in SCID mice.[68] Treatment of the human PCa cell line, LNCaP, with cadmium stimulated cell growth and increased expression of prostate-specific antigen and NKX 3.1, in an androgen receptor-dependent manner.[69] Collectively, these findings support the notion that cadmium may play a direct role in the genesis of PCa and promotion of this cancer to higher grade in the human gland.

Other epidemiology studies, however, had failed to find an association between cadmium exposure and PCa. In a population-based case-control study in Utah, no association was found.[41] In a cohort mortality study on cadmium-exposed workers, no increased risk was noted with five years of follow-up.[70] Another cohort study of 3025 nickel-cadmium battery workers also failed to demonstrate a significant correlation between occupational cadmium exposure and increased PCa risk.[71] In one laboratory investigation, cadmium contents were reported to be similar among normal, hyperplastic, and carcinomatous prostatic tissues.[15]

13.4.3 CADMIUM IS A PROVEN CARCINOGEN FOR THE RAT PROSTATE

In rats, cadmium is a proven carcinogen of the prostate. Cadmium caused malignant transformation of rat ventral prostate (VP) epithelial cells in culture.[72] *In vivo*, the heavy metal ion is cytotoxic to a wide variety of body cells in the rat and yet it is carcinogenic to selected organs including the prostate.[73,74,75,76] The incidence and the site of tumor development appear to be highly dependent on the rat strain and route of cadmium administration. Administration of cadmium, in doses between 2.5 and 5.0 μmole/kg body weight (b.w.), as a single subcutaneous injection, to Wistar rats induced a 34% tumor incidence in the VPs, but not in the dorsolateral prostates (DLPs) of treated animals.[77] However, when cadmium was given as a single subcutaneous injection of 1 to 4 μmole/kg b.w. to Noble (NBL/Cr) rats, a proliferative lesion, termed intraepithelial hyperplasia, was observed mostly in the DLPs of 60 to 80% of the treated animals.[75]

Exposure of NBL/Cr rats to cadmium via drinking water at 25 to 50 ppm caused a 50% incidence of proliferative lesions in both VP and DLP of the exposed rats.[76] Most of the proliferative lesions described in these studies were intraepithelial atypia, adenoma, or microscopic cancers that developed over a period of up to 72 weeks. None of these epithelial lesions involved stromal invasion. When cadmium was injected directly into the VP, there was a high incidence of PIN and cancer within a relative short duration of 270 days.[78] Interestingly, in a more recent study[79] oral administration of cadmium to rats through drinking water increased testosterone (T) levels and down-regulated metallothionein expression in the rat VP. These changes are opposite to those induced by other routes of cadmium administration and are believed to increase the risk of the rat gland to prostate carcinogenesis. Lastly, cadmium was also effective in enhancing the potency of other chemical carcinogens such as DMBA in the induction of cancer in the VP.[80] Of interest to note, the half-life of cadmium in rats was estimated to be over 6 weeks following a single injection of radioactive cadmium into the prostate.[81] This is in agreement with the observed accumulation of this heavy metal ion in the human prostate and its long half-life in the human gland.

13.4.4 MECHANISMS OF CADMIUM-INDUCED CARCINOGENESIS

Although little is known about the mechanisms of cadmium carcinogenesis, several mechanistic pathways have been proposed.[82,56] First, cadmium accumulation is believed to alter intracellular Zn concentrations (see Section 13.3), which, in turn, may affect the regulation of nucleic acids metabolism, activation of transcription factors, and normal operation of a large number of enzymes.[83,84,85,86] In this regard, it is of interest to note that the ratio of cadmium to zinc is often greater in PCa tissues than that found in non-cancerous tissues.[26] Second, cadmium may have direct genotoxic effects, since chromosomal aberrations have been observed in lymphocytes of workers exposed to cadmium[87] and in prostatic epithelial cells exposed to the heavy metal ion *in vitro*.[72] Yet, in a number of genotoxicity testing systems, cadmium has been showed to be only a weak mutagen.[88,89] Alternatively, cadmium may be genotoxic via indirect mechanisms such as induction of oxidative stress and free radical formation.[90,91] The latter premise is supported by the observation that cadmium-induced proliferation of human prostatic epithelial cells in culture could be blocked by the antioxidant trace element, selenium.[92] Cytotoxicity-induced regenerative cell proliferation has also been proposed as a probable cause, since severe tissue injury is a prerequisite of tumorigenesis in the rat testis.[77] More recently, it has been shown that disruption of proto-oncogenes and tumor suppression gene expression may be an important causative factor of cadmium carcinogenicity, since it has been demonstrated the metal ion induced expression of *p53*, *c-jun*, and *c-myc* in prostatic cells *in vitro*[93] and *in vivo*.[94] Lastly, recent evidence clearly indicates cadmium as a bona fide endocrine disruptor of cellular estrogenic and androgenic responsiveness and may exert major impacts on PCa development and progression due to its estrogenicity or androgenicity.

13.4.5 CADMIUM IS AN ESTROGENIC/ANDROGENIC ENDOCRINE DISRUPTOR — RAMIFICATIONS IN PROSTATE CARCINOGENESIS

It is now firmly established that cadmium is an estrogen mimic as well as an androgen agonist. Early studies[95] demonstrated cadmium could induce estrogen-regulated genes such as progesterone receptor, pS2, and cathepsin D in a breast cancer cell line (MCF7). Furthermore, cadmium was able to substitute Zn in the zinc fingers of the estrogen receptor (ER)-α.[96] Subsequent studies firmly established that cadmium directly interacted with the ligand-binding domain of ER-α and transactivated estrogen-regulated genes.[97,98] The binding of cadmium to ER-α was found to be of high affinity [Kd at 5X10(-10) M], sensitive to antiestrogen blockade, and involve binding to specific conserved cysteine groups on the ER molecule.[97] Cadmium also interfered with the binding of ER to the estrogen responsive element (ERE).[98] Due to its high potency as an estrogen mimic, cadmium was effective in stimulating breast cancer cell growth, enhancing uterine wet weight, promoting mammary gland development, and inducing expression of estrogen-regulated genes in castrated rodents.[99,100]

Intriguingly, cadmium has also been shown to disrupt androgen action in the male reproductive tract including the prostate. The metal ion binds androgen receptor (AR) with high affinity[101,102] and mediates AR-activation of an androgen responsive element (ARE) in a PCa cell line (LNCaP) and in a liver cancer cell line (HepG2).[102] In addition, it specifically inhibits type I 5α-reductase activity,[103] which has been found recently to be up-regulated in PCa specimens.[104] Based on this body of knowledge, it is logical to speculate that cadmium may have significant impacts on normal and aberrant growth of the prostate by acting as an estrogenic or androgenic mimic. In this regard, it is well recognized that the development and progression of PCa is etiologically linked to altered hormonal milieu involving estrogen and androgen.[6,12] Since cadmium has been shown to accumulate in the prostate with advancement of age due to its very long half-life in the organ (see Section 13.4.3), the probability that it may exert oncogenic action via endocrine disruption is undoubtedly worthy of future investigation. In this context, it is worth mentioning that exposure of Noble rats to combined androgen and estrogen for an extensive period of time induces pre-malignant and malignant lesions in 100% of the treated animals,[105,106] while exposure of Noble rats to a single dose of cadmium induces a high incidence of prostate tumors in their prostates.[75] Taken together, these studies support the premise that cadmium-carcinogenicity in the rat prostate may be mediated by the combined estrogenic and androgenic action of the citation.

13.4.6 INTERPLAY BETWEEN CADMIUM AND OTHER HEAVY METALS IN PROSTATE CARCINOGENESIS

Interestingly, in animal studies zinc has the ability to modify the carcinogenic potential of cadmium.[73] Administration of zinc apparently potentiated or inhibited, dependent on dose and route of administration, the carcinogenic effects of cadmium in the rat ventral prostate. In the human prostate, there seems to have a distinct antagonistic effect between zinc and cadmium.[26,65,66,107] Marked reduction in tissue zinc contents and elevation in cadmium contents were consistently observed in prostatic cancer specimens. These findings suggested that a high zinc content may confer protection against cadmium-carcinogeneity/toxicity to prostatic cells. Conversely, zinc deficiency, at bodily or cellular level, may exacerbate the cytotoxic effects of cadmium in the prostate.

Information on the interactions between cadmium and other heavy metal ions are scarce and not directly obtained from studies in prostatic tissues. However, recent studies suggested that increased dietary selenium or calcium might offer protection against cadmium-induced cytotoxicity in ringed seal and laying hens.[50,108] One possible explanation for the protective effects of selenium against cadmium-induced damages may be related to its antioxidant action, since cadmium is known to promote a prooxidant state in most tissues.[90,91] Furthermore, as part of the effort to elucidate the impacts of mixtures, the Agency for Toxic Substances and Disease Registry (ATSDR) recently found no evidence of synergistic activity with a mixture of Cd (II), chromium [Cr (III)], and lead [Pb (II)] on metal activation of gene expression.[109] Future studies on potential synergistic or agonistic effects of various metal ions, in addition to Zn, on the impacts of cadmium in the prostate are certainly warranted.

13.4.7 Metallothioneins and Cadmium-Induced Carcinogenicity

Metallothioneins (MTs) have been regarded as one of the most unusual classes of proteins,[110] and their potential roles in carcinogenesis remain elusive.[111] MTs are widely distributed among plants and animals. In humans, there are as many as 17 genes coding for MT, whereas in rodents, two prevalent forms, MT-I and MT-II, are expressed. These polypeptides are characterized by their low molecular weights (~60 a.a.), high cysteine content (one third), a lack of aromatic residues, and a strong affinity for selected metal ions (zinc, copper, cadmium, and mercury). Although MT is mainly a cytosolic protein in quiescent cells, it is translocated to cell nucleus during cell replication and differentiation.[111] MTs have been implicated in a multitude of cellular functions including those related to regulation of essential metal (zinc and copper) homeostasis and trafficking, detoxification of heavy metal ions, and scavenger activity against free radicals, electrophils, and oxidants.[112] Recently, MT-3, a new isoform, has been identified in brain extracts of Alzheimer's patients and shown to inhibit growth of rat cortical neurons.[113]

Much remained to be learned about the interrelationships between MTs and cadmium-induced carcinogenesis in the prostate. In rats, it has been demonstrated that MTs are expressed at significant levels in the dorsal (DP) and lateral (LP) lobes of the prostate.[114–119] However, MT expression in the VP was hardly detectable using conventional methods such as immunocytochemistry, *in situ* hybridization, and Northern blotting.[115,117,118] Furthermore, MT expression was initially reported to be non-inducible by cadmium in rat VP.[117] Coincidentally,[73] Waalkes and co-workers observed a high incidence (> 30%) of tumors developed in the VPs, but not in the DPs or LPs, of Wistar rats treated with a single dose of cadmium at a young age. However, a recent study[119] demonstrated enhanced expression of both MT-I and MT-II in rat VPs following a cadmium challenge.[119] Nevertheless, the levels attained in the VPs of the treated animals still fell short of those expressed in the DPs and LPs of untreated rats.[119] In support of a protective role of MT against cadmium-induced cell death, it has recently been showed that ribozyme-mediated degradation of MT increased rat epithelial cells' susceptibility to cadmium-cytotoxicity.[120] Findings from other studies have added to our understanding of the relationship between MT and cadmium-carcinogenicity. When NBL/Cr rats were treated with a single injection of cadmium at young age, 60 to 80% of the animals developed intraepithelial proliferative lesions, mostly in their DLPs, while administration of cadmium via drinking water induced lesions in both VP and DLP.[75,76] Taken together, these findings have refuted the original hypothesis that rat VP is most susceptible to cadmium-carcinogenicity due to low MT expression levels.

Studies in human tissues have shed new light on the relationship. Expression of various MTs is up-regulated in cancers of the breast, colon, kidney, liver, lung, nasopharynx, ovary, testes, thyroid, urinary bladder, and the prostate. In contrast, it is down-regulated in neoplasms of the liver. Up-regulation of MT-IIa in cancer cells may offer survival advantage, since ribozyme-mediated down-regulation of MT-IIa caused significant cell death in prostate and ovarian cancer cells.[121] In contrast, MT-III has been shown to inhibit PCa cell growth and increased drug resistance.[122] In addition to divalent cations such as zinc, cadmium, and copper, p53[123] androgen[118] and estrogen[124] have been implicated in the induction and overexpression of MT in epithelial cancers.

In the prostate, immunoreactivity of MT is most intense in the peripheral zone, moderate in the transitional zone, and weak in the central zone, hence MT distribution parallels susceptibility of these regions to proliferation.[125–127] Furthermore, expression of MT was correlated to tumor grade, with the highest concentrations found in the highest grade tumors.[126,127] Based on these findings, it is logical to postulate that prostate carcinogenesis is perhaps associated with increased expression of MT, which could be enhanced by steady accumulation of cadmium in the prostate with advancement of age.

13.5   COPPER, NICKEL, AND ARSENIC

Copper and nickel are commonly found to co-exist with cadmium as environmental pollutants.[55] It is, therefore, conceivable that the reported effects of cadmium on the prostate may, in part, be due to the adverse action of copper or nickel contaminants. However, epidemiological data in support of this hypothesis are non-existent, and not a single study had focused on the toxicity/carcinogeneity of these two compounds in the human prostate. In an animal study, nickel chloride added to the drinking water in 5 and 50 ppm were shown to have no effects on the morphology and ultrastructure of the rat prostate.[128] Among all the other metal ions only arsenic has been found to associate with prostate cancer in epidemiological studies.[129–132] The American Council on Science and Health has recently reviewed the carcinogenic risk of arsenic and found evidence that chronic exposure to inorganic arsenic at concentrations around several hundred microgram per liter may cause cancers in various organs, including the prostate, and therefore recommended drinking water arsenic concentrations to be kept below 50 μg/L.[133] Experimentally, arsenic (5 μM) has been shown to exert direct transforming potential on the nontumorigenic human prostate epithelial cell RWPE-1.[134] Paradoxically, low levels of inorganic arsenic were found to be effective in promoting cell death in a variety of prostate cancer cell lines via activation of p38, JNK, and caspase-3[135] and induction of apoptosis.[136] In the clinical setting, low levels of arsenic have been evaluated for their efficacy in treating solid tumors including those derived from the prostate.[137]

13.6 SUMMARY

From this literature review it has become apparent that information on the effects of metal ions on prostatic functions is sketchy. Although cadmium has been identified as a potential environmental carcinogen for the human prostate, its mode of action remains largely unknown. Zinc ion, on the other hand, appears to be needed to maintain normal prostatic functions, and zinc transporters seem to play a major role in maintaining intracellular zinc contents. Since metal ions bind to many common cellular proteins, it is conceivable that zinc homeostasis may influence accumulation rates of various metal ions in the prostate. Among the various heavy metal ions, cadmium undoubtedly has the strongest association with prostate cancer. The recent discovery that cadmium is a bona fide estrogenic/androgenic disruptor raises new questions to its mode of action. Chronic exposure to low levels of arsenic is definitely an emerging threat to prostate health. Future studies that focus on synergism/antagonism between cellular zinc and the various heavy metal ions will help decipher the true significance of environmental metal ions in the development of prostatic diseases in the human male.

REFERENCES

1. Ho, S.M, Lee, K.F., and Lane, K., Neoplastic transformation of the prostate, in *Prostate: Basic and Clinical Aspects*, Rajesh K. Naz (ed.), CRC Press, Boca Raton, FL, 1997, 73.
2. Petrovich, Z. et al. [Authors are Ameye, Baert, Bichler, Boyd, Brady, Bruskewitz, Dixon, Perrin, and Watson], New trends in the treatment of benign prostatic hyperplasia and carcinoma of the prostate, *Am J Clin Oncol*, 16, 187, 1993.
3. Blumenfeld, W., Tucci, S., and Narayan, P., Incidental lymphocytic prostatitis. Selective involvement with nonmalignant glands, *Am J Surg Pathol*, 16, 975, 1992.
4. Epstein, J.I., Adenosis (atypical adenomatous hyperplasia): histopathology and relationship to carcinoma, *Pathol Res Pract*, 191, 888, 1995.
5. Bostwick, D.G., Qian, J., and Frankel, K. The incidence of high grade prostatic intraepithelial neoplasia in needle biopsies, *J Urol*, 154, 1791, 1995.
6. Taplin, M.E. and Ho, S.M., Clinical review 134: The endocrinology of prostate cancer, *J Clin Endocrinol Metab*, 86, 3467, 2001.
7. Lobel, B. and Rodriguez, A., Chronic prostatitis: what we know, what we do not know, and what we should do!, *World J Urol*, 21, 57, 2003.
8. Krieger, J.N. et al. [Authors are Riley, Cheah, Liong, and Yuen], Epidemiology of prostatitis: new evidence for a world-wide problem, *World J Urol*, 21, 70, 2003.

9. Nelson, W.G., De Marzo, A.M., and Isaacs, W.B., Prostate cancer, *N Engl J Med*, 349, 366, 2003.
10. Pavelic, J., Zeljko, Z., and Bosnar, M.H., Molecular genetic aspects of prostate transition zone lesions, *Urology*, 62, 607, 2003.
11. Lijovic, M. and Frauman, AG., Toward an understanding of the molecular genetics of prostate cancer progression, *J Environ Pathol Toxicol Oncol*, 22, 1, 2003.
12. Ho, S.M., Estrogens and anti-estrogens: Key mediators of prostate carcinogenesis and new therapeutic candidates, *J Cell Biochem,* 2004.
13. Vallee, B.L., Biochemistry, physiology and pathology of zinc, *Physiol Rev*, 39, 443, 1959.
14. Bedwal, R.S. and Bahuguna, A., Zinc, copper and selenium in reproduction, *Experientia*, 50, 626, 1994.
15. Lahtonen, R., Zinc and cadmium concentrations in whole tissue and in separated epithelium and stroma from human benign prostatic hypertrophic glands, *Prostate*, 6, 177, 1985.
16. Feustel, A., Wennrich, R., and Dittrich, H., Zinc, cadmium and selenium concentrations in separated epithelium and stroma from prostatic tissues of different histology, *Urol Res*, 15, 161, 1987.
17. Leake, A. et al. [Authors are Chrisholm, Busuttil, and Habib], Subcellular distribution of zinc in the benign and malignant human prostate: evidence for a direct zinc androgen interaction, *Acta Endocrinol (Copenh)*, 105, 281, 1984.
18. Liu, Y., Franklin, R.B., Costello, L.C., Prolactin and testosterone regulation of mitochondrial zinc in prostate epithelial cells, *Prostate*, 30, 26, 1997.
19. Colvard, D.S. and Wilson, E.M., Zinc potentiation of androgen receptor binding to nuclei *in vitro*, *Biochemistry*, 23, 3471, 1984.
20. Fahim, M.S. et al. [Authors are Wang, Sutcu, and Fahim], Zinc arginine, a 5 alpha-reductase inhibitor, reduces rat ventral prostate weight and DNA without affecting testicular function, *Andrologia*, 25, 369, 1993.
21. Zaichick, V.Y., Sviridova, T.V., and Zaichick, S.V., Zinc concentration in human prostatic fluid: normal, chronic prostatitis, adenoma and cancer, *Int Urol Nephrol*, 28, 687, 1996.
22. McCallum, K.A. et al. [Authors are Kavanagh, Farragher, and Blacklock], Ratio of post-prostatic massage urinary zinc concentration to initial urinary zinc concentration. An improved method of assessing prostatic function, *Br J Urol*, 62, 565, 1988.
23. Whelan, P., Walker, B.E., and Kelleher, J., Zinc, vitamin A and prostatic cancer, *Br J Urol*, 55, 525, 1983.
24. Chirulescu, Z. et al. [Authors are Chiriloiu, Suciu, and Pirvulescu], Variations of zinc, calcium and magnesium in normal subjects and in patients with neoplasias, *Med Interne*, 25, 257, 1987.
25. Feustel, A., Wennrich, R., and Schmidt, B., Serum-Zn-levels in prostatic cancer, *Urol Res*, 17, 41, 1989.
26. Ogunlewe, J.O. and Osegbe, D.N, Zinc and cadmium concentrations in indigenous blacks with normal, hypertrophic, and malignant prostate, *Cancer*, 63, 1388, 1989.
27. Tvedt, K.E. et al. [Authors are Halgunset, Kopstad, Haugen], Intracellular distribution of calcium and zinc in normal, hyperplastic, and neoplastic human prostate: X-ray microanalysis of freeze-dried cryosections, *Prostate*, 15, 41, 1989.
28. Lekili, M., Ergen, A., and Celebi, I., Zinc plasma levels in prostatic carcinoma and BPH, *Int Urol Nephrol*, 23, 151, 1991.

29. Uzzo, R.G. et al. [Authors are Leavis, Hatch, Gabai, Dulin, Zvartau, and Kolenko], Zinc inhibits nuclear factor-kappa B activation and sensitizes prostate cancer cells to cytotoxic agents, *Clin Cancer Res*, 8, 3579, 2002.

30. Vartsky, D. et al. [Authors are Shilstein, Bercovich, Huszar, Breskin, Chechik, Korotinsky, Malnick, and Moriel], Prostatic zinc and prostate specific antigen: an experimental evaluation of their combined diagnostic value, *J Urol*, 170, 2258, 2003.

31. Hochachka, P.W. et al. [Authors are Rupert, Goldenberg, Gleave, and Kozlowski], Going malignant: the hypoxia-cancer connection in the prostate, *Bioessays*, 24, 749, 2002.

32. Fuchs, O. et al. [Authors are Babusiak, Vyoral, and Petrak], Role of zinc in eukaryotic cells, zinc transporters and zinc-containing proteins. Review article, *Sb Lek*, 104, 157, 2003.

33. Costello, L.C. et al. [Authors are Liu, Zou, and Franklin], Evidence for a zinc uptake transporter in human prostate cancer cells which is regulated by prolactin and testosterone, *J Biol Chem*, 274, 17499, 1999.

34. Iguchi, K. et al. [Authors are Usui, Inoue, Sugimura, Tatematsu, and Hirano], High-level expression of zinc transporter-2 in the rat lateral and dorsal prostate, *J Androl*, 23, 819, 2002.

35. Franklin, R.B. et al. [Authors are Ma, Zou, Guan, Kukoyi, Feng, and Costello], Human ZIP1 is a major zinc uptake transporter for the accumulation of zinc in prostate cells, *J Inorg Biochem*, 96, 435, 2003.

36. Iguchi, K. et al. [Authors are Otsuka, Usui, Ishii, Onishi, Sugimura, and Hirano, Zinc and metallothionein levels and expression of zinc transporters in androgen-independent subline of LNCaP cells, *J Androl*, 25, 154, 2004.

37. Hasumi, M. et al. [Authors are Suzuki, Matsui, Koike, Ito, and Yamanaka], Regulation of metallothionein and zinc transporter expression in human prostate cancer cells and tissues, *Cancer Lett*, 200, 187, 2003.

38. Henshall, S.M. et al. [Authors are Afar, Rasiah, Horvath, Gish, Caras, Ramakrishnan, Wong, Jeffry, Kench, Quinn, Turner, Delprado, Lee, Golovsky, Brenner, O'Neill, Kooner, Stricker, Grygiel, Mack, and Sutherland], Expression of the zinc transporter ZnT4 is decreased in the progression from early prostate disease to invasive prostate cancer, *Oncogene*, 22, 6005, 2003.

39. Hale, L.P. et al. [Authors are Price, Sanchez, Demark-Wahnefried, and Madden], Zinc alpha-2-glycoprotein is expressed by malignant prostatic epithelium and may serve as a potential serum marker for prostate cancer, *Clin Cancer Res*, 7, 846, 2001.

40. Rishi, I. et al. [Authors are Baidouri, Abbasi, Bullard-Dillard, Kajdacsy-Balla, Pestaner, Skacel, and Bagasra], Prostate cancer in African American men is associated with downregulation of zinc transporters, *Appl Immunohistochem Mol Morphol*, 11, 253, 2003.

41. West, D.W. et al. [Authors are Slattery, Robison, French, and Mahoney.] Adult dietary intake and prostate cancer risk in Utah: a case-control study with special emphasis on aggressive tumors, *Cancer Causes Control*, 2, 85, 1991.

42. Kolonel, L.N., Yoshizawa, C.N., and Hankin, J.H. Diet and prostatic cancer: a case-control study in Hawaii, *Am J Epidemiol*, 127, 999, 1988.

43. Platz, E.A. et al. [Authors are Helzlsouer, Hoffman, Morris, Baskett, and Comstock], Prediagnostic toenail cadmium and zinc and subsequent prostate cancer risk, *Prostate*, 52, 288, 2002.

44. Leitzmann, M.F. et al. [Authors are Stampfer, Wu, Colditz, Willett, and Giovannucci], Zinc supplement use and risk of prostate cancer, *J Natl Cancer Inst*, 95, 1004, 2003.

45. Hoover R., Tobacco and geographic pathology, in *Lung Biology in Health and Disease Pasthogenesis and Therapy of Lung Cancer*, Harris, C.C. (ed)., Marcel-Dekker, New York, 1978.

46. Lloyd, O.L., Respiratory-cancer clustering associated with localised industrial air pollution, *Lancet*, 1, 318, 1978.

47. Commission of the European Communities, *CEC Criteria, Dose/Effect Relationships for Cadmium,* Persamon Press, Oxford, 1978.

48. National Institute of Occupational Safety and Health C. I. B., *Cadmium,* 42, DHHS (NIOSH), Publication Number 84-116, 1984.

49. Thorpe, EPA Electronics and Computer Industry Notebook Section Vb, 1999.

50. Sonne-Hansen, C. et al. [Authors are Dietz, Leifsson, Hyldstrup, and Riget], Cadmium toxicity to ringed seals (Phoca hispida): an epidemiological study of possible cadmium-induced nephropathy and osteodystrophy in ringed seals (Phoca hispida) from Qaanaaq in Northwest Greenland, *Sci Total Environ*, 295, 167, 2002.

51. Nordberg, G.F., Application of the "critical effect" and "critical concentration" concept to human risk assessment for cadmium, *IARC Sci Publ3*, 1992.

52. Friberg, L. et al. [Authors are Piscator, Nordberg, and Kjellstrom], *Cadmium in the Environment,* 2nd edition, CRC Press, Boca Raton, FL, 1974.

53. Piscator, M., Role of cadmium in carcinogenesis with special reference to cancer of the prostate, *Environ Health Perspect*, 40, 107, 1981.

54. Waalkes, M.P., Coogan, T.P., and Barter, R.A., Toxicological principles of metal carcinogenesis with special emphasis on cadmium, *Crit Rev Toxicol*, 22, 175, 1992.

55. Faroon, O.M., Williams, M., and O'Connor, R., A review of the carcinogenicity of chemicals most frequently found at National Priorities List sites, *Toxicol Ind Health*, 10, 203, 1994.

56. Waalkes, M. P., Cadmium carcinogenesis in review, *J Inorg Biochem*, 79, 241, 2000.

57. Waalkes M.P. and Rehm S., Cadmium and prostate cancer, *J Toxicol Environ Health*, 43, 251, 1994.

58. Ekman P., Genetic and environmental factors in prostate cancer genesis: identifying high-risk cohorts, *Eur Urol*, 35, 362, 1999.

59. Sharma-Wagner, S. et al. [Authors are Chokkalingam, Malker, Stone, McLaughlin, and Hsing], Occupation and prostate cancer risk in Sweden, *J Occup Environ Med*, 42, 517, 2000.

60. Elinder, C.G. et al. [Authors are Kjellstrom, Hogstedt, Andersson, and Spang], Cancer mortality of cadmium workers, *Br J Ind Med*, 42, 651, 1985.

61. van der Gulden, J.W., Kolk, J.J., and Verbeek, A.L., Work environment and prostate cancer risk, *Prostate*, 27, 250, 1995.

62. Elghany, N.A. et al, [Authors are Schumacher, Slattery, West, and Lee], Occupation, cadmium exposure, and prostate cancer, *Epidemiology*, 1, 107, 1990.

63. Garcia, S.A., Antona, J.F., and Urrutia, M., Geochemical prospection of cadmium in a high incidence area of prostate cancer, Sierra de Gata, Salamanca, Spain, *Sci Total Environ*, 116, 243, 1992.

64. Ross, R.K., Paganini-Hill, A., and Henderson, B.E., The etiology of prostate cancer: what does the epidemiology suggest?, *Prostate*, 4, 333, 1983.

65. Feustel, A. and Wennrich, R., Determination of the distribution of zinc and cadmium in cellular fractions of BPH, normal prostate and prostatic cancers of different histologies by atomic and laser absorption spectrometry in tissue slices, *Urol Res*, 12, 253, 1984.

66. Habib, F.K. et al. [Authors are Hammond, Lee, Dawson, Mason, Smith, and Stitch.] Metal-androgen interrelationships in carcinoma and hyperplasia of the human prostate, *J Endocrinol*, 71, 133, 1976.

67. Brys, M. et al. [Authors are Nawrocka, Miekos, Zydek, Foksinski, Barecki, Krajewska], Zinc and cadmium analysis in human prostate neoplasms, *Biol Trace Elem Res*, 59, 145, 1997.

68. Nakamura, K. et al. [Authors are Yasunaga, Ko, Xu, Moul, Peehl, Srivastava, and Rhim], Cadmium-induced neoplastic transformation of human prostate epithelial cells, *Int J Oncol*, 20, 543, 2002.

69. Martin, M.B. et al. [Authors are Voeller, Gelmann, Lu, Stoica, Hebert, Reiter, Singh, Danielsen, Pentecost, Stoica], Role of cadmium in the regulation of AR gene expression and activity, *Endocrinology*, 143, 263, 2002.

70. Kazantzis, G., Lam, T.H., and Sullivan, K.R., Mortality of cadmium-exposed workers. A five-year update, *Scand J Work Environ Health*, 14, 220, 1988.

71. Sorahan, T. and Waterhouse, J.A., Mortality study of nickel-cadmium battery workers by the method of regression models in life tables, *Br J Ind Med*, 40, 293, 1983.

72. Terracio, L., Nachtigal, M., Oncogenicity of rat prostate cells transformed *in vitro* with cadmium chloride, *Arch Toxicol*, 61, 450, 1988.

73. Waalkes, M.P. et al. [Authors are Rehm, Riggs, Bare, Devor, Poirier, Wenk, and Henneman], Cadmium carcinogenesis in male Wistar [Crl:(WI)BR] rats: dose-response analysis of effects of zinc on tumor induction in the prostate, in the testes, and at the injection site, *Cancer Res*, 49, 4282, 1989.

74. Waalkes, M.P. et al. [Authors are Rehm, Riggs, Bare, Devor, Poirier, Wenk, Henneman, and Balaschak], Cadmium carcinogenesis in male Wistar [Crl:(WI)BR] rats: dose-response analysis of tumor induction in the prostate and testes and at the injection site, *Cancer Res*, 48, 4656, 1988.

75. Waalkes, M.P., Anver, M., and Diwan, B.A., Carcinogenic effects of cadmium in the noble (NBL/Cr) rat: induction of pituitary, testicular, and injection site tumors and intraepithelial proliferative lesions of the dorsolateral prostate, *Toxicol Sci*, 52, 154, 1999.

76. Waalkes, M.P., Anver, M.R., and Diwan, B.A., Chronic toxic and carcinogenic effects of oral cadmium in the Noble (NBL/Cr) rat: induction of neoplastic and proliferative lesions of the adrenal, kidney, prostate, and testes, *J Toxicol Environ Health A*, 58, 199, 1999.

77. Waalkes, M.P. and Rehm, S., Lack of carcinogenicity of cadmium chloride in female Syrian hamsters, *Toxicology*, 126, 173, 1998.

78. Hoffmann, L. et al. [Authors are Putzke, Kampehl, Russbult, Gase, Simonn, Erdmann, and Huckstorf], Carcinogenic effects of cadmium on the prostate of the rat, *J Cancer Res Clin Oncol*, 109, 193, 1985.

79. Zeng, X. et al. [Authors are Jin, Zhou, and Nordberg], Changes of serum sex hormone levels and MT mRNA expression in rats orally exposed to cadmium, *Toxicology*, 186, 109, 2003.

80. Shira,T. et al. [Authors are Iwasaki, Masui, Mori, and Ito], Enhancing effect of cadmium on rat ventral prostate carcinogenesis induced by 3,2'-dimethyl-4-aminobiphenyl, *Jpn J Canc Res*, 84, 1023, 1993.

81. Aughey, E., et al. [Authors are Scott, King, East, Harris, and Boddy], The distribution and retention of 113 cadmium in the rat following injection into the prostate, *Br J Urol*, 47, 185, 1975

82. Ho, S.M., Metal ions and prostate cancer, in *Endocrine Disruptors: Effects on Male and Female Reproductive Systems*, 1st edition, Rajesh K.Naz (ed), CRC Press, Boca Raton, FL, 1999.

83. Bray, T.M., and Bettger, W.J., The physiological role of zinc as an antioxidant, *Free Radic Biol Med*, 8, 281, 1990.

84. Zeng, J., Vallee, B.L., and Kagi, J.H., Zinc transfer from transcription factor IIIA fingers to thionein clusters, *Proc Natl Acad Sci USA*, 88, 9984, 1991.

85. Oteiza, P.I. et al. [Authors are Olin, Fraga, and Keen], Zinc deficiency causes oxidative damage to proteins, lipids and DNA in rat testes, *J Nutr*, 125, 823, 1995.

86. Ames, B.N., Micronutrient deficiencies. A major cause of DNA damage, *Ann N Y Acad Sci*, 889, 87, 1999.

87. Bauchinge, M. et al. [Authors are Schmid, Einbrodt, and Dresp], Chromosome aberrations in lymphocytes after occupational exposure to lead and cadmium, *Mutat Res*, 40, 57, 1976.

88. Beyersmann, D., and Hartwig, A., Genotoxic effects of metal compounds, *Arch Toxicol Suppl*, 16, 192, 1994.

89. Misra, R.R., Smith, G.T., and Waalkes, M.P., Evaluation of the direct genotoxic potential of cadmium in four different rodent cell lines, *Toxicology*, 126, 103, 1998.

90. Snow, E.T., Metal carcinogenesis: mechanistic implications, *Pharmacol Ther*, 53, 31, 1992.

91. Rikans, L.E. and Yamano, T., Mechanisms of cadmium-mediated acute hepatotoxicity, *J Biochem Mol Toxicol*, 14, 110, 2000.

92. Webber, M.M., Selenium prevents the growth stimulatory effects of cadmium on human prostatic epithelium, *Biochem Biophys Res Commun*, 127, 871, 1985.

93. Achanzar, W.E. et al. [Authors are Achanzar, Lewis, Webber, and Waalkes], Cadmium induces c-myc, p53, and c-jun expression in normal human prostate epithelial cells as a prelude to apoptosis, *Toxicol Appl Pharmacol*, 164, 291, 2000.

94. Zhou, T. et al. [Authors are Zhou, Song, Eguchi, Lu, Lundin, Jin, and Nordberg], Cadmium-induced apoptosis and changes in expression of p53, c-jun and MT-I genes in testes and ventral prostate of rats, *Toxicology*, 142, 1, 1999.

95. Garcia-Morales, P. et al. [Authors are Saceda, Kenney, Kim, Salomon, Gottardis, Solomon, Sholler, Jordan, and Martin], Effect of cadmium on estrogen receptor levels and estrogen-induced responses in human breast cancer cells, *J Biol Chem*, 269, 16896, 1994.

96. Predki, P.F. and Sarkar, B., Effect of replacement of "zinc finger" zinc on estrogen receptor DNA interactions, *J Biol Chem*, 267, 5842, 1992.

97. Stoica, A., Katzenellenbogen, B.S., and Martin, M.B., Activation of estrogen receptor-alpha by the heavy metal cadmium, *Mol Endocrinol*, 14, 545, 2000.

98. Guevel, R.L. et al. [Authors are Petit, Goff, Metivier, Valotaire, and Pakdel], Inhibition of rainbow trout (*Oncorhynchus mykiss*) estrogen receptor activity by cadmium, *Biol Reprod*, 63, 259, 2000.

99. Johnson, M.D. et al. [Authors are Kenney, Stoica, Hilakivi-Clarke, Singh, Chepko, Clarke, Sholler, Lirio, Foss, Reiter, Trock, Paik, and Martin], Cadmium mimics the *in vivo* effects of estrogen in the uterus and mammary gland, *Nat Med*, 9, 1081, 2003.

100. Safe, S., Cadmium's disguise dupes the estrogen receptor, *Nat Med*, 9, 1000, 2003.

101. Wilson, E.M., Interconversion of androgen receptor forms by divalent cations and 8 S androgen receptor-promoting factor. Effects of Zn^{2+}, Cd^{2+}, Ca^{2+}, and Mg^{2+}, *J Biol Chem*, 260, 8683, 1985.

102. Ye, J. et al. [Authors are Wang, Barger, Castranova, and Shi], Activation of androgen response element by cadmium: a potential mechanism for a carcinogenic effect of cadmium in the prostate, *J Environ Pathol Toxicol Oncol*, 19, 275, 2000.
103. Sugimoto, Y. et al. [Authors are Lopez-Solache, Labrie, and Luu-The], Cations inhibit specifically type I 5 alpha-reductase found in human skin, *J Invest Dermatol*, 104, 775, 1995.
104. Thomas, L.N. et al. [Authors are Douglas, Vessey, Gupta, Fontaine, Norman, Thompson, Troyer, Rittmaster, and Lazier], 5alpha-reductase type 1 immunostaining is enhanced in some prostate cancers compared with benign prostatic hyperplasia epithelium, *J Urol*, 170, 2019, 2003.
105. Bosland, M.C., Ford, H., and Horton, L., Induction at high incidence of ductal prostate adenocarcinomas in NBL/Cr and Sprague-Dawley HSd:SD rats treated with a combination of testosterone and estradiol-17 beta or diethylstilbestrol, *Carcinogenesis*, 16, 6, 1311, 1995.
106. Ho, S.M. Sex hormone-induced prostatic carcinogenesis in Noble rats involves genetic damage and cell proliferation, in *Hormonal Caracinogenesis*, Vol. 2, 1996.
107. Feustel, A. et al. [Wennrich, Steiniger, and Klauss], Zinc and cadmium concentration in prostatic carcinoma of different histological grading in comparison to normal prostate tissue and adenofibromyomatosis (BPH), *Urol Res*, 10, 301, 1982.
108. Nolan, T.D. and Brown, D., The influence of elevated dietary zinc, selenium, and their combination on the suppressive effect of dietary and intraperitoneal cadmium on egg production in laying hens, *J Toxicol Environ Health A*, 60, 549, 2000.
109. Mumtaz, M.M. et al. [Authors are Tully, El Masri, and De Rosa], Gene induction studies and toxicity of chemical mixtures, *Environ Health Perspect*, 110 Suppl 6, 947, 2002.
110. Fischer, E.H. and Davie, E.W., Recent excitement regarding metallothionein, *Proc Natl Acad Sci U S A*, 95, 3333, 1998.
111. Cherian, M.G., Jayasurya, A., and Bay, B.H., Metallothioneins in human tumors and potential roles in carcinogenesis, *Mutat Res*, 533, 201, 2003.
112. Maret, W. and Vallee, B.L., Thiolate ligands in metallothionein confer redox activity on zinc clusters, *Proc Natl Acad Sci U S A*, 95, 3478, 1998.
113. Uchida, Y. et al. [Authors are Takio, Titani, Ihara, and Tomonaga], The growth inhibitory factor that is deficient in the Alzheimer's disease brain is a 68 amino acid metallothionein-like protein, *Neuron*, 7, 337, 1991.
114. Bataineh, Z.M. et al. [Authors are Heidger, Jr., Thompson, and Timms], Immunocytochemical localization of metallothionein in the rat prostate gland, *Prostate*, 9, 397, 1986.
115. Umeyama, T. et al. [Authors are Saruki, Imai, Yamanaka, Suzuki, Ikei, Kodaira, Nakajima, Saitoh, and Kimura], Immunohistochemical demonstration of metallothionein in the rat prostate, *Prostate*, 10, 257, 1987.
116. Suzuki, T. et al. [Authors are Yamanaka, Tamura, Nakajima, Kanatani, Kimura, and Otaki], Metallothionein of prostatic tissues and fluids in rats and humans, *Tohoku J Exp Med*, 166, 251, 1992.
117. Coogan, T.P., Shiraishi, N., and Waalkes, M.P., Apparent quiescence of the metallothionein gene in the rat ventral prostate: association with cadmium-induced prostate tumors in rats, *Environ Health Perspect*, 102 Suppl 3, 137, 1994.

118. Ghatak, S. et al. [Authors are Oliveria, Kaplan, and Ho], Expression and regulation of metallothionein mRNA levels in the prostates of noble rats: lack of expression in the ventral prostate and regulation by sex hormones in the dorsolateral prostate, *Prostate*, 29, 91, 1996.

119. Lee, K.F., Lau, K.M., and Ho, S.M., Effects of cadmium on metallothionein-I and metallothionein-II mRNA expression in rat ventral, lateral, and dorsal prostatic lobes: quantification by competitive RT-PCR, *Toxicol Appl Pharmacol*, 154, 20, 1999a.

120. Lee, K.F., Lau, K.M., and Ho, S. M., Generation and characterization of hammerhead ribozymes targeting rodent metallothionein and I and II ribonucleic acid, *Toxicol Appl Pharmacol* 161, 3:294, 1999b.

121. Tekur, S. and Ho, S.M., Ribozyme-mediated downregulation of human metallothionein II(a) induces apoptosis in human prostate and ovarian cancer cell lines, *Mol Carcinog*, 33, 44, 2002.

122. Dutta, R. et al. [Authors are Sens, Somji, Sens, and Garrett], Metallothionein isoform 3 expression inhibits cell growth and increases drug resistance of PC-3 prostate cancer cells, *Prostate*, 52, 89, 2002.

123. Fan, L.Z. and Cherian, M.G., Potential role of p53 on metallothionein induction in human epithelial breast cancer cells, *Br J Cancer*, 87, 1019, 2002.

124. Harris, H. et al. [Authors are Henderson, Bhat, and Komm], Regulation of metallothionein II messenger ribonucleic acid measures exogenous estrogen receptor-beta activity in SAOS-2 and LNCaPLN3 cells, *Endocrinology*, 142, 645, 2001.

125. Suzuki, T. et al. [Authors are Umeyama, Ohma, Yamanaka, Suzuki, Nakajima, and Kimura], Immunohistochemical study of metallothionein in normal and benign prostatic hyperplasia of human prostate, *Prostate*, 19, 35, 1991.

126. Zhang, X.H. et al. [Authors are Jin, Sakamoto, and Takenaka], Immunohistochemical localization of metallothionein in human prostate cancer, *J Urol*, 156, 1679, 1996.

127. Jasani, B. and Schmid, K.W., Significance of metallothionein overexpression in human tumours, *Histopathology*, 31, 211, 1997.

128. Battersby, S., Chandler, J.A., and Morton, M.S., The effect of orally administered cadmium on the ultrastructure of the rat prostate, *Urol Res*, 10, 123, 1982.

129. Barthel, E., [Cancer risk in pesticide exposed agricultural workers (author's transl.)], *Arch Geschwulstforsch*, 51, 579, 1981.

130. Chen, C.J. and Wang, C.J., Ecological correlation between arsenic level in well water and age-adjusted mortality from malignant neoplasms, *Cancer Res*, 50, 5470, 1990.

131. Wu, M.M. et al. [Authors are Kuo, Hwang, and Chen], Dose-response relation between arsenic concentration in well water and mortality from cancers and vascular diseases, *Am J Epidemiol*, 130, 1123, 1989.

132. Lewis, D.R. et al. [Authors are Southwick, Ouellet-Hellstrom, Rench, and Calderon], Drinking water arsenic in Utah: A cohort mortality study, *Environ Health Perspect*, 107, 359, 1999.

133. Brown, K.G. and Ross, G.L., Arsenic, drinking water, and health: a position paper of the American Council on Science and Health, *Regul Toxicol Pharmacol*, 36, 162, 2002.

134. Achanzar, W.E. et al. [Authors are Brambila, Diwan, Webber, Waalkes], Inorganic arsenite-induced malignant transformation of human prostate epithelial cells, *J Natl Cancer Inst*, 94, 1888, 2002.

135. Maeda, H. et al. [Authors are Hori, Nishitoh, Ichijo, Ogawa, Kakehi, and Kakizuka], Tumor growth inhibition by arsenic trioxide (As2O3) in the orthotopic metastasis model of androgen-independent prostate cancer, *Cancer Res*, 61, 5432, 2001.

136. Uslu, R. et al. [Authors are Sanli, Sezgin, Karabulut, Terzioglu, Omay, and Goker]. Arsenic trioxide-mediated cytotoxicity and apoptosis in prostate and ovarian carcinoma cell lines, *Clin Cancer Res*, 6, 4957, 2000.
137. Murgo, A.J., *Oncologist,* 6, Suppl 2: 22-28.

Index

A

AAH, *see* Atypical adenomatous hyperplasia
Abortion, TCDD and, 230
Acrolein, 85
Agency for Toxic Substances and Disease
 Registry (ATSDR), 419
AhR, *see* Aryl hydrocarbon receptor
Ah-responsiveness, modulation of by ER, 256
Alcohol consumption, sexual performance and,
 366
Alcoholism drugs, 366
Alzheimer's disease, 69, 419
Amenorrhea, 75
American Council on Science and Health, 420
American diet, zinc deficiency in, 414
Anabolic steroids, 298
Androgen receptor (AR), 105, 351, 418
 estradiol and, 395
 -to-estrogen balance, 307
 failure to activate, 352
 mRNA, 394
Androgen responsive element (ARE), 418
Androgens and antiandrogens, environmental,
 313–343
 antiandrogenic effects of PBDE-71, 333–335
 antiandrogenic effects of phthalate esters
  during development, 330–333
 developmental effects of p,p DDE' in male rat
  and rabbit, 329
 dicarboximide fungicides, 321–327
  dose-response developmental effects of
   procymidone in male rat, 326–327
  dose-response developmental effects of
   vinclozolin, 323–324
  procymidone, 325–326
  pubertal effects of vinclozolin, 324–325
  vinclozolin, 321–322
 in vitro effects of prochloraz, 329–330
 in vitro effects and short-term *in vivo* effects
  of p,p' DDE, 328–329
 in vivo developmental effects of prochloraz in
  male rat, 330
 in vitro and *in vivo* androgenic effects of pulp
  and paper mill effluents, 316–319
 in vitro and *in vivo* studies with feedlot
  effluents and trenbolone, 319–320

mixtures of antiandrogens, 335
procymidone, 327–328
 developmental effects of linuron in male
  rat, 327–328
 linuron, 327
Andropause, 357
Antiandrogenic chemicals, 314, 315
Antiandrogens, *see* Androgens and antiandrogens,
 environmental
Antiestrogens, 186, 275
Antifungal drugs, 366
Antihypertensives
 ED and, 360
 libido and, 365
Antioxidants, 156
AR, *see* Androgen receptor
ARE, *see* Androgen responsive element
Aroclor 1254, 34
Aromatase activity, inhibition of, 231
Aromatic hydrocarbon receptor, 351
ARs, *see* Androgen receptors
Arsenic, contaminants, 420
Arthritis, 69, 366
Aryl hydrocarbon receptor (AhR), 114, 252
 agonist(s)
  antiestrogenic activity of, 258
  PCB, 260
 identification of, 252
 -mediated antiestrogenicity, mechanisms of,
  264
 -mediated transactivation, 254
 pathway, 233
ATSDR, *see* Agency for Toxic Substances and
 Disease Registry
Atypical adenomatous hyperplasia (AAH), 412
Audio-visual sexual stimulation (AVSS), 349, 350
AVSS, *see* Audio-visual sexual stimulation

B

BD, *see* 1,3-Butadiene
Benign prostatic hyperplasia (BPH), 380, 412
 heavy-metal–ion influences on, 411
 onset of, 383
Bile-duct hyperplasia, 116
Biochanin A, potency of, 143

431

Printed and bound by CPI Group (UK) Ltd, Croydon, CR0 4YY

23/10/2024

01778238-0013